New Vibrational
Flower Essences
OF BRITAIN AND IRELAND

**ROSE TITCHINER, SUE MONK,
ROSEMARY POTTER, PATRICIA STAINES**

FOREWORD BY JULIAN PERRY
ILLUSTRATED BY HANNAH GIFFARD

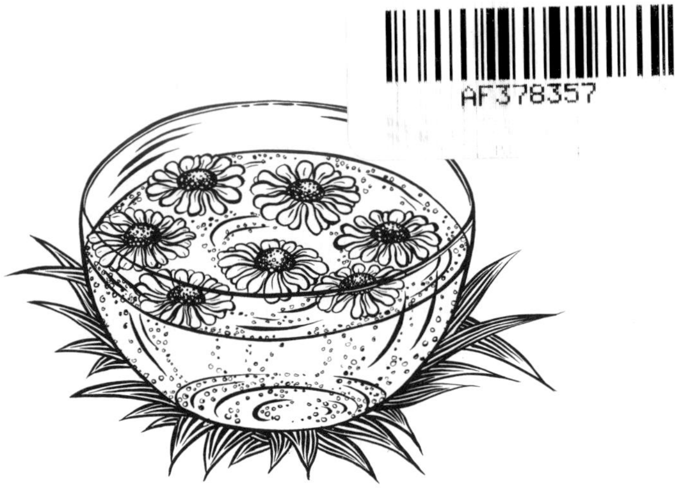

*Waterlily
Books*

WATERLILY BOOKS
The Duke Chediston Green Halesworth
Suffolk IP19 0BB

First published in Great Britain by Waterlily
Books 1997

ISBN 0 9530158 0 7

Typeset by T&O Graphics, Bungay, Suffolk.

Printed in Great Britain by Biddles Ltd,
Guildford, Surrey., and King's Lynn,
Norfolk

DEDICATION

*This book is dedicated to the expression of
love in everything – May that love be
recognised and celebrated by all.*

New Vibrational Flower Essences

OF BRITAIN AND IRELAND

Contents

Footnote: Chapter 1 was written by Rosemary Potter, **Chapters 2,3,4 & 5** were written and compiled by Rose Titchiner, **Chapter 6** was written by Patricia Staines, **Chapters 7,8,9 & 10 (The Repertory and Sets of Essences)** were compiled by Sue Monk, **Chapter 11 (The Cross-Reference Index)** was compiled by Rosemary Potter, **The Appendix** was compiled by Vivien Williamson.

Acknowledgements

ACKNOWLEDGEMENTS FOR COPYRIGHT PERMISSIONS

We would like to thank the following authors and publishers for permission to reproduce material from the books listed below:

Extracts included in Chapter 1

from *The Hermetic and Alchemical Writings of Paracelsus The Great*
edited by Arthur Edward Waite reproduced by kind permission of Shambala Publications

from *The Collected Writings of Edward Bach* by Dr Edward Bach
reproduced by kind permission of The Flower Remedy Programme

from *The Medical Discoveries of Edward Bach, Physician*
by Nora Weeks
from Heal Thyself by Dr Edward Bach
and from *The Twelve Healers & Other Remedies* by Dr Edward Bach
reproduced by kind permission of C. W. Daniel Co Ltd

from *Wings of Light* – White Eagle
reproduced by kind permission of The White Eagle Publishing Trust

Extracts included in Chapter 3

from *The Golden Web* © Gwennie Armstrong Fraser 1995
and from *Nature Spirits and Elemental Beings* © Marko Pogačnik 1995
reproduced by kind permission of Findhorn Press

Extracts included in Chapter 5

from *Dowsing For Health* © Arthur Bailey 1990
reproduced by kind permission of Quantum (W.M.Foulsham & Co Ltd)

Extracts included in Chapter 6

from *The P'taah Tapes – Transformation of the Species*
channelled by Jani King
and extracts included throughout the book
from *P'taah – The Gift* channelled by Jani King
reproduced by kind permission of Triad Publishers Pty Ltd (Australia)

Extracts included throughout the book

from *To Honor the Earth* © Dorothy Maclean 1991
reproduced by kind permission of the publishers Harper Collins

We would also like to thank Paul Tuttle (NWFFCM) and Raj for their kind permission to transcribe material from the Raj Tapes (channelled audio tapes)
Quotes from this material appear throughout the book.

Further details of all the books and tapes mentioned above may be found in the Reading List at the back of this book

GENERAL ACKNOWLEDGEMENTS

The Team, (Rose, Sue, Pat and Rosie) would like to thank:-

Richard Barnes without whose continual help and patient support this book would never have gone to print; for setting us a timetable to work to, arranging the printing and typesetting and helping to pull the book together.

Richard Osbourne (of Brightstar Creative Consultancy) for all the loving care and attention he put into designing the beautiful cover, page layouts, bookmarks and advertising flyer for the book, for his endless patience with our alterations and for all the enthusiastic encouragement he gave to us when we were flagging!

Viv Williamson (of Sun Essences), who so generously allowed us to use her beautiful photographs for the cover of the book and the inside pages, for stepping in at the last minute to compile and type the appendix and descriptions of contributors and for all her support and encouragement and friendship.

Hannah Giffard for freely giving of her time to lovingly draw the illustrations and motifs for the book and for providing the original inspiration for writing this book.

Ken Millie (of T & 0 Graphics) for amazing speedy typesetting, and for all his skill and care in making it all fit and look good on the page.

The Contributors – the essence makers, therapists and others from all over Britain and Ireland who have contributed the bulk of the written material for this book, many of whom have taken considerable time to write about their experience and understanding.

PERSONAL ACKNOWLEDGEMENTS

Rose Titchiner – my thanks go to my husband and friend Mark, for the love and support he has given me throughout the $2\frac{1}{2}$ years I've been working on the book – and for his much valued, constructive suggestions; to my children Jude, Dulcie, Beth and Gabriel for their love, patient support and light; to Sue, Pat and Rosie, without whom this book would never have come to fruition; for all their loving support and enthusiasm, for the many long hours of painstaking work, and for being such wonderful and inspiring friends. To my mother Prue, who has always encouraged me and who passed on to me her love of flowers, gardening and the earth; to my sister, Belinda, for her support and encouragement and for sharing her experience of self publishing; to Sally Stockley, for showing me my connection to spirit and the power of intuition and spiritual healing, for her friendship, support and healing over the years; To Tara Devi, Rosemary Hawkins, Bee Springwood and Rachel Charles, for empowering counselling and friendship; to Raj and to my father, and all those in spirit who love, support and guide me.

Sue Monk – My thanks to the Universal Family of Light, for their love, encouragement and guidance always; to my husband Tom and my children Rosemary and Richard, for their love, support, patience and teaching; to Anne Billings, for her acknowledgement of the voice within; to Ian Stothers for his unstinting help and advice in encouraging my overstretched computer to behave; to Ray, Sebastian and all those who have helped and shared with me and continue to do so on the healing pathway.

Rosemary Potter – my love and thanks go to Allan, Ben, Harriet and Samuel for their continuous support and patience throughout the period of my being involved with the writing of this book; to Rose, for her generosity in giving me the opportunity and challenge; to Sue, for her patience and advice; and to Patricia, for her loving encouragement, and our lengthy telephone calls supporting each other when the going got a little tough. Also, to my dear friends Tamisha, Gay, Paul, Deborah, Jasmine, Christine, Pat, Julie and Lauren for their love and support, sharing their time with me at much welcomed 'retreats'; and to all my friends from the GVM at Norwich with whom it all began!

Patricia Staines – This book would not have come into being had it not been for Rose Titchiner's vision, her commitment to this project and her generosity in sharing it with myself and others. It has been a wonderful experience to work with such open-hearted people. I have received loving support from Rosie Potter, who, when life became so busy, with her gentle encouragement helped me through. I would life to thank Sue Monk for her quiet knowing, that all would be well in the end, and Rose Titchiner, for many supportive phone calls, soul searching and unconditional love. I would also like to thank my husband Ric, for the very difficult job of coping with my tantrums with love and understanding; Ben, my son, for his encouragement and belief in me and Kerensa, my daughter, for being a mum to me just when I needed it. This acknowledgement would not be complete without mentioning the great gift I have been given, as P'taah would say – I have been given 'the jewel in the centre of the lotus flower' and I have managed to take it, thank you P'taah.

Foreword

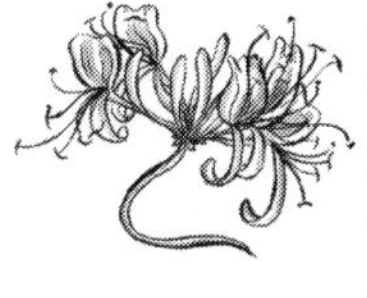

As we are living in times of rapid transformation there can never be enough information portraying the wonderful array of natural healing essences available to each of us. It seems that as we move into these times of enormous change we are blessed with tools to assist us to make the transition.

This book is a much needed contribution to this growing awareness of nature's gifts to all. Further it is particularly germane to the time in that up until now there has been a gap in the market dealing with flower essences indigenous to Britain and Ireland. Flower essences seem to be springing up all over as we plug into the consciousness of Mother Earth and hear the prompts of the realms of Light to take note of what has always been around us but yet did we not see.

The task undertaken by the authors of this book has been great indeed for not only have they taken it upon themselves to gather such a wide range of information and diversity of viewpoints regarding individual essences, but they have gleaned most valuable information for those wishing to take it upon themselves to conduct their own research and experiments. This work is indeed a compendium, a cornucopia of insight and inspiration into the world of healing essences, not just arising from the indigenous flora of the British Isles but from those other 'contemplative' sources that have been channelled through people living in the same regions.

It is not before time that the collective consciousness has arisen to embrace the significance of the natural world in the role of healing. The term vibrational medicine is emerging into common parlance and interest in flower essences has literally exploded over the last year with sales rising by over 80%. Partly due to an increase in stress levels but mainly, I feel, due to the shifting consciousness, the high street shopper is not only becoming more aware but actively seeking healing and calming remedies to smooth life's path. Articles are appearing in popular magazines proposing the use of flower essences to deal with diverse problems and allowing the individual to take back their power and to spare them a long queue at the doctor's surgery!

Public interest aside, the uprising of vibrational medicine represents the birthing of a new paradigm, one that bridges traditional science and spirituality. This bridge is not only vital now but for many the only plausible route by which they can safely embark on a journey of discovery into new realms of possibilities. This schism between science and spirituality, between the sacred and the profane, has been an artificial divide, fostered by the patriarchal power structures and by those who feared the integration of the sacred feminine and the acknowledgement of the imminent Divine. It is essential now, for the sake of the planet and of all of us that we reintegrate the Divine and the material with our transcendent experiences. The use of vibrational essences, of liquid consciousness, can provide enormous assistance in this regard, infusing our whole being with healing vibrations of love and wholeness. In this way the connection to the Inner Presence that is so fundamental to our journey can be wholly nurtured by this approach.

May the authors and all the contributors be blessed for their work and service in bringing forth their guidance and energy from the Heart. In so doing, all who read this work will be encouraged to spread their own light and to know that, whether we manifest as a human being or as a flower, we are all part of the One Life on a path of expansion and discovery.

Julian Perry, 12th March, 1997

Introduction

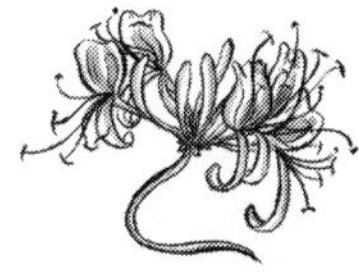This is a book about healing through Love. Throughout the process of it's creation we have been continually called upon to understand more of the nature of what is truly healing, personally, in each of our lives, and in all aspects of the production of this book.

We find healing when we choose Love over fear, and when we honour our integrity and choose what is truly loving, both for ourselves, and for those around us. In order to be able to choose Love instead of fear, we need to be able to trust that we will be supported in that choice. We need to know that whenever we make the choice for Love we are choosing what is real, what is Good/God in everything. Our disease and unhappiness arises when we choose to be motivated by fear and do not allow ourselves to experience Love in some aspect of our lives. Our rational (but frequently fear-based) mind, needs to see a logical and predictable outcome to the choices we make, and, if we listen to it, we will remain in fear, in a place of limitation, in which we do not allow ourselves to experience the infinite healing power of Love. With courage, we can choose Love, and grow to understand that Love is our true nature and the essence of all that is, and that any choice made for Love will be supported in ways beyond that which our rational mind can ever reason.

Flower essences inspire us to heal through their gift of Love. Their healing vibrations are of the many aspects of Love. They illumine those areas of our lives in which we do not recognise Love and they inspire us to return to Love, which is our true expression.

We have tried throughout this book to avoid defining things too closely, and instead to present people's actual experiences, in such a way that readers are called on to reflect upon their own experience. We hope that this is an empowering book that will encourage those who use it to follow their own intuition and integrity, and to continue to question and inquire further.

We have tried to remain true to ourselves, and to the process of the book as it developed. Self-publishing, although challenging gave us the freedom to follow our instincts. It has taken 2½ years to complete this project, It has been wonderful to work together. The book has provided us with a catalyst for much growth and change, since we have found ourselves continually challenged to honour our integrity and what is truly healing and loving, both personally and in relation to the project. So many people have contributed to the book in so many ways and it has come to fruition as a result of great co-operation, partnership, and persistence.

There is a vast amount of information contained in these pages which may at first seem bewildering. In the Repertory there are frequently several different descriptions given for the qualities of an essence made from the same flower (ie: Dandelion). If this seems confusing, we would encourage you to look for what rings true for you, for what most attracts you. Each essence maker works with different facets of healing and will draw on different qualities of the healing energy of each plant. In the Repertory the common healing themes for each plant may be identified within the individual descriptions, and if the reader is drawn to a particular essence maker's description they may go on to look at the more detailed information provided in Chapters 8,9 and 10, in which individual essence maker's sets of essences are described in full. These chapters provide a clearer indication of the healing energy of each essence maker and the plants that they are working with. The Cross Reference Index provides the reader with an opportunity to look up particular issues and identify which essences which relate to those issues.

From our experience we would say, that when choosing vibrational essences, each person needs different energies at different phases of development, and that what might be right for one person is not necessarily right for another. We all need to recognize and trust our own intuition and discernment as to what is most appropriate for each of us, at any one time.

We intend this book to be a validation of the personal healing contribution of each of the many essence makers, therapists and healers who have been working in the field of vibrational flower essence making in the British Isles and Ireland since the 1930s. Each healer draws to them those who need their particular energetic healing note. We see no need for competition in the world of healing. Everything has it's own order and timeliness – one thing does not deny another. Our understanding is growing at an ever increasing pace – this book is intended as a step along the way to greater understanding, healing and unity.

Rose, Sue, Rosie and Pat.
August 1997

THE AUTHORS

ROSE TITCHINER (Light Heart Flower Essences)

Rose Titchiner is a healer, flower essence therapist and essence maker. Light Heart Flower Essences are an extension of her healing and are created in partnership with nature and spirit. She lives in Suffolk with her husband and the younger three of their four children.

SUE MONK (Sue's Flower Essences)

Sue Monk is a flower and gem essence therapist, essence maker and healer. She seeks to encourage others to find their own connection to the light and love within, thus fostering self-reliance and helping to bring forward the knowledge that will help each person realise their mission in life in the best possible way. She lives in Cambridgeshire with her husband and two children.

ROSEMARY POTTER (Gaia Essences)

Rosemary Potter is a Reiki Master, teacher and healer, a flower and gem essence therapist, and aromatherapist. Her interest in flower remedies and natural healing began approximately 20 years ago when introduced to the Bach Flower remedies, in particular, Rescue Remedy. She describes essence making as an "adventure, a joyful, exciting journey of discovery, never ceasing to surprising and delight." Her approach to her healing work is to offer her clients a gentle and supportive space, where their treatments can be viewed as an unfolding process, a journey of exploration for both client and therapist. She lives in Suffolk with her husband and three children and is part of the East Anglian Flower & Vibrational Essence Forum (see Appendix).

PATRICIA STAINES (Loving Nature Flower Essences)

Pat Staines is a flower essences therapist and Reiki Master/teacher, she developed her love for healing whilst using and then later making essences.

The healing and revealing properties of flower essences in her own life led to her completing a two year vibrational medicine course which helped her to further develop her intuition so she could help others. In her practise in Suffolk she combines Flower Essence Therapy with Reiki healing.

CONTRIBUTORS TO THE BOOK

PETER AZIZ (Habundia Essences)

Peter Aziz is a hereditary Shaman of 25 years training. He has also trained in Kinesiology, Iridology, Body Electronics and Homoeopathy. His Shamanic art centres around the use of plant spirits and he now works with them mainly in the form of flower essences. He has made local headlines several times for producing miraculous cures. He works as a healer and also runs courses in Shamanic healing. He practises in Devon, Somerset and Gloucestershire.

DR ARTHUR BAILEY (Bailey Flower Essences)

Dr Arthur Bailey qualified as an electronics engineer at the University of London. As a senior university lecturer, he started investigating dowsing and presented a paper on his research results to the Annual Oxford Symposium on Archaeology. Later, he became President of the British Society of Dowsers for six years. From this background he then developed his series of Flower Essences, the first ones being produced in 1967. Since taking early retirement he has devoted himself to refining and expanding the series.

DAWN CAROL (Living Rainbow Aura Essences)

Dawn Carol has dedicated her life to helping others. She is used for healing in whatever way is appropriate to those who come to her for help. Love is the key word to describing what Dawn is all about. Her essences are an extension of her work which are quite simply tools for healing. Dawn lives in a sacred manner honouring all life forms, praying the prayers of the people and being used to teach. Grounded spirituality, colour, music, spirit and the archangels are important components of her life. Dawn Carol is in her truth.

IMELDA CARROLL (Ard Na Neantog Flower Essences)

Ard Na Neantog is a co creative permaculture garden run by Imelda Carroll and the local Si (Gaelic for nature spirit). Imelda has been gardening in Donegal since 1990 and opened a partnership with the Si in '94. Since then the acre of land situated on a peninsula in the north west of Eire has thrived, in spite of wild, salt laden winds and has produced food and healing herbs for Imelda, her partner Jasper and their two girls, Aoife and Grainne, as well as a surplus to sell, barter and share.

ROISIN CARROLL (Ogham Oils and Essences)

Roisin Carroll is the creator of Ogham Oils and Essences. A teacher by profession she is founder member of the Irish Institute of Reflexologists and the Irish Association of Colour Therapy. In 1986 she opened the footprints School of Reflexology in Belfast, Northern Ireland, followed six years later by the opening of the Rainbow School of Colour Therapy in Dundalk Ireland.

One day while playing golf, she had an encounter with a Hawthorn tree. The hawthorn told her how the essences of its vibrations would help to heal the physical body. Since she had been effectively using the Bach Flower Remedies on herself and her clients, she recognised the significance of this insight. So, alongside teaching these subjects, she was developing and researching Irish oils and their healing medicine. Recognising the need for bringing these oils and essences to the greater public, she then began to assemble a team to make the products and supply them in the market place. She was greatly assisted by her husband and six children. The resulting oils and essences were made available by her company, Celtic Tree Oils, Ltd., starting in 1992.

Her current project is expanding her education material into a book called The Crane Bag: Celtic Tree Oils and Essences Based on the Ancient Ogham. A set of cards is also being developed to accompany the book and provide a divinatory tool.

BRIDGET AND ALFRED CRAIG (Bridget's Flower Essences)

Bridget Craig and her husband are primarily engaged in applying what she has come to understand constitutes a quite new healing system in which she employs the use of flowers in a quite different way. The healing system comprises of eight distinctly different flowers, each of which possesses a quite unique energy system. She has discovered that each of these particular energy systems can be used to restore and balance the energy flow between both the physical and non physical energy systems which together, determine, govern and control the internal body environment, hence, the effectiveness of the Immune Defence System, consequently the quality of life itself.

MARION DAVIS (Real Life Remedies)

Marion Davis started working as a healer in 1989. She made remedies for her patients (with flowers she picked from her garden), to help them with their healing process. Demand for them grew and they became a business in their own right. Reflecting back to early childhood, she remembered picking flowers, (many of them the same as the ones she now uses), to make potions in play. She is presently working towards expanding her own knowledge and wisdom, and helping others with their growing process so that they may achieve their goals in this life time. She enjoys many creative activities – singing dancing, drawing and painting, sewing and gardening. She has three sons and lives with her illustrative partner Brian.

ROSIE DEVITT (Rose Devitt's Flower Essences)

Rosie Devitt is a family person who is married with four grown up daughters. She has a wide range of interests including art, music and poetry. She keeps up a daily practise of yoga and meets regularly to meditate with friends. Her love of nature is life long, and venturing into flower and gem essence making has been like a home coming.

DAVID EASTOE Dip HE (Petaltone Essences)

David Eastoe Dip HE specialises in developing new and different ways of working with plant energy medicines and has discovered remarkable properties for healing the auras of people, animals, buildings and landscapes. David began his spiritual training in 1974 with Tibetan Lamas and has recently completed 10 years research on esoteric healing, including use of plants, sound/music, colour, crystals. David lives in rural Somerset, travelling to offer workshops and demonstrations of his discoveries, in the use of Petaltone Essences, Space Clearing and Sound Healing.

DOCTOR HELEN FORD

Dr Helen Ford describes herself as a holistic physician, meaning that her work takes account of the mind, body and soul of each individual, as well as their relationship with the whole, of which we are all part. She began her conventional medical training (rather unconventionally), with an open history scholarship to Cambridge, which was followed by a double first in natural sciences. Once qualified her experiences within medicine led her to a gradually expanding awareness of the underlying causes of disease, and she began to make increasing use of her own natural abilities as 'sensitive' and healer to treat illness at the level of the subtle bodies by means of healing, crystals, homoeopathy and a variety of Flower and Tree Essences, including those she has made herself.

SIMON FRANCE (Aquarius Flower Essences)

Simon France is a flower remedy developer living in Northumberland. His route to flower remedies was through astrology, which he still practises. He is a member of Aquarius Flower Remedies

KESTRAL GERRARD (Lords and Ladies Essences)

Kestral Gerrard is a healer and teacher with a deep connection to the natural world. He uses sound healing, holistic aromatherapy, regression and higher perception guidance to help people to release mental and emotional blocks, restrictions and conditioning and to integrate mind, body and spirit. He runs workshops on shamanic practices, runes, regression, sound and higher perception. He lives and works in Glastonbury, Somerset.

RICHARD GONZALEZ (Veda Essences)

Richard Gonzalez Lic M.H. is a student of the way of nature; and all its relationships: He works largely with plant medicines and semi-precious stones in his healings, Richard's medicine demonstrates a facet of compassion; a necessary energy in human relationships.

CAROLE GUYETT

Carole Guyett is a herbalist and flower essence practitioner. She likes to work with the spirit of the plant in order to help people envoke their healing power from within, through self-love. Carole lives in Southern Ireland with her husband and two sons.

MARY HARRIS (Earth Essences)

Mary Harris was born in Norfolk and having followed a successful business career in London returned to Norfolk with her husband when the first of their two children was born ten years ago. Mary joined the alternative healing profession five years ago as a result of her own quest for 'good health', and now in order to help others to achieve their best potential, practises in flower essence therapy, psychic healing, massage and aromatherapy. Mary is overjoyed that her 'garden' passion has been enhanced by the gift of 'Earth Essences' as she believes that flower essences are invaluable in gently bringing a heightened awareness, and in effecting and supporting the necessary subtle energy alterations in the healing and growing process.

KAY HARRISON (Artemis Essences)

Kay Harrison has trained in Aromatherapy, Crystal Healing, Health Kinesiology, Reflexology and Shamanic Counselling. Her 'Artemis' Essences evolved as part of her training with crystals under the direction of Sue and Simon Lilly of 'Green Man'. Kay works from Exeter as a therapist and teacher. She is increasingly specialising in emotional stress and finds the Essences an invaluable support for her work.

JUDITH HOAD

Judith Hoad has over thirty years experience in using native herbs and Flower Essences. She qualified in Shen Tao Acupressure in 1991, aged 53. Having empowered herself to gain experience and qualifications she offers healing opportunities to people seeking them in treatment sessions, (by appointments), and in workshops. Believing that non-conventional medicine can empower us to make choices, she also believes that choosing to pay what we wish – and can afford – also empowers us. After she has chosen to give her best attention, loving expertise and generous time to someone, she expects that person to make what is for them an appropriate payment in the same way. She therefore names no fixed fee for her workshops or treatment sessions.

JEAN JACOB (Jean Jacob's Flower Essences)

Jean Jacob is a registered healer, she makes her own flower essences, 80 in all. She uses them mainly for meditation and spiritual attunement. She is an Associate Master in Ikebana from which she has gained insight of flowers and the Higher Realms. She practises astrology, trained by the White Eagle school to give insight into the path of the soul. Colour and crystals are also used in healing, She lives alone in a thatched cottage where she has created a Japanese garden and runs a small boarding cattery.

COLIN KINGSHOTT (Silvercord Essences)

Colin Kingshott is an international facilitator of vibrational medicine and since a child has had a symbiotic relationship with natures expression. His work is now focused upon devic consciousness. He has recently moved to Devon with his wife Diana where they research, produce and teach about essences. They also have schools in Iceland and Sweden for the purpose of co-creating with the intelligence called nature and its expression, flowers.

SHIMARA KUMARA (Crystal Herbs)

Originator of Crystal Herbs, now in partnership with Colin Burbridge and Catherine Keattch due to expansion; healer, channel, founder of the Golden Age Reiki Academy, co-creator of Guild of Vibrational Medicine, Golden Age Reiki /Ray Master. International workshop leader/lecturer, presenter at Mind, Body, Spirit exhibition, London. Writer, broadcaster and founder of the Golden Light Foundation, a charity which takes healing and natural medicines to war torn, traumatised areas and is currently working with refugees in Croatia/Bosnia and medical teams in Chernobyl using donated remedies from Crystal Herbs.

PHILLIPPA LEE (Aquarius Flower Essences)

Phillippa Lee works as a healer and flower essence practitioner in Hexham, Northumberland. Phillippa's focus is in the area of emotional pain and transformation.

SIMON AND SUE LILLY (Green Man Tree and Flower Essences)

Simon Lilly trained in Fine Art, learned Touch for Health and other kinesiology techniques and is qualified in Colour Therapy and Crystal and Gem therapy. When he moved to Devon he began making his own Flower Essences and developed Green Man Tree Essences. His recent work has focused on exploring the energies of trees and the potential for communication and teaching between human and tree spirits. For this, he works with his wife Sue using shamanic and Tree – taught techniques in small groups around the country.

Sue Lilly has been working within the field of complementary medicine for over twenty years using astrology, crystals, colour and kinesiology. Her interest in the patterns of people's lives and how they interact with other patterns from nature has formed the basis of her work with trees and tree essences.

MARION LEIGH (Findhorn Flower Essences)

Marion Leigh joined the Findhorn Foundation in 1976 where she was active in communications and networking with other groups and communities. She returned to her native Australia to strengthen her experiences in these fields, also working with the Australian Bush Flower Essences; and qualified as a homoeopath. In 1992 she returned to Findhorn and pioneered the Findhorn Flower Essence range, based on flowers indigenous to the region and a continuation of that tradition of attuning to the angelic realms informing the nature kingdom that first made the Findhorn Community famed around the world. She subsequently formed a business developing, researching and teaching flower essence therapy and communication with nature.

MARIA MAW (Unitive Flower Essences)

Maira Maw lives in North Wales with her two young children and studies with 'New Light' in Manchester. She is particularly interested in energy patterns, their interactions and expression. Her Unitive Flower Essence range has developed from a life-long love of wild flowers combined with a Biophysical training in research and synthesis of new ideas.

As a therapist (and for her own personal growth) Maira also uses Unitive kinesiology and Astrological counselling. The fundamental aim of her work is to integrate all aspects of life, promoting coherence and unity.

BRIDGET MEAGHER (Ballybane Flower Essences)

Bridget Meagher, is a qualified medical herbalist and mother to two boys. She is living in West Cork, Eire, her home for the past 10 years. It was here she discovered the Irish Flower Essences.

She is a working herbalist treating a wide variety of chronic and acute cases. After years of travel she now runs courses in Herbal remedies for the home, and guided herbal walks.

She would eventually like to set up an alternative hospital where different disciplines work together healing patients.

MARK MORDIN

Mark Mordin has studied, practised and taught alternative medicine for over twenty five years, beginning in the Middle East and continuing through a fourteen year stay in India, where he also studied yoga, meditation and tropical horticulture in depth. Returning to England , he opened his practice and continued to learn. He holds diplomas in sixteen different forms of therapy and has studied several others.

His practice is loosely based around the energetic systems of Oriental medicine, but with a lot of input from western therapies. He uses body work and nutrition to work upon structure and function via both 'energetic' and 'physiological' systems.

YANA NILSSON (Glastonbury Holy Thorn Essences)

Yana Nilsson is a qualified practitioner in Flower and Gem Essences, Transpersonal Psychotherapy and Aromatherapy in Dorset. She lectures for the Chalice Foundation in Exeter and works with earth energies and sacred sites around the world.

Over the past 20 years her love for and affinity with the Nature Kingdoms, her practise of meditation and spiritual and personal development have been greatly enhanced by the use of Flower Essences. She has found them to be gentle yet highly effective catalysts for change, working on many levels of the subtle bodies which in turn affect the mental emotional, physical and spiritual bodies.

She has a strong affinity with Glastonbury, the Chalice Well Gardens and the legends of Joseph of Arimathea and feels very honoured to have been used as a channel in the making of the Holy Thorn Essences.

ANN PARKER

Ann Parker, a health Kinesiology practitioner and authorised teacher, became interested in Flower Essences in 1984. She started to retail the Bach Flowers and in 1990 started to make up specialised bottles for clients. Ann now has over 2000 essences from all over the world. For Health Kinesiology, muscle testing determines what to do. For clients unable to visit for H K Ann uses dowsing to find which essences are needed to create the right vibrational resonance to promote healing and harmony on the physical, emotional mental and spiritual levels so the client experiences a sense of well being.

JULIAN PERRY (Silver Star Essences)

Julian Perry worked for ten years in the NHS as a clinical scientist but left in 1990 to focus more intently upon the spiritual path. He lectures and runs workshops encouraging people to access their own Divinity, working with the Mother energy to facilitate awakening. Interest in energy and vibrational medicine has blossomed in recent years and he initiated the creation of a series of essences within the 'Silver Star' group that has been running for over twelve years.

Julian is now deputy director of a charity dedicated to bringing a wide range of complementary healing practises into prisons where he also applies his own skills in vibrational medicine.

FREYA SHERLOCK (Middle Earth Essences)

Freya Sherlock lives and works with her husband and three children on their growing family farm in West Cork, Ireland. Together they endeavour to farm their animals consciously and with compassion. They have found their organic garden to be a source not only of excellent food, but of wondrous remedies too; be it the essences, or substance of a plant, they use both for the welfare of the family and animals alike. Freya passionately loves nature and delights in the co-creative process of working with nature's intelligence to sustain a garden and farm.

GAY SLATER

Gay Slater has been using Reiki and chakra healing for several years in conjunction with homoeopathy and flower and gem remedies. She incorporates different techniques such as fascial unwinding and creative visualisation. She used to practise as a chartered physiotherapist before taking on more holistic therapies 10 years ago. Gay has recently started working in a team for the Complementary Medical Services for prisons. She also has a private practice in Sevenoaks, Kent.

RIC STAINES (Loving Nature Flower Essences)

Ric Staines is a Reiki master, horticultural lecturer, broadcaster and journalist who has been interested in the natural world all his life. More recently he has developed the first validated course in Holistic Horticulture. He lives in Suffolk and helps his partner Patricia Staines to make and develop Loving Nature Essences. He also runs workshops in Holistic Horticulture.

VAL ST. CLAIR (Church Farm Rose Essences)

Val St Clair works with the subtle vibrational energy zones and centres within and around people and places. Disturbances in the subtle patterns of these vibrations can cause a disruptive effect both physically and emotionally. Val offers guidance/diagnosis for life/health issues through intuition and insight. She uses flower essences to support her work. Val's work often includes investigating 'paranormal' situations. She is s full member of the H.P.A.I. Val co-founded Church Farm Roses which she was inspired to prepare as part of her work.

JANE STEVENSON (Sun Essences)

Jane is a healer and practitioner who has dedicated over 14 years to treating people with Flower Essences. A childhood spent in Cornwall developed a very strong connection with nature and even today she is at her happiest sitting in the middle of a field surrounded by flowers and trees. Her interest in complementary medicine began when her infant daughter was successfully treated for asthma by a naturopath. Now a young grandmother living in Norfolk, she is an experienced and respected dowser who has achieved much success with clients using this method of diagnosis. Having a strong affinity with animals she finds dowsing an ideal way to tune into their individual needs and has been asked to help with a multitude of problems ranging from a cat with cystitis to a depressed turkey, (it was probably near Christmas!).

PETER TADD.

Peter Tadd is a clairvoyant therapist, healer and lecturer living with his wife and young family on the coast of West Cork, Ireland. His innate abilities have served his full time profession since 1978. His work takes him throughout the United States, Canada and Europe where he has colleagues in both traditional and non-traditional methods of healing. His communication with the natural world has been enhanced by North American Indian traditions and his travels to ancient sites. He is a practising Buddhist.

ANDREW TRESIDDER

Andrew Tresidder is a teacher and maker of flower essences, and practises as a G P in Somerset.

ELLIE WEB (Harebell Remedies)

Ellie Web is the founder and developer of Harebell Remedies. As well as making and supplying essences to individuals and practitioners, she also practises from home using dowsed combinations of her remedies as a way of supporting people through personal change. With a training in body-work, psychotherapy and the experience of being a single mother in a rural area, she hopes her work promotes the belief that contact with nature is essential to our balance and well being. Ellie lives with her younger daughter and three cats.

VIVIEN WILLIAMSON (Sun Essences)

A primary school teacher by profession and mother of three sons, her love of flowers and trees goes back to family outings and holidays during childhood. She founded Sun Essences in 1990 having been involved with Flower Essences since 1981. A Reiki healer she has explored Herbal Medicine, Hypnotherapy and N.L.P. as a healing path. However, after experiencing an ever deepening connection with nature she decided to concentrate solely on making essences of the highest possible quality and seeking excellence in the manufacture and distribution of Flower Essence products, including a selection of flower slides and photographs.

JULIAN WINSLOW (Wight Flower Essences)

Julian Winslow works as a gardener at Ventnor Botanic Gardens on the Isle of Wight. He has worked with and used herbs for more than ten years which has evolved into making, using and supplying flower and gem essences. This is along with yoga, meditation, music, jewellery making and writing has become part of his own process and the realisation of simple uncluttered joy. It is this that he hopes to give to others on their journey back to spirit, that journey being the cause of all life's symptoms.

IAN WOOD (Middle Earth Flower and Rose Essences)

Ian Wood is an astrologer who was involved in making flower essences in the West Country during the summer of 1988. He is now living in West Cork, teaching astrology and doing chart reading. He also works with gems using Indian Astrology.

DISCLAIMER

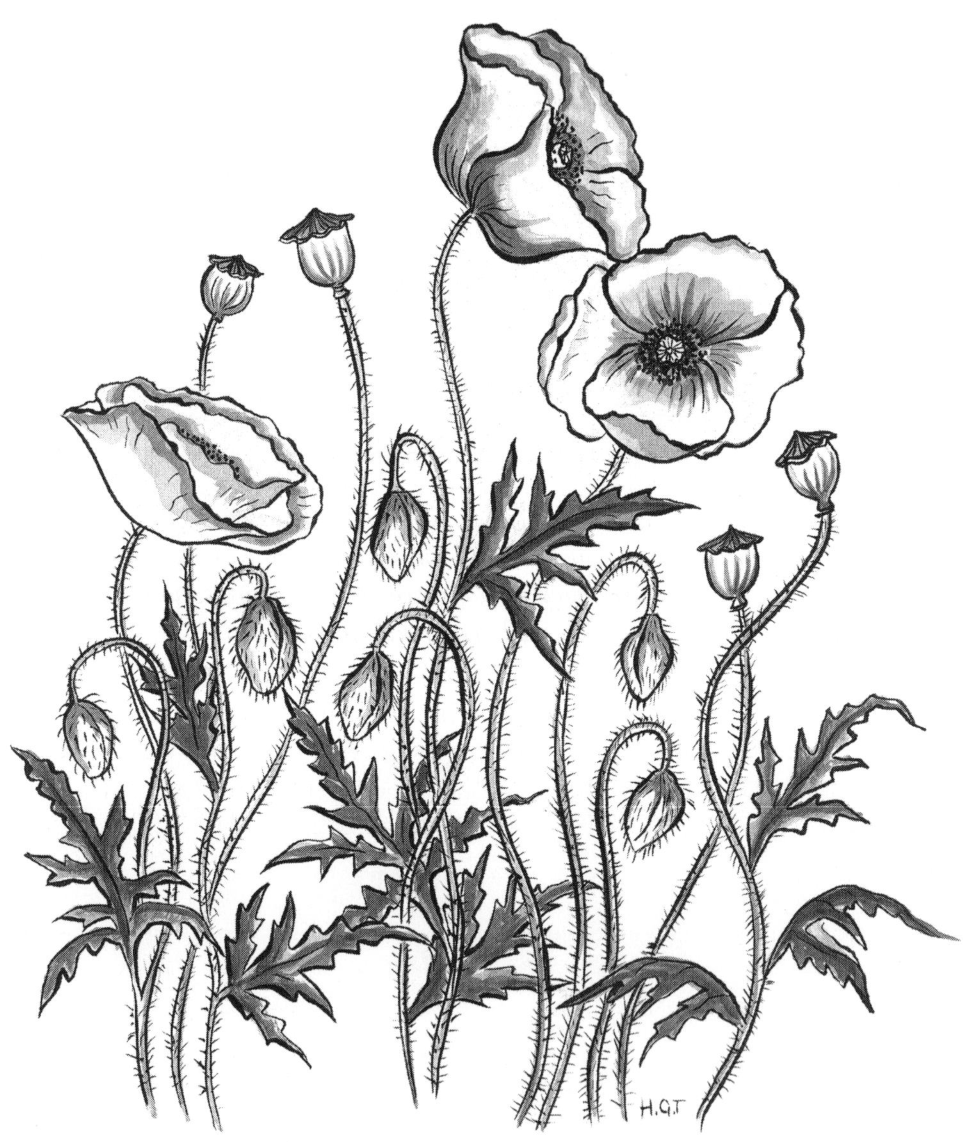

Chapter 1

A brief history of flower essences and their development

"Just as God in His Mercy has given us food to eat, so has He placed amongst the herbs of the fields beautiful plants to heal us when we are sick. These are there to extend a helping hand to man in those dark hours of forgetfulness when he loses sight of his Divinity, and allows the cloud of fear or pain to obscure his vision" – Dr. Edward Bach

What are Flower Essences? How do they work?

What pleasure flowers bring us. The sight of flowers in bloom is a breath of joy that can lift the spirit and touch the soul. What else can replace words so gracefully as the gift of flowers in celebration, love, thanks and memory.

Every human sentiment has been ascribed a floral symbol developing into a perfect language of flowers through which we can express our emotions. The Rose for example, honoured as the queen of flowers in Greek mythology and one of the oldest flowers in cultivation, would have been given as a token of beauty, youth and a declaration of love; the response perhaps being Honeysuckle, meaning 'devotion and affection,' or Lavender, signifying 'constancy and loyalty'.

Certain plants became symbols for man to express his beliefs, privilege, authority and also his religions – the Lotus flower for example, having deep religious significance with its history of symbolism going back 5000 years. The Iris was considered to be a symbol of power where, in Ancient Egypt, it was placed on the brow of the Sphinx and throughout history has remained a 'royal' symbol, the three large petals symbolising faith, wisdom and valour.

Some plants came to represent the sacred emblems of saints, prophets, religious festivals and holidays, even today we use special plants at festivals and celebrations throughout the year. In China and Japan which are particularly floral conscious countries, flowers came to represent the seasons and months of the year. Many plant names can be traced to the tales and traditions of ancient civilisations, the folklores being handed down with many still remaining today, an illustration being that of the humble Red Clover which was favoured by the Greeks and Romans as a symbol of good and evil, a five-leaf clover being unlucky but a four-leaf clover representing 'good-luck'.

The Development of plant medicine

Throughout the history of mankind, we have lived happily with trees, plants and flowers, the use of which was well known, revered and utilised for many purposes. Nature has provided us with food and shelter, healed our wounds both physical and emotional and has given us decoration, beauty and aroma. The peoples of ancient civilisations valued and honoured the plant kingdom, being in total communion with it, aware not just of its functional uses and its beauty but respecting its healing capabilities.

In ancient Egyptian medicine, illness meant imbalance in the body which could be restored by the use of flowers, herbs and plants which they used with great skill, blending magic, prayers, spells and sacrifice. Records show a complex system of medicine which was effectively able to deal with the most commonplace conditions that disrupted life. Archaeological evidence from ancient Mesopotamia shows revealing insights into their pharmacopoeia, in particular, the herbs and plants they used in their everyday treatment of ill health. Although both these civilisations had in part a scientific system of medicine that they used in conjunction with more holistic methods, it is interesting to note there was a strong shift in attitude away from the scientific towards a system based on practicality and experience. Similar threads can be seen weaving their patterns through the rich medical cultures of early Indian, Chinese and Greek medicine, their pharmacopoeia also showing extensive leanings towards plant substances.

The common link between wellbeing and maintaining equilibrium within the body occurs throughout this early period and beyond with similar patterns of thought appearing, winding and meandering through different cultures – the growths, the breaks and re-emergences occurring through the ages.

Greek influences

Hippocrates (c460-375BC) is often referred to as the 'Father of Medicine'. He advocated treating the human body as a whole, complete organism – a precur-

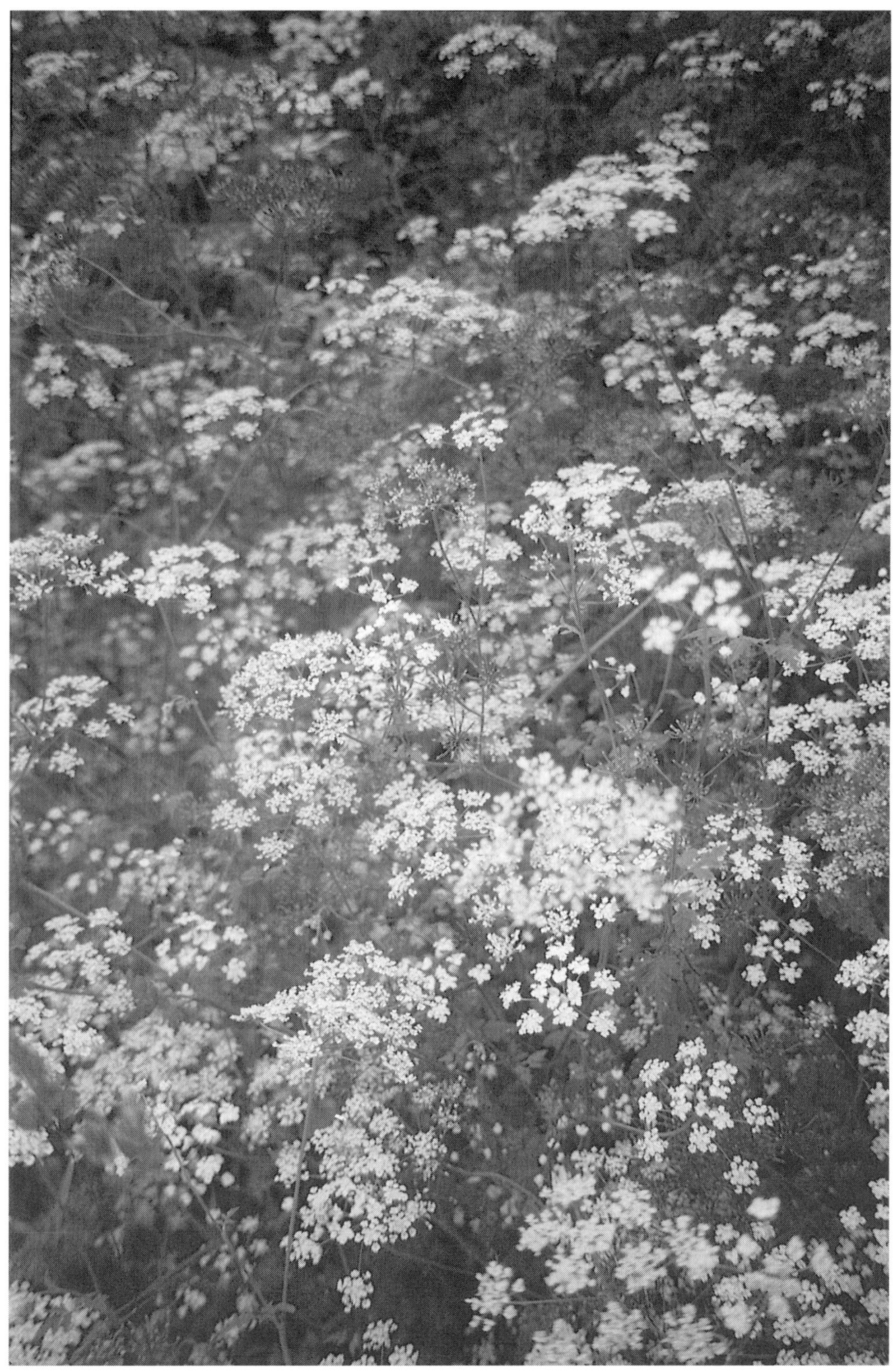

sor to what we would now refer to as 'holistic healing' and placed great emphasis on diet and prophylactic methods. He believed it was vital not just to treat the symptoms of disease but to find the cause. His writings are of great importance as he used and wrote about a great number of plant medicines.

Galen of Pergamum who was born cAD129, was greatly influenced by Hippocrates. He wrote more than 500 works, studying anatomy and physiology and establishing a basis for further research – his system to well-being was holistic taking into account environmental influences, nutrition, digestion and breath to maintain a balance in the system.

The work of Culpeper and Hahnemann

In England the use of plants, herbs and flowers continued with the work of Nicholas Culpeper (1616-1654) who was a well-known astrologer-physician. Although his way of combining astrology and medicine was unorthodox and greatly condemned by his immediate contemporaries in the medical world, the legacy of his herbal remedies are as important today as they were during his lifetime.

Allopathic medicine has its roots in herbalism with large numbers of orthodox drugs being derived from plants, for example, opiate painkillers extracted from the opium poppy and the heart drug, Digoxin, from the foxglove. Until approximately 50 years ago, nearly all pharmacopoeia entries which describe the manufacture of drugs indicated a herbal origin. Modern drugs are now of course, chemical copies, but being deprived of the 'life-force' of the real plant and its true healing properties.

It is in the late 18th century that we see the emergence of homoeopathy – Samuel Hahnemann, a German doctor (1755-1843) discovered the principle that 'like cures like,' similar to today's vaccines. Hahnemann realised that many of the symptoms suffered by his patients during illness were actual visible signs of their body's defences fighting the disease. Boosting these defences by giving his patients minute quantities of a herb or substance would produce in healthy people, exactly the disease he was endeavouring to cure. Hahnemann worked with the Doctrine of Signature, a system of relating the healing properties of plants to where they grow, their conditions, their shape and colour. Willow for example, is a tree that grows traditionally in damp places and is used to ease conditions like rheumatism that are worsened by damp weather. Hahnemann believed in treating the whole person and not the disease.

The emergence of flower essences

"Health is our heritage, our right. It is the complete and full union between soul, mind and body; and this is no difficult far-away ideal to attain, but one so easy and natural that many of us have overlooked it" – Dr. Edward Bach

It is said that the ancient esoteric civilisations of Lemuria (approximately 500,000 years ago) and Atlantis (approximately 150,000 years ago) developed and used flower essences extensively. In Lemuria, the people lived and worked in harmony with nature, mankind benefitting from a partnership of mutual co-operation with the plant kingdom. Flower essences were used primarily for spiritual growth, the Lemurians being so sensitive that they did not have to physically ingest the essence of the plant, being in the plant's presence was sufficient to receive it's healing effects. Later, during the Atlantean civilisation, flower essences were used as a system of medicine for they lived less in harmony with nature and disease had become more prevalent.

The Swiss alchemist and mystic Paracelcus (1493-1541) is credited with collecting dew from blossoms to treat emotional imbalances in his patients. Although a rebel in his life, frequently upsetting authority, he was individual and indeed an innovator, the importance of his lengthy writings cannot be underestimated. He wrote on the Doctrine of Signature;

"God has enriched the light of Nature with such ample gifts that even one who is not addicted to the light can know all things that are therein. Is not this a great thing which external signs offer to man's knowledge?"

Following on from Hippocrates and the early Greek traditions was the belief in the 'elements', a prominent alchemist system which Paracelsus followed, whereby the qualities within nature, of earth, air, fire and water and the balance of their resulting 'humours', played an important role in maintaining good health within the body and mind.

Another significant alchemical principle was the search for the 'quintessence' of life, that which could be extracted from all living things. To produce this, involved the refining of substances taken from nature in order to enhance their healing powers on both physical and psychological levels. Paracelsus believed in the divinity, the spirit of man, knowing that illness could not be present as long as there was harmony between the mental and spiritual facets of an individual. He speaks in his writings of, *"the quintessence of nature. the force, the virtue, the medicine, enclosed within all things, the life spirit"*

"the Life of things is none other than a spiritual essence, an invisible and impalpable thing, a spirit and a spiritual thing"

Dr. Edward Bach

It is to the more modern times of this century that we move to the pioneering work of Dr. Edward Bach (1886-1936). He was indeed an extraordinary man, the legacy of the flower remedies he left has certainly paved the way for future research and development, his methods of working and making essences, a foundation for others to follow in his footsteps.

A highly intelligent and intuitive man, a doctor and bacteriologist and like many who had gone before him, 'unconventional' and 'innovative' in his approaches to health and healing with similarities in his philosophies to other famous physicians.

Dr. Bach's research and work with intestinal bacteria led him to prepare nosodes – (vaccines) which could be given orally. The results for those with chronic disease were remarkable and are still relevant and in use by homoeopaths today.

Dr. Bach became increasingly dissatisfied with conventional treatments, he felt that they concentrated too much on the physical body. He knew, like Paracelsus and Hahnemann before him, that in order to have complete health and well-being, the emotional and spiritual aspects of a person must not be ignored – he recognised how destructive emotions such as fear, anger and depression could be. A turning point in his life occurring at the age of 43 when he gave up his successful Harley Street practice as he knew that his future research was to find remedies from amongst the wild plants and herbs of nature. Through his perceptive observation of human suffering, Dr. Bach went on to find a complete range of flower remedies which he declared to be complete and final before he died. Before finding some of the plants, he would experience extreme states of mind for which the particular remedy was required and would be drawn to the correct plant which would subsequently ease his physical and mental distress. The philosophy behind Dr. Bach's methods takes into account the whole being – body, soul and mind – and is intended for anyone, regardless of social, cultural or time factors.

After the early death of Dr. Bach, his close friends and colleagues Nora Weeks and Victor Bullen were entrusted with the continuation of his work at the Bach Centre, Mount Vernon. It was Dr. Bach's wish that his system of healing should be shared amongst everyone – the simplicity of the system being fundamental. Some of Dr. Bach's early work and writings are still intact, held in the archives of the Bach Centre, and although he destroyed many of his old papers and research notes, the weight and depth of knowledge contained in his modest books 'Heal Thyself' and 'The Twelve Healers and Other Remedies' is enormous.

For many years until the 1970's, the Dr. Bach remedies stood alone. Gradually interest in flower remedies has grown with inspired makers from all around the world. Today, in addition to the original 38 remedies of Dr. Bach, there are now hundreds of remedies all of which are relevant to our rapidly changing world and addressing mankind's emotional, spiritual and physical needs.

Flower Essences – 'Tools for transformation, catalysts for change!'

"The Happy soul does not die of disease. Disease is the result of inharmony. Preserve harmony in your souls and it will be in your lives; your bodies will know no disease because every cell will be under the control and direction of God in you". – White Eagle

Hipprocrates, Paracelsus, Hahnemann, Dr. Bach and other great healers, all shared the philosophy that illness was the result of imbalance, which could show upon the body as physical and emotional pain and suffering.

Energy or life-force is within all living things, that innate quality that constitutes 'life'. Eastern medicine has always recognised this life-force and has worked with the energy. To the Chinese, it is known as 'chi' which flows through meridians, channels forming a network of energy throughout the body. In India the energy is known as 'prana' meaning 'breath of life'. Illness or dysfunction is seen as an energy blockage.

When we are born, we are generally strong in life-force, but our health and well being is influenced as we grow by the difficulties and experiences we encounter. Our resistance to illness and our body's vital energy can be weakened by negativity in the form of anger, fear, frustration, hate, resentment, etc., becoming trapped within the body. Flower essences renew and restore the energy to its trueness activating our life-force which is the 'real' healer.

The human body and all life forms are surrounded by an aura, a field of bio-magnetic energy, which mirrors physical vitality. The aura and the other bands of energy surrounding the human body, known as 'the subtle bodies' (see Chapter 2) play an important role in maintaining good health. The subtle bodies vibrate at high frequencies and therefore the energy directed towards them needs to vibrate at these frequencies too. Flower essences contain the high frequency energies that are needed containing unique energy patterns and healing characteristics. Flower essences are the electromagnetic patterns, the etheric imprint of the flower. The positive energy/vibration of a flower essence counteracts the negative state within us, working at the levels of the subtle bodies readjusting disturbed emotional patterns. Today, the original Kirlian Photography which was able to capture plant and human energy fields on film is being further expanded and researched to include the energy fields of flower essences.

Our lives are constantly moving, changing and growing, occurring on an individual, collective and global scale. It has been said that our only confirmation of life is growth, sometimes the growths and changes seemingly occurring in a positive way to enhance our lives, whilst at other times our resistance causes us pain. Flower essences gently alleviate the pain and support the changes and growth, they can be likened to a candle being lit within us shifting our consciousness and allowing us to see the lessons to be learnt from our misperceptions and imbalances and also helping us to become more perceptive to the changes and obstacles, those opportunities for growth that come our way.

Flower essences do not contain any part of the plant as such and although sharing a 'natural' heritage with herbalism, homoeopathy and essential oils, they are made differently. Herbal remedies are made from many different parts of the plant and are usually ingested in the form of tinctures and teas. Homoeopathy as discussed earlier, is based on the 'law of similars' and involves using various natural substances which are repeatedly diluted and then 'succussed' or shaken to produce a remedy for internal use. Essential oils are pure plant concentrates, mainly distillations of the aromatic oils from numerous parts of the plant and containing therapeutic properties that have an impact not only on the physical body but on our emotional and mental states too.

Flowers are the highest concentration of the plant's life-force at the peak of its growth. In the making of a flower remedy, when the flowers are infused into natural spring water, the energy, the vibration of the plant is encapsulated, becoming 'liquid energy. Unlike allopathic medication such as anti-depressants or tranquillisers, which will force change on our brain chemistry to affect our emotional state, flower essences gently encourage change, allowing a 'partnership' of desire and commitment to begin. With the taking of flower essences, healing takes place at a gentle and subtle pace which our 'higher self' guides. By taking responsibility for our own healing process, our lives becomes a process of continued learning where the obstacles and challenges continue, but our perception, ability and the way we choose to deal with them is changed as we are able to observe from a calmer and more balanced body and mind.

Many people are becoming more aware that for everyday, commonplace emotional disturbances, allopathic medication is not the answer, often having unpleasant side effects. The resurgence of interest in complementary therapies, shows the desire to find another way – the tide of events going full circle. The pace of modern life leaves little time for nurturing ourselves or others, with increasing stress in the workplace a common thing as society strives inanely to more materialistic goals. As stress, trauma, emotional disturbances take hold, our bodies and minds are not able to function properly, we become more anxious which in turn effects our immune system and we lay ourselves open to illness – we invite it in! Therefore it is important to redress the ingrained imbalances which may originate and be linked to shock and trauma that occurred, even many years ago. The emotions that we carry for many years, as well as other disturbances such as surgery, physical injury, environmental pollution, dietary neglect and abuse and long periods of taking medication, will detrimentally affect our subtle bodies, filtering into and penetrating the very cells of our physical body which can then become unbalanced. Our life-force is affected; when we are well, our life-force is strong, when we are low, our life-force is weaker.

In flower essences mankind has been given a wonderful gift – the means to transform, to return to our natural heritage for our healing. By making use of what nature has provided us with, we can thereby ease the journey our souls have chosen to experience.

"Mankind is often stretched upon a cross in physical life, but as a result of crucifixion the fragrant rose is born within him. The rose stands for the heart of love. Would you withhold from humanity the sweetness and perfection of the rose?" – White Eagle

Chapter 2

Subtle Energy and Developing Awareness

"God-Goddess, the Mind of Creation, the All That IS, you may say is another description of love and that is the glue which holds the multiverses together. Without this energy force, this Light of Creation, there is no life, no existence. Every cell, every molecule, every sub-atomic particle shines with its own God-light. As you honour who you are as an embodiment of God-light, how can you not honour every thing and every one in your universe as a non-separate part of that same Light" –

P'taah – from 'The Gift' channelled by Jani King

Much of the information given in this book relates to the understanding that there is more to life than meets the eye! We exist in a period of tremendous change and transformation which is affecting all levels of existence and awareness. All our beliefs, structures and limited views of who we are and what we are a part of, are coming up for examination. In these often confusing times flower essences offer us a tool to help us to recognize what is true about ourselves and the world we inhabit.

The intention of this chapter is to look at the different areas of subtle energy that we may become aware of and interact with (consciously or unconsciously), while working with flower essences. None of this information is gospel! Our understanding and perception is expanding all the time and it is hoped that the readers will use their own discernment to determine the validity or usefulness of this information.

Simon France contributed the description of the Universal and Human Energy Field and the seven chakras, Gay Slater the information on pendulum dowsing and Maria Maw the description of muscle testing (Kinesiology)

As we work with flower essences and seek to find healing in our lives, we may

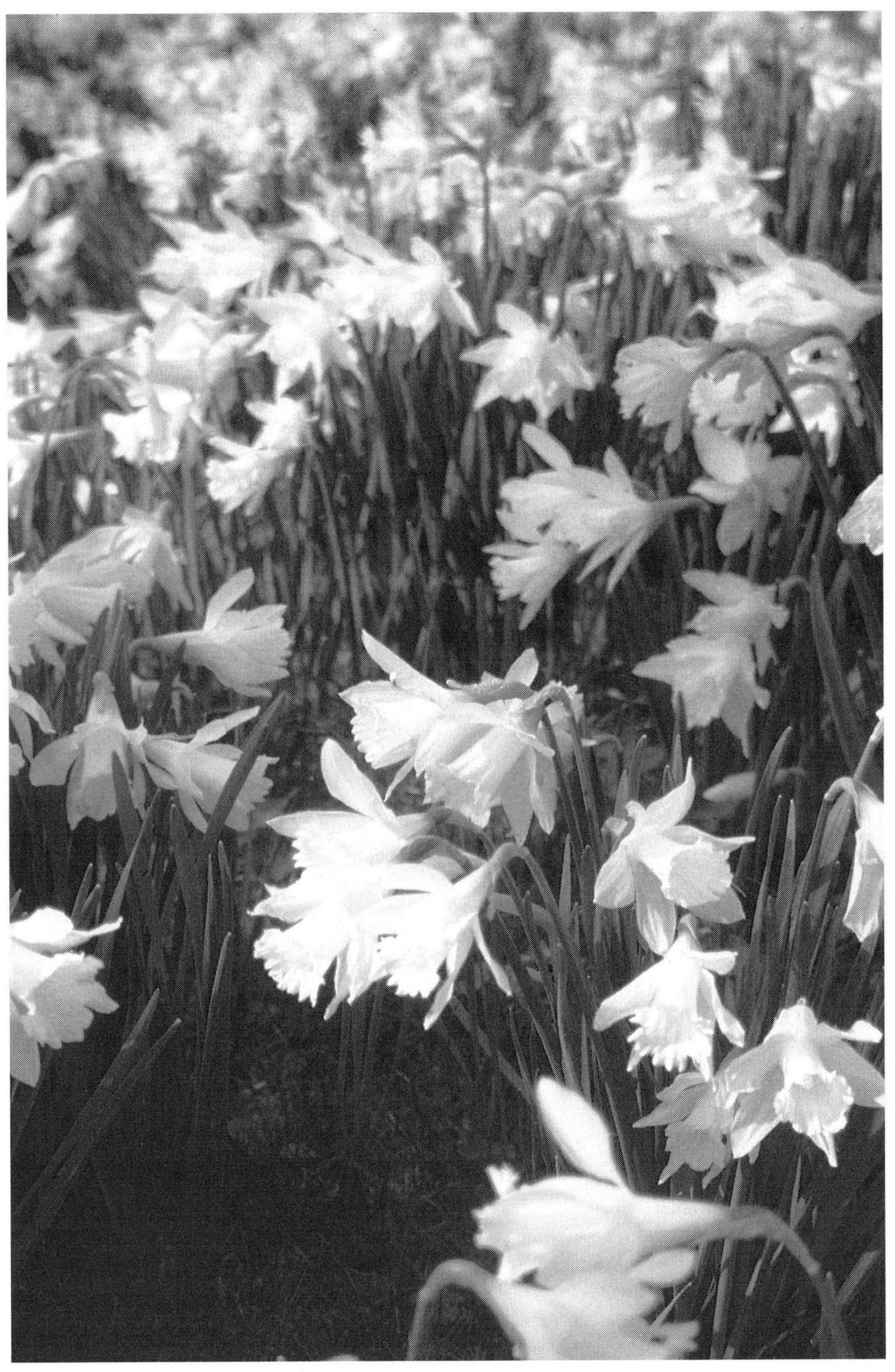

become aware of, or read about the universal and human energy field (or human aura) and the chakras. The following is a description of these:

The Universal Energy Field (Simon France)

"Everything is energy: it permeates all space, all animate and inanimate objects and connects everything together. This is what is referred to as the universal energy field. Not only are we a part of the universal energy field but so is every sentient being: everything needs to draw upon universal energy in order to exist and without it there would be no life forms".

The Human Energy Field or Aura

There is more to life than what can be seen with the eyes. The physical reality we perceive with our five senses is only one dimension; beyond lie many more. Likewise, there is more to our physical body than meets the eye. Surrounding our physical form is a field of energy, the human energy field. The vibrational rates of this energy field are so fast that they function beyond the speed of light, in realms that physical science is only just starting to penetrate but which have been explored and documented over many thousands of years by various esoteric/mystery/spiritual schools. Our physical body is enveloped in an invisible form of energy matter which extends out as far as the tips of the fingers of our outstretched arms.

This energy field does more than envelop our body; it actually interpenetrates the physical form. Our physical form is in fact part of the human energy field, where the energy has slowed down and contracted to such an extent that it no longer vibrates at frequencies beyond the speed of light. The further the energy field extends beyond the physical body, the quicker and more subtle are the vibratory rates. The outer edge of our energy field is the most rarefied, vibrating at very high frequencies, while the areas closer to the body vibrate more slowly.

The human energy system consists of seven layers beyond the physical form. The first layer closest to the body, extends an inch or two beyond and is referred to as the etheric body; at this level it is vibrating only slightly above the speed of light and is not difficult to perceive. Beyond the etheric there are six other bodies, the emotional, mental, astral, etheric template, celestial and causal, all vibrating at increasingly faster frequencies. Each succeeding layer completely interpenetrates all the layers below it, including the physical. The subtle bodies are not a remote or occult concept but an integral aspect of our physical bodies. In fact many alternative/complementary therapies work on the human energy field to effect healing. These include acupuncture, radionics, homeopathy, crystal healing, vibrational essences and spiritual healing.

Each of these seven layers or bodies is concerned with different aspects of our being. The bodies which are close to the physical transform the universal energy to a vibration which is slow enough for the physical body to use for growth, nurturing and sustenance. The bodies further away deal with the spiritual aspects of our being, while the bodies in the middle of the spectrum are concerned with our emotional and mental activities.

Chakras

The chakras are an extremely important part of the human energy field. When in good health they are highly charged and vital and can be imagined as swirling vortices of energy within the aura.

Chakra is a Sanskrit word meaning 'spinning wheel', for this is exactly what a chakra is – a spinning vortex of energy in the human energy field. This is a description of the seven major chakras, although there are many smaller chakras to be found in the aura. The major chakras can be said to be the organs of the subtle bodies, playing a vital and influential role in our well-being at all levels.

The centre or heart of each chakra is attached to a central column of energy running the length of the body, in the same location as the spinal cord. The chakras penetrate the physical body and extend out, in a cone shape, to the edge of the human energy field. They resemble whirlpools spinning in the energy system affecting all of the subtle bodies.

The first, or root chakra, is located at the base of the spine, extending down between the legs. The second, or sacral chakra, is located about two inches below the navel. The third, or solar plexus chakra, is located at the solar plexus, where the bottom of the ribs join. The fourth, or heart chakra, is found in the middle of the chest. The fifth, or throat chakra, is located at the level of the throat. The sixth, or brow chakra, is situated in the middle of the forehead, just above the bridge of the nose. The seventh, or crown chakra, is right at the top of the head, extending directly up.

Function and Purpose of the Chakras

The primary function of the chakras is to transform the energy coming to us from the universal energy field to frequencies our body can accept. Chakras stepdown the high or spiritual energies of the cosmos; otherwise we would overload and burn out. The energy we receive from the universal energy field is called prana or life force and without it we could not live. The chakras are also the points through which energy leaves our bodies. Thus our thoughts, intentions and actions pass out through the chakras, in the form of vibrations, into the energy field where they can influence other beings, events or situations.

Each chakra is like a radio tuned to receive a different frequency, or to be more precise, a range of frequencies. They pick up vibrations of similar frequencies from the universal energy field and feed them into our being. There is an in-built filter system within the chakras which screens out negative or harmful energies, although in unhealthy chakras this natural immunity functions less well. The universal energy field contains everything we could possibly need or know and when the relevant chakra is mature enough the information will flow through the chakra, influencing our being accordingly.

The chakras are dynamic centres within the human energy field working through all seven layers of the subtle bodies. The chakras are the passageways through which energy can pass from one level of the subtle anatomy to another. If they are blocked or unbalanced, the necessary exchange of energy between the various layers of the human energy field is impaired.

It is widely accepted in holistic medicine that any physical disease is a result of imbalances first appearing within the subtle anatomy. We create our ill health, as well as our health, through our actions, thoughts, emotions and belief systems. If disease is not treated in the subtle bodies, it will at some point work its way down to the physical level of our being. This principle is also true of the chakras: blocked or unbalanced chakras will result in the dis-ease manifesting within the corresponding area of the physical body. Treating dis-ease at the higher and more subtle levels of the chakra is much easier and less drastic and invasive, than having to deal with the imbalances when they have manifested in our physical form.

Key concepts associated with each chakra

The following list contains Key concepts for each of the seven major chakras. It is by no means complete but it is presented to give the flavour of each chakra.

ROOT: *the ability to be here on planet Earth; being properly grounded, realistic and able to concentrate; orientation; patience; aggression; safety and survival; action; instincts.*

SACRAL: *sexuality; creativity; power and control in relationships; money; seat of emotions.*

SOLAR PLEXUS: *personal empowerment; making choices; self-esteem and assertion; confidence; intuition; being responsible for one's own life.*

HEART: *love; the ability to give and receive love; unconditional love; compassion; open-heartedness, loving oneself; heart's desire.*

THROAT: *communication; the expression of will power; personal expression, truth; creativity.*

BROW: *Knowledge; reasoning, development of the intellect; wisdom, learning, insight, clairvoyance; understanding.*

CROWN: *faith and belief; the meaning of life; spiritual orientation; enlightenment; acceptance; completion; alignment with the higher forces."*

Minor Chakras

In addition to the 7 major chakras it is recognized that there are 21 minor chakras located at the following points: one in front of each ear, one above each breast (where the clavicles meet), one in the palm of each hand, one on the sole of each foot, one just behind each eye, one related to each gonad, one near the liver, one connected with the stomach, two connected with the spleen, one behind each knee, one near the thymus gland and one near the solar plexus. Although these chakras do not appear to have such an obvious role as the seven major energy centres, many of them have recognized roles: those who use their hands in their healing work will necessarily develop the chakras in the palms of their hands and in order for us to be fully grounded we need to open the chakras in our feet.

There are, in addition, many smaller vortices situated all over the body (ie: in the fingertips) and it has been suggested that the smallest of these may correspond to the acupuncture points used in Chinese medicine.

Higher chakras

Over the years many healers and psychics have reported their experience of seeing or sensing further chakras extending above the crown chakra. There are many differing opinions as to the number, positioning and role of these chakras. Some of the essences in this book are described as having a healing purpose related to these chakras. Healers and psychics have suggested that our chakras are developing and changing in accordance with our spiritual awakening. We feel it is inappropriate to give any information on the nature of these chakras in this book; their existence is recognized, but little is documented and we feel that it is up to individual therapists and healers to recognize their own experience in relation to chakras and to value their own intuition and guidance when working with chakras and subtle energy centres.

(For further reading on chakras, subtle energy and healing – see reading list at the back of the book)

INTUITION, GUIDANCE, DOWSING AND KINESIOLOGY

When working with flower essences, whether making them or using them, we often need to use our intuition to receive answers to questions which arise, such as: "How many drops do I put in this bottle?", "Which essences shall I use," "Is this is the right day to make this essence?", "Is this the appropriate method to use?". Sometimes we have more detailed questions to ask and are seeking information and guidance relating to the qualities of an essence we have made, or we may be looking for deeper insights into an emotional issue we are facing, or seeking inspiration when preparing a talk or an article for a magazine.

Whilst we can draw on other people's opinions and experience, sooner or later we need to know what is real for ourselves. As we heal our own lives and help others to uncover their healing, we discover that the most empowering and healing thing we can do for ourselves is to learn to listen and know what's true for us, as individuals and to act from that understanding.

So, what is intuition? what is guidance? – Fundamentally speaking, intuition is the way in which we directly connect to the reality of life, from the standpoint of who we are and where we are, as individuals. It is our personal way of connecting to what might be termed: Universal Consciousness/the Source/The Flow/God and finding whatever it is that we need to know at any time. We all have this connection, it is our birthright. We don't need to be special, psychic, or highly developed to have complete access to whatever we need to know at any time; all we have to do is to learn to listen and feel and with experience, to trust our sensing and intuition.

Many people use their intuition on a regular basis without even recognizing it as such. Business managers, stockbrokers, people working in the creative arts: film makers, sculptors, commissioning editors etc… regularly make choices and decisions based on 'hunches', or inspiration. Everyone can be fully intuitive once they learn to recognize the signs and learn to ignore the limitations of the left brain/rational mind. As we learn that intuition can be relied on, it can become a way of connecting with whatever we need to know, in any situation we find ourselves in, throughout our lives.

The question is:- how do we recognize intuition? The most easy first step in recognizing and trusting our intuition is to take a frequently occurring event, one in which we can hazard a guess as to its outcome and can fairly swiftly find out whether our guess was correct. I first began to test my intuition by trying to work out whether someone would answer the phone when I was calling them. I tried to feel whether they were there, or not and could immediately find out if my sensing had been accurate. I have played this game for years as a way of strengthening my recognition of this internal yes/no feeling.

Obviously everyone has a different internal intuitive response which they will recognize with a little practise. For me, it's always an open/closed feeling, or a stop/go feeling, almost like a traffic lights, but not visual. As I practised recognizing this feeling, I noticed a third response which was in between the yes/no; a kind of 'maybe' feeling, which could move to either yes or no; like an orange traffic light! I have learnt from experience that this feeling means 'ask further'. Often this feeling is related to situations where a question of timing or approach might be relevant, eg: when asking whether it is appropriate to phone someone, the answer might be 'maybe' and further questions might draw the answer, "not now, phone this evening, they are out, or busy". When asking whether to put a particular essence into a treatment bottle and receiving a 'maybe' response, further questioning might indicate that this essence is appropriate for this person, but to use it topically, or to add it to a later bottle after the current issues have been addressed.

Intuition is merely an internal recognition of the same information that we can receive by using dowsing or muscle testing/kinesiology. The more we use intuition, the more we can trust it. The main thing our rational mind can't stand about intuition is the fact that we have to make a decision first and find out later whether we were 'right'. The rational mind likes to have everything sewn up first before making a decision. If we listen to our rational mind it will come up with innumerable arguments and reasons why we should not follow our intuition, many of them fear based and if we listen to this 'rational' mind we will then often find it impossible to hear and act on our intuitive feeling. The best tactic is to let our rational mind have its say (which may be lengthy!), to recognize and acknowledge it, but to not let ourselves become involved, to stay in the role of the observer. Sometimes it helps to write down all our fears and arguments until they stop, as this can be immensely revealing as to where our resistance and fears lie and can help us know ourselves better and understand what motivates or inhibits us.

When we are asking a question where we have a lot hanging on the answer, ie: when making decisions where the outcome may profoundly affect us, or those around us; then the rational mind may shout so loud, with so many arguments and fears, that we may be unable to hear the answer. If we do hear the answer we may not have the courage to act on it. The same is true for dowsing. In this situation it is almost impossible to hear a true answer (except in emergencies when what we need to hear seems to be yelled so loud that we can't ignore it). When faced with weighty decisions it is best to first get out into the open all our thoughts and fears and really examine all the nuances, undercurrents, arguments and anxieties, either by writing it all down, or by talking at length to someone who will listen without judgement or comment. Often this process in itself may reveal to us the leading edge of our answer and we will find ourselves now ready to hear that answer and act on it with surety.

The hardest thing about following our intuition is that we have to act first and find out later! Julia Cameron, in her book 'The Artist's Way' (Pan Books 1995) says that she tapes the following sentence to her writing desk: "Leap and the net will appear", to help remind herself that Life/the Universe supports us when we follow our intuition.

When first learning to recognize our intuition it is best to use it for the seemingly smaller questions and decisions in our lives – those daily choices – "Shall I go shopping this morning, or leave it till this afternoon? … Do I feel like doing this piece of work today, or another?". What we begin to realize is that our 'gut feelings' are inextricably linked to our intuition. In fact, 'gut feelings' – the actual physical feelings in our solar plexus are a direct and accurate indication of whether or not we are connecting with our intuitive response, or our rational/ego mind. When we experience a feeling of peace or calm in the area of our solar plexus, then we can be pretty sure that whatever we are sensing is accurate.

This 'gut feeling' sense comes even more into play when we develop our intuitive connection to the point where we begin to hear more than just 'yes', or 'no', or 'maybe'. Often after we have become familiar with our intuitive response and have come to trust it and use it increasingly in our daily lives, we may get to the point where we are asking questions that demand more than a yes or no response and we may also realize that, in many ways, we are receiving more detailed answers. We may find that a phrase or a sentence unexpectedly drops into our minds, or a stream of thoughts appear which reveal, perhaps in much detail, the answer to our question. Sometimes an answer arrives in other forms: from something we hear on the radio, in a line from a song, or we might idly pick up a book or a magazine and find our answer written there. The more this happens, the easier it is to trust that we will always find the answer that we are looking for.

There are three things to bear in mind when asking for answers to questions:-

The first is to be specific; this is very important as the question is the leading edge of the answer. If we can formulate a clear question we are already halfway to the answer. Those who use dowsing or kinesiology will know the importance of accurate questions. It is important to work out just exactly what is the question we need to know the answer to.

The second is to expect an answer.

The third is to not stipulate that the answer be 'right', to not be hung up about whether the information we receive is true or not, because by doing so we limit what we can hear or experience. In order to experience a greater possibility than that which we can reason with our rational mind, or see with our limited perceptions, we need to allow ourselves to hear and experience whatever guidance or revelation we receive, without censure or judgement. Ironically, we are more likely to come up with the truth if we can remove our anxiety as to whether or not the information we receive is accurate, or not; because this anxiety, this desperation to 'hear true', comes from our rational/left brain, which can completely inhibit our ability to hear anything which might be received by our intuitive/right brain. After the experience we can then try to ascertain how much of what we have received rings true for us. Then is the time to ask more questions until we feel that we are happy with the answers we have found. Sometimes an answer can be challenging and it can take some time and much further questioning before we feel at home with the answer.

I find the following passage provides an extremely clear explanation of how we may determine the validity of any information we receive, either from our own internal listening, or from external sources.

"It isn't as though you have a lot of choice as to what you are going to listen to:- you're either going to hear the voice for truth, or you're going to hear the voice of the ego — the voice for fear. These are the only two choices you have. When you listen to the voice for fear (or the voice of the ego) you are miserable. It's what you have been listening to all along, until somewhere along the line you realize that there is a voice for truth — whatever you might call it — God, an angel, the Holy Spirit; but once you find out that there is an alternative, then it behoves you to enquire of the voice for truth.

Now, the real question then is — not how do you distinguish between the various spirits, but how you distinguish between the voice for truth and the voice for fear. And that's where simple honesty comes into play — What are the fruits of what you're hearing? — The voice for the ego will tell you: "Save your own arse… Take care of number one… Be alert for the dishonesty of others… The world is an unsafe place to be… Love is not called for here… Love is not called for there…" etc… etc… You can tell the difference, if you are willing to be honest and one of the best ways to be honest, one of the ways to bring forth the 'environment' of honesty, is to enquire of your guidance without having an investment in the answer. If you have an investment in the answer, you are quite likely to hear your own little ego voice answer you.

An answer that you have an investment in, is brought forth by what the Course (A Course in Miracles) calls a 'pseudo' question. It's a question that isn't really a question, but a request for confirmation of what you already believe, or what you want to be true; but when you ask with the intent to hear whatever the truth really is, in spite of what you want the truth to be, you will be in that place where the answer can be heard from the Holy Spirit – from the voice for truth.

Most people find that when they are hearing the voice for truth, there is no sensation whatsoever in the pit of their stomach, in their solar plexus, but when the ego is responding, there is that queasy sensation that children experience when going down a fast elevator and that is usually an excellent guide as to what is the source of the information that you're hearing.

There isn't you and your ego and you are not your ego. You are the Christ… you are the Divine One that you are, either seeing everything clearly, or through a glass darkly… When you are seeing through a glass darkly, you are experiencing through the lens of ignorance. That perception of everything and the thoughts that accompany it, are nothing more than the manifestation of the ignorance of who you are – and that is called the ego – that is the Christ dreaming a dream – it's not another presence.

…So, these two voices aren't really two voices, they are two different ways of perceiving one thing – Reality. The ego can't do anything to you. The ego is really just a faulty way of perceiving and either you are perceiving, by means of ideas, ignorantly, or you are perceiving by means of whole vision, Reality; and thus there are only two things for you to function with and one of them is an illusion.

…It's a simple matter of whether you're going to listen to the voice for ignorance and believe all of its limitations, or whether you are going to engage in curiosity about the truth and care to listen for the voice for truth and make commitment to that and enjoy the bubbling forth of a spring within that nourishes the experience of your divinity, in every aspect."
Raj – Leiston Abbey, October 1996

The best time to ask questions that require a more detailed answer than 'yes' or 'no', is perhaps before we go to bed at night. Sometimes the answer will come before sleep, on waking in the morning, in the shower, or during the course of the next few days. If we gets into the habit of having a pen and paper handy at all times, or a pocket dictation recorder, then we can write down , or record, all the insights and inspirations that arise. The important thing is to start writing, or recording, whatever we have picked up, without judgement or censorship, or worries about grammar, or completed sentences, until we reach the very end of the flow of ideas. If other thoughts, anxieties, preoccupations come up as well, we record these too, until these too have run their course. It doesn't matter if it doesn't all seem to relate. We can aim to treat this as an 'emptying' exercise in which we allow all our thoughts and feelings, conscious or unconscious, to flow out onto the page, or find voice. Often we will be surprised by the insights and unravelling that will occur in this process, along with often very detailed answers to the questions we have asked.

This gathering of guidance, intuitive insight and intuition bears particular relevance when we are attempting to discern the qualities of an essence we have made. We will find that if we ask specific questions, ie: "What are the physical qualities of this essence?", or, "What is the deeper and more fundamental picture that lies beneath this particular emotional pattern?", we may find that we can receive quite detailed information and that we can go on to ask further questions until we are satisfied that we have understood what we need to know for the present.

Pendulum dowsing and muscle testing (kinesiology) are both very valuable ways of accessing the same information that we receive when using our intuition. They are both immensely helpful in clinical practice, offering us another means of obtaining accurate information and diagnosis. I feel it is important to include some information about them in this chapter, since many flower essence practitioners and essence makers use these skills in their daily work. Since I am lacking in sufficient experience or knowledge of either practice, the following descriptions were generously contributed by Gay Slater and Maria Maw.

Pendulum Dowsing – for Flower Essences and more:
(contributed by Gay Slater)

"The ancient art of Dowsing has been used over the centuries to assist people to connect to the Source, or the Universal Mind, in order to obtain information that their rational minds could not work out. The uses of dowsing have been many, from locating underground water or geopathic stress, to detecting mineral deficiencies or food intolerances in a person or animal. We can use dowsing to ascertain which flower remedies to use, how to apply them, or how frequently to take them.

THE PROCESS

Pendulums are made of varying materials, e.g.: glass, wood metal, quartz or other materials. The principle is to use an object that is uniform in shape that can be suspended by a chain or thread from the fingers and thumb. It should be heavy enough to hang vertically and swing in an even circle. Take up the pendulum and mentally ask to be shown a 'yes' swing. Wait for the pendulum to start moving and note the direction, either a back and forth motion or a rotation clockwise or anti-clockwise. In the same manner, ask to be shown a 'no' swing. This will then become your basis for asking any questions mentally asked by you.

Before you start, it is wise to sit down and centre yourself, so as to be in a calm state of mind so as not to influence the outcome with your preconceived expectations. Be detached, yet focused. If you feel your mind may affect the answer, you may just ask the pendulum if this is so. If you get a 'yes', then re-phrase the question so that you can be sure that the answer is from a higher source and then re-check.

It is most important to ask if it is appropriate to dowse for the answer to this question, before you get down to detail. Sometimes it is in the highest wisdom that it is not the right time to know this, or it is not appropriate for you to know this about this person. Perhaps, even, there is a better way for you to find out.

THE QUESTIONS

First you need to be clear in your mind what it is you need to find out. Typically it may be to see if flower remedies are appropriate to use at this time, then how many should be given in the first bottle and then, which ones are best to use. Next it is useful to find out how many drops it is in highest wisdom to use how often in a day, on how many days of the week and for how many weeks – perhaps whether orally or topically, on chakra points or in the bath. Also useful is to find out what supportive measures can be taken, whether adjustments to diet or lifestyle, to reduce stress, or perhaps some additional therapy such as healing or counselling.

Using charts can provide a quick way of working through hundreds of remedies, some of which you may even never heard of. One way is to use a semi-circular chart, divided into concentric arcs, with different groups or sets of remedies listed in each of the arcs. The pendulum is held over the centre of the radius and will swing in a straight line towards the group that is most appropriate to your question. (see diagram)

Another concentric layer of the chart could contain the numbers 1 to 15, to be used to determine how many remedies, frequency of dosage and for how long to take them etc… Each person will need to develop their own way of using and constructing a chart, if they feel drawn to using this way of obtaining guidance. The diagram is really a prototype for you to develop.

PENDULUM DOWSING - SAMPLE PRACTITIONERS CHART

WHICH TREATMENT?

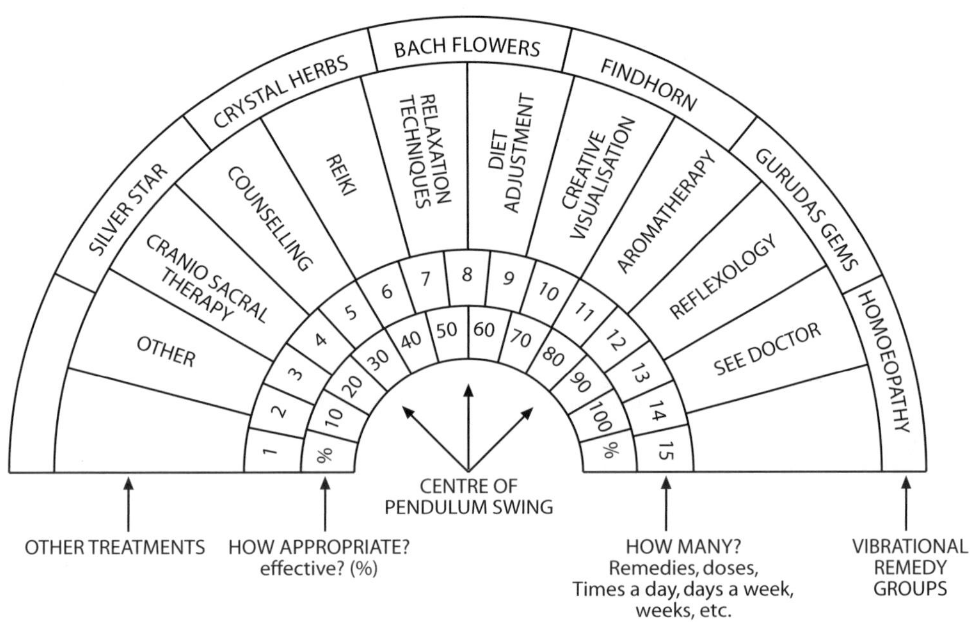

WHICH REMEDY?
or food, vitamin etc.

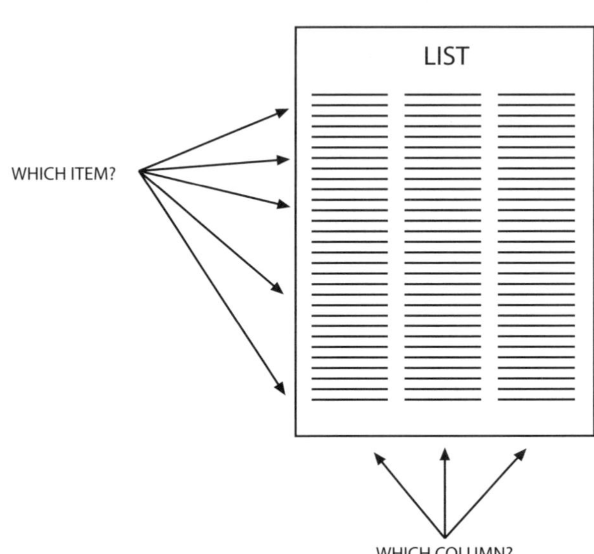

Having ascertained which set of remedies is to be used and how many individual reme-dies, then take a list of the remedies in the chosen set and simply use the directional swing of the pendulum to show you in which column is the first item to be found and then ask for the exact location of the item in the column, in the same manner. Proceed like this for each remedy needed.

A further concentric arc could have different supportive measures in it , such as healing, perhaps with a section marked 'other', as this gives space for something not on the list to come to mind. Your intuition and higher guidance is the means for formulating the ques-tions and receiving the answers via the small muscles in your hand and together with the intellect, evaluate the answers. Occasionally the pendulum gives a different swing from normal. This may mean that the answer is not a clear-cut yes or no. It may be a condi-tional yes, in which case further questions should be asked.

EVALUATION

With the information you have now received, you may find that on looking up the reme-dies that have been given, you can now see evolving a clearer picture of the person need-ing the remedies. You can see by the nature of the remedies selected, that a certain area of the person is being addressed, whether on a physical, emotional, mental or spiritual level. Your intuition will guide you once more to supportive ideas as you read about the appro-priate remedies. You are then in a better position to discuss and gently find out more about the issues concerning them at that time. This time spent with your client is most valuable, as it is helping them to externalize what needs to be changed for their onward growth and healing so as to heal the Earth. When the client has left, or when you have finished assem-bling the remedies, always pause to give thanks for the many loving sources of energy that have been sent to you, to work in this way.

OTHER USES

The uses of the pendulum are as broad and far reaching as the scope of the imagination. Care must be taken only to ask for appropriate information. Questions about the future are inapt, as we have free will and therefore this determines future events and cannot accurately be predicted. Also information should not be sought for personal gain and advancement at someone else's cost. You can seriously affect your own dowsing ability and even your health if you abuse this gift.

Dowsing is a stepping stone, for you to make better contact with your intuition and the higher dimensions and eventually to find that you can communicate directly with your higher self and other sources of light as you increasingly find that you are getting the answers before you pick up the pendulum. Trust this guidance and continue to ask ques-tions and you will receive all the help that you need from both the energy sources of the Earth and also from other higher dimensions.

All is one".

MUSCLE TESTING

(contributed by Maria Maw)

"Muscle testing is a method of accessing information directly from the body and it utilizes the body's nervous responses to different stimuli. It usually involves applying light pressure to an extended arm. The amount of resistance in the arm indicates the body's nervous reaction, or energy response, to a given stimuli.

Our bodies' energy levels respond rapidly to certain experiences, substances or information. Muscle testing picks up not only on dramatic changes in energy levels, but also very subtle ones of which we are consciously unaware. As a tool it can be used alone by a therapist to test for reactions to substances, or in conjunction with a Question and Answer technique. Here the test provides 'yes' (strong response), or 'no' (weak response) to a series of questions aimed specifically to access more detailed information".

SELF TESTING USING FINGER TESTING:

This is a kinesiology method of muscle testing oneself which does,not require the assistance of a partner. Finger testing can be used to obtain positive or negative responses to questions (as one does with standard muscle testing and dowsing)

CREATING A CIRCUIT:

For **right handed people:** place together the tip of your **left** little finger and the tip of your **left** thumb.

For **left handed people:** place together the tip of your **right** little finger and the tip of your **right** thumb.

When you join your thumb and little finger, you close an electrical circuit in your hand and when testing you will be using this circuit.

These fingers can touch in whatever way is most comfortable – finger pad to finger pad, tip to tip, or thumbnail resting on top of little fingers nails.

TESTING THE CIRCUIT:

To apply pressure to the circuit in order to obtain positive or negative responses:

Place the thumb and forefinger/index finger (of the opposite hand to the one you are using to create the circuit), inside the circle created by the circuit fingers. The thumb and forefinger should touch the circuit fingers – don't attempt to join the testing fingers.

Testing for a positive answer:

With the fingers in this position ask a yes/no question to which you know the answer is yes, ie: Is today Monday?, then, pressing the circuit fingers together at the tips, apply the same degree of pressure with your testing fingers against the circuit fingers, attempting to push apart the circuit fingers. Your test fingers should look like scissors opening as you try to push apart the circuit fingers… If there is a positive answer to your question you will find it hard to push apart your circuit fingers. Apply steady, even pressure with your test fingers, equal to the pressure of your pressed circuit fingers (don't use a pumping action to try to push apart your circuit fingers).

Testing for a negative response:

Repeat the above procedure, but this time asking a question to which you know that the answer is no. Apply equal pressure again – a negative response will show if the circuit breaks and the circuit fingers weaken and easily open. Each person has a slightly different negative response and their circuit fingers will either separate a lot, or only open a short distance. Keep checking until you are familiar with your particular positive and negative responses. It helps to rest your forearms on a table or in your lap so that you are not creating muscular tension in your arms while you are testing.

Finger testing tips:

Always centre yourself before testing each question and be aware of when your concentration is affected by external or internal distractions. As with dowsing it is often hard to obtain an accurate answer to those questions where we have a lot hanging on the answers.

In this case it may be best to ask someone else who is not involved, to test for the answer, or to wait until one can approach the question with equilibrium. Not all questions are meant to be answered at the time that we choose to ask them. Sometimes we have to wait for things to be revealed.

Don't try to test your circuit fingers before you have joined them with sufficient pressure to create a circuit. This is especially useful to remember if you are doing a lot of testing and are going too quickly or not concentrating.

The question is the leading edge of the answer – it is important to ask accurate questions if you want accurate answers. It is also important to focus on the question as you ask it. It's no use asking what essences to put in a dose bottle while trying to decide what to cook for supper! It is also essential to have an open mind about the answer. If you don't want to accept a particular response to an answer you will block the true response with your will.

Chapter 3

Consciousness in Nature – Communion and Partnership with Nature

"We wish always to bring you closer to the core of life, the divine essence of life! At the depths of our being light shines forth from the centre to infuse and penetrate all life. Stand bathed now in this peace and illumination! Let your spirit and divine nature be revealed until all is united and merges with the Divine!…" Landscape Devas, from The Golden Web, by Gwennie Armstrong Fraser

"We rejoice at human co-operation. We have always been willing to do so and rejoice now because you are reaching out to us. The initiative must come from your side; we do not force ourselves on you. we have always been part of life on Earth and of human endeavours, even when you have been unaware of it." Landscape Angel and Devas from 'To Honour the Earth' by Dorothy Maclean and Katherine Thormod Carr

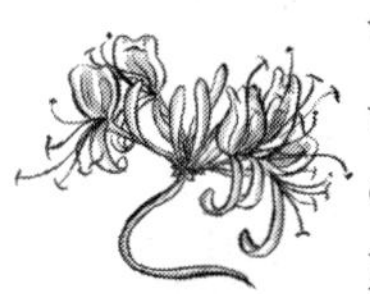

Whenever we spend any time working with flower essences, particularly when making essences and discerning their qualities, we are connecting with the conscious healing energy of Nature and are in partnership with that consciousness, whether we are always aware of it or not. In making essences we partner our own healing energy and intent, with the healing (Unconditional Love) energy of Nature, and sometimes too, with the healing energy of those in spirit who choose to assist in this healing partnership.

As we reach out to connect with the plants and trees that we feel drawn to work with, questions may arise as to the reality of Nature, its consciousness, and our relationship with Nature. Most of us have grown up with the mythology of fairies, elves, dwarfs etc. We may also have read psychic and spiritual development books with descriptions of the different orders of Nature spirits and elementals, including descriptions of their 'visible' forms. Many of these descriptions, although perhaps originating from someone's actual experience, present anthropormorphic traditional mythological visual images of Nature Beings. Marko Pogačnik, in his book, 'Nature Spirits and Elemental Beings' (Findhorn Press 1997), expresses his concern about these limiting descriptions:

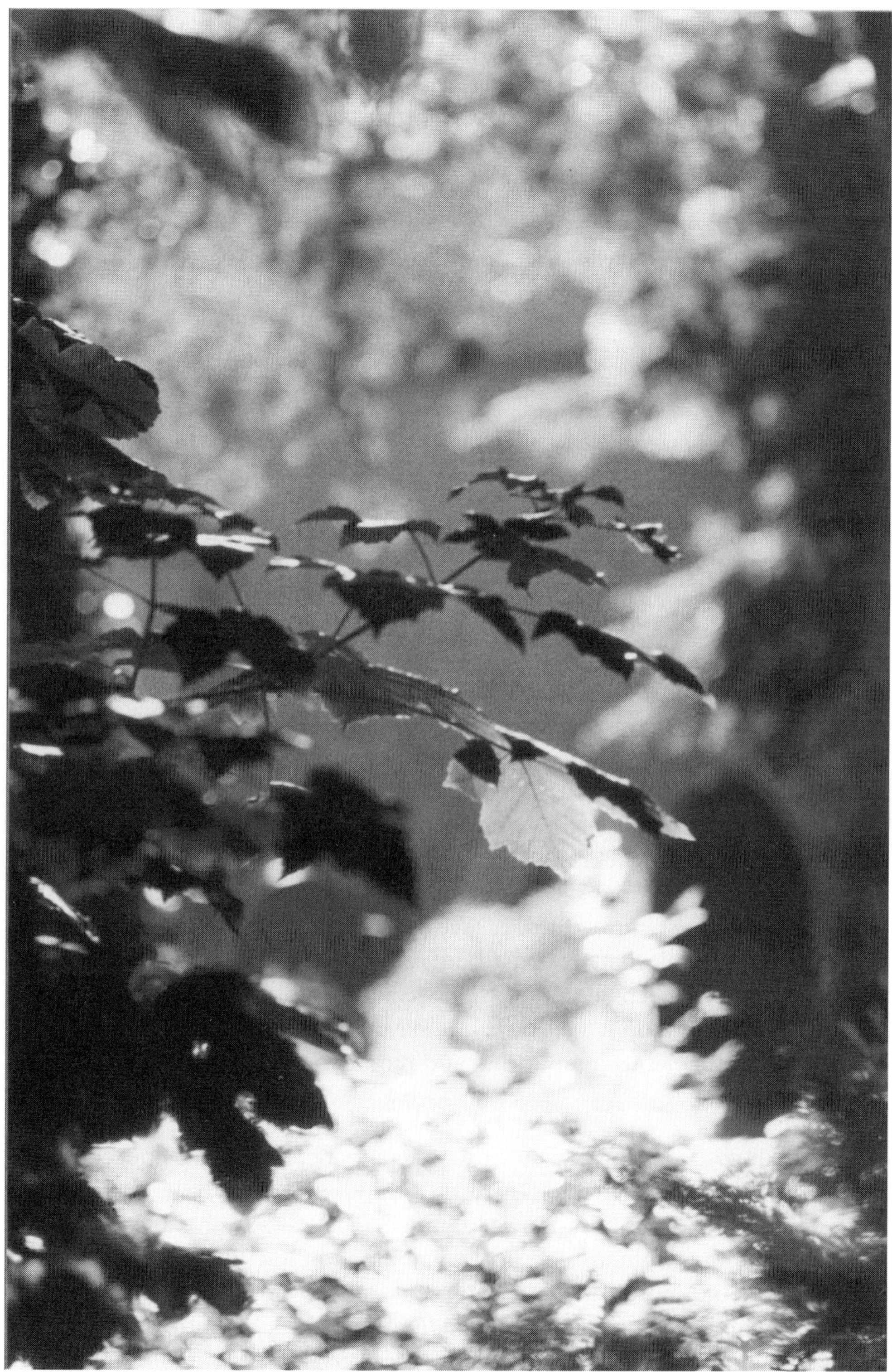

"In my opinion it is not right to force the world of dwarfs, nixies (water elementals) and fairies into visible forms related to our physical reality. Many people believe it would only need a refinement of our sense of vision to be able to see the ethereal forces of the elemental world, as if normal sight could be upgraded to clairvoyance…

In my experience this idea of clairvoyance is based on unfounded pre-conceptions. It rests on the assumption that the human viewpoint is the reference point for all of creation, without giving any consideration to the unique differences in the elemental world. Human beings have developed a very definite, refined outer physique, but we display to only a tiny extent how our inner thoughts and feelings operate. In contrast, the elementals are free of any pre-determined form. They can change their appearance to show what is happening inside themselves, which is very different from our human ways. Whatever form we perceive them in, it is either a mirror that reflects our stored archetypal memory of how we imagine them to be, or it derives from the language of pictures used by the elementals themselves to draw our attention to a certain message they want to deliver. They are without definite form unless we project our archetypal or imagined forms on them. One of these imposed makeshift images is the little gnome with his red pointed cap, his long white beard and leather trousers. Lovers of nature superimpose this picture onto the being of earth spirits. In turn this picture influences clairvoyants, who then claim it as the definite, indubitable truth."

Since we are in a time of tremendous evolutionary change as well as growth in consciousness, a time in which we are all becoming more awake to the multi-dimensional reality of existence, it seems important that we approach our growing consciousness with an open mind. Much of what was previously thought to be the rule, whether it be in relation to scientific understanding or healing and psychic teachings, is now being replaced by new understanding and experience. Every day old rules are being discarded as new discoveries are made as to the true nature of things. We each need to value our own real experience and not think that we must be wrong if our experience does not tally with what we have been taught, or what we have read in a book. If we don't see Devas or fairies, but nonetheless feel we have a meaningful or profound experience of Nature – let us honour that and remain open to further expansion of our own experience of who we are and what we are a part of.

The true, but at present mostly unseen, energetic, intelligent and conscious being in Nature, is far greater than anything that can easily be described in words. In general this is because we human beings still perceive and experience ourselves and the world around us, from a limited three dimensional perspective; whereas the mostly unperceived reality of the world we inhabit is wondrous and multi-dimensional, complex, fluid, formless, but intricately ordered, intelligent and infinitely conscious. Our language can seem very limited when we try to put into words revelations as to this multi dimensionality. Perhaps the nearest human expression of these dimensions is the aboriginal 'Dreamtime'.

There are, however, some descriptions of the consciousness in Nature that do not burden us with anthropormorphic or mythical images. Some of these can be found in the writings of Dorothy Maclean, Gwennie Armstrong Fraser, Marko Pogačnik and Machaelle Small Wright (see Reading List at end of book). Much of the text in their books is from their own direct experience of communion and communication with the consciousness in Nature. The following passages are taken from Gwennie Armstrong Fraser's book, 'The Golden Web' (Findhorn Press 1995). In the early part of her book Gwennie describes the interrelated, interactive consciousness of all existence, and then goes on to describe the Devic level of consciousness, (The quotes in bold italics are from the Devas themselves):

"When I first heard Nature speaking to me through the Devas, the archetypal patterns and energies within the natural world, my love and experience of Nature since childhood came sharply into focus again with new meaning. I was not seeing the presences but hearing them. This brought the reality of other realms through into my own life with a single, profound realization: that human life is part of a much greater field of consciousness, that Nature has its own levels of consciousness and intelligent forms, and that a flow of consciousness exists between humanity and Nature that allows mutual awareness and communication.

The Devic level of consciousness is a force of light and energy which exists throughout Nature. Devas belong to the plant, vegetable and mineral kingdoms and they exist in all places and in all things. They are essential energies composed of great light, and they are highly refined and pure in nature. Deva is a Sanskrit word meaning 'Shining One'. The Devas may be described as beings of light since they are bodies of light and energy which encompass the growing formations of trees, plants, rocks, and also the elements. Devic consciousness thus embraces both organic and inorganic matter.

The Devas govern the formation, details and components of each individual species. They therefore represent the myriad forms of Nature and are beings which exist in light form to nurture the growth of all living systems. As such they are life-giving and they have their own consciousness. Since Devas are involved in life formation, their nature is precise and exact. They bring together and focus the life energy of individual species, which is like a concentrated pattern and imprint. They are essential energy forms which contain the collective pattern of an entire species. These essential energies can be described as Devic essence, for they represent the total nature of a species and everything pertaining to a particular species is contained and gathered within the Devic energy and light body. Their consciousness is therefore highly evolved and represents the uniqueness of living forms.

The Devas always describe themselves in terms of light and they continually refer to the light of their realms…

All of Nature is an ocean of life forming energy, and we are the tides and forces at work within the ocean, working to give it life, shape and form, and creating the seasonal and cyclical patterns. All life contains a basic energy or life-force. Each species, each individual plant, each detail of a stone, or a flower, or a grain of rock -the flow of water itself – is a moving interaction between these basic forces. We communicate to you a basic notion of energy. But it is important to understand that this energy is not a singular, independent entity – it is united and interwoven with All the energy at work in creation. Therefore we draw from the sea of light, the ocean of creation, to distil our imprinted patterns to an essence. This is the impulse of life which gives form to a particular plant or stone.

We are ceaselessly at work, shaping the flow of life. It builds. We are at work within an ancient matrix of energy which has already formed the landscape as you know it. We continue to build the detail, the cloth of the land which characterises the life of Nature which surrounds you. Everything is a manifestation of this force of life, an outward expression of essence, light and energy. We are the forces of subtle energy which govern the fabric and formation of life.

It is exquisite, intricate, detailed work. It is born of light, a light of distilled, pure energy. This is our source, to which we all belong. By the source we mean the greater essence from which we are derived and from which we receive our motivation and pattern to fulfil. The laws of nature are complex, but we best describe it to you as a pattern of interwoven threads. Each strand is a strand of light and energy which weaves the cloth. It is so intricate that humankind has little conception of what lies beyond the outward form of Nature. But we are here, at work, ceaselessly creating life. We draw essence together – this is radiating energy which amasses and forms. Do you see? It is a shaping THROUGH energy. We draw together qualities.

And thus when you see us, if you do see us, you would see us as shimmering light, shimmering energy. You would be amazed by the beauty of our realms. You would know in an instant our luminosity, lightness and perfection. We reach forward to you in ways that you CAN perceive. Therefore perception of beauty, appreciation of form, quality, content – all these things bring you to an awareness of the fabric and substance of life, of which we are the central force. All of Nature is created by this central force, this central energy and light. It is the breath of life that sustains us all. Therefore we wish humankind to know us more closely, to realize our interconnection, our interdependence and our need to respect and mutually benefit one another. In this, reality has to be recognized and understood for what it is, a much more complex and detailed web of relationships than has been understood.

We do not wish to give confusion or speak in terms you do not understand. If you see beauty in all Nature's forms, and know that beyond physical matter lie energy and patterns of light which shape life, you have a basic understanding of what our life forms are. We have consciousness, different to yours, but capable of transmission. Thus we speak through to those who are receptive and can receive the vibration of energy to which our realms are aligned. We leave you with our light, our joy, our blessings upon you."

Through ignorance and limited perception, much of humanity has been arrogant in its relationship with Nature. We have mostly behaved as if we have owned the earth and have acted toward it with little sensitivity, respect or appreciation. How often have we attempted to inform the earth or our plants, of our intention to interfere in their realm? How often have we asked permission to enter a wild place, or pick a wild flower? The natural world gives unconditionally and always seeks to heal and redress imbalance. It welcomes our cooperation and the opportunity to work together for the greater good. We are constantly partnered with nature and always have been. Our physical form is Nature – our blood and cells are formed, maintained and nourished by the elements of this world. Everything we touch or interact with is formed from Nature – our houses, clothes, cars, computers, food, books, the air we breathe, the water we drink, the electricity we use. We cannot live without our relationship with Nature and now, with growing understanding we are beginning to recognize the unity and consciousness of all things – the Divine Reality.

If we wish to develop greater awareness of, and communion with, the conscious reality of Nature, we need to allow in a greater experience of the world around us, to let go of any fixed or limited perceptions we may hold as to the nature of the world and our part in it. There is so much to see and experience when we stop for long enough to just 'be with' the world around us, with curiosity, appreciation and an open mind – to see with new eyes, to smell, to touch, to taste, to listen and hear, to love and to feel. The natural world is all around us, even in a city, and we may have an equally powerful experience of Nature from 'being with' a pot plant, a bunch of flowers from a flower stall, or a favourite tree in the park, as from spending time in a place of great natural beauty and wilderness.

This chapter ends with a quote from the Devas themselves (from Gwennie Armstrong Fraser's book 'The Golden Web'):

"The first way in which people can increase sensitivity to us is to seek us. Stepping into Nature itself is a conscious wish to spend time in our realms. This consciousness reaches us… We reach forth to all who come to us, and who respect and cherish the greater pattern of life to which all belong.

We speak in many ways! Our messages are also carried in sunlight, in droplets of rain, in the magical world of wildflowers, the depths of the forest and the waterfall pools. We are everywhere and everywhere we shine forth our gifts to life! Recognition of beauty and of the essential nature of life is the true priority. Nature shines and radiates! The gifts and blessings are there for all who have use of senses and direct them towards us. Love of Nature is the great gift you give to us. It is an exchange. Thus sensitivity is not a limited activity, for it is placing an awareness into our realms. We acknowledge and respond. Communication is made in all forms possible – it showers life all around you! This must be communicated. For Nature touches and blesses all, and all are welcome…

In stepping close to the world of detail and beauty, Nature's essence is revealed to you. These steps are part of learning and exploration. Each step changes awareness, within and around you. Awareness of the grain of a leaf, or the scent of a flower, or the inner pattern at the heart of a flower, brings you into our realms and awakens your heart to beauty in the world around you."

Chapter 4

Making Vibrational Flower and Plant Essences

"Do you truly appreciate the wonder of a plant? On the inner levels where energy is particularly clear and powerful, we hold the pattern in consciousness. On the outer levels, these different energy patterns appear: each leaf distinct and beautiful, each flower exquisitely planned and executed, each seed carrying its own life message. Each flower has a flavour, scent and power of its own. Some plants heal a wound, some help the eyesight, some balance the emotions. You are each intimately related to plants and to all creation on Earth and beyond. This is the miracle of the oneness of life".

(Rue Deva – 'To Honor the Earth' – Dorothy Maclean)

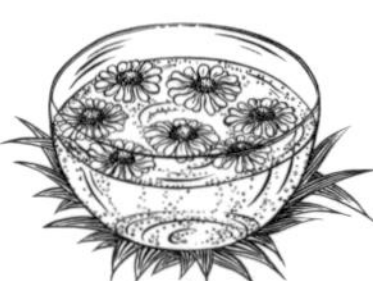

Essence making and the use of flower essences is very much a journey of the soul; an opportunity to listen to our hearts and discover what is true for us. Whilst there are basic methods that we can follow or adapt according to our intuition, there are no rules.

This chapter outlines the many different approaches to flower essence making – from Dr Bach's Sun Method to channelled essences. The aim has been to take an impartial and quite detailed look at how essences are being made and what we understand to be occurring when we make an essence. The information is based on current information and understanding and therefore may soon be replaced by the writing of other authors on this subject, since understanding and awareness are developing at a phenomenal rate at this time.

It is possible for anyone to make a flower essence. One does not have to be 'special' to connect with the consciousness of nature with the intention of creating a tool for healing. The most important requisites are our best intentions and attention, respect for the consciousness of nature, open hearts and minds and a willingness to see beyond our current perceptions of ourselves and the world about us.

As Ellie Web says:

"I really believe that everyone is able to make an essence and that in doing so we learn a

valuable skill, that of using our intuition. Of course some people are already more in touch with that side of themselves, so for them it is easier and some people are simply not drawn to doing anything like this. For anyone who says "Oh I would love to be able to do that", I would say try it!"

Making a flower essence offers us the opportunity to develop a deeper understanding of our own consciousness and the reality of the interconnected conscious mind of all creation – a recognition of God/Love/the Source in all. We can make an essence for ourselves or our family and deepen our connection to the natural environment around us. Even in an urban environment, a much loved houseplant or a wasteland buddleia may contribute to an essence for our healing.

Co-creation with nature

No description of essence making would be complete without considering the unconditional gift of love from the plants and the nature devas, our partnership with them and also with those others in spirit who help and support us in this work. A potent healing essence is developed from this co-creative partnership and through the intention to bring the conscious experience of love, healing and enlightenment into the world.

For centuries our relationship with the natural world has been one of dominion and psychic separation as we harnessed or destroyed Nature for our own purpose. A few cultures such as that of the Native American chose to maintain a partnership with Nature and the spirit within Nature, in which they took only that which they needed and then only with permission and thanks. Making essences offers us the opportunity to begin to glimpse the true reality of the consciousness of Nature and of ourselves and the potential for tremendous healing and creativity that can be generated by a partnership between Nature and Mankind.

Making a flower essence, if only once, can alter forever how we perceive the beings with whom we share this planet. It can be such a revelation to 'be with' a plant or tree, to allow ourselves to experience more of the reality of their Being and to make an essence with the co-operation of that Being, whose healing vibration can then be held to assist those in need of inspiration. Whilst making flower essences, many essence makers have had a powerful experience of the energy and consciousness of the plants and of the plant and nature spirits or devas and have become aware of a web of interacting and communicating energy patterns extending throughout all life and through many dimensions – to quote Simon Lilly (of Green Man Tree Essences):

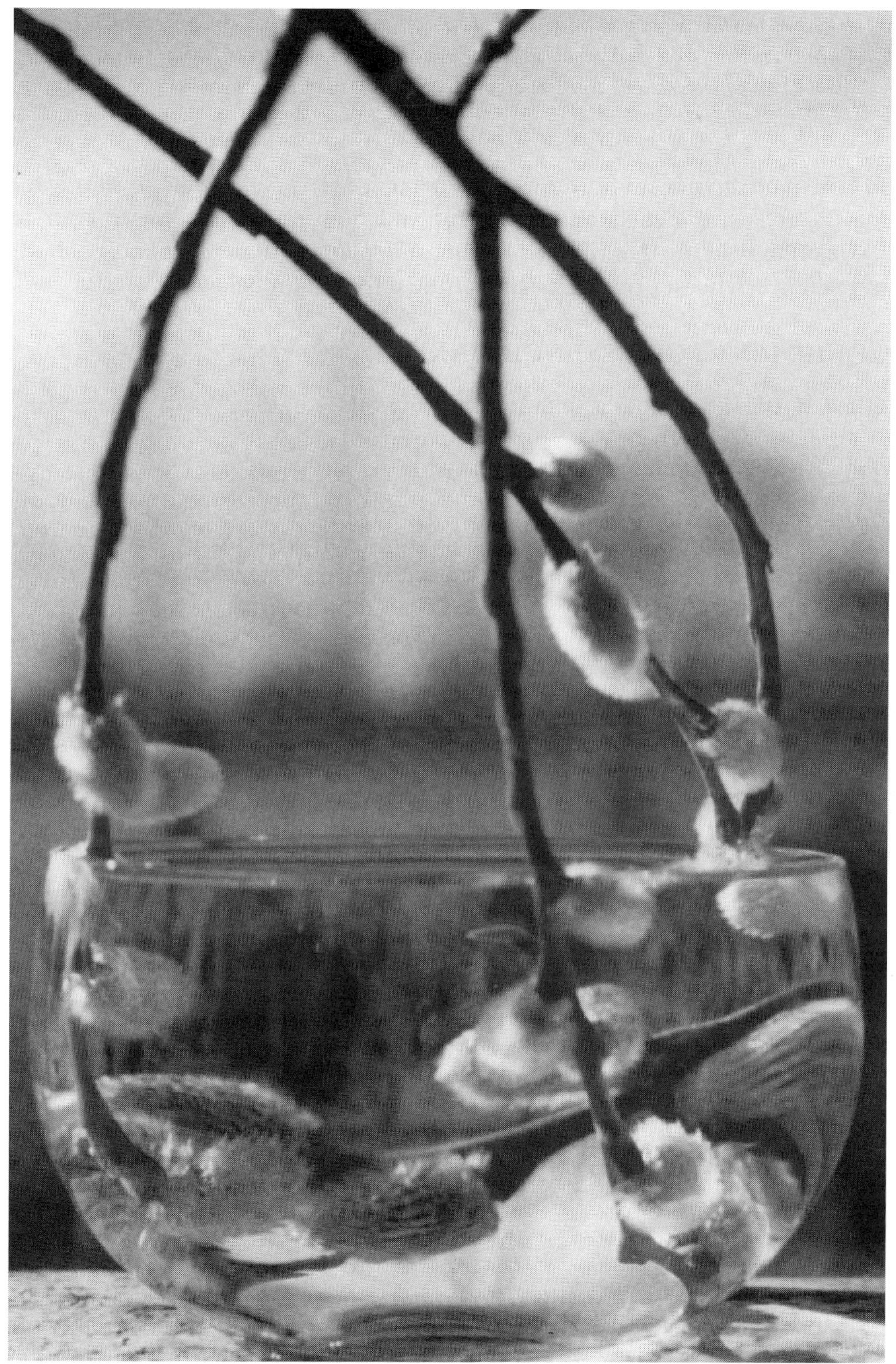

'Considering the actual process of making essences is so simple, it is amazing what a shift in consciousness can often occur. Almost immediately it is possible to feel a shift from everyday awareness to one where energy-flows and the interconnectedness of life becomes more apparent'

(Those who are new to flower essence making may wish initially to skip reading the following details on equipment and preparation and may prefer to move on to read the descriptions of choosing plants, attunement and methods of making essences, prior to looking at the information below.)

EQUIPMENT FOR ESSENCE MAKING:

Glass bottles (for mother tincture, stock and dose bottles):

These can be large; ie 100-500ml for storing mother essences, or as small as a 10ml dropper bottle used for storing stock essences. Dose bottles are generally 25-30ml dropper bottles. These can be used direct from the manufacturer although some recommend rinsing first with spring water.

A small amount of mother essence goes a very long way so it is worth considering not using the largest size bottles if one is only going to be using the essences to treat family and friends, especially if the cost of brandy is a consideration! Most essence makers use amber glass bottles for storage but some prefer to use clear or green or blue. One essence maker suggested that the chemicals used in the manufacture of some blue bottles might adversely affect the essences. Some makers prefer to use corks instead of lids for mother essence bottles.

(For information on re-cycling and cleansing bottles see under 'Preparation' further on in this chapter)

Essence making bowls, ie – Glass bowls, glasses, or glass tumblers:

Preferably not heat proof glass. Most essence makers use clear glass with no designs or marks on the surface, some say the best glass to use is lead crystal or, better still, a quartz bowl or half of a quartz geode. It is up to the individual to choose, according to what is available and what feels most appropriate to them at the time.

Spring Water, purified water or distilled water

If there is a spring nearby, of unpolluted, good quality water, then perhaps this is the best source of water for essence making; otherwise, most people use whatever is the best bottled natural mineral water available. (Jean Jacobs uses tachyon water for her Ascended Masters essences.) Peter Aziz uses fresh dew, collected before dawn, to make some of his essences.

Alcohol for preserving the mother tincture

Brandy, or vodka of whatever quality feels best. Some essence makers use other alcohol such as whisky. Viv Williamson and Jane Stevenson (Sun Essences) use Absolute Alcohol for preserving those mother tinctures that they will use for dropping onto pillules.

Non alcoholic preservatives

Mother essences can be preserved with cider vinegar or glycerine or honey as an alternative to alcohol. (see page 76 for non-alcoholic ways of preserving dose bottles)

Stainless steel or enamel pan and lid, (for boiling method and for sterilizing equipment)

It is best to keep a pan solely for this purpose. If using a cooking pot it really needs thorough cleaning and rinsing, followed by 20 minutes boiling before it can be used for essence making or sterilizing equipment.

A jug, preferably not plastic, for pouring the newly made essence into the mother bottles for storage.

Clean cloths to wrap cleansed bowls and jugs

Unbleached filter papers (to filter debris from mother essence)

Scissors or secateurs

Soft string (For tying down branches or stems)

Labels and pen

Notebook

It helps to record details of essence making along with any impressions received whilst making an essence as these can often aid us in understanding the qualities of an essence.

PREPARATION:

Cleansing bowls and equipment

There are many different approaches to cleansing the bowls and equipment used in essence making. The purpose of cleansing is to remove any energetic traces of previous essences from essence making bowls and to sterilize mother, stock and dose bottles to minimize the development of bacteria and viruses in stored essence and treatment bottles.

Boiling:

Many essence makers sterilise their bowls, jugs and bottles by washing and rinsing them first and then boiling them in a steel or enamel pan kept for this use. Some recommend 20 minutes of boiling, but practise has shown that many glass bowls will crack with this kind of treatment and so it's best to bring the bowls to the boil slowly and then simmer gently for 10 minutes before carefully draining. Even using this gentler approach the bowls can crack. Another disadvantage to boiling is that the bowls and bottles can become coated with a film of lime if the water is hard. We recommend that only rubber droppers and plastic lids be boiled and that glass bottles and glass pipettes should be sterilized in the oven, or steam sterilized and that glass bowls should be either steam sterilized or cleansed using one of the other methods given below. This way breakages and chalky bowls and bottles can be avoided.

Oven sterilizing

Clean and rinse glass bottles (and glass pipettes) in hot water, shake out water, (if sterilizing pipettes – place these inside the bottles) and while bottles are still warm, lay them on a clean wire rack in a moderate oven. Remove after 15 minutes and lay to cool on a clean tea towel. (Old treatment bottles can be recycled in the above manner – soak in hot water to remove labels before washing and rinsing thoroughly – lids and rubber droppers can be boiled for 10 minutes while the bottles and pipettes are sterilizing in the oven.)

Steam sterilizing:

Electric steam sterilizers, of the type sold for sterilizing baby bottles, can be used to prepare bowls and bottles for use. This method is used by Viv Williamson and Jane Stevenson (Sun Essences)

Cleansing with crushed quartz crystals:

Gurudas recommends cleansing used bowls with crushed quartz crystals wrapped in a piece of pure linen. This piece of linen and crystals is then briefly dipped into pure spring or distilled water along with the bowl to be cleaned. The bowl is then dried and the quartz is cleansed by dipping again in distilled water.

Cleansing bowls with salt:

Bowls may be cleansed with salt (after thorough washing and rinsing). Rub some clean sea salt, kept for this purpose, around the bowl, then rinse thoroughly before blessing and using.

Cleansing bowls and bottles with sound:

Richard Gonzalez has developed a way to clean bowls and bottles using sound:

"When cleansing bowls or stock bottles, I have found the quickest and most effective method to be with the use of sound. I use Tibetan gongs or chimes to clear unwanted vibrations from vessels and also to raise their vibration to receive the fluid"

Cleansing bowls and bottles with the smoke from burning sage leaves:

Richard Gonzalez also recommends surrounding the bowls and bottles to be cleansed, with the smoke from burning sage leaves. He has found this to be an effective way of cleansing.

Cleansing bowls by blessing and prayer:

Many essence makers like to offer up their bowls for blessing and spiritual cleansing before they begin to make an essence. It is a good way to focus and to connect with Spirit and one's higher intent. There are no rules about this: each essence maker has their own way of connecting with spiritual inspiration and what matters is that the whatever we do has meaning for us and is not simply an adopted ritual. Some essence makers like to hold their bowls in sunlight, or in visualized spiritual light as they make their connection and ask for help in their work.

Pat Staines uses the following approach to prepare her bowls, after rinsing and immediately prior to use:

"I hold the bowl, with my left hand underneath and my right hand on top, covering the bowl. Having stilled myself, I focus on my heart centre and ask that the highest vibration and the purest white light cleanse the bowl of any adverse vibrations".

Many essence makers use dowsing or muscle testing to check whether their bowls are cleansed and ready for use.

Once sterilized or cleansed, bowls and jugs can be wrapped in clean linen or cotton cloths and stored, ready for use at any time.

Whilst all the above are optimum methods of cleaning equipment, sometimes conditions call on us to be spontaneous and make use of whatever is available at the time. At these times, I feel **pure intention** can raise the vibration of the materials we are using and the resulting essence may be as good, if not better, than any made with scrupulous attention to physical detail.

CHOOSING PLANTS, ATTUNEMENT AND ASKING PERMISSION

Choosing plants:

There are many ways in which we are drawn to particular plants to make essences. Sometimes we may go out with our bowl intending to make an essence from one plant and end up being almost irresistibly drawn to make an essence from a completely different plant that we may have hardly noticed before, but which now seems radiant and fascinating. Often a plant may call to us over a long period of time; it may be a plant we have had a long association or friendship with. We may have received part of the picture of the healing qualities of the plant before we come to make the essence. Sometimes we make an essence and then realize that it relates to issues we are currently facing ourselves, or a client arrives and it becomes obvious that this is exactly what they require.

Essence makers may look for a plant to treat a particular person or issue, or may wish to replenish the supply of an essence and are looking for suitable plants.Sometimes a plant may appear in meditation or a dream.

Clairvoyant Peter Tadd describes how plants may call us:

"Flower essences are a product. They start with the plant's devic form working through the flower of a single species. Along comes an intuitive person who is interested in creating a flower essence. The plant probably has known about this idea even before the per-

son was ' conscious' of it him or herself. I feel that plants are broadcasting to us all the time".

Viv Williamson and Jane Stevenson who work together to make the Sun Essences describe how they are drawn to the flowers they use:

"We now understand that we are called to flowers that are correct for Sun Essences to make. We make a point of checking which flowers have recently held our attention in one way or another – colour, shape, feeling an unusually deep response to them etc. and as a rule we will be drawn to the same ones. Then, when the time is right (which may not be that year) we will be guided to the right place to make them".

With the level and spread of environmental pollution in the British Isles and the scarcity of wild places that are protected from human interference it is often difficult to find ideal locations for making flower essences. Many essence makers choose to use plants that reflect the environment in which we live, as Simon Lilly says:

"There are no truly unpolluted areas on this planet. Even an apparently natural location will have residues of pollutants, so I tend to focus on other aspects: – if a tree is healthy, mature and in flower, it is showing that it is balanced in whatever environment it happens to be in. It could be argued that the experience of a tree in a polluted environment is of more use to us as it teaches us energetically how to cope with and transmute pollutants. The main point is to have a clear energy pattern of the plant".

and Marion Leigh gives this example:

"In front of the house in the village of Findhorn where I was staying, was a large grassy common area, blanketed in daisies. One morning a team of council gardeners appeared with lawnmowers and without a thought I rushed down to ask them to wait until I had picked some of the flowers. They watched bemused as I silently attuned, asked for permission, gave thanks and proceeded to pick daisies and float them in my glass collection bowl. I could just imagine what they would be saying during their tea-break – another one of those loonies from the Findhorn Foundation communing with the flowers!

My doubts about including this flower essence into my repertory arose because of it's very public roadside location, but it came to me that this was the very reason for including it. Sure enough, when I tuned in, what I received confirmed that the essence of daisy would be for those seeking calm amidst the storm and hustle and bustle of daily life".

Our choice of plants may be confirmed by intuition, dowsing or muscle testing.

Attunement:

Most essence makers, in their own way, try to open their perception, to attune, to the conscious energetic being of the plants they wish to create the essence with. The simplest approach is to be still and open one's awareness to both internal and external perceptions.

Often attunement occurs over a period of time as we make a connection with a particular plant or group of plants. We may already have established an internal dialogue. Most essence makers like to sit quietly next to the plant they are preparing to make an essence from and try to focus on the energetic presence of the plant, to sense its overall healing quality and to make friends with it and appreciate it's unique beauty and purpose.

Ellie Web describes her approach:

"Making a mother essence is a meditation. We need to have a clear consciousness and a pure intention. One cannot make an essence when one is stressed or in any kind of negative state. This does not mean that we must be perfect! But we should have at least enough well-being to put our day to day troubles aside and sometimes, often, always! the essence we are making will have a timely message for us.

When I'm making an essence I sit and meditate for a few minutes, quietening my mind and slowly tuning in to the energy of the plant. I notice all I can about the flower, it's signature, it's body language, it's relationship to the environment, I am open to communicating with it, being aware of anything I feel this particular plant says to me, translating the essence of the flower into my own language. If I can, I write a few words about it. This synthesis is happening at an unconscious level too, so I don't worry if I can't, the words may come later.

Some essence makers feel drawn to call on Angels, devas, fairies or other beings involved with the plants, or with healing energies and guidance, to ask for their help in making an essence. Others feel that if this energy is called into the flower essence it may overlay it with layers of additional vibration which may affect the purity of the essence. Simon Lilly says:

Any process of blessing, summoning of archangels etc. will probably impress individual characteristics into the essence and this may enhance the efficacy for some people who are also aligned to those forces summoned/prayed to/meditated upon, but I prefer to allow the essence vibration and it's source/spirit/deva/awareness to keep itself discreet.

There is, however, a vast difference between calling in the energetic vibrations of those in spirit to imprint an essence and asking for help and guidance from spirit whilst we are making an essence. Many essence makers consciously work together with spiritual companions when they are making essences without invoking their energy into the essence itself.

Asking permission:

Once still and receptive, we can use our intuition, dowsing, muscle testing, or whatever means works best for us, to ask permission to use this plant's energy to make an essence for healing.

Sometimes the answer is no; this is not the right plant, the right time or day; at other times, the answer is yes and we can go on to ask which flowers wish to be used, how many, which colours, how long to leave the essence etc. . . Experience has shown that if the answer is "yes" to making the essence but one still feels uncomfortable, then the next questions to ask are whether the time is right and if so, where to make the essence, which plants, which approach to use, which parts of the plant to use. It helps to keep an open mind and not get too fixed an idea about how essences need to be made, as our awareness is continually expanding and presenting us with new possibilities. If we go to make an essence on a day when we have other jobs to do, distractions from children, mental or emotional concerns, or a fixed idea that this is the day, or the plant, or the way to make an essence, we will find it hard to hear our guidance and respond appropriately. Many essence makers have said that they wait until they know it is the right day, the right place and the right plants and only then do they make an essence. This means that sometimes they may have to wait a considerable time to make some essences if the opportunity is not presented during the flowering period of the plant in that year. One essence maker has spoken of waiting three years to make some essences. This approach requires trust that everything has it's time.

Peter Aziz says:

When a relationship has developed with the spirit of the plant, I wait for the spirit to call me to prepare the essence. They usually call me the evening before, so that I can be prepared and they give me a vision of where I can go. They then wake me at dawn and call me to the spot, where I prepare the essence.

METHODS OF MAKING FLOWER ESSENCES:

Our methods of making flower essences have developed mainly from the work of Dr Edward Bach in the 1930s. He devised two ways for preserving the vibrational healing energy of flowers:- The Sun Method and the Boiling Method. These methods were later developed in Gurudas' book 'Flower Essences and Vibrational Healing'

Since that time, both here and abroad, many people have made flower essences and have adapted Dr Bach's original methods according to their own intuition and circumstance. Some essence makers prepare their essences in the rain, some by moonlight, others float only a single flower in their bowl and a few people are moving away from picking flowers altogether and are devising ways of obtaining flower essences without removing parts of the plant.

The following descriptions of these different methods are intended to provide a base from which people can work – In no way are they fixed rules, – merely starting points.

Sun Method (Dr Edward Bach's method)

Choose a clear, bright, sunny day with no clouds in the sky. Begin making the essence before nine in the morning. Fill a sterilized, thin glass bowl (of about ½ pint capacity) with pure spring water, if possible from a spring nearby. Hold the bowl under the flowers to be picked, or carry the flowers to the bowl on a leaf so as to avoid touching the blooms. The whole surface of the water should be covered by flowers. Place the bowl beside the parent plants, but avoiding letting any shadows fall on the bowl, either your own, or from plants or grasses. Leave the bowl in the sun for 3-4 hrs or less if the sun is very hot and the flowers begin fading. If the sun becomes clouded during this time the remedy should be discarded. When the remedy is ready, remove the flowers from the bowl using a stem from the plant, rather than your fingers. Pour the essence into a sterilized amber glass bottle to halfway, filling the remainder of the bottle with brandy (to preserve). This is called the mother essence and is further diluted to create the stock and treatment bottles used in flower essence therapy.

As Julian Barnard says (in 'The Healing Herbs of Edward Bach' published by Bach Educational Programme 1988):

> *"When the remedy has been prepared you will sense the vitality and see that the water has been subtly changed"*

The Boiling Method (Dr Bach's Method)

Dr Bach mostly used this method for potentizing essences in the winter months when he felt there were not enough hours of continuous sunlight to adequately imprint the energy pattern of the flowers into the water.

Choosing a bright day, pick the flowers for this remedy before 9 am. Three quarters fill a clean enamel, or stainless steel pan with the flowers and stems of your chosen plant. The stems should be about 15 cm long. Cover the pan with the lid and take it home immediately (so that the flowers retain their vitality). Cover the stems and flowers with 2 pints of pure spring water and bring to the boil, without the lid on. If necessary, use a twig from the plant to press the flowers and stems down, as you simmer the remedy for 30 minutes. At the end of this time replace the lid and leave the essence outside to cool. When cold, remove the stems from the pan using a twig from the plant instead of your fingers. Filter the essence, using unbleached filter paper and then half fill a sterilized amber glass bottle with the essence, filling the remainder with brandy (to preserve). This is now the mother essence.

Most essence makers stick to the above guidelines if they are trying to replicate any of Dr Edward Bach's original thirty eight flower remedies and they try wherever possible to choose plants growing in similar habitats to the plants he originally used.

Tasting the original mother essence and giving thanks:

After making an essence, most essence makers taste a small amount of the mother essence from what is left in the bowl after they have filled the mother bottles. Often this can give us a real taste of the quality of an essence, particularly with wonderfully fragrant flowers such as cowslips or lilac.

Any remaining drops left in the bowl can be given back to the earth or the plants, while giving thanks for their healing gift and for the participation of the devas and those in spirit who have helped in the making of the essence.

Gurudas' Method

Many British and Irish essence makers have been influenced in their work by Gurudas' book 'Flower Essences and Vibrational Healing', (see reading list) and the information he gives on making flower essences. Gurudas' basic methods derive from the work of Dr Edward Bach, but the information in his book, much of which he received during trance channelling sessions with the mediums Kevin Ryerson and John Fox, explores these methods in much greater detail and adds new developments to the original methods. The main details and developments that he introduced were as follows:

Water:

Although Gurudas recommends using unpolluted local spring water, he feels this is hard to obtain and advises the use of distilled water.

Brandy:

He recommends using the least processed brandy available to preserve the essences and to use less brandy in the mother essence bottles; perhaps as little as 25% brandy, except where the essence has an intense life force ie: with roses, in which case, he recommends using 50% brandy to prevent the formation of bacteria or virus in the bottle. He suggests pouring the brandy into the bottles first before the mother essence to prevent the vibrations from the essence permeating the brandy bottle.

Moon Essences:

He mentions making essences in moonlight, leaving the bowls for 3-4 hrs.

Quartz cleansing:

Gurudas gives a method of cleaning bowls with crushed quartz crystals. (as described earlier in the chapter)

Amplification or enhancement techniques:

Gurudas introduces a number of ways in which the vibrational energy of flower essences can be amplified. The most frequent methods used are those involving pyramids and crystals. He describes placing bottles of essences under pyramids made from gold, silver or copper; with arrangements of clear quartz crystals and lodestones around the outside of the pyramid. He suggests that by doing this, the energy and clarity of individual essences can be maintained and enhanced.

Quartz or silver cutting tools:

Gurudas advises using a silver instrument or a piece of quartz to remove flowers from the plant as he says this stabilizes the life force of the flowers.

NEW APPROACHES AND DEVELOPMENTS IN ESSENCE MAKING:

Many British and Irish essence makers have used the above methods when making flower essences, but have adapted or developed them according to their intuition and circumstance. The following are some of the new developments and approaches used by these essence makers.

Weather and Timing:

Most essence makers don't discard an essence if the sun becomes clouded during the making; they simply leave it for a longer period to receive sufficient light. Many feel that making an essence at the 'right time' (in instinctive, spiritual terms) is more important than whether the weather or time of day is perfect. There are now many who make essences on overcast days, in light drizzle, overnight, or over the period of a day and a night. Some feel that by pure intention and co-operation with devas and angelic beings we may make essences indoors without the presence of physical sunlight. Dawn Carol talks of using 'spiritual sunlight'.

Peter Aziz states:

"I consider the co-operation of the spirit far more important than any physical circumstances, so I don't worry if clouds pass across the sun. If the plant spirit wants to come into the water, it will do so, even if the circumstances are far from ideal; though I do listen carefully to the needs of the plant and co-operate as much as I can. Different plants will ask for different types of water, different lengths of time in their preparation and different phases of the moon".

Peter Tadd has this to say:

"Plants, unlike minerals or animals are direct products of natural sun light and are unique in their relationship to the sun in two ways: first, what is commonly known as photosynthesis, the very basis of organic life and secondly, their energetic relationship to what is known as ether, or chi. The same kind of etheric forces which compose the energetic body of the plant is found in the 'physical' ether of the chakras and the outer edge of the aura of animals and humans. This is very important to us in again a couple of ways: first, when we tune into that level we feel instantly 'better' and a sense of lightness and connectedness to life and secondly, it is the etheric bridge that makes it possible to communicate with plants and flower essences.

I believe Dr Bach is right about the preparation of essences. When the weather is sunny we are experiencing an atmospheric high pressure and we naturally feel strengthened by the sun's rays. When it is cloudy we find our energies rather low. This exactly corresponds to the human aura and is why, at the end of the last century, it was fashionable for sensitives' to refer to the aura and the human atmosphere: for example: emotional depression appears as a grey, dense cloud in the aura".

Lunar Essences:

There are now an increasing number of essences being made by moonlight and starlight. Two sets of essences in this book are made in this way: 'Moon Flowers (Aquarius Flower Remedies) and Church Farm Roses. Essence makers choose this method for the different qualities imparted to the essence by the moon and stars.

Astrological influences:

Some essence makers consider carefully the astrological influences at the time of making an essence. Jean Jacobs feels that plants should be picked on their correct planetary day: ie: Monday – Moon. Tuesday – Mercury. Wednesday – Mars. Thursday – Jupiter. Friday – Venus. Saturday – Saturn. Sunday – Sun.

Whilst it is possible to plan the astrological timing for making an essence; essence makers have often made an essence at an intuitively chosen time and have later found that there have been unusual and powerful astrological influences at that time.(see the Church Farm Roses story at the end of the chapter)

Richard Gonzalez suggests:

"The time that a remedy is created at will undoubtedly affect its vibration and potency: where the planets are – the phases of the moon, if in the day or the night; all has its effect; but to try and work it out mentally, can send you mad. It is much easier to become sensitive to the plants involved and to our intuition… If sensitivity is involved, I have found all difficulties in finding the 'right time are immediately solved".

Saturated Essences:

Vivien Williamson and Jane Stevenson make two saturated essences: one from Copper Beech leaves and one from a mixture of autumn leaves. To do this they completely fill a bowl of spring water with leaves and stand the bowl outside for 1-3 days, before filtering and bottling with brandy. This forms the mother essence.

Alcohol Essences:

Both Arthur Bailey (Bailey Essences) and Andrew Tresidder make some of their essences by infusing the plants in alcohol instead of spring water. Arthur Bailey puts the flowers, leaves or fruit straight into vodka and stands these for varying lengths of time before straining out the plant matter. The mother tincture is then ready. The lengths of time depend on the essence; for example: Bistort may be left 15 minutes, whereas Pine Cones may be left for 24 hours. Arthur decides this by intuition and dowsing.

Cutting, picking and handling flowers:

One of the questions which arises when making an essence, is whether to directly handle the flowers that we pick to put in our bowls. Dr Bach felt that one should avoid touching the blooms with one's hands and he suggested covering ones hand with a leaf. Gurudas recommends cutting the flowers with a silver instrument, or a piece of quartz, before placing immediately on the water, as he says this stabilizes the life force of the flowers, preventing their critical essence from returning to the earth

Many essence makers now feel quite comfortable about picking by hand the flowers they use and directly touching the flowers before laying them in the water, although most still use a twig or plant stem to remove the flowers from the finished essence.

Dawn Carol says:

"I always use my hands to pick the flowers as this is the way that spirit and the devas prefer. It means that there is a good exchange of energy between the devas and myself – it means that they can receive direct confirmation of my healing intent and purpose and of course, my love. It also means that I can tell which flowers they wish me to have because if I am meant to have them they break off easily and if I am not, there is absolutely no way the stems will break; and in this way the devas have a more direct way of guiding my hands".

No-pick Essences:

There is a shift in approach away from picking parts of plants for use in the making of essences. Essence makers in different parts of the world are developing new ways to make essences which do not involve physically interfering with the life flow of the plant.

Andreas Korte, a German essence maker and researcher, who makes essences in Europe, Africa and America, places half of a clear crystal geode, filled with spring water, within the energy field of the flower and leaves it within the energy field until it becomes potent. The energy field of a flower or fruit can be likened to the aura and can be sensed intuitively by holding ones hand above the flower, or by using a pendulum. The crystals in the geode focus and hold the energy pattern of the flower, which is then imprinted into the water by the action of sunlight.

In the Himalayas, Drs Atul and Rupah Shah make their essences by placing a glass bulb over a flower and then gently pouring water over the flower into the bulb. The essence is fixed in the water by sunlight

Living Essences

Vivien Williamson and Jane Stevenson (Sun Essences) make some of their essences without picking the flowers they use. These they call 'living essences'. They dip the living flower into their bowl of spring water and hold it in place with a forked stick. This is left to stand for between 2-8 hours. They also make other essences in the same way , but, in addition to a single dipped spray of living flowers, they float some picked blooms on the surface of the water.

Other essence makers use a similar approach when making some of their essences – Light Heart Flower Essences 'Pussy Willow' essence was made by tying a single spray of willow catkins to the top step of a wooden stepladder, on which was placed the glass bowl of spring water; the catkins and ends of the stems were immersed in the water for the time it took for the essence to potentize.

Patterned Essences:

Viv Williamson and Jane Stevenson also make what they call patterned essences'. They have felt guided to lay the flowers in patterns on the water in their bowls. This is usually when the species of the plant has different coloured blooms. These essences are mostly used topically and are designed to impress a new pattern onto the energy system.

Laser essences:

Colin Kingshott uses a laser in place of sunlight to imprint some of his essences, particularly those made from poisonous plants, as he says:

"In this method there is nothing intrusive being passed to the water except the transference of the flower's vibrational signature and the water then becomes structured and retains the flower's signature".

Channelled Essences, imprints in essences, quality of essences

In a sense, all flower essences are 'channelled' essences, in that we ask that the vibrational healing essence of the flower be drawn into the water in our bowls and held there indefinitely for healing inspiration. Some essence makers specifically ask the devas of the plants they are working with, that the flowers in their bowls may serve as a focus for the channelling in of the archetypal healing energy of that group of plants, for example: when making a dandelion essence we may ask, for the greatest good, that the archetypal healing energy of all the dandelions across the world be drawn into the water through the medium of the flowers in our bowl.

Many healers channel their own healing energy into their flower essences, either consciously or unconsciously. Sometimes this comes about as a result of their strong intention that the essence should have a specific healing purpose, which they have envisaged and which they perceive to be needed at this time.

It has been noticed that essences often carry an underlying imprint of the state of mind (sometimes the unconscious state of mind) of the essence maker at the time of making the essence. Obviously the most inspirational, vibrant and deeply healing essences are those made with the most loving clear intention, the most humility and the most clarity of mind that we can muster. This may mean, that we realise, after honest reflection on the energy of some of our essences, that whilst we may have the correct description of the quality of an essence, the essence itself may need re-making at a time when we are in a clearer state. There is nothing wrong in this, we do not need to feel bad if we have to re-make an essence – by acknowledging our human-ness we drop our 'front' and allow in greater love, healing and truth. It is through our vulnerability and honesty that we allow growth and change to occur.

"The most direct route to enlightenment is right through the centre of our humanity".
– Rajpur (from the Raj tapes)

Inspired by the possibilities of imprinting essential healing energies into vibrational essences many healers have felt drawn to make 'channelled' essences either with, or without flowers, by calling in the energy of those in spirit, ie: archangels, angels, the White Brotherhood etc., the energy of living masters, elemental energies or stellar energies. This can be a very powerful way of making this healing energy freely available to anyone, at any time. Again, it is the responsibility of each essence maker to approach this work with the greatest love, humility and honesty, to ensure that each essence carries the clearest healing energy possible and if necessary, to re-make an essence if they have inner doubts as to the vibrational quality of that essence.

Enhancing essences:

A number of essence makers feel drawn to use various approaches to amplify or enhance their essences. The most common approach is to place essences, often surrounded by an arrangement of crystals, under a pyramid form kept for this purpose. The suggestion is, that this will amplify the energy of the essences and cleanse the essences of any 'negative' influences they may have picked up during their making, handling and storage. Others use devices such as 'stargates', which are geometric structures, often large enough to sit under, which are designed to focus energy in a manner similar to pyramids.

There has been some discussion about the effects of amplifying and cleansing essences using devices such as pyramids and stargates. Some feel it is an essential part of their essence making practise and contributes to the energy and clarity of their essences, while others feel that the use of such technology is inappropriate and detrimental to the subtle energies of flower essences.

The clairvoyant Peter Tadd, who has devoted much time to discerning the energy and healing qualities of individual flower essences, for U.K. flower essence distributors and for essence makers in different parts of the world, has looked at what happens to flower essences when they are enhanced in different ways.

The conclusion he has drawn is that:

"When we make a vibrational flower essence we contact a particular form of life that is very conscious, highly subtle and remarkably sensitive to environmental conditions and the essence takes on the sensitivity of the plant and is affected by the process and the intention of the essence maker.

We need to respect the basic truth about plants. plants have evolved from this earth and this solar system. Their relationship to the sun's energy in photosynthesis is unique. The sun is our star and not other stars.

Pyramids are unique structures of pre-Atlantean origins, probably from peoples who travelled from distant star systems and have been used for rituals of initiation and preservation. Pyramids are about cosmic and terrestrial numeric values and for our species, geometrically represent the process of post-Atlantean human incarnation and dis-incarnation. These initial rituals were about the human journey of the soul into earth form – representing involution and in Egyptian times, out-of-body initiations or after-life journeys. Their main influence on the human chakra system is on the root, or muladhara. This is very different to plants, which are basic to evolution.

Plants essentially are spatial, elastic, levitational and heliotropic. Where some might argue that this represents a balance to the forces of the pyramid (and other modern enhancements), I would ask the reader to consider the differences between implicit and explicit forces. Plants are living examples of the basic vibrations of life force and ether. They are living forms of sacred geometry. Their 'power' derives from their subtle and implicit forces. In us their main influence is on the lateral points of the sacral or sadisthana chakra.

It is the plants internalised geometries which permit photosynthesis to occur. They are 'living' qualities of the cell when compared to that of the solid structures of the mineral kingdom and/or set geometric patterns. David Spangler agrees: "The cell is a living crystal. It possesses a highly structured internal order, yet this geometry is organized around information rather than around position, as in a crystal lattice". (David Spangler, Reimagination of the World, Bear & Company 1991, page 62). I firmly believe and have witnessed that certain 'enhancements' are a superimposition of first chakra levels of order on to second chakra dynamics of growth and interaction. The dynamics include free will, balance and individuality.

For some reason the use of pyramids in areas where they are historically situated around the Atlantic ocean, retain these ancient resonances. This is strangely not true for the developers on the Pacific rim, where pyramids are a new geometric form. It is possible that this is the result of the earliest civilization, (in Pacific areas), of Lemuria, whose basis of life science was on integration with and not control over, natural forces. They never developed technologies that we know as modern science. Modern science is a result of an overmentalized solar plexus or manipura chakra. The result of this imbalance is to establish a feeling of individuality which is exaggerated and incorrect. The devic world is calling on us in many ways and now especially through our communication with flower essences, to see and really know that we are co-equals".

Looking at other methods of enhancement, such as channelling the essence maker's own healing energy and intentions and channelling the energy of other beings: angels, the White Brotherhood, guides etc., Peter Tadd says that he has noticed that:, *"the essence can develop many different layers of energy and that in some essences this can become quite chaotic and can interfere with a clearer healing energy"*.

We need to be sensitive when making an essence, to the influences we introduce into the process, the imprints we are overlaying into an essence, both through technology, through ritual, or the calling in of the energies of other entities. It is not that ritual or channelling cannot both be very powerful means of contacting and using healing energy, but we need to be clear about when it is appropriate to use such methods and also, as to whether we are actually making a clear connection with the energy we intend.

It is up to each of us to continually question and monitor our approach to our work, to see clearly when our ego self is clouding the picture, to understand why and to deal with any issues such as the need for recognition or approval which cause us to be motivated from the standpoint of an insecure ego. We also need to be clear as to whether we are following other peoples' guidance, or our own inner voice and to try to not be too rigid in our perception of the 'correct' way to make and use flower essences.

Combination Essences:

Many essence makers have combined essences after making to create a blend that can be used to address life issues and experiences; ie: for grief, for addictive patterns, for shock etc. Some essence makers are now making blended essences by placing together in the same bowl of spring water the different flowers or flowers and gems needed to create the blend. This is then left to potentize, before bottling as the mother tincture of that blend.

Bottling mother essences – proportions of alcohol:

Most essence makers in the British Isles and Ireland add at least 50% alcohol to their mother essence bottles to prevent the growth of bacteria and viruses.

Marion Davis adds a high proportion of alcohol to her mother essence bottles and adds sugar to some mother essences to improve their keeping quality.

Some essence makers leave the mother essence to stand in a quiet, dark place for a few days after initial bottling, to allow the essence of the flower to imprint thoroughly into the liquid, before diluting to stock bottles; again leaving the stock bottles to sit undisturbed for a few days (sometimes next to the mother) before using.

Viv Williamson and Jane Stevenson mix the mother essences which go into each of their combination blends and leave these to stand for some time before dilution directly into their 50ml dosage bottles. The strength of these dose bottles is weaker than a stock bottle and so the essence will lose effectiveness if further diluted.

Dilution of mother essences to stock bottles and sucussion:

There are many different opinions as to how many drops of mother essence should ideally be put into a stock bottle. Dr Bach used 2 drops of mother essence in a 30ml bottle of brandy. Several essence makers have said that they like to add more drops to stock bottles – some put 2 drops in a 10ml stock bottle of alcohol, some recommend not diluting further than stock potency and using stock bottles for treatment purposes. Gurudas recommends 7 drops in a stock bottle regardless of whether the bottle holds several drams or several ounces, because he says that vibrational essences work partly from the influence of the seven dimensions and that this amount enhances the flower essences' clinical effectiveness.

Arthur Bailey has developed a method of twice diluting his essences to arrive at stock potency.

"Originally we used the Bach methods of dilution down to stock bottle, but after some checks by dowsing, it was discovered that greater potency could be obtained if a different method of dilution was used.

Instead of diluting straight from the 'mother tincture' to the stock bottles, a two-stage dilution was evolved. This has proved beneficial in giving greater potency to the finished stock essences. It appears that some potency is lost if too great a dilution is achieved in a single stage. The reasons for this are not clear, but it may well be related to the way that water 'inherits' the information from the original herbal extract.

We also give a few sucussions to the first dilution tincture bottles after preparing them from the mother tinctures. This is not essential, but it does give a rather more 'solid' feel to the final product.

The two-stage dilution corresponds approximately to a 2C homeopathic dilution for each stage. That is an approximate 10,000 to 1 dilution from Mother tincture to Stock bottle. (two stages each of about 100:1). The first dilution from Mother tincture we term our Daughter tincture. The second stage of dilution is the finished Stock bottle".

Several essence makers feel that it is beneficial to sucuss their mother and stock bottles after bottling. Ellie Web sucusses her essence bottles by hand – she says:

"I wish I had a gentle version of a sucussion machine, as is used in homeopathy. I've never seen one, but they sound a bit harsh. I do think this method of shaking with impact does help to activate the flower essence and it would save me hours of walking around my rug, slapping the bottoms of bottles. This, of course, is all part of my focussing ritual. When the bottle is opened the essence should be clear and lightly fizzy".

Alcohol-free essences:

There is an increasing demand for alcohol-free essences, either for those with alcohol intolerance or for babies and children. Some of the methods currently being researched are:

Vegetable glycerine: (where the mother, stock and dose essences are all preserved with vegetable glycerine)

Vegetable glycerine is suitable for use in treatment bottles for diabetics. Richard Gonzalez uses three parts of vegetable glycerine to one part of distilled water for his mother tincture bottles. To prepare stock bottles he uses half and half – distilled water and vegetable glycerine with a few drops of mother essence.

Liquid honey as a preservative

Liquid honey has been suggested as a non alcoholic preservative for flower essences but we have been unable to find anyone using it for this purpose. It would seem likely that the honey would need to be warmed and diluted with spring water in order to satisfactorily mix in the flower essence. It might be a good idea to experiment with the proportions of honey and water so as to avoid possible fermentation.

Essences in cider vinegar:

Cider vinegar has been used as a preservative in stock and dose bottles for many years but is not as palatable as glycerine or honey. The general recommendation is to use undiluted cider vinegar in stock bottles and one part cider vinegar to three or four parts spring water in dose bottles.

Salt-water as a base for dose bottles:

Arthur Bailey is researching using salt-water as a preservative in dose bottles. He suggests using a 5% solution of sea-salt in water.

Storage of Essences:

Most essence makers store their mother essences in glass bottles in a quiet place away from electrical or human disturbance. and strong smells and with the bottles not touching each other, sometimes individually wrapped in paper. Suitable places for storage might be a quiet cupboard, or wooden trunk or chest of drawers, or in cardboard boxes in an undisturbed, cool, dry place. Some like to place quartz crystals in the storage area to help maintain the potency of the essences. Richard Gonzalez wraps his mother tincture bottles in silk bags, both as a way of protecting the essence from outside influences, but also as a means of preventing the energetic frequency of the individual essence from influencing essences stored next to it.

Stock essences are generally stored in small glass dropper bottles (between 10-30 ml) and kept in boxes with card dividers, again to prevent the bottles touching each other. These can be kept in drawers in a quiet place, free from strong smells, heat and other interference.

Some essence makers don't allow other people to hold or handle their mother essence bottles, or their stock bottles prior to sale as they feel the essences can be influenced by the energy of others and that this will alter the energy pattern of the essence.

Further information about the preparation of stock and treatment bottles and the making of pillules, sprays, oils creams and homoeopathic potentization of essences can be found in Chapter 5.

CONTRIBUTORS' EXPERIENCES

MAKING ESSENCES:

Viv Williamson and Jane Stevenson (Sun Essences)

Making a 'Patterned' essence (Hawthorn)

"Throughout the spring of 1995 all the colours of the hawthorn blossom, from red through to pink and white, communicated their unsurpassed brilliance. Both Jane and I received this message and we acknowledged it; however, no opportunity was presented to make a Hawthorn essence until 1996 when we were planning to make an Oak essence.

Jane and I had to travel some miles to our planned location. We stopped near a church to a blaze of every shade of hawthorn imaginable and also to a massive stand of about six low-hanging oaks, all in perfect bloom. Of course we moved no further and once the Oak essence was prepared, we concentrated on the Hawthorn.

Feeling very connected to the Hawthorn, we picked all possible shades of blossom and began, for the first time, to create a pattern with the flowers on the surface of the water – white flowers in the middle, then pink and red around the edge. Then a powerful message suggested we break the red circle and arrange the white and pink flowers to reach the edge. Two bowls were made: one a floated essence, the other a saturated essence and these two would be mixed together.

The picture of this remedy came through as letting love and light into a troubled emotional heart (note the pattern of the flowers) Hawthorn is a heart remedy in many ways, used by homoeopaths for such and having a herbal history for being a heart tonic. This essence has proved itself of great value topically, particularly around the heart area".

RIC STAINES

Protection – (The story of the Birds Foot Trefoil essence)

"What follows happened in the summer of 1994 whilst we were on holiday in Ireland. We made a number of essences from the flowers of the fields and bogs and on this particular day I was drawn to make one on my own. I collected the bowl, water and scissors and walked up the lane beside the house.

I was drawn into the field above the yard where we had already made an essence. It was a beautiful sunny morning and the field was alive with wild flowers. I stood quietly, taking in the beauty and energy of that place. A flower caught my attention and as I looked, many others of that species stood out from the mass of colour. I knew this was to be my essence for today.

I collected enough flowers to fill the bowl and then placed it in the centre of the group of plants I had been drawn to. I sat and meditated for a while, feeling the pleasure of the energies for this contact. I was then called to return to the family waiting in the house, but before I left I needed to protect my essence. I spent a few moments to protect the bowl and it's contents by encircling it in white light. When I was satisfied that this had been done I thanked the energies and left.

After returning to the house we all went out intending to return at lunch time, but we were so entranced by the place we visited we stayed longer. We finally returned home late afternoon. As soon as we had got in I remembered my essence, so I took leave of the others and once again walked up the lane.

You can imagine how my heart leapt, when on approaching the gate to the field where my precious essence lay, I noticed that the gate had been moved. Not only had it been moved, the muddy entrance was now covered in hoof prints. "Oh No – they have moved the cows into my field" I thought. I now had visions of cows with cut feet, Pat's best essence bowl shattered, even dying animals – what had I done?

My fears continued as I climbed the gate and slowly, oh so slowly, edged my way round the little knoll to look over the field. As I lifted my eyes a strange sight appeared – there were some cows spread out over the field, but the main group were where my essence should be and there wasn't a flower left in the field. As I approached the main group of cows I could not believe my eyes. There in the middle of the group was a circle of wild flowers, completely untouched, about six feet in diameter and right in the centre of the flowers was my essence! – completely safe, just as I had left it, except it was now the centre of attention of about ten cows. They looked on in mild amusement, but made no effort to move or to eat the flowers in the circle, which by now were the only ones left in the field.

I slowly moved forward and picked up the bowl, gave thanks to the energies, the white light and the devas and made my way home. Before leaving the field I glanced back to see the contented cows just finishing the last wild flowers in the meadow. I will never forget this experience all my life".

VAL BOULTING

The making of Church Farm Rose Essences

"On the eve of June 23rd, three of us set off for the mountains. As we drove we were witness to an extraordinary sight. It was just beginning to get dark, the sun was sinking and as it moved downwards a rainbow formed around it. There was no rain, or threat of rain and yet there it was. I have never seen this phenomenon before. I am told esoterically it is a sign of hope. We were also informed that the full moon that night was special, in that it only appeared in that astrological order once every seven years and that it relates to destiny.

We reached Church Farm about nine. Working intuitively, we set up the crystal grid on a bed of peppermint and thyme. The grid of seven clear terminated quartz crystals in place, we began to choose the first roses. We were intuitively led to each rose and asking its permission, we plucked its head, using, as instructed, a piece of clear quartz crystal, letting it fall gently into a crystal bowl of pure spring water and then thanking the bush for releasing its flower.

The first rose was Iceberg, which we were told later is to do with influence. We felt this had to be placed in the centre. Six more roses were chosen and placed in bowls around the central bowl, all inside the grid where I had also felt inspired to place my piece of rock from the tomb of John the Baptist. The roses in position, we stood in silent meditation, each in our own way asking for a blessing from the divine source, leaving the whole evening's work in the hands of our creator. As we finished, I looked up into the sky. The moon was magnificent, a cross of white light went right through her as she sat on a formation of clouds that looked like a praying figure. (We have a photograph of this) As we stared in wonder, we saw a shooting star move straight across the moon, bright pink like a silent firework.

Following direction, we left the roses in the moonlight for the next three hours, except Iceberg, which we left until noon the next day, being instructed to add eight drops of this essence to each of the other six. We then continued the preparation in the usual way, adding 50 parts of brandy to 50 parts of essence. Church Farm Roses work numerically with the number eight, so eight drops of the mother essence are added to each pot of cream."

JULIAN WINSLOW (WIGHT FLOWER REMEDIES)

Making an essence from the flower of Agave americana – Ventnor Botanic Garden, Isle of Wight.

"Accidents, contrary to popular belief, don't happen: and it was no accident that at the time I started making flower essences one of the Agaves in the garden started to flower. Because of the climate in the south of the island, especially on the cliffs where the Botanic Garden is situated, we are able to grow flora which would be killed by frost in other parts of the country.

The Agave is a particularly amazing plant which looks to me like many saw-toothed sea mammals bursting out of the ground. Its life cycle is amazing in that it can take up to thirty years to flower and then seeds and dies – some orgasm!

This particular plant was about 15 years old, but had been moved twice in its life; not something a six foot wide succulent plant usually does! This, in conjunction with the very hot summer, probably stimulated the flower. The flower spike itself terminated at about 18 feet and was spectacular in its growth rate. The spike was so charged with energy it was interfering with the air around it. Emitting from it was a deep resonant hum like an organic power station.

Being physically able to make the essence was a feat verging on a circus act. This consisted of me climbing a ladder, champagne glass of spring water in one hand, a pair of scissors in the other, supported by the front end loader of a small tractor and two bewildered but congenial fellow gardeners.

Our efforts were not in vain. As I cut the first flower it slowly tilted its head towards the water, nectar flowing from it in a slow motion dance and joined the water in a spiralling embrace. The feeling I got at that moment was a beautiful release, like the kiss of the first light of dawn as it is squeezed from the womb of the night. The action of the essence was given to me concisely and clearly, it was so loud and clear that it was almost a shock:- **strength in the face of adversity**".

PATRICIA STAINES

Making the Redshank essence

"I had this experience with Redshank when I was in the vegetable garden. There was a large patch of wonderful wildflowers and amongst them was a large specimen of Redshank. I was gardening away when I had this feeling that I must turn around – it was quite overwhelming – it was like something insisting that I did. When I eventually did, I saw this Redshank. Its leaves were a beautiful dark green, with a deep red spot in the middle of each leaf and the flowers were like tight little knots.

I had the feeling that I needed to make an essence from this plant. It was several days before I could make this essence, so I would go out and look at the Redshank and wait to hear what the properties of this essence were for and what it could be used for. Over a number of days certain things were communicated to me from the Redshank – little snippets of information – things like: "bitterness", "help with the pancreas", "useful with people with diabetes", "bitter and sweet", "self-punishment".

At this time I was treating a woman with diabetes and I felt that I was being given an essence to help with this condition. After making the Redshank essence I gave it to this woman to take as part of her treatment. She experienced a powerful release of buried feelings of bitterness, which was followed by a great improvement in her condition".

MARIA MAW (UNITIVE FLOWER AND LIFE ESSENCES)

Group Essence making:

"In the past the impulse to make a flower essence has been intuitive. For example, I felt drawn to a particular flower and would muscle-test if it was appropriate to make an essence that day. However, most essences are now made in workshops for which I test the day and the time. When the group has come together and we are clear of our intention, we muscle-test our way to the group of flowers to be used. Most flower essences need bright sunshine for their preparation but occasionally an overcast day has been tested as appropriate.

The group forms a circle around the flowers and we sit silently communing with them, making our intentions known. Each person picks whatever flower heads they feel drawn to until there are enough floating downwards on the surface of a half an inch depth of spring water, in a clear glass bowl placed amidst the plants. We remain silent for a few more minutes in order to leave our blessings and to hold the space for the next few hours, during which time every one of us needs to put our awareness into what is happening for us physically, mentally, spiritually, internally and externally. Often my feelings change dramatically during this time".

DAVID EASTOE (PETALTONES FLOWER ESSENCES)

Making the essence 'Golden Light'

"This essence was made in an incredible natural power spot in Buckinghamshire. I left the flowers to 'cook' in their bowl in the sun, at the edge of some woods, in a large, recently cut cornfield. Returning at sunset to collect and bottle with my equipment, and quietly moving through the woods, I discovered a middle-aged couple having a cuddle only a few feet away from the bowl! They stood and embraced for ages, whilst I hid in the woods, not wanting to disturb them, or to be seen either. Eventually, after what seemed an hour, they strolled back across the field to their car. Waiting for them to depart, I was mystified to see the man go to the rear of his vehicle and get something out of the boot. It turned out to be a trumpet which he proceeded to play, with some emotion, to the setting sun, while his wife or lover sat in the car and I began bottling the essence!!"

MARY HARRIS (EARTH ESSENCES)

Choosing plants

"The trees and plants from which I make the essences are indigenous to this country and thrive on cultivated land. They are subject to the same pollutions and vibrations that we are now.

Each tree or plant that may provide an essence is brought to my attention. I watch and listen for at least a year as it tells its story, reveals its secrets. I note the confirmations that are given on all levels. When the time is right to make an essence, I just know, it is not planned. I am drawn to it and my own energy vibrations are attuned to that purpose on waking. Everything is always right. As I prepare to make the essence, I am filled with a knowing of its purpose; a clarification of all that I have felt over the period of time of getting to know it.

The final confirmation comes when the latest essence to be made proves to be the very one that is needed next".

SIMON LILLY (GREEN MAN TREE ESSENCES)

"In general plants make themselves known to me, that is, I notice them in passing or begin thinking of a particular tree or flower that I have seen around. With tree essences however, the logistics of collecting flowers can sometimes pose problems if the tree happens to be large with flowers only on the top branches. It is then sometimes the case that I have to search for another tree of the same species in flower with lower branches, or growing on a slope etc., so that collection is possible".

SUE MONK

"I usually make an essence when I am specifically drawn to it, usually by the colour or the signature; occasionally by specific channelling, ie: "You need to make it". I don't always know what, or who the essence is for until it has been made. Quite often it is for me, or for a client who might already be seeing me, or who might ring up the next day, or even the same day; or it might be for a relative. Thus the essences are made according to need".

SIMON LILLY

Attunement

"When we are essence making, a particular state of mind is entered that feels similar to a deep meditation but is a spontaneous response to the activity of collecting the flowers. There is a short linking/flowing with the plant or the plants to be employed and a statement of intent, with an asking for permission – this is usually given, ie., it is felt as an acceptance of purpose or a feeling of "yes" in the mind. Occasionally there is a feeling of resistance, or even a clear "no", in which case alternative plants are sought, or collection delayed.

I do not, when making essences, communicate directly or perceive spirits, though they make themselves felt – as a sense of presence, or a change of air movement or increased stillness etc. There is not particular attunement with the plant or essence whilst it is being made. I feel that the less I can be involved energetically, the better for the clarity and purity of the essence. The essence is, after all, of the plant, tree or whatever; not of me meditating, musing, daydreaming, chatting to, or otherwise interacting with the plant. There is no way of avoiding some energy interaction (as that is all everything is anyway – interacting energies), but I prefer to keep it to the minimum in the making stages".

SUE MONK

Attunement

"I meditate for a short time before going out to make an essence and when starting to make it. I call upon the devas of the particular plant to help me and also the Universal Family of Light. I ask that the essence be made in the best possible way to assist humanity and I give thanks for the privilege of being allowed to make it. I also ask which colours and/or blooms I specifically need, as the colour combination is sometimes important. I try to do this as much as possible by intuition or by allowing the blooms to 'jump out' at me".

ROSIE DEVITT

Devas and nature spirits

"I am aware of devic entities and nature spirits. They sometimes appear to help me with my inner work and I love to feel close to them. I 'see' them within sometimes and at other times simply feel their being with me. I try to keep in close contact with them while I am collecting flowers and following through each part of the process of making an essence".

ANDREW TRESIDDER

Weather

"Today I was blessed with sunlight – but making essences doesn't always happen in fine weather. Sometimes the bowls potentize in the porch – but never in driving rain. Last night was nearly full moon and was right for an aqueous essence of Pink Rose, which sat for twelve hours in moonlight… Sunlight is not essential – an essence will still potentize in dull weather or overnight, or even, if protected, in stormy weather; but obviously the healing vibration may well vary in minor, or sometimes major respects. Sometimes the overnight essence may be more appropriate than a daytime one would be".

ELLIE WEB

Weather and quality of light

"Living in south west Scotland I would not make many essences were I to wait for com-pletely flawless sunny days! I certainly do not discard an essence just because of a little cloud or even a light shower. What makes a good flower essence is a certain kind of day; it has a special quality, of course sunshine is important but in this part of the world there is a certain brightness which somehow makes things more potent".

FREYA SHERLOCK

Making 'inspirational' combination essences

"I enjoy making combination essences that respond to one's needs in that moment. This involves taking a walk through the garden or around the countryside and putting into the glass bowl of spring water whatever I feel drawn to, or called by. It could end up a collection of flowers, buds, leaves, mosses, grasses, ferns, or even impressions… such as mentally imprinting into the bowl the energy of a waterfall, a morning star, or a particular tree or rock, or a passing flight of birds. Quite simply, anything whose energy I feel drawn to, will in some way be put into the water. In this way, I make a 'meal' of essences, each meal imparting its own distinct goodness and inner nourishment".

ANDREW TRESIDDER

Alcohol essences

"Today I felt inspired! A beautiful sunny October day! There was a wonderful sunrise which saw me standing beside a giant puffball (an essence I recently made on the hill behind), and a stunning full moon appeared at 7 p.m. In turn I was drawn to three different plants in the garden: a red fuschia with a double purple corolla, a red begonia and a yellow abutilon. It felt right to make each essence an alcoholic one – a single flower (in this case) floating in about 200ml of vodka in a glass bowl. The abutilon, however, chose not a bowl but a flask shaped tumbler which echoed its own shape. After about six hours in strong sunlight the essences felt 'right'.

After making a hundred or so aqueous essences, alcoholic ones began to appear. This method, using vodka instead of spring water seems to give a different vibration. It seems especially suited to fruits and berries, but I have also made flower, bud and even leaf alcoholic essences".

Chapter 5

Discerning the Qualities of Flower Essences

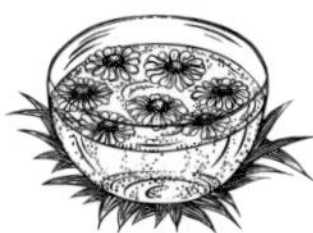

Perhaps the most important thing to understand about descriptions of the qualities of flower essences is that one description is not 'right' and another 'wrong'. When looking through the Repertory of the book, readers may perhaps feel bewildered by the number of different descriptions of the qualities of essences made from the same plant (ie: Dandelion). However, often on closer study we will find that there is often a common underlying theme than runs through these descriptions, or that there is a particular area of healing which each of these descriptions illumines in a different way. There is no conflict in this; – the reason for this being that each essence maker has their own particular healing energy and purpose and will be drawn to make essences which relate to their healing gift. Their descriptions will reflect the particular aspects of healing which they resonate with. Each flower has a range of healing qualities which we can work with within certain boundaries. Together with the consciousness of the plant, the plant devas and those in spirit who help with this work, the essence maker (consciously or unconsciously) co-creates healing essences.

Each plant has a field of healing qualities which we can work with. The boundaries of this field define the individual expression of each plant. Some of the healing qualities within this field are shared within the same species and some relate to the environment of the individual plant within that species, eg: there are certain qualities shared by all Dandelions, but a Dandelion growing in a dry, rocky place will have a different energy to that of a Dandelion growing in a lush meadow.

There are several ways in which an essence maker will arrive at an understanding of the qualities of an essence they have made, but each essence maker's description will reflect in some way their own healing qualities and understanding. It is as if several people go into a room and then describe their experience of it. One who loves fabric may describe in detail the curtains, cushions and sofa throws; another who loves painting may describe the pictures on the walls; someone else may talk of the atmosphere of the room; another the

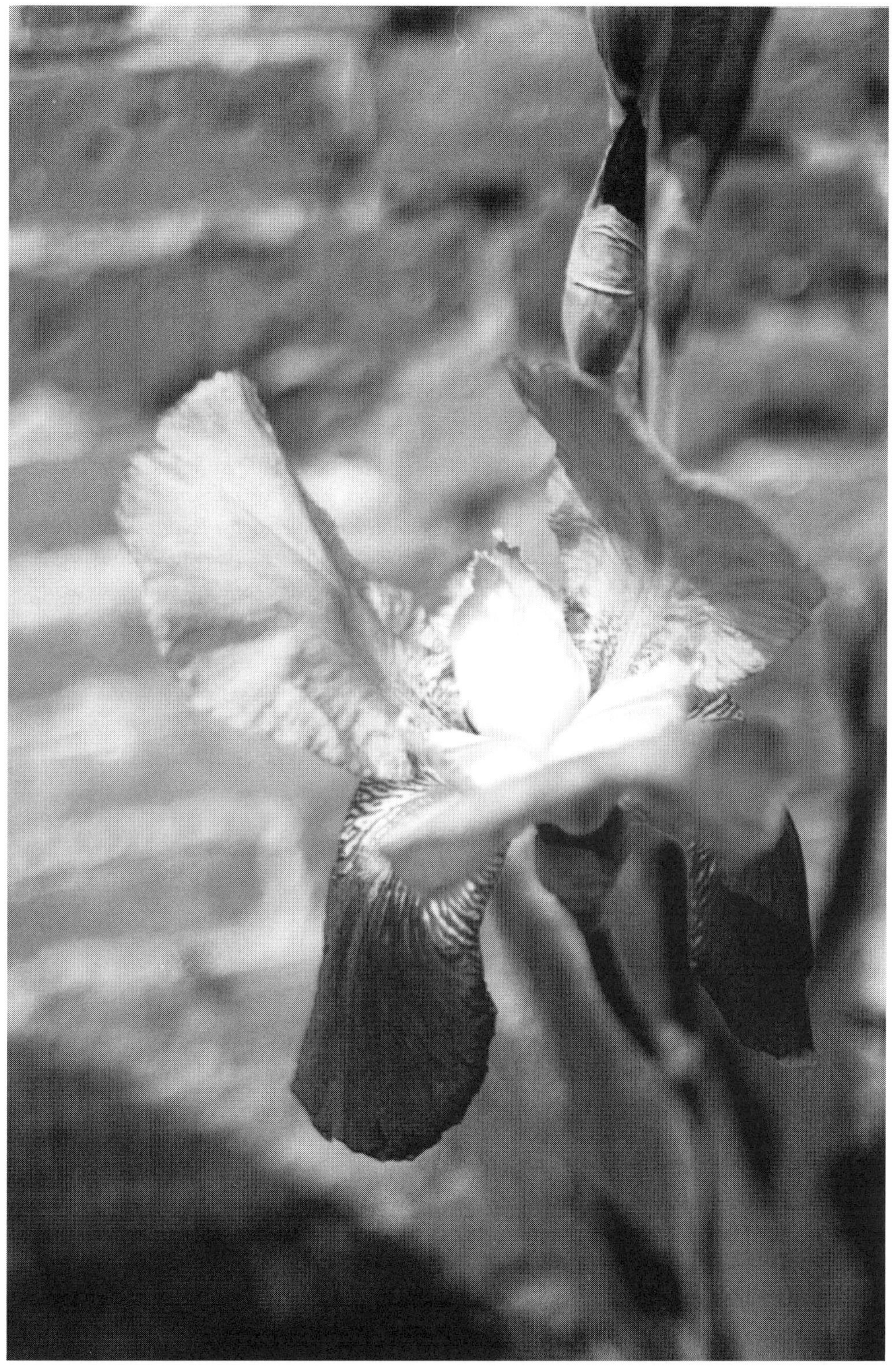

architecture; someone else may comment on the tidiness or disorder of the room! It is the same room, but within it's boundary of four walls there is so much to see and describe. So it is when discerning the qualities of a flower essence – we are drawn to the aspects of healing which relate to each of us, both as healers and also in relation to our own personal healing and awakening.

There need be no competition, no right or wrong in this. Each essence maker's essences will attract those who, at any given time, need that specific healing energy. This is not a fixed thing – we are all changing continually and what may be appropriate for us one day, may not another.

Simon Lilly (Green Man Tree Essences) comments:

"It can be devisive to compare the same essence described by different makers and then dismiss one or both because they do not agree completely with one another. Although it is likely that there should be some correlation between descriptions, just because there isn't doesn't indicate inaccuracy. It is always so vital to remember that we are dealing with holistic and fine-level non-biological/non-physical energy fields, ie; 'magic', more than 'science' (as currently defined)

The energy signature and depth of complexity of a plant being is comparable to a human – how many descriptions of the same person will a group of acquaintances give?

We all see the world as it is created through our own sense organs, memories and mental patternings. There is really no harmonious, life supporting way in which the same energy pattern will create the same effect in two individuals and even if the effect is going to be the same, how can we guarantee the experience of the effect will be similar at all?"

Vivien Williamson (Sun Essences) feels that:

"All flowers that grow have the potential to be used to make a healing essence; however it might not be appropriate or practical to potentize them all. It appears that the plant calls to those flower essence makers who are closest tuned to its vibration and in so doing a connection is created through which information about its healing potential is channelled. The flower expresses a general quality or 'tone', but beyond that it appears one can bring some personal flavour to the essence, as the healing energy may be fluid/flexible. Hence the differences in descriptions from different companies and why individual sets of essences seem to have very definite 'characteristics', which are not only like their countries of origin but also resemble the makers themselves. This also means that one can never make the exactly same essence twice and that integrity in making an essence must be of highest importance.

The essences one is drawn to making are often related to the needs of one's personal life journey. Every essence I have made has been of great use to me at the time of making."

Ellie Web (Harebell Remedies) has this to say:

"I do not believe that the message of a particular flower is a fixed thing: that you take this one for this particular set of symptoms or these emotional states and that is it. In a sense there are as many interpretations as there are people to receive the message or even as there are circumstances where a person and a flower meet. Having said that, it does seem that people receive similar messages from the same flower generally, so that is why we say "this is for this" and "that is for that", but it is by no means fixed and, more importantly, there are no 'right' or 'wrong' interpretations.

The messages all have the same purpose or intention anyway and that is to help us to understand ourselves in order that we may come to love and forgive ourselves and cherish ourselves better – that is all, it is very simple!"

Ways of Discerning the qualities of Essences:

There are many different ways in which we can come to an understanding of the healing qualities of an essence we have made. Each person has their own way of uncovering this understanding. We do not have to have 'special' gifts in order to be able to do this. Everyone has the ability to know whatever it is they need to know at any given moment of their lives – nothing is denied us – we only deny ourselves. There are many different ways in which we can access our intuition and guidance (see Chapter 2). The most important thing is the desire to know what rings true for us, and the curiosity, courage and integrity to allow ourselves to uncover and honour our own truth. Ellie Web offers the following advice:

"My method of discerning the qualities of flower essences is not hard to do (see Flower Meditation at the end of the chapter). It takes a leap of faith to start trusting your own intuition; to be open on that level means being positive and very present, aware of the vibrancy of the plant and of your own intention, leaving all judgemental thoughts elsewhere. It's not this terribly important, serious, scary thing. In fact it's fun to relax and enjoy being close to nature. I have never met an unfriendly flower! (though some, of course, are more awesome than others). Generally it is a joyful and moving experience.

To be honest, the difficulty comes when translating what I have received into words. Again, it is simply a matter of trust and I do it the best I can, because if I want to share the essence with others, then I need these words. Making, prescribing and using flower essences is a fine way to develop intuitive skill. This skill is much needed, and funda-

mental in our healing process. I believe that this explains the increasing popularity of the use of flower essences. This other level, this different way of understanding, together with conscious, positive intention is a way to reconnect with Nature, with our own needs and the needs of our planet."

Recording impressions – First impressions:

When making flower essences it really helps to keep a notebook in which one can record any information relating to making essences. Often the first indications of the qualities of an essence come from our initial impressions of that plant, long before we get to the point of making an essence from it. Nowadays I try to record any feelings I may have about plants that I feel drawn to, even if I have no immediate plans to make an essence from that plant. It helps to record any feelings and impressions we may have about a plant, without judgement. We can always decide later which are relevant to our description of an essence. Sometimes a picture is built up over a period of time and it is not until we feel we have amassed all the information that we need, that we realize that what might have seemed an insignificant impression – perhaps a word which kept coming up – is in fact central to our understanding of this essence. It doesn't matter if our impressions seem very individual, nor if they relate to our own experience. We are far more likely to arrive at a true interpretation of the energy of our essences if we follow our own experience rather than re-word someone else's interpretation of the quality of an essence made from that particular plant. Each essence maker draws on their own experience and the facets of healing which they work with, and this will inevitably influence the essences they make, and the way in which they describe them. The vibration of that essence and it's description will contain both the energetic note of the essence maker as well as that of the plant, and it is these energetic notes which will attract those who need this particular energy.

Our association with some plants may go back a long way, to early childhood or even other lives, so we may find, when making an essence that we have already some internal picture of some of the qualities of that plant and that this is our starting point for building a clearer picture of it's healing qualities. Some times a plant may seem to call us over a period of time and we may find ourselves repeatedly seeing it, reading about it, thinking about it's history, fascinated by it. At other times we may be drawn to a plant we have never noticed, or hardly bothered with before. Suddenly it seems to demand our attention and we make a new friend. In this way we form our initial impressions.

Impressions received while making essences and bottling:

As part of the act of making an essence most essence makers make time to still themselves to tune in to the energy of the plant and to 'be with' the plant and observe it in detail. In drawing together an energy picture of a plant we may draw on its physical characteristics: its form, colour, habitat, life-cycle, taste, smell, texture etc...; as well as the non-physical impressions we may receive. Discerning the healing properties of plants by the physical characteristics of that plant was termed 'Doctrine of Signature' by 16th century Swiss alchemist and mystic Paracelsus. This approach has relevance when forming a picture of the properties of an essence but we may need to be watchful of imaginative interpretation of these physical characteristics! Simon Lilly points out the danger in this:

"I have found the Doctrine of Signatures is relevant in many cases, but can only be discerned retrospectively once other information has been gathered. This is perhaps due to lack of personal experience with the system. I often feel that when using this system alone one can be in danger of making anthropormorphic assumptions ie: droopy heads = shyness etc..., where it may not be particularly relevant."

Sometimes two people are drawn to make essences together and this can prove to be a strong healing partnership. Viv Williamson (Sun essences) writes of her experience of this and of the importance of writing down impressions:

"I work with Jane Stevenson, and we now understand that we are called to the flowers that are appropriate for Sun Essences to make. We make a point of checking which flowers have recently held our attention in one way or another – colour, shape, feeling an unusually deep response to them etc., and as a rule we will have been drawn to the same plants. Then, when the time is right (which may not be that year), we will be guided to the right place to make them and, together we will tune in to the energy of the plants as we make the essence. Together we seem to forge a more complete connection with the plants, than alone, and so receive very direct communications as to their healing properties. We have to be careful to write it all down as it comes, or we will completely forget it – remembering only a few words, when in fact two pages of information may have been received."

While making an essence, most essence makers as they go about their day, maintain a mental and intuitive connection with the essence and the plant as it is potentizing. Ellie Web writes about the process of gathering information about an essence and the importance of allowing a description to evolve in its own timing:

"What often happens with me is that during the day when I am making a new essence it is very much in my thoughts, even though I may be doing other things while the essence is sitting in the garden. Slowly it is influencing me. When I go to sit by it and when I actually come to bottle it and later in the evening, or even any time in the next few days it will become clearer to me. What I am saying is that I allow myself to be guided as to when I write about the essence and the affirmations too. Right timing is one of the ways that I make it easy for myself because as soon as it becomes difficult, then I am not enjoying it anymore and I start to build up a resistance and then of course I can not do it, or at any rate I don't want to!"

Once an essence has been potentized and bottled there is often a small amount left in the glass bowl which can be tasted. At this point further impressions may be received through ones physical, emotional, mental and spiritual responses. Simon Lilly expands on this:

"Initially, after preparing the mother essence there is usually some remaining after bottling and this is taken neat. A fair idea of the broad function of an essence can be gained then: what areas of the body are brought into awareness, whether a mood change occurs, whether it is calming, energising, activating and so on. Were one in perfect balance with ones awareness this would be all that was necessary, but few people are familiar enough with their "ground state" to be conscious of all the changes brought about by an essence in this way (and of course the effect would vary from person to person to some extent)."

Further impressions obtained by intuition, guidance/channelling, dowsing, kinesiology, direct testing, blind testing and feedback from users:

Once an essence has been bottled we can continue to build a picture of its qualities. Sometimes a clear picture may form quite quickly, whilst at other times the picture eludes us. This may be to do with a question of timing – perhaps this essence is not for use now, or maybe we need to have certain experiences before we can fully understand the message of this essence and find the appropriate words to express it. Sometimes we inhibit our uncovering the message of this essence by a feeling that we can't do this work, that we are not capable of knowing, not advanced enough etc., or we may feel limited by someone else's description of an essence made from this plant and feel unable to find out what is true for us and this particular essence we have made.

As with all intuitive and healing work we need to be our own judge and monitor. It takes courage and honesty to find out for ourselves not only what our essences are for, but also as to whether they have a good, clear, vibrant energy or whether we feel we should pour some of them away and start again. It is surely better to have a few, very clear and potent essences than fifty that we are not, in our heart of hearts, comfortable with. I am sure that even the best essence makers have 'off' days and have to question their work and throw away essences that are not good enough, or revise descriptions they have written.Whatever means we use to gather information about our essences we need to check our gut feelings as we go along. With dowsing and kinesiology it is just as easy to influence the answers that we are getting, as it is with intuition and guidance. Integrity is the key, plus experience in recognizing when we are hearing or receiving true, and when we are unable to hear clearly because of our own ego issues. (see Chapter 2 for more information on intuition, guidance, dowsing and kinesiology). This doesn't mean that we must discard radical information that we may have received, in favour of what we may feel to be a 'safer', less challenging description. We may know deep down, when we ignore the protestations of our rational mind, that some radical understanding and information we may have received about an essence rings completely true even if we can not prove our intuition at this point. The most important thing is to remain true to ourselves throughout the process and to trust the timing of it all. Often we receive confirmation of our intuition at a later date.

Arthur Bailey describes, in his book, 'Dowsing For Health' (Quantum 1990), how, despite being a very experienced dowser (he had been both Scientific Adviser and past President of the British Society of Dowsers), he was unable to discern, by dowsing, the qualities of the essences that he had made. He was able to choose them for people using dowsing and was always accurate in his choice but had not been able to get a clear picture of their qualities using dowsing, despite whatever questions he posed.

"Over an eleven year period I had come up with about twenty-six new flower essences. I used them on a regular basis, but was still no nearer finding out just what they were for. Then circumstances arose that completely changed my life. I went to York to hear a meditation teacher give a talk. It was called 'Meditation in Everyday Life'.

...I started to work with this teacher who was called John Garrie... One of John's long-term students was a lady called Caroline... I had told her about my remedies, and went to see her in London to discuss them with her.

She was interested in my remedies, and particularly in my lack of knowing what they were for. I remember she fixed me with a searching look and said, "Arthur, you have created these essences, so deep down you must know what they are for. I have worked as a secretary so I can take things down at speed. I will take out the essences one at a time and read out the names. You lie back and relax, and tell me just whatever comes into your mind. I will write it all down and then we will see what you can intuit about them"

I thought I had been well and truly rumbled. I had that uncomfortable feeling that she knew I could give the answers, and worse she would not let up until I agreed. So that was the way it was. I lay back with my eyes closed and listened to her reading out the names.

Much to my surprise words came into my head. Phrases like 'cooling warmth', 'comfortably bewitched', 'breaking through into new levels of consciousness', and so on. When I saw the final list I was amazed. It all made good sense and corresponded well with the patients I had seen. This was the first breakthrough into my understanding the remedies.

I now had a further problem. It is one thing reading about clairvoyance and perhaps half believing it, it is something different to find yourself actually doing it. Once again I had experienced something that my rational mind found quite unacceptable and I went home in a state of shock. I now had a list of what the remedies were for, but I was not at all happy about how I had obtained it, for I hadn't really believed such things could work in this way.

On the positive side I could now talk more freely to other people about the remedies. I did however tend to keep quiet about how I had discovered the information, and was rather embarrassed by it all. If questioned too deeply, I muttered things about dowsing for the answers. Not true, but at that time I could not cope with the information I was being presented with.

There was no doubt that the remedies could greatly help to alleviate symptoms, to make people feel better; that I knew from experience. What I now knew was that they operated in a different way than by just removing symptoms, they helped people at some deeper level.

It was about five years later, owing to the work I was doing with my meditation teacher, that the whole healing pattern suddenly appeared to become clear to me. The essences were for attitudes of mind, how we view the external and inner worlds, not for the emotional states themselves,… but for that which comes before. I realized that the remedies were to help the patient let go of old outmoded belief patterns, desires, rigid ways of thinking. In fact everything that gets in the way of personal freedom and living a free and happy life

At long last I had found the answers that I had been looking for. I realized that I could not have arrived at those conclusions before, because such concepts had not even entered my head. It had been a case of 'knowing in part and seeing in part'."

When attempting to build a picture of the qualities of an essence, essence makers use intuition, guidance, dowsing and kinesiology, direct experience of taking the essence, blind testing, feedback from essence users, as well as drawing on their understanding of the Doctrine of Signature of the plant, colour therapy, astrology, sacred geometry and numerology etc…

Simon Lilly explains the approach that he and his wife, Sue, use for discerning the qualities of the essences they make:

"With Green Man Tree Essences, the techniques used for identifying main areas of function were a combination of dowsing, muscle testing and intuitive listening, (this is sometimes where Signatures become apparent)...

Once the Essence is stabilized in brandy, a few drops are ingested, rubbed on, sprayed around, and further detailed impressions are gathered. We have formulated a code of keys derived from our experiences as colour therapists, and we dowse these and the levels they act on: ie. – from physical to spiritual, and this information tells us the range and action quite precisely. later, in assessing appropriate combinations for individuals, one can see time and time again the relevant essence appearing, giving us some confirmation on the initial analysis. Most of our assessments whether by dowsing or kinesiology, are done blind, by group and number, so usually we don't know what has come up until we check our lists.

Later assessment and confirmation comes from feedback from the users of the essences. We can never be absolutely certain if our description is completely accurate, but in our way of working what is accurate or inaccurate is not ultimately very important because we are assessing for individual need rather than for symptom pictures. The essences selected may give us an idea of what is going on, but at a level of interest or confirmation only.

In fact when we first started making Green Man Tree Essences I was a little reluctant to label the essences at all. However, people need some backup for their gut/intuitive choice and brief descriptions help (as well as hinder), to give confidence.

At the end of the process of key-coding each essence, we tune in again to see if there is any further information available. If there is, it is usually of a more esoteric nature."

Simon Lilly goes on to talk about the ways in which the qualities and actions of an essence, and the issues and patterns relating to that essence are described:

"The problem I have most often found with essence descriptions is that they stress the negative emotion (or perceived negative emotion), involved in a situation. A very common reaction is denial – " I am not envious, hateful etc. etc.!" This type of negative presentation of essence issues leads to a tendency to say " I feel miserable and fearful of...... so I will take...... to get rid of the fear etc., ie. spiritual aspirin. Descriptions which stress the negative emotion don't allow the individual the choice to decide to enhance the positive side. It works like affirmations work – If you are ill you don't work with an affirmation like "I don't want to be ill", or "I am not ill"; you work with "I am well now", "I have boundless energy coursing through me now", or similar.

One essence description may say "hate, envy, jealousy" and another analysis by someone else may say "love, forgiveness, understanding", ie. the other side of the coin. Yet again another analysis of the same essence may say "activates heart chakra, aligns emotional, causal and spiritual bodies", or "strengthens immune system and thyroid and thymus function", or "aids assimilation of the mineral gold". Each analysis is looking at the total landscape of the energy signature of the essence from different windows. The more holistic an approach, the more of an overview one has of any part of life energy patterns (which is after all what all flower essences are), the more synergy (evolutionary advancement of wholes by parts), and the more linkages there are between seemingly disparate or opposite characteristics. If one looks at linguistic root words this is easy to see – it's how the human brain works. The same root for light, bright, white, will be the root for its opposite, dark, dull, black, because in order to define light you have to have a concept of what 'light' isn't, and what isn't 'dark'. This is also the way good affirmations are formed: an affirmation like "I am not ill" has to be interpreted by the mind as a picture of what "I am ill" means, and then crossing that image out with a big scribbly "not" and a negation of the first image set up. It doesn't work well that way."

When looking at feedback from essence users it is important to recognize that each person taking a particular essence will have an individual reaction to it. We are all unique in every way. Some people may experience an aggravation of emotional, mental or physical patterns which will provide them with an opportunity to see clearly what they are doing as they repeat these patterns. For one person this may seem an unpleasant experience and they may feel that the essence is not working, or is making them feel ill; whilst for another they may appreciate the clarity they get from seeing their issues in sharp focus and may consequently find it easier to consciously change their pattern of reaction. One person may experience great inspiration while taking the essence and, as a result, integrate a new approach or response to life. So, when looking at feedback from essence users we need to be careful to take an overview of their responses to taking that essence, and we should bear in mind that symptoms arising from taking an essence do not indicate the energetic healing qualities of an essence, merely the individual's response to the energetic input of an essence.

It is not always necessary to define the qualities of an essence, particularly if it's an essence we have made for our own use or for clients who come to us for healing therapy. In these situations we may perhaps use dowsing or kinesiology to choose which essences are appropriate for someone and we may feel no need to know exactly what are the qualities of those essences, particularly if they prompt an obvious healing response. However, the benefit of having a good description of the healing qualities of an essence is that it enables us to consciously address habitual patterns and issues, and, for those who are not familiar or comfortable with dowsing and kinesiology, it offers a way of identifying the particular qualities of each essence, and thereby choosing which essence we feel is most appropriate for use at any given time.

For those who would like to begin to understand the qualities of essences they have made, but feel they need a starting point – a door into their own understanding, this chapter ends with Ellie Web's (Harebell Remedies) flower meditation: (It is helpful to have a notebook and pen close by so that you when you have completed the meditation, you can record all your impressions before you forget them.)

FLOWER MEDITATION

*(**** denotes pauses)*

Imagine we are entering a large flower garden. It has been opened today especially for us. It is a sunny morning, the birds are singing and the sky is clear

*The gardeners who tend this garden have the utmost respect for nature. the flowers are growing in all their favourite places. there are patches of woodland and open grassy spots. There is a pond and a bubbling stream running into it. There is a walled garden and a rock garden and many hidden circles and niches for the wide variety of wild and cultivated plants that grow here. Let yourself wander happily in this garden for a while. *********** The atmosphere is peaceful and safe. **** There are no harmful influences here **** This garden is protected by a circle of very old trees. **** Your presence is welcome.*

*Communicate your gladness to be here. Allow yourself to express that gladness. Run in and out of the bushes, roll on the grass, paddle in the stream, laugh, cry, pray – whatever you are feeling, acknowledge that and find a way to release it. ***********

*Now turn your attention to finding a special plant which is flowering. Take a moment to feel in which direction you are being drawn and slowly walk along that way, searching from side to side as you go. Take your time, you may know straight away which flower is attracting you, one which you noticed earlier perhaps, trust your first thought. If not, look carefully around you as you go. Look closer, some flowers are very tiny, and not just on the ground, the bushes and trees may be flowering too. ****

Once you and your flower have found each other, sit or lie comfortably (you will have to stand if it's a tree) and take some time to get to know each other. If you know its name, greet it, if you don't, greet it anyway and introduce yourself.

*Really try to imagine what it must be like to be that flower. Feel its vibration, it has a language all of its own. Trace its story, remember back to times when this flower may have been highly valued for its rare beauty, fragrant scent, valuable medicinal properties, or some unique practical benefit. ****** Tell the flower who you are, what it is like to be you, living where you do, in the body that you have, and the life that you are living. **** Share your concern for, and vision of the future. ***********

*Letting your mind wander in this way prepares us for moving to a deeper level. **** Close your eyes now and deeply centre. **** Bid your mind be quiet now and concentrate on your breathing. **** Breathe naturally, in rhythm with the day, and with the life force within and around you. **** Feel the earth below you **** and the sky above you ****Feel the vibration that is you! *****

*Now look at your flower. You are very close. Look at what we call the flower's signature; this simply means what it is suggestive of in terms of colour, shape, texture, scent etc... What are its unique features? Do they remind you of anything? Parts of the body? attitudes? life situations? **** What is the plant's relationship with the earth, the sky, with its surroundings? **** In what way is that different from yours? **** What are the words to describe this particular quality/feeling that you observe about this flower? Is it saying something to you? What is it saying? *****

*Take your time. Can you translate the flower's essence into your own language? **** It does not matter if you cannot, the words may come later. Be a little creative, or at least do not block what is your natural thought/response/feeling at this moment. A kind of synthesis is occurring between you. The actual physical making up of a flower essence is an attempt to preserve this alchemy for other times or places when you might need it. ********

*Prepare to take your leave of your flower. Thank it for giving its special gift and promise to keep it with you in spirit for a long time to come. Say goodbye and wander slowly back to where we started, thoughtful of what you have learned and of the precious gift you may be bringing to share with others. ************

*Back near the entrance, take another moment to search for words to describe what the flower's message is and write it down, or imagine yourself telling a friend about it. ********

*Slowly we all leave the garden now without looking back. Open your eyes and bring yourself back to the room. ******* If there are others who have shared this meditation with you, look at each other and be aware if you can of the flower each person has brought with them.*

Chapter 6

Choosing and using new flower essences

"Righteousness without love makes us hard.
Faith without love makes us fanatical.
Power without love makes us brutal.
Duty without love makes us peevish.
Orderliness without love makes us petty".   *Anonymous*

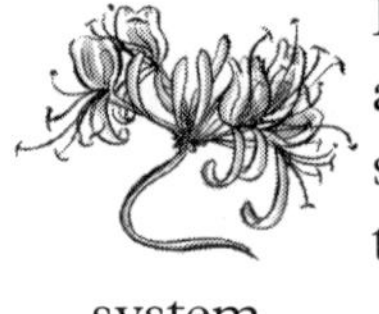 In the following chapter we will explore some ideas about choosing and using flower essences. It is intended to provide the reader with some suggestions and guides, to encourage the reader to develop their own understanding of this wonderful, and easy to use, healing system.

Whilst we do not specifically discuss the metaphysical aspects of dis-ease, this concept is an integral part of our understanding of the function and purpose of dis-easement, and can be yet another pointer to help with the identification of issues and essences. The journey of understanding and development is intended to be a joyful one, inspiring the same feeling we might have, after a long hard working day, when we are at last on our way to the comfort and familiarity of our own home.

Life's Journey

When we start working with flower essences, we embark on a journey of self discovery and self awareness. Once we start this journey, nothing will ever be the same again. When we understand who we truly are, we not only help ourselves, but we help everyone around us. We owe it to ourselves to explore our true nature and discover what we truly are, and that is LOVE.

Flower essences are a tool to help us to get back to love. They are a catalyst for change. When we start working with flower essences, we must understand that we will need to play an active role in our own healing process. Flower essence therapy is not a passive therapy – "take this four times a day and all will be well". Flower essences open up a channel for communication with our core being, by releasing and balancing suppressed emotions, and bringing these into our conscious awareness.

This form of healing is actually revealing what is already there. The suppressed emotions form a veil over the very light of our being and prevent us from radiating our true divinity.

Detecting the different beliefs and upsets that have occurred in the past, that make up this veil, can be exciting, as we get to know who we really are. It can be a wondrous experience as we cleanse the doors of our perception and let go of these old issues and come towards the infinite perception of ourselves and our universe.

As we resolve these limitations and peel back the layers that have served to protect us, we begin to open up, like a flower opens to the sun.

If we consider a Waterlily flower as an analogy for our inner journey: it, in a single season (the lifetime of the flower), grows, develops, rises to the light at the surface of the water, and then each petal unfurls, showing its true glory to the sun. We are like that flower. We remain closed and protected for our early journey through the muddy waters of this lifetime until we come into the light. Then, as time passes, each petal (which has been protected by our inner being) slowly unfurls, allowing our own perfection to shine forth. Flower essences can act as a key to unlock this unfurling process. Perhaps it is no coincidence (or is it synchronistic) that each petal (issue) needs to be brought into the light before those underneath can open. As we unfurl and bring light to each issue, we then move closer to our full potential.

We are constantly creating situations in our lives that reaffirm those old beliefs and patterns which we developed in childhood. Flower essences help to break this cycle of repetitive patterns, including those issues that we have come into this incarnation to work with and resolve. As we identify these issues our life's purpose becomes clearer. We can develop an understanding of our life's purpose by talking with ourselves honestly, and listening to the answers, to effect changes in belief necessary at this time. Our greatest limitation is not that we are inadequate, but the fear of our power. It is our light, not our darkness, that frightens us.

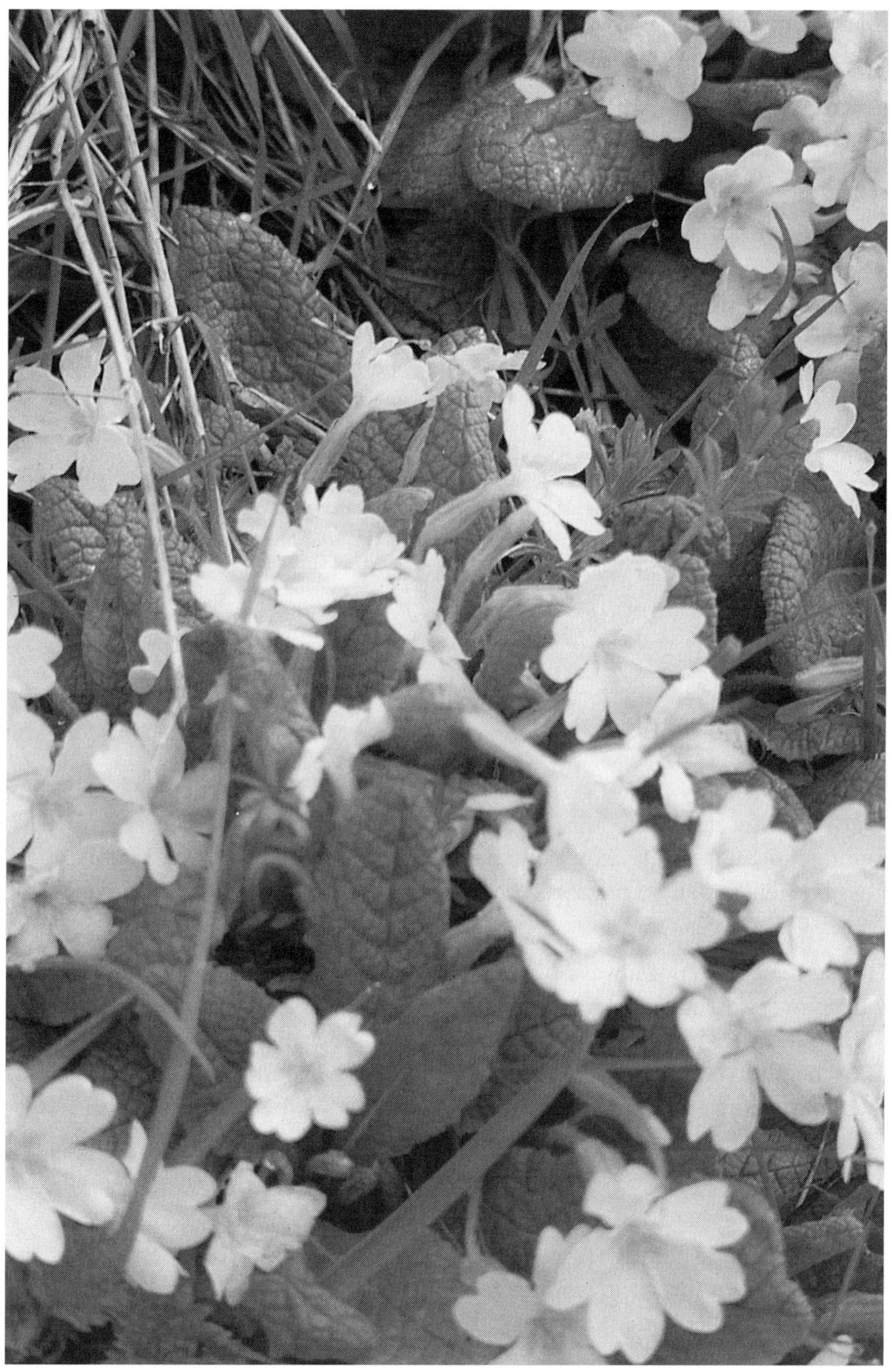

"This coming into the harmony is also called the Goddess arising within the breast of all. Woman is to embrace the attributes, within genetic memory, of enslavement. Man is to embrace the fear of woman, the fear of the power of woman; to know that what he fears within woman is that which he fears within Self. And it is for woman to understand that it is alright to be strong, alright to recognize her own power. So you see, dear ones, coming into this harmony is in truth to be found within the harmony of SELF, through the enhancement of those aspects within SELF which have formerly been unembraceable – to love what you have judged to be unlovable. And so it shall be, because you have sent forth the desire. In this fashion you will understand your own power to manifest exactly what you want. As you are all so desirous of coming into the understanding of non-separation within each and every breast, so you have chosen. It is that you have chosen the broad spectrum game plan, and that is why you have incarnated at this time. You merely get into a muddle now and again in your moment-by-moment life, where you would sometimes seem to lose the plot.

And that is alright, because in this time you will certainly experience what you were afraid to experience before. The fear will be called forth, and the situations will come with amazing rapidity until you have learned the lesson."

P'taah – from 'The P'taah Tapes – Transformation of the Species'
Channelled by Jani King

Getting to where we are now

We are constantly creating situations that reinforce the particular beliefs that we hold. We came into this lifetime with a predisposition to certain beliefs, reinforced by past-life experiences, so, often as not, in our early childhood, these beliefs are again reinforced, continuing our core or soul issues.

These issues are not always obvious. They may well have been buried under our many protective layers. To get to the core issues we may need to address other blockages that are more obvious. This allows the core issues to emerge into the light. Sometimes these inner issues may become apparent much earlier and need to be treated more immediately. This therefore brings the soul's life purpose into expression, bringing it through the higher self and the subconscious, into our conscious awareness, and subsequently into our reality.

Flower essences help us to re-establish contact between our personality and our soul. When this connection is re-made, we are able to communicate wholly once again. When we are separate from the oneness of everything we become lonely and fearful. This adds to our feelings of separateness.

A path to this re-connection is by looking at, or resolving, the key issues in our life, from childhood emotional experiences through adulthood to our now being.

We may choose to look at our life issues – episodes in our lives that have been important milestones. We may be able to identify patterns that re-occur throughout this time. There is often an instance in our childhood, perhaps when we were about three years old, when something happened (the age of three is when it is believed that we come into conscious knowing). It may have been something as simple as being put down while our mother answered the telephone. This perhaps gave us a feeling of being abandoned. If we have come into this life with a predisposition for lack of self-worth, this common event may reinforce this core issue. These feelings can then turn into misguided forms of belief which limit the personality's understanding of the soul's intention. In other words, a minor incident in the past creates a misguided belief about ourselves (a blockage, limitation, or issue). If we have a predisposition or soul issue in this area, we have a deep issue to resolve.

Childhood is therefore often where we may look for indications of our blockages. In adulthood we may be able to look at how we have created more limitations, and reinforced the old beliefs and patterns that we formed in earlier years.

These misguided feelings and patterns build up and become part of who we think we are. We are completely unique. We are not all coming from the same point. Each person's soul issues will be different, because each person's belief structures come from their unique experience. This brings us to who we are in our now moment.

One of the other ways in which we limit ourselves and reinforce these belief structures is by judging our emotional states to be good or bad. These emotions are what they are. We often feel that there is a battle going on between good and bad. We polarize everything, but emotions are JUST emotions. It is the judgement that makes them positive or negative. If we can get an understanding of this it helps us to release our judgement, and therefore our resistance to change. When we take out the judgement, and love ourselves, a transformation occurs. This loving of who we are, warts and all, prevents these diseases about ourselves from manifesting in the physical body.

"There is no difficulty that enough love will not conquer; No disease that enough love will not heal; No door that enough love will not open; No gulf that enough love will not bridge; No wall that enough love will not throw down;

It makes no difference how deeply seated may be the trouble, How hopeless the outlook, How muddled the tangle, How great the mistake, A sufficient realization of love will dissolve it all. If only you could love enough, you would be the most powerful being in the world."
Emmett Fox

Detecting the different beliefs and upsets that have occurred can be fun. It is joyful to at last let go of these issues. Flower essences help us to move through the blockages and limitations to our greatness, and help us to get in touch with the love that is within us all.

WAYS OF SELECTING FLOWER ESSENCES

Initially, by reading the flower essence descriptions, we may choose an essence that resonates with ourselves. We often find that we resonate with many essences and have to begin a selection process. The very act of reading these descriptions and trying to find those which feel most appropriate, not only begins our involvement with flower essences, but also starts us on a voyage of self-assessment, since we need to look more closely at how we are feeling as we try to match the essence descriptions.

When attempting to select an appropriate flower essence from the vast numbers available to us, we need to narrow down the field of choice. One way of doing this is to identify a single issue.

There are a number of ways that flower essences can be selected, the following is a guide that may be helpful in choosing essences.

Selecting flower essences by identifying issues

(The cross-reference index can be used to identify which essences relate to which issues. Further information on these essences may then be obtained from Chapters 7,8,9 & 10.)

Identifying issues

If we find it difficult to identify a specific issue, we need to observe how we are feeling. Some issues are easily identifiable, such as physical illness, grief, anger, jealousy, fear etc. So, being honest and open, without judgement, will ease the identification of the issue, emotion or trait.

Matching issues to flower essences

We can now match this identified issue to one listed in the Cross Reference Index. This may indicate a number of flower essences which address this issue. For example: if we have identified a feeling of abandonment, originating in childhood; we look up abandonment in the Cross Reference Index, and perhaps find a number of different flower essences listed. Each of these essences approaches abandonment from a different angle. (we may also be directed to look at other issues linked to abandonment, eg: loss and separation)

This identification of a feeling or issue can therefore lead us directly to a single appropriate flower essence. However, we may wish to address a number of different aspects of an issue; in which case, a combination of essences that relate to these differing aspects may be useful at this time. Flower essence makers' catalogues or reference material may also be used. (Further information about combinations of essences is given in this chapter, as well as in the Cross Reference Index and Chapter 9.)

Levels

Issues may occur at a range of different levels, so selecting a flower essence for any of these levels may be appropriate. We need to bear in mind that any individual essence may work on a number of different levels of an issue; this includes physical, life, and soul issues. The following couple of examples may help to illustrate this.

In this first example, three essences address the same issue on three different levels:

"I can't make a decision." – I could choose a flower essence for indecision (the presenting, or immediate issue). However, if I go a stage further, to another level, and look at why I can't make a decision, it could be: – "I doubt myself" (invalidate what I know). The appropriate essence when selected would then address this life-time issue. I could go further still, to yet another level, which leads me to: – "I have a predisposition to a lack of trust", (or not trusting my inner guidance). Therefore, taking a flower essence for: 'not trusting in inner guidance', would address my core, or soul issue. This example explains how an immediate issue may be operating at a 'deeper' level..

In the next example we will show how one essence addresses a problem on a number of different levels:

A client comes with herpes as a presenting physical problem. During the discussion, a feeling of being 'unclean' surfaces. On further discussion, a sexual issue is brought to light. An essence is prescribed for the sexual issue, which is then resolved, as is the feeling of being 'unclean', and the herpes clears up.

As we are at the threshold of new understanding this exciting new system of healing, this whole aspect of levels is one that has not been fully comprehended yet. It will be revealed to us as we shift our conscious perception through the new flower essences which are being discovered. It is all part of the evolutionary process.

Combinations, Catalysts and Support essences

Combining flower essences has become a major part of flower essence therapy. In fact, many essence makers now provide a range of pre-mixed combinations to address certain issues. Also being produced, are combination essences specifically for physical symptoms.

The practice of combining flower essences is one that seems to develop with experience. The greater our knowledge of essences, the more adept and skilful we become at selecting them. Individual essences address issues on differing levels, or provide different approaches to an issue.

Initially it may be appropriate to combine a few essences with a close association around an issue. Care must be taken not to muddle the effects by combining too many, or conflicting essences. If several essences are combined, sometimes a release of other hidden issues may occur. If this is suspected, adding an essence to support the person through the catharsis, or release, can be beneficial (a Support Essence). At other times, adding a specific essence to the combination to speed up, or regulate the release may be helpful. These flower essences may be considered to be catalysts, since they can help to shift a major blockage , when the identified essences appear not to be working. This release of a block can cause a shift in our awareness, allowing the flow into consciousness. In these instances, the Repertory may be used to identify Catalyst and Support essences.

Type Essences

Type essences are flower essences which address frequently repeated patterns of a personality type. We may have needed to take a particular essence regularly over a period of time, or we may find that it comes up for us with monotonous regularity. This could be our Type essence. It can be easier to identify it if we keep a journal, or card index of what flower essences we take ourselves, or give to clients (rather than relying on our memory).

If we can persist in the use of a Type essence, the rewards and insights can be amazing. It can be a very quick way of resolving a number of long-term issues which may have clouded the veil surrounding more immediate presenting issues. Another possible way of identifying Type essences is by using astrological information, as Peter Damien does in 'An Astrological Study of the Bach Flower Remedies'. Some, such as Gurudas, consider individual plants to be associated with specific planets or other astrological aspects. Historically, many plants have been assigned to a specific astrological sign, for example: Sunflower – Leo. This can be a means of selecting a Type essence by matching the astrological type of plant to the person.

As with any stage of flower essence work, choosing essences may be done by using intuition, dowsing or muscle testing.

Healing Crisis

When taking flower essences differing responses may occur. There may be an immediate effect, or even a dramatic shift in awareness. However some may be unaware of any change in their emotional state or perceptions, although for most some sort of change occurs.

From time to time during this unfurlment we may be confronted with what could be termed a 'healing crisis'. This may occur when emotional states intensify before being released. If such emotions have previously been suppressed or disowned, then, when they are being drawn into our conscious awareness, they may at times feel overwhelming. It is at this time, if the emotion does not feel transitory, that some action or support may be necessary.

The following suggestions may be useful at these times:

Cutting down the frequency with which you are taking the essence.

Using a support essence, such as one for feeling overwhelmed, a strengthening essence or an essence for clarity.

Writing down, or keeping a journal about the emotions that are surfacing.

Having Reiki/Healing treatments, Counselling etc....

Meditating can help to still and centre the mind, and often allows further insight into blockages.

Asking our guides for help (we need to be very specific about what help we are asking for, we get what we ask for)

By using supportive methods, the healing crisis can be overcome and a great understanding of the emotional issues can be reached.

Intuition

If we open our hearts and listen to our intuition (without judgement), and trust, we will find that we are given the information we need to select essences. (See Chapter 2)

As an example of receiving intuition in choosing essences: I find that during a conversation with a client, a flower essence will drop into my consciousness. I now know and trust that this is the appropriate essence, but the first time it happened it took a lot of trust, (because of my investment in the outcome). Would it work? It did, and subsequent experiences have shown that it does work. I just need to trust; even to the extent that, at times, I cannot work out why I have given a client a particular flower essence until the next time I see them.

The very act of taking flower essences, for whatever reason, helps to clear the direct channel of communication with our higher self. In fact, there are specific essences to help with intuition or communion with our higher self. We have access to all the knowledge we need, and therefore the answer to every question.

In fact, choosing essences by intuition is a good way to practise trusting our own intuition. If we live by our intuition we will truly be on our path, connecting to the divine source/all that is/god, and be truly coming home. (Some people use channelling as a means of ascertaining appropriate flower essences, or to guide them to the appropriate plant for making essences.)

Another aspect of intuition or guidance, is when a plant unsolicitedly attracts our attention. The voices of the flowers and nature surround us all the time and speak to us on many levels. Beyond words they communicate or vibrate their message. We only need to shift our awareness to hear them.

The more we open to Nature's gifts, the more we understand that we are not separate, but are all part of the same life force. So it is not surprising that flower essences hold a key to our reconnection with Nature.

Dowsing and muscle testing/kinesiology

When choosing and using essences, dowsing and muscle testing techniques are often used. These methods can prove useful when selecting essences and may also be used to answer many of the questions relating to dosage, number of drops, combinations, how to take, and for how long. (For further information on these techniques, please refer to Chapter 2.)

Selecting Flower Essences for others

When selecting flower essences for others, be they family, friends, or clients, the following guidelines may be helpful.

A person may come to us with any type of problem or presenting issue, including a range of possible physical symptoms, emotional problems, major life issues, relationship problems etc.. This can appear a very confusing situation, (where's the emergency or crisis essence .... Ah.. that feels better!!) In this situation we need to remember that the basic process of essence selection still applies. The process of identifying appropriate issues by intuition, knowledge of essences, honest discussion, dowsing, or muscle testing, can still be used.

We don't have to have all the answers when we act as a facilitator in the healing process of another. In fact, when they play an active role, it is part of their taking responsibility for their own well-being. It is important to establish trust, treating people as we would like to be treated. It is also important to feel a connection between ourself and the other person. We need to remember that we are both journeying and exploring together and we need to listen with our heart. We learn so much about ourself when we prescribe essences for others. Often an issue which we have just dealt with ourself, will be an issue that is confronting the person who has come to see us. We have an inner understanding of how this issue might feel to that person.

It can be both a great honour and a humbling experience, when someone reveals and shares their inner-most feelings with us. We need to respect them at all times. When people feel safe, they will open up and reveal their true feelings. Their inner knowing tells them it is safe, if we are emanating warmth, security and unconditional love.

We need to listen wholeheartedly whilst facilitating the exploration of the person's feelings and emotions. It is important to ensure that judgement does not cloud our impartiality during a session.

Writing down key words and phrases that come to mind during a session, will help us when choosing appropriate essences. By observing how a person looks and their attitude to life, we may obtain pointers as to what essences to prescribe. If we need more time to decide what to prescribe, we can tell the client that we will forward their prescription in the post. As with all flower essence work, using our discernment and what feel right for us is the key to effective prescribing. Whichever approach we use will be right for us... good luck.

Children

Children can be very open and receptive to taking flower essences. They instinctively know they can help because they have not yet developed fully the blockages, limitations and patterns of adults.

The following event happened at a Natural Healing Exhibition. A young boy of about seven came to a stand I was working on. There was a display of flower essences. The boy instinctively went to an essence bottle and picked it up and asked me what it was for. I explained that it was for people who were feeling very aggressive towards other people. He immediately responded with, "Oh I need that one, I have been wanting to hit my little brother all day", – he had chosen the essence he needed!

Having at our disposal flower essences, which give us the ability to assist in children's spiritual, mental, emotional and physical well-being, is a gift beyond measure. Being able to help clear their emotional dis-easement, from an early age, helps to prevent them from reinforcing any patterns they may be beginning to establish. If a child's development is not hindered by limitations, it can blossom more easily, and therefore speed up the conscious awakening and healing of the planet.

Flower essences can help babies to cope with the transition from the womb to the outside world, by helping to transmute the shock from both birth trauma and change. In this situation, Julian Barnard (of Healing Herbs) suggests putting flower essences on the mother's nipples so that the baby can absorb the essence while suckling. Another way for the baby to absorb essences is through the mother taking the essences herself, which enter her bloodstream and are passed into her milk, and then through to the baby. Flower essences may also be added to the baby's bath water and evaporated into the babies aura.

Animals

Animals also respond to flower essences but selection of an appropriate essence can be more difficult. Animals express their feelings in a number of ways; we need to take care to detect their moods and feelings, as opposed to their instinctive actions. Once we have done this we can choose an essence in the usual way.

A pet can be very close to its human companion, and so it can be useful to treat both, or at least examine the relationship. The dosage and means of application may need to be adjusted to suit the particular animal. Essences may be placed in drinking water or baths, applied topically or evaporated or sprayed into the aura of an animal.

Plants

Plants appreciate the use of flower essences on themselves. Usually applied topically, via a spray atomiser or watering can, they can help to lessen the shock of transplanting, pruning etc.. They can also aid the well-being of a plant affected by pests or disease. It can be helpful to apply essences when watering seeds and transplanted plants. In fact, flower essences can be used to treat plants in any creative way we might think of – the plants will certainly appreciate it!

WAYS OF USING FLOWER ESSENCES

The real beauty of using flower essences is their simplicity. It is impossible to overdose when taking them. They only act where there is an imbalance and they can be used alongside other forms of health care, such as allopathic medicine, homoeopathy and most forms of holistic therapy. They are safe to use for pregnant women, children, plants and animals.

The most common way of using essences is orally. However, there are many creative ways of using flower essences covering a wide variety of different methods and our understanding of the applications of this therapy is growing continually. Flower essences can be added to creams and applied topically; they can be put into bathwater from where they can be absorbed through the skin; they can be added to compresses and placed on inflamed areas of the body; they can be evaporated into the aura, or applied to the chakra points of the body, or even just held in the aura; they can also be used to cleanse rooms by adding essences to an atomiser and spraying a room, or a whole building and they can even be put into cleansing products (as does Marion Davis of Real Life Remedies), or used in any creative way that feels appropriate.

Dilution of flower essences

Flower essences are normally bought at stock dilution from essence suppliers. Essence makers usually give directions as to the dilution to dosage. However, intuition, dowsing, kinesiology and muscle testing can also be used to determine appropriate dilutions.(see Chapter 2)

There are many different approaches as to how the actual dosage dilution is produced from the Mother tincture. As with all aspects of flower essence work, there are no hard and fast rules. There are certainly tried and tested ways that have been used over the years, originating from the work of Dr Edward Bach, and Gurudas. Opinions differ on whether to dilute straight from the mother tincture to dosage bottle, or from the mother tincture, to a stock bottle dilution, and then further diluting to a dosage bottle.

Preparing a dosage or treatment bottle

A suggested basic guideline for dilution for dosage is: 4 drops from a stock concentration bottle, to a dosage bottle (15 – 30 ml) in $^3/_4$ spring water to $^1/_4$ preservative (brandy, vodka, glycerine, cider vinegar etc.). In hot weather it may be advisable to increase the proportion of preservative in the dosage bottle. If preparing a combination dosage bottle (a blend of different essences) put 4 drops of each essence into the dosage bottle. Some essence makers suggest using 7 drops of Mother tincture, added straight to the dosage bottle, as recommended by Gurudas. (For further information on stock bottle preparation and dilution of essences, see Chapter 4)

It is a good idea to label the dosage bottle, with information such as the name, dosage instructions, date, and if you have prepared the bottle for a client, your name and telephone number.

How do we take essences? How many drops? How often?

Directions for taking essences may be found in the essence maker's instructions. If this is not the case, then a suggested guideline is: 4 drops 4 times a day. These are either dropped on, or under, the tongue. It is the frequency of taking the essences, not the amount of drops, that is important. This regular use brings about a catalytic action which increases the strength of the change or shift in awareness. It may be a good idea to establish a routine of when we take doses from our treatment bottle, ie: first thing in the morning before we rise (as we are more receptive then), around midday, and before the evening meal; taking the final dose before going to sleep.

Flower essences may be taken more frequently for an acute state (over a relatively short term), or even a dose whenever needed. However, each prescription is usually taken for a period of two weeks, to a month, depending on the issues being addressed. Often a change can happen immediately, if the presenting symptoms are transitory. Usually, deeper issues take a bit longer to resolve. When first taking essences there can be a feeling of relief to begin with, a feeling of well-being – possibly a connection is made with our inner knowing, that help is at hand. On observation, it is often with the second bottle of flower essences that a real change starts to happen, and feelings that may have been buried begin to surface in our awareness. When the clearing begins to take place, there can be an experience of revisiting an area in our life where deep issues are stored. As we revisit this area, we get an opportunity to resolve and change our perception of where we thought the problem lay.

Combining essences

It is generally agreed that combining essences in a dosage bottle can be helpful. However, the accepted total number of essences that may be combined together in one dosage bottle, varies with each essence maker and therapist (from 3 – 20 essences per dosage bottle!), also the agreed number of drops can vary. Intuition, dowsing or muscle testing are commonly used to discern what is appropriate in this situation.

WAYS OF TAKING ESSENCES

Oral use

There are two main ways of taking essences orally: Firstly, the most common way, is by placing the required drops via a pipette from a dropper bottle, on or under the tongue, making sure that the pipette does not touch the tongue (as bacteria could collect on the pipette and be put back in the bottle). Placing drops under the tongue is thought to aid absorption into the blood stream. In the Bach system, it is suggested that holding the essence in the mouth for about one minute aids absorption.

Secondly, the flower essences can be placed in a glass of water or fruit juice, and then sipped several times throughout the day. It is a good idea to cover the drink with a cloth if it is likely to be kept for more than a day. A non-liquid way of taking flower essences orally, is to use pillules. These are sugar based, and the vibrational frequency of an essence can be transferred by various means to the pillules. Pillules such as those produced by Sun Essences are virtually alcohol free and can provide an alternative to alcohol liquid based essences.

For those sensitive to alcohol such as babies, young children and animals, it may be appropriate to apply essences topically (see section below on Topical use)

Preparations for alcohol sensitive people

When preparing a dosage bottle for alcohol sensitive people there are several methods that can be used:

Prepare the dosage bottle with about $1/4$ cider vinegar (instead of brandy) and fill the remainder with natural spring water.

Prepare the dosage bottle with about $1/3$ vegetable glycerine, topped up with natural spring water.

A dosage bottle of only spring water (plus added essences) will keep for between several days to a week in a refrigerator.

Patricia Kaminski and Richard Katz suggest (in their book 'The Flower Essence Repertory') that the amount of alcohol ingested by dilution from a 30ml stock bottle of spring water (with prescribed essences added) is about one part in 600, and could be considered insignificant. They also suggest it can be further reduced by adding the dose to a half pint glass of water or juice – this brings the amount of alcohol down to one part in 4,800. (For further information about the preparation of non-alcoholic Mother tinctures and stock bottles, see Chapter 4.)

Topical application of flower essences

Baths

One relaxing way of gaining the beneficial effects of flower essences is to put them in the bath. Gurudas suggests that bathing with flower essences immediately distributes the vibrational influence of the essences into the aura, and from there it can be absorbed into the subtle bodies.

When adding essences to the bath, the drops are normally taken from the stock bottle, and added direct to the full bath (making sure the bathwater is not too hot). Some essence makers give instructions as to the use of essences for baths. Their suggestions vary from five to 12 drops. Gurudas suggests that using seven drops helps attunement to the seven dimensions. When no instructions are given, or when using essences from several different essence makers, the appropriate dosage can be intuited or dowsed for etc..

Creams and Lotions

As a means of topically applying flower essences, creams and lotions have been used as carriers. For many years crisis creams containing flower essences have been produced for inclusion in first aid kits. These creams are generally made from non-animal products, to which flower essences are added. Usually a combination of crisis or emergency essences are used. These creams can be applied direct to the affected area, or used as protection for areas of friction. Crisis creams can be used for sprains, minor burns, insect bites, lesions, rashes and areas of sensitive skin.

Church Farm Rose Essences add their rose essences to a vegan base cream, made with glycerine and vegetable extracts. They recommend massaging the cream into the skin, avoiding sensitive areas. It can be applied to the soles of the feet, palms of the hands, over the heart, and on the back and front of the chest, to relieve symptoms.

Marion Davis makes moisturisers and beauty creams containing flower essences, and a number of essence makers produce flower essence creams for eczema.

Massage and Aromatherapy

For the massage therapist and aromatherapist, or anyone involved in bodywork, flower essences can be added to oil blends and used directly on the body. Rosie Potter suggests that using the correct aromatherapy oil, in combination with flower essences, has the advantage of being able to apply the essences where they are most needed, and can provide amplification in an holistic treatment. She recommends that in specific physical conditions such as eczema, psoriasis and other skin conditions, a cream containing jojoba oil, or evening primrose oil, or essential oils that are anti-allergenic, anti-pruritic and emolient, together with flower essence that deal with the presenting issues, can all be combined and varied to suit the individual. One of the emergency or crisis creams can be applied to areas of the body where there are problems, before the massage oil is used, to help with the manipulation. Mark Mordin, a therapeutic body-worker and nutritionist, uses flower essences on purely physical problems, and combines them with his body-work (in addition to using them to treat emotional conditions).

Compresses

Using compresses is another way of applying flower essences to areas of the body that have swellings, sores, lesions, or any form of skin condition. Rosie Potter recommends using a clean, soft, cotton cloth when giving compresses. She suggests adding 10-15 drops of stock essence to a medium sized basin of water, soaking the cloth in this, and then lightly squeezing out the excess water before placing on the skin. For warm compresses, she suggests covering with a thick towel to keep the heat in.

A combination of crisis or emergency essences can be used for this purpose, or a combination of essences, depending on the problem.

Atomisers

The use of atomisers to distribute flower essences is another method suggested by some essence makers. Simon Lilly (of Green Man Tree Essences) suggests adding a few drops of tree essences, to a small amount of water in a clean plant sprayer or atomiser, and using this to spray around the body, or in a room. This can be an instantaneous way of infusing the essence into the aura, which he likens to the experience of walking into a grove of ones favourite trees. He also suggests placing a drop or two onto the palms of the hands, and then quickly passing the hands in a sweeping motion through the aura.

Sun Essences (with their Solar Blends) recommend putting 20 drops of their Crisis essence into a mister bottle of water, and spraying this into the aura, or in a room where there are many people. They suggest that this helps bring a collective feeling of calm. This blend can also be sprayed onto animals fur, or into the atmosphere around them, to help soothe them. Emergency or Crisis blends may also be put into an atomiser and sprayed into the atmosphere of a room, prior to exams.

David Eastoe (of Petaltone Essences) produces an essence called 'Crystal Clear' specifically for cleansing buildings, healing rooms, motor cars, crystals etc.. He suggests using a few drops in a plant mister of water, and spraying this around the area to be cleared. Several essence makers suggest putting essences into an atomiser spray, and using this to spray in treatment rooms after each client, or to spray around the home, or to use in any other creative way that can be thought of.

Auras, Chakras and Subtle Bodies

The healing vibration of a flower essence, matching the vibrational frequency of a chakra, can stimulate healing on an energetic level. Essences are being made for this purpose (chakra essences) and are listed in Chapters 7 & 8. Essences may either be taken orally, to effect this healing, or drops can be placed on the area of the chakra, or rubbed into the hands, and swept through the aura, or held over the chakra points. (Further information on chakras may be found in Chapter 2).

Homoeopathic potentization of flower essences

A number of flower essence therapists are now exploring and researching the use of homoeopathic potentization of flower essences. Dr Maria Maw, (of Unitive Flower Essences) works with homoeopathic potencies of flower essences, for specific clients. Her practise is to give a flower remedy (at standard stock potency) for several days, for a specific emotional issue; this is followed by a break of a few weeks. She then gives the same remedy, prepared at increasing homoeopathic potencies. Each of these potencies is taken for several days, followed by a short break, before increasing the potency. She has found this to be very effective, since the client seems to access deeper levels of the issue with each increase in potency.

Practitioner Anne Parker makes homoeopathic potencies of flower essences using a radionics instrument. She has found that when she uses these potentized essences for her clients, they require fewer treatment bottles than previously, in order to clear confronting issues and patterns, since the homoeopathically potentized essences appeared to work more swiftly than the standard stock potencies of essences.

Some flower essence therapists and essence makers suggest that the basic differences between flower essences and homoeopathic medicines are sufficient to indicate that apparently 'amplifying' the effects of essences by potentization is not appropriate. Some even go so far as to suggest that this could intensify the causal action of flower essences, and produce a less universal 'safe' product. There are also some schools of thought that suggest that 'artificial' methods of potentization, such as the use of radionics machines, do not produce the same product as diluted and sucussed potentizations of essences, since they feel that the very 'essence' of the flower is missing from the radionics potentized essences.

In this area, as in all aspects of flower essence practice, there are no hard and fast rules, and each individual, when working with their own integrity and discernment, will devise whatever method is appropriate to their situation.

Enhancement of essences

After preparation of the dosage bottle, some essence makers and therapists recommend tapping or succussing the bottom of the bottle, to energize and mix the essences. It is also suggested that this process is repeated, to re-energize the essences, before each dose is taken.

Another method of enhancing or re-energizing essences, is to hold the dosage bottle and ask for the highest collective consciousness, of those particular flowers, to activate the essences to the level for the greatest good of all concerned.

Some essence makers use pyramids or stargates to enhance the vibrational frequency of their blends. (See Chapter 4)

Affirmations

There are a number of books that show how the use of affirmations can help release blockages affecting our physical and emotional well-being.

When we use affirmations we are making a definite conscious connection to our healing process. Affirmations work well when used in conjunction with corresponding flower essences. When combining the use of affirmations and flower essences, it is recommended that the affirmation be repeated each time a dose of the flower essence is taken.

When we repeat the positive qualities of an essence we are confirming our intent to let go of some of our belief structures. Affirmations can bring us into the present, into the 'now' moment. Starting an affirmation with, "I am now", is one way of doing this.

For example: "I am now letting go of fear", "I am now feeling worthy of who I truly am", "I am now releasing my resistance to change", "I am lovable in this now moment".

Affirmations can be a form of meditation; they can help to centre and concentrate the mind, and therefore enhance the effect of taking the flower essence.

Conclusion

As we work with flower essences we realize that we can use them in everything we do and at any given time. Their unique breadth of application is wonderful.

We realize that, as with all of Nature's gifts, they are a tool to assist us on our journey home, and, like us, they too are a part of the greater evolutionary process.

I hope, in this chapter, that I have been able to explore the fact that there are no hard and fast rules when working with flower essences, since we are all unique, all going on our individual journey, into our inner knowing of who we are. We can all discover that we are our own master. We know instinctively what is appropriate for us. We have a choice all the time. We can choose the voice for fear, or the voice for love.

Let the flowers and their life force speak for themselves. We only need to be still and listen with our hearts.

> *"We are borrowing from a natural world,*
> *to get back to a natural world,*
> *a natural cycle to get back home".*

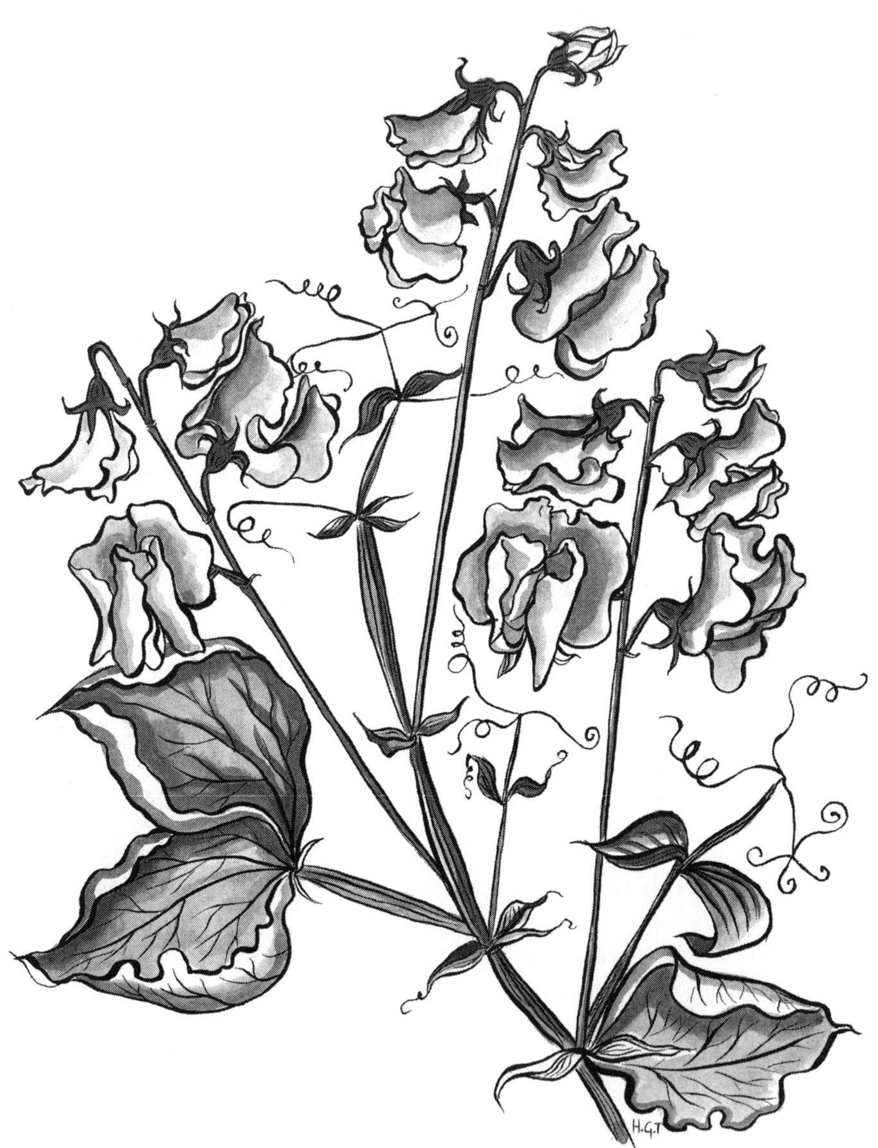

Chapter 7

The Repertory

NOTE: In some instances more details about individual essences can be found in Chapter 8 where the essences made by each contributor are listed in sets.

Key for Contributors:

Artemis Flower Essences	*A.F.E.*
Aquarius Flower Essences	*A.F.R.*
Bailey Flower Essences	*B.E.*
Ballybane Flower Essences	*B.F.E.*
Bridget's Flower Remedies	*B.F.R.*
Carole Guyett	*C.G.*
Church Farm Rose Essences	*C.F.R.*
Crystal Herbs	*C.H.*
Dr Andrew Tresidder	*A.T.*
Earth Essences	*E.E.*
Findhorn Flower Essences	*F.F.E.*
Gaia Essences	*G.E.*
Glastonbury Holy Thorn Essences	*G.H.T.E.*
Green Man Flower Essences	*G.M.F.E.*
Green Man Tree Essences	*G.M.T.E.*
Habundia Flower Essences	*H.F.E.*
Harebell Remedies	*H.R.*
Imelda Carroll – Ard Na Neantog Flower Essences	*I.C.*
Jean Jacob Flower Essences	*J.J.*
Judith Hoad	*J.H.*
Light Heart Flower Essences	*L.H.F.E.*
Lord and Lady Flower Essences	*L.L.F.E.*
Loving Nature Essences	*L.N.E.*
Middle Earth Flower Essences	*M.E.F.E.*
Middle Earth Rose Essences	*M.E.R.E.*
Rosie Devitt Flower Essences	*R.D.*
Silvercord Essences	*S.C.E.*
Sue's Flower Essences	*S.M.*
Sun Essences	*S.E.*
Unitive Flower Essences	*U.F.E.*
Julian Winslow Wight Flower Remedies	*J.W.*

★★Harebell Essences which are particularly good for external use.

Key for Sun Essences:

F – Flowers floated on spring water, in the sunshine
L – Living flowers held in spring water, in the sunshine
B – Flowering twigs boiled in spring water
S – Plant material filling bowl of spring water and left out in all types of weather
C – Flowers cut with scissors
H – Flowers picked by hand
P – Flowers laid in pattern on the water

EXPLANATION OF THE REPERTORY

The purpose of the Repertory section in this book is to illustrate the healing themes of individual plants. Under each plant heading, i.e. – Dandelion, is given the descriptions of the qualities of this essence, from all the individual essence makers who have made this particular essence.

Each essence maker's interpretation of the healing qualities of an essence they have made will inevitably differ from the description of this essence, made from the same plant, by another essence maker; since each maker will focus on those aspects of this plant's healing energy which reflect their own healing path.

The essence descriptions given in the Repertory are brief descriptions of the qualities of these essences. More detailed descriptions can be found in Chapters 8, 9 and 10 in the individual essence makers set of essences.

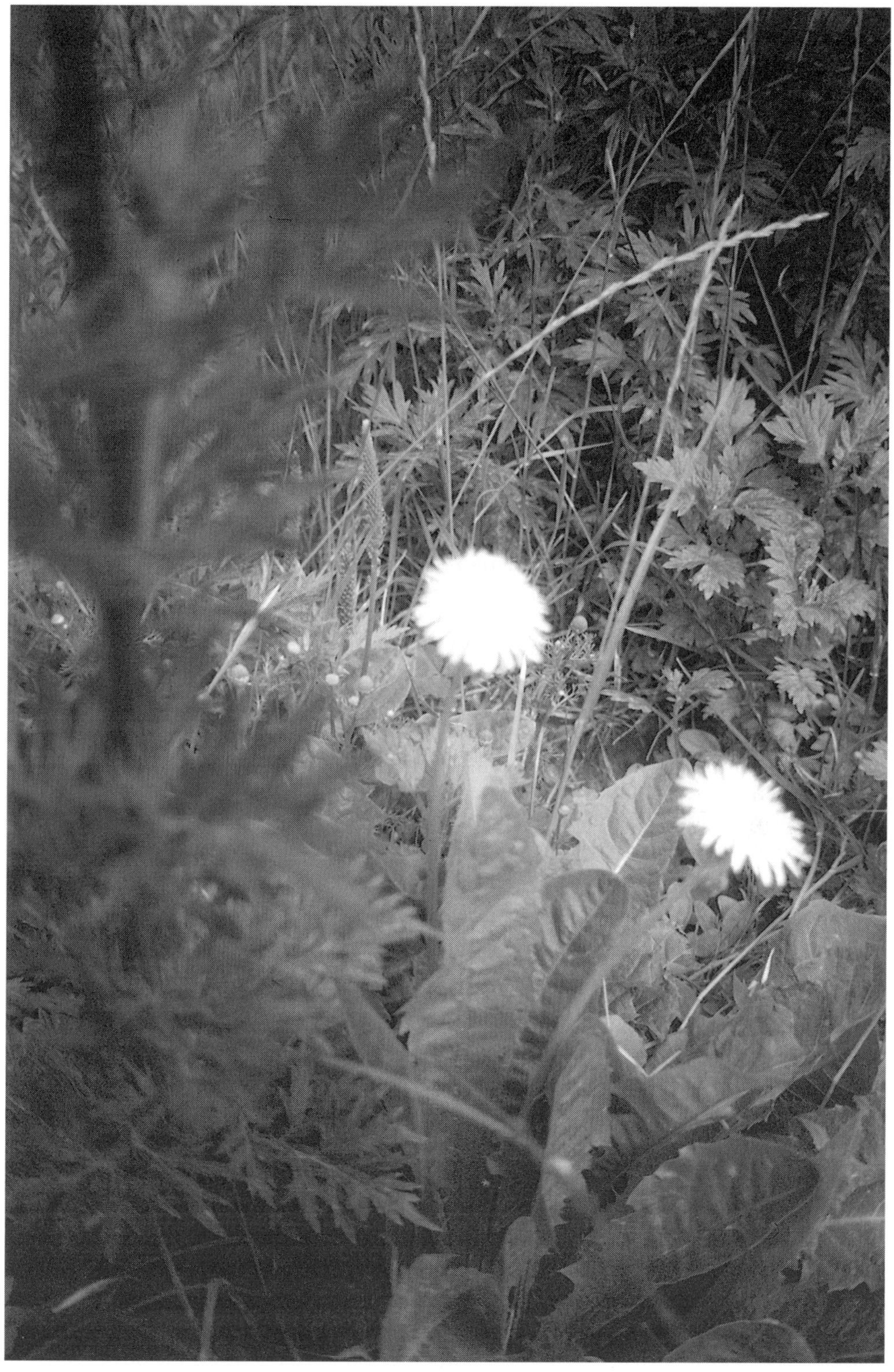

AFRICAN VIOLET *Saintpaulia*

Venus. For group work-spiritual linking. Used by sensitives and those who are reaching out to higher dimensions. Balances the nervous system and disharmonies in the mental body. Connects to the pineal. Crown chakra. *J.J.*

AGAPANTHUS *Agapanthus*

Brings courage and strength to higher purposes. *C.H.*

AGAVE *Agave americana*

Strength in the face of adversity. Patience. Good to use with people who are rehabilitating after a long illness, accident or operation, or those who are weary of life's journey, those struggling to see hope for the future. *J.W.*

AGERATUM *Ageratum*

Brings the soul qualities into the physical, grounding. *C.H.*

AGRIMONY *Agrimonia eupatoria*

Used for the liver, stomach and also for rheumatics, gastro-enteritis and gall bladder problems. The light bringer, will help you to absorb more prana and to bring spiritual awareness so that you may acquire spiritual wisdom. *S.C.E.*

ALDER *Alnus glutinosa*

"Release". Reduces nervousness and anxiety. Brings clarity of mind and eases stress. Increases life energy. *G.M. T.E.*

ALDER (LUNAR)

Alder is the remedy to heal sexual problems that have occurred in past lives. Good for past life sexual servitude, disempowerment through such actions as rape, abuse, incest or prostitution. Alder also treats the guilt and self-disgust of those souls who are aware that they themselves have sexually abused in a previous life. *A.FR.*

ALFALFA *Medicago sativa*

Strength, self-worth, earthing and expressing your spiritual spark. Honouring and communicating your own needs, especially spiritual needs. Rooting. Absorbing vitality from the Earth. *H.FE.*

ALKANET *Anchusa officinalis*

For centering safely in order to change in a deep way. Brings inner strength. There is a sense of opposites uniting in preparation for a transformation.

'I am centered and ready to transform'. *H.R.*

This essence is connected with the energies of transformation. It acts as a catalyst to facilitate deep changes, working from a firmly rooted base. This can help to transform opposing energy patterns that may have been caused originally by incompatible parental energies in childhood. It works on the mother/father within, affecting the internal male/female energies at the same time.

Planets – Pluto, Moon, Saturn

Chakra – 3rd *M.E.FE.*

This is a good essence for healing of wounds; can be used in cream base. Also for ulcers.

'Maybe I should become the decision maker' – self responsibility. *S.C.E.*

ALKANET (GREEN) *Pentaglottis sempervirens*

Calm in a storm.

Alkanet can help one to keep positive and balanced in situations which are chaotic or obtrusive.

Feelings of support and protection help to hold and focus energy, enabling clear communication and a way through difficult circumstances. *L.F.H.* *S.E.*

For being gentle with oneself and others by understanding and accepting who you are and where others are coming from. *L.L.F.E.*

ALMOND *Prunus dulcis*

Growth in children. *R.D.*

Mental maturity, fears of ageing. *C.H.*

AMARANTHUS (RED) *Amaranthus*

Viruses, inflammations. *R.D.*

AMARYLLIS *Amaryllis*

Can be used to perfect the art of meditation, brings calm and stillness, helping to go within. *C.H.*

AMELANCHIER *Amelanchier canadensis*

Smoking, torn tissue rejuvenated, varicose veins. Control of glands improved. Lymphs, pancreas. Clarity of thought. Compulsive gamblers. Courage. Drug addiction symptoms. Selfishness. Will power weak. Stopping smoking. All chakras especially fifth. Throat nadis. *B.F.R.*

ANEMONE *Anemone*

Balancing all chakras. *C.H.*

Anemone pavonina

This helps to balance all the major chakras, with a particular focus on the throat and the brow, to help with communication, including telepathy. It helps with difficulties in communication due to an inability to ground the energy properly and helps us to focus clearly on our needs. *S.M.*

ANGELICA *Angelica*

Angelica allows us to feel a greater degree of protection, guidance and love from the angelic kingdom. It is particularly important at major life passages. PHYSICAL USE: Treats epilepsy and many other neurological disturbances, skin ulceration and eczema. *A.F.R.*

Affinity with angelic forces. *C.H.*

APPLE *Malus sylvestris*

Keynote: Higher Purpose

Helps us to integrate our desires and our willpower to realise positively our goals and visions. By aligning with Higher or Divine Purpose we channel these powerful energies into right action. Indications: blocks to realising inherent power and ability, unable to sustain self-discipline, the glamour of power and superiority, lack of power to act or self-assertion, succumbing to lower desires, unbalanced sexual expression, depletion of sexual creative forces.

Attributes: development and right use of will, removing blockages to positive action, concertedness, inner strength to overcome inertia, self-discipline, humility, obedience to higher will, reforming lower desire to love and selfish will into will-to-serve.   *F.FE.*

Malus domestica (wild specimen)

"Detoxification". Helps the elimination of toxins and brings in spiritual energies. Transforms negative emotions.   *G.M.T.E..*

APRICOT

For arrogance, brashness, egocentric people, selfishness, greed, materialistic. Brings about a softening, gentleness, sweetness and humility and a compassion for others.

G.E.

ARIZONA FIR *Abies lasiocarpa var. compacta*

To help us to celebrate our life and existence as a spiritually based being   *B.E.*

ARTEMISIA *Artemisia*

Helps develop telepathy, for left brain hemisphere damage.   *C.H.*

ASH

This flower essence is for balancing male/female energies in oneself and in relating. Wherever there is an imbalance, disharmony or a need to connect with the anima/animus this essence would be appropriate. Its signature is that the tree contains both male and female flowers.

Planets – Sun, Moon

Chakras – 3rd, 7th   *M.E.FE.*

Fraxinus excelsior

"Strength". Harmony with your surroundings. Feeling in tune. Flexibility and security.   *G.M.T.E.*

AUBERGINE

Lifts the base chakra energy, shifts blockages. Sexually related problems.   *C.H.*

AUBRETIA *Aubrieta*

This essence is for bringing up and clarifying emotions that have been suppressed, so that they can be dealt with. It can throw new light on a situation that one feels trapped in. Deep breathing is facilitated with this essence, therefore useful in such therapies as rebirthing.

Planets – Moon, Neptune, Pluto

Chakras – 2nd, 3rd, 6th   *M.E.FE.*

AURICULA *Auricula*

Balances the emotions. Solar plexus.   *C.H.*

AUTUMN LEAVES

Transition.

The colours of autumn are mixed together to give a Natural Earth Essence that re-connects you with nature and the ever-changing patterns of life. Today people find themselves living many lifetimes within one – dying and being reborn like the cycles of nature. This can be a very difficult process. Autumn leaves can be supportive when going through such periods of profound personal change. *S.*   *S.E.*

AZALEA *Rhododendron*

Orange. Self forgiveness.   *A.T.*

Rhododendron 'Wayford Woods'

Unleashing creative forces to channel and be inspired.   *A.T.*

BABY BLUE EYES *Nemophila menziesii*

For those of us who feel unsafe and insecure in this world due to a lack of emotional support during childhood. Taking this essence helps to restore the soul's original innocence and child like trust.   *A.F.R.*

BALSAM POPLAR *Populus balsamifera*

Cleansing and healing the sexual chakras. Balances the flow of sexual energy. Releases pain and tension from sexual issues.   *H.F.E.*

Childhood emotional issues, any age.   *C.H.*

BANANA *Musa*

Bone marrow.   *R.D.*

BARLEY

Barley grains. Dissolving the belief of needing to rely on the leadership of others for my own truth.   *A.T.*

BASIL

This essence is used when there is a sense of shame, guilt or disgust around sex. It heals the separation experienced between sexuality and spirituality.   *A.F.R.*

Heart and throat chakras, brings clearance of grief, allowing it expression.   *C.H.*

BAY *Laurus*

Bay buds. Unblocking the need to be led. Settling into yourself and distributing the energy evenly.   *A.T.*

Laurus nobilis

"Energy". Deep-rooted vitality. Blocked and suppressed emotions released. Spiritualises physicality.   *G.M.TE..*

BEAKED HAWKSBEARD *Crepis vesicaria*
Connects the solar plexus with the crown chakra, to uplift the emotional body by keeping a spiritual focus. Rising above petty emotions and trusting in one's own destiny.   *H.F.E.*

BEECH *Fagus sylvatica*
"Easy-going". Confidence and hope in oneself and one's life. Relaxation and release of held-in trauma. Confidence in self-expression and speaking out clearly.   *G.M.TE..*

BEGONIA *Begonia*
To move to the next stage of development from a healing plateau.   *C.H.*

BELLFLOWER *Campanula barbata*
Newborns' adjustment to sound. Children's creative expression. Throat chakra. *C.H.*

BELL HEATHER *Erica cinerea*
Keynote: Stability
Helps to access inner strength and resolve to stand one's ground after stress, trauma or conflict.
Indications: Loss of faith in self, lack of confidence, mood swings, easily swayed, apparently victimised by circumstance, loss of direction or purpose, fragile.
Attributes: Tenacity, affirmation, trust inner knowing, faith in oneself, standing up for oneself, resolute in stance and purpose, assertiveness, following one's own path with confidence, resilience, self-recovery.   *F.F.E.*

BELLS OF IRELAND *Moluccella laevis*
Links to Divinity of nature; stress and anxiety.   *C.H.*

BERGAMOT *Monarda*
For cleansing and disinfecting wounds and infections. Use internally and externally as a swab with 7 drops in a small cup of water.   *C.H.*

BETONY *Stachys officinalis*
For nervous asthma, migraine, a nerve tonic. Awakens the kundalini, through creative visualisation this stimulates the energy that is needed for service   *S.C.E.*

BILBERRY *Vaccinnium myrtillus*
Integration of the Self. Calms and brings peace to thought processes. Communication clarified. Increases equanimity and balance in all situations, especially where there are extremes of emotion that may bring conflict. Clarity, discrimination and wisdom brought to spiritual states.   *G.M.F.E.*

BINDWEED *Convolvulus arvensis*
For the ability to face fear. For inner strength to conquer. For resilience.   *E.E.*

Calystegia silvatica
Connecting, binds ideas/people together.
Use to resolve karmic and inner child issues. It is indicated for people who stifle their

emotions – helps them to recognise and come to terms with their deepest emotions. Bindweed encourages the resolution of karmic patterns by forming the connection between current stresses and past life issues. It is also useful for connecting therapist/clairvoyant and client together for more effective work (both would need to use the essence at least a half hour before the session).

Protects by strengthening the silver cord for astral travel. Bindweed strengthens all the subtle bodies and meridians and gives all round protection at all levels. It's associations include the colours gold and yellow, direction North, planets Earth, Moon and Saturn. *A.F.E.*

BIRCH *Betula pendula*

Keynote: Perception

Helps us to broaden our perceptions and transcend limitations of mind. Through expanding our consciousness and seeing our cosmic connections we gain understanding and peace of mind.

Indications: obscured or unclear vision, stuck in thought patterns which hold us back, inability to see beyond ourselves or our concerns, worry, introspection, dulled senses, living in the past or future, escapism or day-dreaming, out-of-body states, 'blind spots', not learning from past mistakes, confusion of mind.

Attributes: bringing in the light of the mind, expanding one's awareness into the cosmos, contacting Universal Mind, direct experience of the infinite here and now, deep mindfulness, realising the inner wisdom of life experiences, focussed and intuitive attitude and power to see the vision and direct one's course to it, cultivating spiritual vision. *F.F.E.*

BIRD CHERRY *Prunus padus*

"Sensuality". Unblocking deep emotional wounds. For those who have become over-defensive of emotional attachments, are sexually or sensually repressed, mentally rigid and overcritical and uncomfortable with physicality. *G.M.T.E.*

BIRDS FOOT TREFOIL *Lotus corniculatus*

Effect of taking essence: Helps change one's perception of Self, recognising one's value oneself. Not needing to get it from others. When own value is recognised it allows achievement without trying, in all areas and hence recognition.

Presenting conditions: Feels lacking recognition. Tries to please by doing too much. Feels small and insignificant and lacks focal point. Disperses energy in many directions 'running around like a headless chicken'. Tries to be all things to all people instead of being true to self. *L.N.E.*

BISTORT *Polygonum bistorta*

For protecting those who tend to "self-destruct" during a period of great change. *B.E.*

BITTERCRESS *Cardamine*

Whole plant excluding roots. For understanding, encompassing and channelling 'the light'. *E.E.*

The keyword for Bittercress is 'steadfastness'. This remedy arises for people who are loyal companions, who stay with their convictions despite upheavals. These are admirable qualities but bring their own stresses usually in the form of pressure to give way (comparable to a great tree in gale force winds, unable to bend as a young sapling might). Along with these qualities may go a sense of being temporarily unsettled by strangers.

U.F.E.

BLACKBERRY *Rubus fruticosus*

Venus. Libra. Brings causal and spiritual bodies to integrate with the physical. Forgiveness and persistence. Conscious manifestation of creative thought. Under armpits for orgone energy which creates vitality. Awakens love when afraid of dying. Overcoming inertia.

J.J.

Opening to and understanding love in its deeper levels. Bramble teaches one to approach love with gentleness, care and respect.

H.F.E.

Grounds ideas into reality. This essence is indicated when a person has lots of ideas but seems unable to find enough will to bring them into reality, perhaps due to the perceived pain of living. Blackberry can harness power and energy and help one to focus on and attain the goal without distraction. *L.F.H.*

S.E.

Blackberry aligns the mind with the will, making it easier to ground goals and ideals in the physical world. It is also given to those who fear death. PHYSICAL USE: helps the blood absorb food throughout the body and purifies the entire endocrine system.

A.F.R.

Lethargy.

R.D.

High level astral protection from psychic attack.

A.T.

Dreams stimulated. Death/dying fears and bereavement depression.

C.H.

This essence helps the fears of a dying person or a fear of death in general; whether it be for the self, or fear that someone else is going to die. It is also good for manifesting thoughts and ideas into the tangible world, or if one is feeling stuck it gets things moving again.

Planets – Saturn, Chiron, Pluto

Chakra – 5th

M.E.F.E.

Strengthening. Use for poor circulation and mental clarity.

It is suggested for: cleaning the blood, improving circulation, balancing blood pressure and increasing the absorption of oxygen throughout the body. It stimulates the adrenals to increase stamina, encourages kidneys and lymph to throw out toxins and the muscles to throw off lactic acid. It is also useful for spleen, liver and urinary problems. Use for mental fatigue, depression and lethargy. It calms the mind for meditation and channelling. Blackberry energises and balances all the meridians and nadis, it opens all the chakras but does not balance them.

Blackberry amplifies other essences in combinations and assists their assimilation. It's associations include the colour red, direction South, planets Venus and Mars, Tarot Emperor.

A.F.E.

Some people go through periods in their lives when the force of physical or mental restrictions are so strong that they are unable to move – they feel debilitated. These restrictions may be imposed by rules, disability or fear, but whatever the limitation, there is a perception of not having any control over the boundaries, or room to manoeuvre. The sense of debility can be accompanied by resistance and struggle or resignation and laziness.

Bramble brings a quiet strength, a freeing of the spirit, a sense of expansion which goes beyond the ordinary perception of existence. *U.F.E.*

For stomach disorders, hypertension, also for coronary disease. Used for skin conditions such as eczema, also mouth and throat infections. For those who like to be by themselves, self protection. *S.C.E.*

BLACK EYED SUSAN *Rudbeckia*

Sun. To confront traumas of the past. Healing forgotten issues which need to be faced. Brings light into darkness. For courage. *J.J.*

Will help to draw to you that which is needed for your growth and change. *C.H.*

BLACK MEDICK *Medicago lupulina*

At night, whole plant. To balance the black/white, positive/negative aspects of the self. For understanding and encompassing power. For fearlessness. *E.E.*

BLACK POPLAR *Populus nigra var. betulifolia*

"Solidity". Creates a powerful peacefulness. A sense of security and inner clarity. Very comforting. Blends all energies. *G.M.T.E.*

BLACKTHORN *Prunus spinosa*

Saturn. Dark night of the soul. Depths of despair. Self opinionated people who are not open.

To open the door where one cannot see the light. *J.J.*

Coping with fears, facing one's dark/shadow inwardly and in external environment. *L.L.F.E.*

Balancing beauty with power. Gives you security in showing your inner beauty, while protecting you and keeping you strong. *H.F.E.*

Brings spiritual understanding to fear. Use at night after taking karmic fear essence during the day for release during sleep. *C.H.*

"Circulation". Helps absorption of nutrients. Stabilises emotions. Brings hope and joy. Strengthens the blood supply. *G.M.T.E.*

For those who are unconsciously seeking support. Life may be experienced as burdensome, there may be deep feelings of resentment, repressed rage or outbursts of extreme anger. There is a sense of physical tension in the body as if creating an additional support structure to the skeletal system and this may result in back problems especially lower back.

Blackthorn helps the recognition that it is not only OK but desirable to be supported by others and by the Universe and that by opening to receive we also give. *U.F.E.*

The remedy for the depths of despair – the "Valley of the Shadow of Death". *B.E.*

BLACK TULIP *Tulipa 'Black Swan'*

Clears the third eye. Clarity, originality. Honouring one's own creative perception, expression and vision, regardless of outer pressures to conform. *H.F.E.*

BLEEDING HEART *Dicentra formosa*

Non-attachment.

This essence is useful when there has been neediness or co-dependence within a relationship. If the partnership ends, the pain of lost love is often experienced as unendurable. Bleeding heart helps one to work through the grief and begin the process of healing the self. *L.F.H.* S.E.

Heart disease, blood pressure. R.D.

Bleeding heart is a very powerful heart cleanser and strengthener for those who must learn the deeper spiritual lessons of love and freedom. This essence promotes the ability to love unconditionally. PHYSICAL USE: alleviates heart disease, regulates blood pressure and is a tonic for muscle tissue. *A.F.R.*

For those too emotionally attached. Heart chakra, heart diseases. *C.H.*

BLUEBELL (WILD HYACINTH) *Endymion nonscriptus*

Cooling and calming; good after any injury or trauma, but generally brings forth feelings of content and of deep well grounded joy★★.

'I can always find a cool, quiet, happy place'. *H.R.*

Venus. Female depression. Post natal especially with fear and guilt. Helps self-love and kindles re-growth for brighter future. Brings joy and colour where there is grief.

J.J.

Mixed colours. Tranquillity.

The fresh, uplifting quality of a Bluebell Wood is embodied in this healing essence. The fragrance, colour, stillness and perfect peace can reconnect you with your higher self and the tranquillity this brings is useful in times of stress. *L.F.H.* S.E.

Creative expression, singing, music, chanting, sound therapy. Throat chakra. *C.H.*

For attuning to devic energies when working in the garden or working with nature.

M.E.F.E.

There are times in life when everything seems to be happening at once. This can feel tremendously exhilarating and/or dangerously overwhelming – a bit like riding rapids. There can be a sense of needing to be in control, which brings frustration, as usually events are moving so rapidly that we have no control and yet, there is another level of control which is required in order to be alert and open to all the experiences and opportunities. This brings a certain amount of inner tension such as a cat poised to leap, but the tension may need to be held over a long period. The whole situation can become quite stressful.

Bluebell brings a suppleness to the experience – stamina without rigidity. It's soothing effect in high energy situations also makes Bluebell a useful remedy for over-exposure to the sun. *U.F.E.*

Keywords – 'No one is more powerful than thou'.

Negative aspects – Always weepy. Over eager. Scattered thoughts. Recovery from bad judgement. Lacking vitality.

Positive aspects – Quality time with your children. Feeling happy and content. Recognising a reincarnation.

Physical attributes – Lassitude. P.M.S. *B.F.E.*

Hyacinthoides non-scripta

Where there has been depression, when one feels to be falling apart inside. *B.E.*

Scilla nonscripta

Used for glue ear, throat, thyroid gland. For independence, but fearful of the unknown and for unsolved problems.   *S.C.E.*

BLUE GERANIUM

Effect of taking essence: Acceptance of change, especially in menopause, going with the flow of life's cycles and rhythms.

Can remove resistance to the change from life creation to creating a life. To help mentally adjust to this new life opportunity. Helps the passage through menopause.

The physical changes that come about at menopause (the change of life) can be helped with this essence.

Presenting conditions: Emotional and physical upset predominantly due to the change of life during menopause, i.e. hormonal imbalance, erratic periods. Where there is a resistance to letting go of the fear of not being a woman.   *L.N.E.*

BOG ASPHODEL *Narthecium ossifragum*

For the "willing slave", those who are always wanting to help others yet ignoring their own needs.   *B.E.*

Effect of taking essence: Balances up male sexual drive (the male impatience) the change from need, to a loving expression. Also aids diversion of male sexual drive to other creative activities. A lifting of the kundalini energy from base/sacral chakras to the higher chakras (heart/throat etc.). It can balance the need for release. It can aid in spiritualizing sex, allows openness, removes shame and guilt.

Presenting condition: Preoccupation with sex. Very needy demanding affection, comfort, release.

Looks to others for gratification and reassurance of worthiness.   *L.N.E.*

BOG HYPERICUM *Hypericum elodes*

Effect of taking essence: Aids transitions. Helps to move through the pain and fear of showing who we truly are.

Pain and suffering can come from resistance. This essence will ease the flow of life past or through the resistance to bring joy.

Presenting conditions: Hiding behind a mask. Fearful of showing true self to the world. Anxiety, unease, or general sadness about inability to move through fear, so hides behind a mask.

Particularly when pressures build in our everyday lives.

The sadness of hiding – not being able to reveal inner self with joy.   *L.N.E.*

BORAGE *Borago officinalis*

'For courage' and 'brings good cheer'. Essentially a tonic. Borage strengthens and opens the heart, eases the emotions.**

'I feel joy in my heart. I am encouraged and cheerful'.   *H.R.*

Lightness of heart.

Use borage when there is great heaviness and sadness in the heart. It can break through the dark to discover an inner lightness which brings support, optimism and renewed courage. *L.F.H.*   *S.E.*

Borage is for courage. It can be used for any situation that is difficult to face. Borage stimulates love and compassion, bringing joy, optimism and light into life.

Physical use: stimulates adrenals, circulatory system, skeletal structure and thyroid. *A.F.R.*

Strength, courage, happiness. *R.D.*

Opens the heart chakra, bringing joy. *C.H.*

This essence lifts the spirits up; it can turn feelings of discouragement into enthusiasm. Borage makes the heart grow glad, as it expands the heart energies. It gives strength and courage when facing challenging circumstances.

Planet – Jupiter

Chakra – 4th *M.E.F.E.*

It is a common condition of Western culture that people fear not having enough and in particular not being able to provide themselves with what they need. There is a loss of trust in the Universe, family, community, environment that one's needs will be met. 'Modern' people live with an increasing sense of isolation where they cannot depend even on close family for support.

Borage helps to open the mind to the experience of trusting that one's needs will be provided for. It brings about an increasing sense of 'togetherness', whether with family, friends, community, God or environment and can ease sore throats caused by the stress of not being able to ask for what one needs. *U.F.E.*

BOX *Buxus sempivirens*

"Clarity". Strengthens the mind and will. Clears the head. Eases irrationality and confusion. Links you with your Higher Self. *G.M.T.E..*

BRACKEN

Pteridiurn aquilium (Aqueous extract)

Psychic sensitivity blocked from childhood, with consequent fear of "coming up front" to one's psychic potential. *B.E.*

Pteridium aquilium (Alcoholic extract)

Leaves. Where there has been an habitual playing of the "child" role in life. *B.E.*

BROMPTON STOCK *Matthiola*

To help those new to spiritual ideas, insight and initiation. Crown and ajna chakras. *C.H.*

BROOM *Cytisus*

Mars. Fire/Air. Renewal. Sweeping all out-moded and unneeded dross. Opening to the golden light. Perseverance. Protection. Helps depression. *J.J.*

Cytisus scoparius

For perseverance through difficulties. Keeping busy and motivated. 'Sweeping clean'. Renewing faith. Steadies the heart.

'I have a strong calm will. I can start afresh'. *H.R.*

Keynote: Clarity

Broom stimulates mental clarity and concentration, facilitating ease in communication and creative thought when in a state of bewilderment.

Indications: Memory loss, dullness, feeble-mindedness, bewilderment, confusion, lack of integration, co-ordination or communication.

Attributes: Mental clarity, concentration, communication, integration, decision making, self-expression, guidance, intuition, creative thought, clarity of purpose.

F.F.E.

BROOM *Genista*

Heals differences in relationships, particularly parent/child. Helps sinus symptoms.

C.H.

BUDDLElA *Buddleia*

Rebuilding after a storm; the first to take root and flourish in the rubble. Can be applied after any trauma or shock, particularly abortion or miscarriage. Can also be used in cases of infertility. *J.W.*

Helps one to feel spiritual contact in the darkest of situations. *C.H.*

This essence is the 'rainbow bridge' remedy. It enables us to link up with angelic forces and spirit guides, specifically for helping to clear up past life emotional wounds, which are hindering our development.

Planets – Sun, Moon, Chiron

Chakras – 2nd, 3rd, 6th *M.E.F.E.*

Buddleia davidii

For pineal gland, eyes, blood cells. To focus the mind and help you to meditate.

S.C.E.

BUGLE *Ajuga*

Helping to develop unconditional love. Manifesting inner creativity onto physical level. *L.L.F.E.*

BUTTERBUR *Petasites*

Overcoming anxiety. Release of excess energy. *L.L.F.E.*

Being dependent on external events or validation is not a recommended route to happiness. It's more likely to bring frustration, resentment and an ever increasing lack of trust. Happiness can be viewed as isolated incidents brought on by external events, or a deep continuous undercurrent of inner well-being. Happy people tend to be very open and trusting; they derive pleasure from simple things and are slow to criticize either themselves or others.

Butterbur helps to open the senses, to allow experiences of pleasure from sight, sound, taste, touch and smell. These 'gladden the heart' and open the way for an increasing sense of trust. *U.F.E.*

Petasites hybridus

For blocked-off self love and not realising one's own inherent "goodness". The remedy for poor self-esteem. *B.E.*

BUTTERCUP *Ranunculus*

For when we feel low self-worth. This essence shows the soul the radiant light
shining from within. *A.F.R.*

Self confidence. *R.D.*

Whole plant. To bring awareness of one's environment. For adaptability. For
resilience. *E.E.*

Recognition of self worth from within, not from others' perceptions. *C.H.*

This essence helps you to discover your hidden talents, whatever they may be. Once
you have done this it enables you to share these gifts with others. This is extremely
useful if you are in a situation with a group of people and you feel a need to
contribute. It will help to overcome shyness as you will know what it is you have to
offer.

Planets – Mercury, Saturn

Chakra – 2nd *M.E.F.E.*

There are times in life when there is nothing to achieve by 'doing'. It is necessary to
wait – for events to unfold, for lessons to be learned. These periods of waiting can be
frustrating and it takes great patience and insight to appreciate their value and
intrinsic part in the process of life.

They are a phase of transition, a period of seeming inactivity which can bring
feelings of 'nothing is going to change', associated with a slump in energy and
general despondency. It can be tempting to 'give up', to become disillusioned or to
fight and attempt to provoke events.

Buttercup facilitates a settled energy state whilst awaiting the next phase of
development. It brings the qualities of acceptance and joy in the 'here and now'. *U.F. E.*

Ranunculus acris

For being in touch with the inner child, relaxed, well grounded and appreciative of
life's riches. 'It is safe to feel pleasure, joy and abundance now'. *H.R.*

Links to the fairy kingdom. To be childlike and open. Opens third chakra to light.
Reveals the key to nature. *J.J.*

For where there is a jaundiced view of the world and difficulty in letting the
"sunshine" in. *B.E.*

Comforting, use if feeling overwhelmed.

It is useful for all types of stress as it opens and strengthens the solar plexus chakra.
It could be used to encourage a gentle de-tox and for general pain relief. It is
recommended for removing stress from the site of an injury and is indicated for
teenagers to bring some stability to their rioting hormones. Gives psychic protection
by re-establishing boundaries, realigns the subtle bodies bringing them back into
balance. Associations include the colour gold, direction East, planets Sun and Moon,
Tarot 5 of Cups. *A.F.E.*

For pain relief, pancreatic disorders, central nervous system. To enhance feelings of
security, for loneliness or feelings of being alone. *S.C.E.*

Ranunculus bulbosus

Recognising one's own uniqueness.

This essence is indicated when there is a lack of self-esteem. Buttercup warms and nourishes the being with golden light. It brings an understanding of how special and unique life is, no matter how humble it may seem. *L.F.H.*   *S.E.*

BUTTERFLY BUSH *Buddleia davidii*

When life is empty and barren. Feelings of inertia, without purpose. In need of motivation.   *J.J.*

CALENDULA *Calendula*

Releasing sadness by understanding its cause. Earths and balances emotions.
L.L.F.E.

This essence is concerned with cleansing the mind to bring clarity in areas of visualisation. The heart/mind link is enhanced allowing one to visualise, without clouding by a overly intellectual approach. Inspirational information in the form of vision can then occur.

Planets – Jupiter, Uranus

Chakras – 4th, 6th   *M.E.F.E.*

CALIFORNIAN POPPY *Escholtzia californica*

Aligns the mental, causal and spiritual bodies. Gives astral, psychic and spiritual balance. Solar plexus. Psychic vision. For those who can be pulled in the wrong direction who need the spiritual path, not psychic deception.   *J.J.*

This essence encourages a balanced psychic opening, aligning heart with spirit, giving a strong sense of inner knowing. PHYSICAL USE: treats multiple sclerosis and other nerve diseases, strengthens the eyes and the middle ear.   *A.F.R.*

Inner balance, psyche.   *R.D.*

Spiritual and psychic balance. Helps assimilation of gold therefore good for nervous diseases and multiple sclerosis.   *C.H.*

Romneya

Opening to higher self. Self beyond gender. Joy, gentleness and love. Enhances meditation.   *J.W.*

CALLA *Calla palustris*

After physical abuse or cruelty this essence helps restore dignity and self-worth. *C.H.*

CAMELLIA *Camellia*

Loving attitudes, links to earth energies.   *R.D.*

To open, develop and balance heart chakra.   *C.H.*

'CAMPANULA' *Glomerata superba*

Frankness and honesty in expression. Eliminates need for secrecy.   *C.H.*

CAMPHOR *Cinnomonum camphora*

Toxicities removed from subtle bodies allowing vibrational remedies, homoeopathy etc to work more effectively. Camphor and coffee no longer impede life-force through body, but camphor essence won't prevent long term effects of those substances on the physical. Activates meridians. *G.M.F.E.*

CAMPION *Silene*

Most pregnancy and birth problems. *C.H.*

CAMPSIS *Campsis*

Aligns and balances all the chakras. For right/left brain imbalances, dyslexia, learning difficulties, neurological disorders and diseases of the nervous system. Helps with psychic development and intuition. *G.E.*

CANNA *Canna 'President'*

To build stamina and strength. *C.H.*

CANTERBURY BELL *Campanula medium*

Throat chakra. Inner hearing, in combination with other essences for clairaudience. *C.H.*

CARNATION *Dianthus*

Attunement with devic orders and fairies. Crown chakra. *C.H.*

CASTOR OIL PLANT *Ricinus communis*

Helps repair brain neurones, brain disorders. Motor neurone and Alzheimer's disease. *C.H.*

CATALPA *Catalpa x erubescans*

"Joy". Stabilisation of emotions, helps find peace of mind. Reduces anxiety, increases self confidence in what one can achieve. Joy. *G.M.T.E.*

CATMINT *Nepeta*

Brings alignment between the heart and throat chakras. *C.H.*

CATS EAR (LUNAR)

This is the remedy for past life deceits and misunderstandings, for those who have in a previous life uttered falsehoods. Certain roles in society require one to be economical with the truth or twist facts to suit one's own position. Karma inevitably has to be encountered from such actions and cat's ear is the essence to help untie such past life actions. It can also be used in past life relationship therapy. *A.F.R.*

CEANOTHUS

Throat chakra, related problems, thyroid. Unconditional love. *C.H.*

CEDAR *Cedrus*

Stimulates hair growth, scalp disorders. Colon, intestinal tract. *C.H.*

CELANDINE

Stimulates metabolism. *R.D.*

Vocal cords, throat chakra, thyroid. Helps access information including contact with spiritual guides. *C.H.*

Throat chakra essence. For difficulty in self-expression, suppression of self, introversion.

Encourages greater and clearer communication, speaking one's truth, diplomacy. For diseases of thyroid, mouth, vocal cords, trachea, cervical vertebrae, nervous system, speech impediments. *A.F.R.*

This essence is connected with the throat. It is good for singers, lecturers and all occupations that require transfer of information as it is the communication remedy. It is good for communication on all levels including that with spirit guides and also communication of energies between partners, as it stimulates the tantric experience.

Planets – Mercury, Venus, Uranus, Neptune

Chakra – 5th *M.E.F.E.*

Celandine people are alert; they are acutely aware of sensory information – like seeing a movement from the corner of the eye. But this can also make them 'jumpy'/nervous. A high degree of alertness can bring a self confidence and full participation in life but it can also come with fear and a constantly taut state of being.

Celandine helps facilitate a 'relaxed' state of alertness, a poised rather than tense state of being, able to respond to changes in senses and details. This facility comes with an opening of the way internally and externally. *U.F.E.*

CENTAUREA *Centaurea dealbata*

For cleansing of the higher chakras i.e. throat and above. *C.H.*

CENTAURY *Centaurium erythraea*

For chronic fatigue syndrome, M.E. and for loss of appetite. Stimulates the feminine intuitive energy and will help you to express this. *S.C.E.*

CHAMOMILE

Brings the gifts of serenity, emotional balance and a sun-like disposition.

Physical use: augments the entire nervous system and strengthens the ductless glands. *A.F.R.*

For calmness, serenity, releasing anxiety. Solar plexus. *C.H.*

Brings energy and activeness in a relaxed way, without causing stress. Helps to develop self-discipline. *L.L.F.E.*

Chamaemelum nobile

Calms and soothes. Release of anxiety and fear. Helps deep relaxation, meditation and acceptance of a situation. For high strung, over responsible states.★★

'I let go of worry and return to calm'. *H.R.*

Serene, sunny disposition, emotional balance. For those easily upset, moody and irritable, unable to release emotion and tension. Meditative states made more easy. Emotional tensions eased. Nervous system, endocrine system enhanced. Mental clarity and logical functioning. *G.M.F.E.*

Used for nausea, eczema and as a sedative. Will help to gain insights into conscious levels of past lives.
S.C.E.

Cotula anthemis

Calming.

Chamomile is useful when there is emotional turmoil which can create stress, sleeplessness and digestive problems. This essence can ease the tension and bring relaxation deep within the body. *L.F.H.*
S.E.

CHARLOCK *Sinapis arvensis*

For the "Peter Pans" of this world who cling to childhood states. They want to be liked and so often become an habitual victim.
B.E.

'CHEIRANTHUS' *Erysimum 'Wenlock Beauty'*

For strengthening/cleansing of the spleen.
C.H.

CHERRY LAUREL *Prunus laurocerasus*

"Balance of mind". All problems with the mind and head. Imagination and inspiration used practically. Helps maintain molecular and genetic integrity of the body. Subtle perceptions accessed. High level protection and support.
G.M.T.E.

CHERRY PLUM *Prunus ceracifera*

"Confidence". Wisdom and security of the inner self helps remove fears. Tense muscles and rigid mental concepts are eased. Opening up on emotional levels. Helps shyness.
G.M.T.E.

CHICKWEED *Stellaria media*

Moon and Saturn. Sharing, uniting kindred spirits to show us all is one. Balances higher and lower energies. Forgiveness over prejudice. Helps to balance 3rd, 4th and 5th chakras to resonance. Star to guide us to the light.
J.J.

Being happy with yourself, so you do not need the understanding and appreciation of others and do not need to attract 'draining' relationships.
H.F.E.

When there is a perception of frequently having to move from one environment to another, to adapt one's behaviour and deal with very different issues, a great deal of stress can arise, often manifesting as worry.

Chickweed helps to integrate the different environments and needs, to bring the perception that all the environments are part of one larger whole. There comes an increasing sense of being part of a larger community where the self need not be divided and all needs are interconnected.
U.F.E.

CHICORY *Cichorium*

White chicory. Victims of sexual abuse, purity.
C.H.

Cichorium intybus

This essence is for the liver, gout, also rheumatoid arthritis and is used for gall bladder and gallstones. For those mentally stressed due to lack of relaxation. *S.C.E.*

CHIONODOXA *Chionodoxa*

Hope, joy and upliftment. *C.H.*

CHRYSANTHEMUM *Chrysanthemum*

This essence is for when we identify too strongly with the material world and lose touch with our spiritual self. Chrysanthemum is also given for fear of death. *A.F.R.*

Helps to bring those of differing ideas more together into harmony. Liver and kidneys cleansed and strengthened. *C.H.*

CINQUEFOIL

Solar plexus. Good for stubbornness. *C.H.*

Potentilla reptans

Painful menstruation, piles, sore throat. For high ideas and goals in life, don't burn yourself out. *S.C.E.*

CISTUS *Cistus*

Cleanses pancreas. Useful in a fast. *C.H.*

CLEAVER *Galium*

For releasing the need for emotional control, possessiveness and taking advantage of others. *C.H.*

Galium aparine

For the lymph system, cystitis, psoriasis and to lower arterial blood pressure. Will help you to connect with nature in a spiritual way, allowing you states of higher awareness. *S.C.E.*

CLEMATIS *Clematis*

Insight, wisdom. *R.D.*

Clematis 'Nelly Moser'

Cleanses and opens the 8th chakra, just above the crown. *C.H.*

COLTS FOOT *Tussilago farfara*

Allows those to speak that have been held in the silence of winter. Helps with expression of deep or past emotions, while also being grounding and supporting. For any ailment that prevents vocal or facial expression, including sore throats. *J.W.*

Working with and attunement to animals. Shamanically working with animal allies. Brings a loving attitude. *L.L.F.E.*

This essence comes up for people who 'don't get angry' or are not easily angered. This may be because they were told as children that it was unacceptable to express anger and any provocation will result in guilt, shocked silence or tears. Its as if anger is completely bypassed, almost obliterated from their experience. Anger is a valid emotion and can be expressed safely and respectfully. If it is never expressed or recognised it tends to become repressed and will often result in physical aches and exhaustion and a general numbing and sluggishness of the nervous system.

Coltsfoot helps to free the congestion of past repressed anger in a safe way and allows for a freer expression of healthy anger and assertiveness thereby facilitating a sense of equality and will. This results in a release of associated physical problems and an increased alertness to the fast pace and rapid changes of modern life.   *U.F.E.*

COLTS FOOT (LUNAR)

Coltsfoot aids the process of deep karmic release where there is a sense of something forcing its way to the surface. When such patterns rise from the subconscious it can be as if something large is pushing or welling up inside, stretching or pulling apart the tightness or rigidity that has for so long held it all down and there can be a sense of disgust, regret, guilt, shame or other negative emotions around the patterns as they force their way out. Coltsfoot relaxes that tightness or rigidity, which is most likely fear and thereby affords a greater ease of passage for the release into consciousness of the deep karma.   *A.F.R.*

COLUMBINE *Aquilegia vulgaris*

Venus. Opens the 8th/9th chakras. Known as the gift of the Holy ghost, it raises one to higher consciousness.   *J.J.*

Activates higher chakras located above crown chakra. This greatly enhances the healing and integration of higher faculties and functions. Aids in the rebirth and complete healing of the Self. Inspirational.   *G.M.F.E.*

Helps activate brow and crown chakras. Attunement to angelic kingdom.   *C.H.*

To relax the nervous system, for hysteria, liver jaundice, gall bladder conditions. For trust in and honouring of your intuitive, inner feelings and connecting with your wisdom.   *S.C.E.*

COMFREY *Symphytum officinale*

'For mending'. Helps repair natural cycles. Good for injury, tiredness and memory loss'.★★

'I am relaxed, integrated, in rhythm, united and whole'.   *H.R.*

Saturn. Integrates mental and nervous system. Good for memory. Balances left and right brain. Muscular degeneration. Releases sub-conscious tension.   *J.J.*

Nervous system.   *R.D.*

Nerve endings, nervous system diseases. Memory, left-right brain balance.   *C.H.*

Root chakra essence. Grounds, stabilises and balances. Helps develop and initiate any project, develops strength of character, stability, releases past-life talents, will to live, creativity. Increases our desire to be here on earth. Treats diseases of bowels, rectum, anus, urethra, adrenals, difficulty with any of the eliminative processes. *A.F.R.*

A calming essence for gastric conditions. Also a very good essence for painful joints. It has anti inflammatory qualities. Can be used in cream base for eczema and psoriasis. For the over emotionally dependent, 'I like to be loved'.   *S.C.E.*

Keyword – 'Transformation'

Negative aspects – Environmental chaos. Wintery feeling inside. When words are inadequate. Fear of giving self time out.

Positive aspects – 'I understand the Great Unknown'. Preparation for a winter hibernation. Helps lift the Spirit. Regaining faith.

Physical attributes – Pains in the joints. Profuse menstruation.   *B.F.E.*

Positive: For dynamic patience and stillness and being present in the fullness of now. For meditation, receiving and communicating information, grounded spiritual and psychic development, deep connection with the earth and the natural world and trusting our own unique healing, developmental and creative process. For creating the time and space to heal and be creative, curiosity and joy, mental and creative work.

Indications: For feeling limited or restricted by circumstance, fighting or resisting being where you are, inattention and avoidance of being in the now, daydreaming, impatience with the healing process, living for the future, unwilling or unable to experience meaning or good in the now, unable to be still or meditate, not benefiting from experience because of avoiding connecting with situations – sometimes as a result of unresolved previous trauma and fear.

Physical: For recovery from injury to brain, spine, nerves, skeleton and muscles, degenerative conditions of the spine, recovery from paralysis and muscle wasting, recovery from surgery, building fitness and strength, osteoporosis, co-ordination of left brain/right brain, recovery from strokes and comas, dyslexia, improving mineral absorption and stimulating the creation of healthy collagen and connective tissue. May help in the treatment of M.S., M.E. and motor neurone disease. Improves memory and detailed memory recall. Regulation of natural cycles.

May help reduce excessive and prolonged bleeding and may help reduce bleeding in general: from wounds, nosebleeds etc. *L.H.F.E.*

COMMON MOUSE-EAR *Cerastium fontanum*
Whole plant. For scrutiny. To bring understanding of the 'whole'. *E.E.*

COMMON SPOTTED ORCHID *Dactylorhiza fuchsii*
Opening the crown chakra, channelling, contacting devas and angelic kingdoms in a balanced and earthed way. *H.F.E.*

COMMON VETCH *Vicia sativa*
For circulation problems, also for the heart. For feelings of frustration and limitations, for unwarranted criticism. *S.C.E.*

COMPACT RUSH *Juncus conglomeratus*
Life not feeling fulfilled, life seeming to pass one by. This essence assists new beginnings, new energies and new insights. *B.E.*

CONEFLOWER *Echinacea*
Immune system. *R.D.*

Echinacea 'The King'
Powerful flower, created in Lemuria to symbolise the descent of man into matter. Works powerfully on the physical body, helps strengthen heart, lungs, kidneys and abdomen. Helps purify the blood and helps cells to better communicate with each other. *C.H.*

CONVOLVULUS *Convolvulus*
Brings alignment to the crown and higher chakras. *C.H.*

COPPER BEECH *Fagus sylvatica*

Grounding.

A Natural Earth Essence. Copper beech can help to clear the bodies energies, enabling one to feel balanced and grounded. It can renew the life force and strengthen one's connection to the earth. Useful in spray around feet. *S.*   *S.E.*

Fagus sylvatica var. purpurea

"Depression". Relieves depression and brings a deep, enlivening sense of peace and detachment from worries. Energises emotions in a positive, non-aggressive way.

G.M.T.E.

CORAL BELLS

Spiritualising sexual/sacral energy.   *C.H.*

COREOPSIS *Coreopsis*

Helps spiritualise the intellect.   *C.H.*

CORN

Allergies to corn. Detachment and rationality to emotions.   *C.H.*

CORNBINE *Convolvulus arvensis*

An excellent essence to combine with others for constipation, blood, fevers. For emotional traumas, excessive worry and for letting go.   *S.C.E.*

CORNCOCKLE *Agrostemma*

Helps draw in energy through 9th and 10th chakras.   *C.H.*

CORNFLOWER *Centaurea cyanus*

For being comfortable with one's individuality. Protects sensitivity and special gifts. Heals damage from institutions.

'I belong to myself and I like myself'.   *H.R.*

Frees from conditioning. Gives confidence to self.   *J.J.*

A useful essence for skin conditions, it aids digestion and can be tried for stimulating the hair follicles. 'Let me show you how creative and expressive I can be'.   *S.C.E.*

COSMOS *Cosmos*

Linguistic abilities.   *R.D.*

Cosmos gives clear articulation of thoughts, especially when speaking. Cosmos can be given to shy, introverted or procrastinating individuals, such people could express themselves more clearly.   *A.F.R.*

Cosmos dipinnatus

Aligns the mental and etheric bodies and combines the heart and throat chakras for easier expression. For nervous speech problems when too much information is not absorbed.   *J.J.*

Dark pink and maroon blooms. Clear interaction.

When an individual is overwhelmed by too many negative thoughts, interaction can become defensive and confusing to others. Cosmos cleanses and clarifies the mind processes, enabling communication to be kind and of greater integrity.   *L.F.H.*   *S.E.*

COTONEASTER *Cotoneaster*

Berry. Lights a match to spirituality.   *A.T.*

COWSLIP *Primula veris*

Strengthens the solar plexus and settles the emotions. For when you are feeling vulnerable.

Comforts and uplifts the emotions.   *H.F.E.*

Helps children understand relationship and environment problems, helps parents understand children.   *C.H.*

Connecting with the inner child. Accessing inner truth and innocence. Communicating inner truth.   *L.L.F.E.*

Anorexia nervosa. Bacterial inflammation. Eczema. Liver imbalance. Psychosomatic illnesses. Solar plexus imbalance. Cannot make decisions. Confusion. Inability to cope with life. Over-analytical mind. Self-critical. Liver, nervous system, solar plexus, stomach. Works on all chakras especially eleventh, breast bone and liver. Helps to impart wisdom.   *B.F.R.*

Positive: Soothing, comforting, gently renewing and restoring. Brings a sense of the 'Divine Mother', a sense of being supported, an awareness that we are not alone. Calming. For self-nurturing. Helps us to give up our burden to God/the Mother/the Source, to cease struggling and listen to our heart and the still voice within. Helps us to ask for and accept, help and guidance: "Show me the way". Comforts and soothes babies and young children, brings a sense of security.

Indications: For those who have been stretched to the limits of their physical and emotional endurance, who have struggled long in difficult and dispiriting circumstances, who are weary and feel alone in their struggle. For those facing long illness, disablement or death, particularly those living alone; for when we feel alone in our troubles and feel the need for support, when we need mothering, especially if we were deprived of maternal support in childhood. For when we seek attention and sympathy from those around us, sometimes by becoming ill, or by acting the victim ("Poor me"). Cowslip helps us to recognise this desire and encourages us to listen to, love and support ourselves and make positive steps to meet our own needs. For mothers and carers who need to nurture and care for themselves and worry and over-anxious states. For babies and young children who have been traumatised by a difficult birth, separation from the mother, illness or invasive medical treatment and children who have been deprived of mothering.

Physical: Exhaustion, weariness. Solar plexus and heart. Digestive problems, particularly those aggravated by worry and exhaustion. Colic. Difficulty assimilating food (particularly for babies with digestive problems). Sleep difficulties when we are over-tired or anxious (combine with Dandelion and Red Clover).   *L.H.F.E.*

CRAB APPLE *Malus*

Final piercing of the web of illusion.   *A.T.*

CRACK WILLOW *Salix fragilis*

"Spiritual sun". Letting go, allowing things to happen. Sense of oneness with the world. Communications with the Higher Self, the planet and the energies of the sun.

G.M.T.E.

CRANESBILL *Geranium*

Helps one become single minded, spiritually and mentally.   *C.H.*

Geranium pratense

Used for problems with the veins and for the capillaries. For protection from over involvements, to develop compassion and sensitiveness.   *S.C.E.*

CREEPING BUTTERCUP

Keywords – 'Secrets, Binding'.

Negative aspects – When life is disintegrating. Perplexed. Unsure. Pensive parents. Attention seeking in children.

Positive aspects – Brings lovers together. Transmutation. Feminine principle. Getting to the mountain. Remembrances.

Physical attributes – A rescue remedy for children specifically.   *B.F.E.*

CREEPING JENNY *Lysimachia nummularis*

For muscular pain, rheumatic joints. For low self esteem, to help with confidence and self expression.   *S.C.E.*

CROCUS *Crocus*

Useful for babies in first few months to protect fontanelle.   *C.H.*

CROCUS – YELLOW *Crocus balansae*

Venus. Saffron for the navel centre for digesting higher knowledge and processing it.

J.J

CYCLAMEN *Cyclamen*

Helps the individual to absorb higher energies, especially the new rays currently being directed to earth, consciousness raising, transformation of DNA pattern. 1990s essence.   *C.H.*

CYMBIDIUM *Cymbidium 'Cambria'*

For defiance in the face of undermining influence. Overcoming frustration, lack of confidence and fear of disapproval. Embracing the tiger within.

'I am confident and strong. I confront and overcome'.   *H.R.*

CYPRESS *Cupressus*

Overcoming loneliness by connecting to inner self. Bringing oneness (oneness opposite to loneliness).   *L.L.F.E.*

DAFFODIL *Narcissus*

Venus. Cleansing, removes lack of self-worth. Crown chakra. Raises consciousness, for meditation. Links to the higher self. Good to take when dowsing. Good for emergency in accidents. *J.J.*

Daffodil works on all 7 main chakras in the body and also those in the hands and feet. It concentrates mainly on the brow, heart and solar plexus chakras, helping to 'see' intuitively. It removes fear so that 'second sight' can develop freely. This allows us to perceive that what we need is around us already.

'Those who have eyes to see, let them see'. *S.M.*

Vitality, blood pressure. *R.D.*

Increased sensitivity, inner hearing, higher self attunement. *C.H.*

Crown chakra essence. Useful for searching for meaning, crisis of belief or faith, psychosis, perfectionist, elitism. Encourages enlightenment, knowing, acceptance, fulfilment, completion, alignment with higher forces. Treats disease of the nervous system, synchronisation between the left and right hemispheres of the brain. *A.FR.*

For connecting with one's higher self in a powerful and fearless way. Helps to establish a strong inner connection so that one is able to resolve issues in which fear has previously blocked progress. *M.E.FE.*

Double daffodil.

Abundance.

This essence can allow one to let in feelings of joy and happiness. It releases an often long-term, rigid and constricted attitude, opening the heart to the rich abundance of life. *L.FH.* *S.E.*

Narcissus ajax

Aligns mental body with Higher Self. Useful in deep meditation techniques and for listening to guides or the Self. Works with the crown chakra to pass information to the conscious mind.

Useful in deepening daily meditation practices. *G.M.FE*

Narcissus pseudonarcissus

A 'spring clean' essence, helping to banish winter blues. Useful anytime for depression, self doubt and low self esteem.

'I love and trust myself. I am open to the sky and to the sun'. *H.R.*

Appreciation of one's talents.

Wild Daffodil is indicated when ones talents seem insignificant or do not appear to fit into society. This essence can help the recognition of their worth. Once they are used with this positive attitude they can blossom and grow with abundance. *L.FH.* *S.E.*

DAHLIA *Dahlia*

Transmutes sexual energy to higher expression. Base and sacral chakras. *C.J.*

DAISY *Bellis perennis*

Venus, Moon, Mars. Balances 1st, 2nd and 3rd chakras. Aligns the subtle bodies.
Alleviates stiffness to be vibrationally flexible. Releases joy through simplicity.
Stabilises spiritual seeking.
J.J.

All kinds of emotional release. Helps person to speak and express their emotions.
L.L.F.E.

Spiritualises intellect. Scattered information brought into clear focus. Understanding
from an intuitive level. Stabilises those who are constantly seeking but not finding.
Clarity and understanding, especially in spiritual areas. Relieves hiccups and shallow
breathing.
G.M.F.E.

The signature of the daisy is perfect for its use when unveiled. Each yellow dot in the
centre is in fact a flower in it own right, each individual is brought together to form
the whole; the perfect metaphor for all creation. The image I was given when
connecting with the plant was of a telephone exchange, all the different lines coming
in and getting connected. The essence can be used to bring many diverse energies or
information together to form a coherent whole and understanding. When we are
confused, it is usually not because of information we don't have, it's because we need
to put what we do have in order so we can discern the pattern.
J.W.

Keynote: Innocence

Daisy allows us to remain calm and centred amid turbulent surroundings or
overwhelming situations, creating a safe space in which to be vulnerable.

Indications: Being overwhelmed, fear of losing control, distraction, confusion, easily
swayed, inconsistency, indifference, 'up in the clouds', fickleness, oversensitiveness.

Attributes: Calm and centred amid intense activity, lightness, presence, being or
staying on purpose, protection, ability to enjoy, rediscovering innocence, playfulness.
F.F.E.

Daisy helps when we feel intellectually scattered; it brings clarity and understanding
to what is trying to be learnt. Daisy is a good essence for students of any kind.
Increases humility by opening the high heart chakra, located where the breast bones
meet below the throat.
A.F.R.

Intellectual relaxation.
R.D.

Whole plant. For connection (especially to the Earth). To bring a sense of purpose
and belonging.
E.E.

Brings clarity to thoughts, inner knowing.
C.H.

This essence is useful if you need to collect scattered information into a cohesive
form to make sense of it. It works by spiritualising the intellect allowing one to gain
an intuitive grasp of what is going on. It gives one a clarity of mind which helps you
to understand what your feelings are on a particular topic.

Planets – Mercury, Saturn

Chakras – 3rd, 7th
M.E.F.E.

There is a time to act and a time to be still, but it can be very confusing knowing
which is which; one can feel frequently out of synch with events.

Daisy helps those who have a fear of being still and it facilitates appropriate
responsiveness, but most of all Daisy develops a trust in the connections of life.
U.F.E.

DANDELION *Taraxacum*

Jupiter. Letting go of fear, releases stress. Good for mental body, aligns etheric, mental and causal bodies. Muscle relaxant when stress in the mental body lodges in the muscles. *J.J.*

This is a wonderful essence for stress. It is for when we overdo it and are unable to sit still and reflect. Dandelion helps us to listen to the body and emotions.

Physical use: many uses including alleviation of muscular degeneration, fevers and leukaemia. *A.F.R.*

Muscular relaxation. *R.D.*

Releases muscle tension caused by mental stress. *C.H.*

Oversensitivity, emotional imbalance. *L.L.F.E.*

This essence helps to relieve deep physical and emotional tensions that are manifesting as muscular tensions in the body. The essence can be taken in liquid form both aurally and in a bath. It can also be mixed with a massage oil to be applied directly to the tense region. It is also helpful in removing deep emotional blockages that may exist.

Planets – Sun, Jupiter

Chakra – 1st *M.E.F.E.*

Sometimes the difficulties of life can become so overwhelming that any joy or spark of creativity becomes lost. Life, or even one's own body may feel dirty.

Dandelion acts as a purifier; it clears a path through the turmoil, so that a love of life can be seen and felt even amidst the stress and destruction. *U.F.E.*

Taraxacum officinale

For relaxation of mental stress and muscle tension (especially neck and shoulders). To stop being overwhelmed and let go of irrational fears. Trust in our ability to cope with life.★★

'It is safe to relax. I trust in my own calm strength'. *H.R.*

Dynamic, effortless energy, lively activity balanced with inner ease. For those overly tense especially in muscles, overstrung and hard-driving on themselves. Relaxation of stress and muscular tension. Useful for poor posture. *G.M.F.E.*

Centreing. Understanding one's emotions and the cause of one's reactions. Helps release hatred and resentment. Allows one to receive nourishment and find the space for healing.

Good for liver, pancreas and solar plexus. *H.F.E.*

Relaxes tension in the body.

Dandelion is helpful when one's body has become tense due to an over stressed life-style. This essence can help one to 'go with the flow', feel more relaxed and be able to cope better with the ups and downs of everyday life. *L.F.H.* *S.E.*

Helps to release knotted energies in our bodies and minds. Helps to release forgotten feelings and emotions which have perhaps led to frustration, moving forward to a state of directed clarity in which choices can be made in the light of self honesty. *J.W.*

Flower, stem and leaves. To balance the male and female aspects of the self. For acceptance.

For tolerance. For flexibility. *E.E.*

Positive: For the Knowledge that we are invulnerable. For true protection that comes from knowing that nothing can harm us. For deep peace and relaxation and the recognition of God/Good in All, letting go of defence and releasing fear, feeling relaxed and secure within the light of one's eternal being.

Indications: For tension, inability to relax, for fearful defence, locked in fear, trauma, negativity, fear of losing control, or of being overwhelmed by fear or negativity (one's own of someone else's). Vulnerability.

Physical: Solar plexus. Sacral. Muscles. For releasing tension, fear or strong emotion held in the physical body, pain of unknown origin and dis-ease arising from tension, trauma or fear.

Shock. Trauma recovery – Post traumatic shock syndrome. Panic attacks.

L.H.F.E.

DAY LILY *Hemerocallis*

Symbolising rebirth, it helps give an understanding of external life. *C.H.*

DEADLY NIGHTSHADE *Atropa bella-donna*

Powerful third eye stimulator. Psychic purge. Clears one from psychic interference. To be used in single dose as required, rather than repeatedly. *H.F.E.*

The dark blanket of a night sky calling for a time of rest. For quiet introversion, turing to look inside and calmness of mind. For rest and reassurance. For those who only give out and take no time for themselves, those with troubled sleep or who cannot relax. For overexcitement or hyperactivity. *J.W.*

DEADNETTLE *Lamium*

Helps activate chakras above the crown, especially the 13th. Spiritual energy. *C.H.*

DEEP PINK ROSE

This essence is a 'love' essence and works on the heart, opening it up to a feeling of warm intoxicating and spiritual love. Continued usage of this flower will gently unfold the heart, just like the flower itself opening and move one towards a state where one feels love for all people and all things. It is the essence of universal love.

Planets – Moon, Venus, Neptune, Chiron

Chakras – 1st, 4th *M.E.R.E.*

DEEP RED ROSE

Works on lowest section of heart chakra to draw up and transmute negative energy from solar plexus. *C.H.*

The essence of 'pure' passion. It grounds and purifies passionate feelings of the heart. It is useful in allowing us to express sexual feelings in a pure way, through the heart. It releases negative mental thought forms connected with blockages and frustrations of these energies.

Planets – Sun, Venus, Mars

Chakras – 1st, 4th *M.E.R.E.*

DELPHINIUM *Delphinium*

Brings awareness of the need to be a channel for expression of one's individual spirit. Throat chakra. *C.H.*

Delphinium 'Lord Butler' and 'Blue Nile'

A combination of two delphiniums, for those who have fear/anxiety lodged in their heart. It works on the throat and heart chakras to enable the fear to be released through communicating effectively. Also for those who have trouble sleeping when the cause is anxiety, allowing to come to the surface that which is needed and giving the strength to make the necessary changes.

'Open your heart to release what you no longer need'. *S.M.*

DEUTZIA *Deutzia*

Angels of perfume ray operate with this flower, helps attunement to them. *C.H.*

DIASCIA *Diascia*

Helps those striving towards unconditional love. For distant and earth healers. *C.H.*

DIGITALIS

Helps soften those who are hard hearted. Heart disorders. N.B. This essence does not contain any sap from the plant or flower. *C.H.*

DILL *Anethum graveolens*

Brings light to problems. Depression. Obsession with death. *C.H.*

DIPLADENIA *Dipladenia*

Yellow. Attunement to angelic realms. *C.H.*

White. Grounding spiritual ideas and visions. *C.H.*

DOG ROSE *Rosa canina*

For coughs, colds, constipation, gall bladder problems, general exhaustion, bladder and kidney conditions. For those who are over emotional. *S.C.E.*

DOG'S MERCURY *Mercurialis perennis*

Astral projection, path workings and underworld journeys. *H.F.E.*

Releases blocks in root and sexual centres. *L.L.F.E.*

DOG TOOTH VIOLET *Erythronium revolutum*

Eczema, eye problems, hair loss, hearing loss and inner ear problems, motion sickness, periodontal diseases, scalp problems, skin conditions, smallpox, internal ulcers.

Claustrophobia, fear from past lives, self righteousness, universal emotionalism. Works on all chakras. Spiritual quest. *B.F.R.*

DOG VIOLET

Keywords – 'Down Trodden'.

Negative aspects – For despair and violence especially toward children. Reluctance. Overload.

Positive aspects – Oneness; Joy enters one's life like a beam of sunlight.

Physical attributes – Some cancer conditions, head problems, congestion in chest, sore feet.   *B.F.E.*

DOUBLE SNOWDROP *Galantus nivalis "flore-plena"*

For when there are frozen attitudes and approaches to life. This remedy brings openness; a lighter touch.   *B.E.*

DWARF ELDER *Sambucus ebulus*

Enhances lunar qualities, intuition, subtle power and magnetism.   *H.F.E.*

EARLY PURPLE ORCHID *Orchis mascula*

For unblocking the energy centres in the body and protecting any vulnerable spaces so created.   *B.E.*

Keywords – 'Shape Shifter'.

Negative aspects – Temper tantrums in children. For children who tell tales. For children who bully. Misrepresentation. Self obsessed. Overload. Bad spellers. Do not want to be alone.

Positive aspects – Clinging to Life. Feeling of unconditional love. Helps physically disabled people to respect themselves. Surprise out of the blue.

Physical attributes – Insomnia. Serous back injury. Trauma. Pain in the right pelvis in women.   *B.F.E.*

ELDER *Sambucus*

Venus, Mars. Protection for fear of psychic possession. When one feels invaded.   *J.J.*
This essence allows one to travel safely and gently into the dark depths of the subconscious, allowing these areas to be lit up and brought to life. For very deep emotional blockages that need healing slowly and gently.

Planets – Moon, Venus, Uranus, Pluto

Chakras – 3rd, 4th, 7th   *M.E.F.E.*

Sambucus nigra

For protection in situations that are potentially abusive. When we feel invaded or wronged and also feel helpless.

'It is safe to trust. I confront my own fear. I can say no'.   *H.R.*

Wisdom to rise above apparent opposites and encompass dualities.   Recognising the importance of all things, each in its own cycle.   *H.F.E.*

Keynote: Beauty

Elder stimulates the body's natural powers of recuperation and renewal. It helps us to contact and radiate the beauty and joy of our inner eternal youth.

Indications: Feelings of unworthiness or self-consciousness, dislike of oneself or body, feelings of ugliness or heaviness, feeling old, dullness, overidentification with one's image, subdued or held-in personality, masking of the true self, lack of personal vitality or aliveness.

Attributes: Invoking recuperative powers of the body, self-acceptance, enthusiasm, youthfulness, acknowledgement of the process of ageing, lightening-up, new

energisation on cellular level through increased inflow of pranic energy; revealing and radiating our true being and beauty, joyful expression of the physical body.   *F.F.E.*
"Self-worth". Calms aggression, brings stability, love and forgiveness. Balances self-image. For times of transformation and change. Good for fretful children.   *G.M.T.E.*

ELDERFLOWER *Sambucus nigra*

Integration of the shadow side.

Elderflower can help one to come to terms with the dark side that is within us all, which for many can be a daunting challenge. This flower can encourage deeper understanding of the self, so a balance may be found. *F.H.*   *S.E.*
Circulation, mental abilities, past life recall.   *R.D.*
Helps the individual to trust that all their needs will be provided for. Inner security.
C.H.

For coughs, colds and as a tonic; for hayfever. For excessive worry, or mental confusion, a need for your own space.   *S.C.E.*

ELEAGNUS *Eleagnus*

Of use wherever the aura has broken down by debilitating illness, accident, drug abuse, etc. It can also be used to help protect yourself when entering atmospheres of an unbalanced nature which you don't wish to absorb.   *J.W.*

ENGLISH ELM *Ulmus procera*

"Enthusiasm". Desire to progress, move on. Re-energises the mind when fatigued and balances the heart when feeling drained or over-emotional. Clarity for decision making and study.   *G.M.T.E.*

ERTHRINA

Liver cleanser. Tonic for nervous system.   *C.H.*

EUPHRASIA

Keyword – 'Intuition'.

Negative aspects – For children who cry wolf. When one feels like a servant. 'On the verge of murdering someone' feeling. Let down by one's best friend.

Positive aspects – Sheer joy. Intuition working well. Encourages psychic signals. Good for single parents. For parents who feel they are neglecting their children. For children who are going through a 'rite of passage'.

Physical attributes – Itchy eyes and sinus problems/hay fever.   *B.F.E.*

EVENING PRIMROSE *Oenothera*

Communication.   *R.D.*
For tension at time of full moon, P.M.T., rebalances hormones.   *C.H.*

Oenothera hookeri

Nurturing.

Evening Primrose is indicated when there is an avoidance and fear of deep personal contact, which can inhibit sexuality and the ability to love. This may be due to emotional deprivation experienced in the womb, at birth or throughout early infancy.

This flower can help resolve these internal issues by encouraging the beginnings of self-nurturing. *L.F.H.*   *S.E.*

This essence can be given to anyone who has experienced, whilst in utero or early infancy, lack of emotional support, rejection, neglect or abuse by the mother. Fear of commitment, coldness or emptiness within are classic symptoms of this early pain. Evening Primrose literally rebirths the soul, providing all emotional nutrients that were lacking at incarnation.   *A.F.R.*

Oenothera biennis

Stimulates digestion through interaction with the solar plexus chakra and can help with disorders from indigestion to constipation. Can also calm anxiety.   *J.W.*

Sedatory, balancing.

Helps to promote emotional stability and is especially useful for relationship traumas, divorce, bereavement etc. Assists you to become emotionally self sufficient. Used regularly it releases tension in the uterus easing pre-menstrual syndrome and period pain, this may also eventually help to reduce the size of fibroids. Evening primrose also stimulates the nervous system and so may well be of long term benefit for Multiple Sclerosis. It is also indicated for an over-active thyroid, but it is definitely contra-indicated for ME and Post Viral Syndrome because of its strong calming effects. It does not combine well with other essences. Associations include the colours gold and yellow, direction West, planet Sun, sign Libra and Tarot Art. *A.F.E.*

A very good essence for skin conditions (ectopic eczema especially in children). Epstein Barr virus, also for hyperactivity. To halt depression, for sharing, communicating and expressing yourself.   *S.C.E.*

EXOCHORDA *Exochorda x macrantha 'The Bride'*

Circulatory system. Fatigue. Motion sickness. Confusion. Joy. Mental clarity. Self nurturing.

Breasts, pelvis, stomach. All chakras especially sixth, shoulders and wrists. Throat nadis. Spiritual quest.   *B.F.R.*

EYEBRIGHT *Euphrasia*

Increasing perception and psychic abilities. Helps to see what needs to be done in one's life.   *L.L.F.E.*

Euphrasia officinalis

'For gladness'. Good for a weak brain and memory. Can help us to get things into perspective.

'I honour my feelings. I am glad to see the truth'.   *H.R.*

Imparts an ability to see beyond the immediate, to have an overview, as if standing on a mountain top.   *J.H.*

Euphrasia nemorosa

Clear sight.

Eyebright is indicated when there is a need to live life through someone else, which can be confusing. A sense of identity is lost and it then becomes difficult to see one's own path. This essence can bring a wider viewpoint, so one can clearly see the self, others and new opportunities. *L.F.H.*   *S.E.*

FENNEL

This essence is of value in calming the mind. It helps to clear muddled thoughts, thus allowing the mind the clarity needed to focus and concentrate. This remedy can be very useful in meditation, as it brings the background 'babble' of thoughts under control.

Planets – Mercury, Pluto, Chiron

Chakra – 5th   *M.E.F.E.*

FEVERFEW *Tanacetum parthenium*

Adaptability.

In extreme and difficult situations this essence can help one adapt very quickly, encouraging the quality of flexible thinking. It brings out strength and tenacity when needed, e.g. travelling, moving house, stressful work situations. *L.F.H.*   *S.E.*

Helps disturbed sleep caused by insecurity.   *C.H.*

FEVERFEW (LUNAR)

This is the remedy for past life confusion, uncertainty about meaning, direction, purpose or identity. Souls in need of feverfew are seeking to transform this karma into clarity; they are moving out of the dark maze into the simplicity and truth of light. However, it is very hard for them to accept that life can be sharp, focussed, single pointed. For these souls to hold a vision, to be committed, to know their path is one of the greatest challenges of the life. To step out of the maze is the most exciting and frightening action to take, bringing intensity, polarization and crisis. Their past confusion is the safety net, the escape hatch in case living in the reality of light and truth is too difficult. Feverfew aligns these souls with their true destiny, allowing them to contact their own personal power which has been unused in previous lives.   *A.F.R.*

FIELD MAPLE *Acer campestre*

"Aching heart". A balance to those hearts reaching for love. Understanding and contentment when overwhelmed by a sense of responsibility or remorse for mistakes, accidents etc. Heart chakra aligned to higher love.   *G.M.TE..*

FIELD PANSY *Viola arvensis*

To bring awareness of energy fields and energy interaction. To cleanse the aura. *E.E.*

FIELD SCABIOUS

Keyword – 'Balance'.

Negative aspects – Depression when life feels incomplete. Illusion. Fear of growing old. Fear of life.

Positive aspects – Raised consciousness. Regain intelligence. Communal healing. Spellbinding.

Physical attributes – Delayed menstruation. Good for the onset of clinical depression.   *B.F.E.*

FIG *Ficus*

Releases hidden blocks and fears in subconscious, memory and psychic development. *C.H.*

FIGWORT *Scrophularia nodosa*

Overcoming judgement towards gross matter. Recognising materiality as an aspect of spirituality. Loving material existence and seeing it as a vehicle for spirit. *H.F.E.*

FIRETHORN *Pyracantha atalantoides*

This remedy is concerned with balancing up the "fire" energy within a person. This unbalance can be due to long-suppressed emotions. *B.E.*

FIVE LEAVED RED CLOVER *Trifolium pratense*

The essence of the magical dynamics of fire, will, direction, inner strength, purification.
(Caution: This essence is volatile and is shaped by your thoughts. Always take it with a clear intention in mind.) *H.F.E.*

FLANNEL FLOWER *Fremontodendron*

Specifically for skin rashes caused by allergies and also for shingles, especially when it is around the solar plexus area. *C.H.*

FLAX *Linum*

Throat problems, throat chakra, for speaking up in group situations. *C.H.*

Linum usitatissimum

Such a gentle essence that it can be used quite effectively to remove heavy metals from the body. Gentle upon the stomach and for eczema and shingles. To calm down over activity and increase your own perception and for those who hide in a crowd. *S.C.E.*

FLEABANE

Lethargic and apathetic states. Gives life and vitality in gentle way. Overcoming parasitic auric energy (draining people etc.). *L.L.F.E.*

Pulicaria dysenterica

Earths solar energy, to give strength and stability; this gives immunity against parasites on many levels. Provides the quiet vitality that allows one to build health. *H.F.E.*

FLOWERING CURRANT *Ribes*

To gain confidence and overcome fear of facing oneself. Third chakra. Releases overall fear.
Will provide inner strength. *J.J.*

Ribes sanguineum

Is warming and opens the heart, expands and softens the lungs. Strengthens the naturally flowing breath.★★

'My heart is warm and open. My breath and love flow freely'. *H.R.*

Relaxation of tense muscles. Calms anxious, nervous and fearful states. Cleanses and harmonises the functions of the mental, astral and causal bodies which helps to heal conflicts that have arisen between one's beliefs and ideas and the appropriate life-purpose. Stabilisation of emotions, peace and joy. *G.M.F.E.*

For those who have lost heart but still keep going. Often they feel that they are facing inevitable defeat. *B.E.*

FLOWERING RED CURRANT

Keyword – 'Survival'.

Negative aspects – Mood swings. Overly arrogant. Restlessness. Worries on money matters.

Positive aspects – One's presence is felt from afar. Empathy to new surroundings. Nine lives like a cat. Reconciliation. First Spring Day feeling. 'Sweet success comes my way'.

Physical attributes – Diarrhoea. Shakes, blows to the extremities. *B.F.E.*

FORGET ME NOT *Myosotis*

Spiritual relationship of all things. Good for memory. Pineal gland stimulated. Maintains emotional balance. Aligns mental and emotional bodies so that lower influences are closed.

Opens the crown. Used for accidents and emergencies. Connects to spiritual guides. *J.J.*

This essence helps us remember those in other realms, those who have died and those who are incarnating. It makes us aware of karmic relationships and so widens consciousness and self-responsibility. PHYSICAL USE: increases communication between the cells in the brain, which in turn allows the brain's electrical messages to reach different parts of the body faster and more effectively. *A.F.R.*

Keywords – 'Forget me not'.

Negative aspects – Nervous about life. Remorse with tears, inadequacy.

Positive aspects – 'I can deal with delicate situations'. 'This phase of my life is complete'.

Physical attributes – Pain in lower back. *B.F.E.*

Anxiety, sleep disturbances, memory, clarity of mind. *C.H.*

This essence is useful for people who have a bad memory. Continued use will improve the memory so that it can be relied on again. It is particularly useful in connection with remembering dreams as it helps to bring up problems that are trapped in the subconscious (forgotten). These problems are then worked out in the form of dreams which will be easy to remember, particularly if the essence is taken before sleeping.

Planets – Moon, Mercury, Saturn, Uranus

Chakra – 7th *M.E.F.E.*

As the name says it is very easy to forget about oneself to become distracted by the needs of others.

Forget-me-not encourages the user to take some time alone and to enjoy the release of external pressures. In so doing there will be a greater ability to think problems through and to focus on tasks despite sudden disturbances. *U.F.E.*

Myosotis arvensis

For remembering reality. Grounding and emotional balance. Release of negative thoughts (often through dreams).

'There is wisdom in my subconscious and answers to all my fears'. *H.R.*

Awareness of karmic connections in our personal relationships and with those in the spirit world. Deep mindfulness of subtle realms. For those with soul isolation, lack of awareness of spiritual connection with others. Blocked communication from other dimensions. Memory, clarity of thought, release of negative thought patterns. Faster reaction time. Enhances functions of subconscious and dream state. Integrates crown chakra activities of meditation, dreams and visions. *G.M.F.E.*

FORSYTHIA

Used for sugar addiction. Restores the flow of energy. *J.J.*

Bereavement. Helps us to see higher aspects. *C.H.*

Forsythia suspensa

Balancing energy levels. Brings more awareness of how we gain and lose energy. How to absorb or use it better.

'There is an abundance of energy. I choose how make use of it'. *H.R.*

FOUR LEAVED CLOVER *Trifolium repens*

The essence for connecting with Nature Spirits. Puts you in touch with the hidden secrets of nature and expands awareness into new dimensions. The essence of Magic. *H.F.E.*

FOXGLOVE (PURPLE) *Digitalis purpurea*

For letting go. Releasing anxiety about one's material situation, or what is to come. Seeing the light at the end of the tunnel. Letting go of the material illusion. Aids transition into other planes.

Good for trancework and inner journeying. Good for the heart and gallbladder.

H.F.E.

For feeling wounded or betrayed. Learning to take some responsibility for whatever has hurt us.

'I accept and 'own' my pain. It is an essential part of my growing'. *H.R.*

For those who feel confused in life and suffer from woolly thinking. Foxglove helps to bring the needed stillness of the mind. *B.E.*

Digitalis purpurea and alba

Venus, Mercury and Saturn. Feelings of being hurt. When there are deep wounds in the heart. Often confused thinking. Wanting a way out. Alba – contacts to the psychic. *J.J.*

FRENCH MARIGOLD *Tagetes patula*

Sun. Mental/causal bodies. Psychic abilities, clairaudience.   For those who are closed off from the world. For the need to listen.   *J.J.*

Each of us has inside a great inner knowing – a being that knows why we came to be here, that knows why the call to Earth was made. That inner being is our Self – it has the wisdom that we need from day to day, based on many experiences. With this wise being we can realise that we already know the answers from inside ourselves; that has always been the case. French Marigold helps us to access more clearly this deep, loving voice within that knows and loves us – that **is** us, that helps us to find our way out of the maze of all the things that we create and co-create.

When we have listened to ourselves, we are more able to listen to others and to 'hear' them correctly. French Marigold is for listening and understanding the truth on all levels. This includes clairaudience and physical hearing.   *S.M.*

French Marigold develops psychic abilities. It is further used for hearing difficulties or understanding what others are trying to say. It is useful for schizophrenia and autism.

Physical use: eases inflammation in the inner ear and pancreas, treats muscles which are attached to the bones, such as tendons and eases genetic deterioration of the spine and viral inflammations.   *A.F.R.*

Inflammation e.g. Inner ear.   *R.D.*

Inner hearing, psychic abilities. Inflammation, viruses.   *C.H.*

FUCHSIA *Fuchsia*

Pale pink sepals, purple corolla. Opening up of heart centre to allow unconditional love to flow.   *A.T.*

Red sepals, double purple corolla. Brings deep peace and a remembering of the secrets of life.   *A.T.*

White. Gentle emotional release.   *C.H.*

Red, white/blue, pink or combination. All work to bring attention to underlying emotions.   *C.H.*

This essence helps in the understanding and awareness of blocked emotions. This can be blocked emotions that are causing tension and psychosomatic illness. It is also good for anyone wanting to change a low opinion of themselves.

Planets – Moon, Saturn, Neptune

Chakras – 3rd, 4th   *M.E.F.E.*

Keywords – 'I have no regrets'.

Negative aspects – 'I don't like myself'. Coming to terms with loss either physically or emotionally. Flighty unreal ideas. Fear comes easily. Disobedience in children.

Positive aspects – Co-operation in children. Set one's personal boundaries. Allows one's truth to blossom. 'I need to give to me'. Vision to go on.

Physical attributes – For infertility. Music therapy.   *B.F.E.*

Fuchsia 'Little Jewel'

A wonderful essence for dislodging and releasing blocked energy. Fuchsia opens up the heart chakra, bringing out all which has been locked inside. The floodgates will open releasing any pent-up emotions which are causing blockages preventing spiritual attunement. Once these emotions have been recognised they can be treated and worked through; this is a very important part of the learning process.   *C.H.*

Fuchsia magellanica

Repressed emotions which cover up deeper issues.   *J.J.*

Helps the soul to encounter and transform deep, hidden and painful emotions which are often covered up by a hyper-active emotional front. Powerful remedy to aid deep cathartic release.   *A.FR.*

Dissolving the weakness of the disbelieving self.   *A.T.*

FUMITORY *Fumaria officinalis*

A cleansing essence, good to use before other essences. Awakens deep intuition, which leads to empathy with others.   *S.C.E.*

GALTONIA *Galtonia*

Brings to a head unresolved issues in relationships, especially when having a sexual base.   *C.H.*

GARLIC

Garlic is used to alleviate fear. It is useful for periods of low vitality when there is openness to disease and attack on all levels.   *A.FR.*

Cleanser and purifier at many levels. Anger and fear.   *C.H.*

GAZANIA *Gazania*

Helps open and cleanse crown chakra. Good to help visualisations with white light.   *C.H.*

GEAN (WILD CHERRY, MAZZARD) *Prunus avium*

"Soothing". Focuses energy in physical body and stimulates self-healing. Calms the heart and mind. Creates a smooth flow of energy. Helps reduce pain.   *G.M.T.E.*

GERANIUM (CRANESBILL) *Geranium*

Geranium atlanticum

For bringing a cherished and well grounded plan through to reality, e.g. starting a business, giving up smoking, getting into print, learning to paint, drive, sing etc. 'I now allow this plan to manifest'.   *H.R.*

Geranium 'Scarlet Eye'

For those still in the dark, gloom, possibly even despair, but recognising the need to contact their spirituality. Like a person in a darkened room, moving around, bumping into things but unable to find that light switch. This is their essence. Their fingers will find the switch and their whole being will be flooded with light and love, which in turn will illuminate the world.   *C.H.*

GERANIUM *Pelargonium*

This essence from mixed zonal geraniums relaxes the body. It activates the throat, heart and base chakras to release unwanted energy, helping the life force to enter. It aligns all the major chakras and nadis temporarily, allowing the light to enter again where there has been darkness and lack of direction. Good for depression and releasing negative energy. *S.M.*

Pelargonium roseum
Venus. Calming, soothing. For those needing to open to love. Heart chakra. *J.J.*

GEUM *Geum*
Energy. For those whose confidence was damaged in childhood. *C.H.*

GIANT REDWOOD *Sequoiadendron giganteum*
"Weight of responsibility". For those who are too hard on themselves or on others. A sense of balanced responsibility, tolerance and relaxation that allows wisdom the space to develop. Relieves tension in pelvic and abdominal muscles. *G.M.T.E.*

GLADIOLUS *Gladiolus*
Helps to become stabilised in spiritual intent, when drawn back into ego dimensions. Crown chakra. *C.H.*

GLASTONBURY THORN
"Out of the woods". A clearer direction is found. What feels right to do and be emerges from indecision and chaos. This brings immediate relaxation and release from tension, increasing subtle information and intuition. Claustrophobia. *G.M.TE.*

GOLDEN CROCUS *Crocus domesticus*
Self-image improves, forgiveness and tolerance within oneself. Ability to express one's own feelings, if needs be forcefully. Integrity of one's own energy and protection. Healing from past hurts. Fears and anxieties ease. Joy, wisdom and personal power are strengthened. For under-dogs and scaredy-cats! *G.M.F.E.*

GOLDEN ROD *Solidago*
Golden Rod is given when we are too easily influenced by social pressure and family ties in our desire for love and acceptance. This essence strengthens the sense of individuality. *A.F.R.*
Spiritual guidance through increased connection with higher self. *C.H.*
Works on ego bringing it into balance by either stabilising an overemphasised ego or increasing self confidence and self worth when these are lacking. *L.L.F.E.*

GOLDEN SAGE *Salvia officinalis var. Icterina*
Motivating.
Reduces mental clutter so use before meditation. Provides motivation and a sense of purpose. Ideal for the stress of exams/interviews etc. Encourages self forgiveness and improves self esteem. Golden sage is recommended for nervous, introverted, shy people. It is indicated for: flatulence and digestive disturbances, shingles and chickenpox, tension or sick headaches, neuralgia, balancing blood pressure and as a gentle de-tox. Golden sage is very grounding, it balances the meridians, opens the solar plexus chakra and strengthens the subtle bodies.
Associations include the colour pink, direction East, planets Venus and Mars, Tarot 3 of Swords. *A.F.E.*

GOLDEN SAXIFRAGE *Chrysosplenium oppositifolium*

Integrating the sun into the feminine soul. Understanding the feminine aspect of the solar energy. Opening the heart to give freely.   *H.F.E.*

GOOSEBERRY *Ribes uva-crispa*

Sense of ease and relaxation of cares. Improves attitudes to the world outside. Enjoyment of life and living. For those who wish to save the world single-handedly. For those who fear getting involved. Improves poor circulation in hands and feet.

G.M.F.E.

GORSE *Ulex europaeus*

Keynote: Joy

Gorse is a light bringer, stimulating vitality, enthusiasm and motivation at times of apathy and low immunity, bringing light-heartedness and enjoyment of life.

Indications: Apathy, burn-out, low immunity, listlessness, lack of motivation or joy, unable to join in or to share oneself.

Attributes: Renewal of life force, vitality, motivation, enthusiasm, living in the moment, enjoyment and celebration of life.   *F.F.E.*

Gorse is given to those who experience deep depression, despair, hopelessness and resignation. Gorse brings the qualities of faith, hope and joy back into life.   *A.F.R.*

"Integration". Eases restlessness, frustration and jealousy. Joy from emotional security and growth. Helps integrate new forms of energy or knowledge in a useful, personal manner.   *G.M.T.E.*

Gorse is about endurance, knowing no fear and concentration. This remedy can help to strengthen these faculties in times of need such as undertaking a major task which requires stamina, fearlessness and singlemindedness. However, Gorse will also help to lighten up individuals whose life situations have required that they are permanently in this state which then causes undue stress.   *U.F.E.*

Positive: For understanding that true forgiveness is the act of letting go our judgement of ourself and others. A phoenix remedy to build a new way of relating from a centre of unconditional love, understanding and compassion for ourselves and others and the recognition of God/Good in all.

For compassion and healing our desire for justice. For the recognition that each and everyone of us is worthy of love at every moment of our lives, regardless of what acts we have committed.

Indications: For when it is hard to forgive ourselves, or others, and for healing conflict and pain in our personal relationships. For hurt feelings, often held for many years, aggressive defensiveness, and for those judged by others to have committed an act that is unforgiveable; helps them to release their judgement of themselves and nurture love for themselves as they begin to heal their life. For whenever we feel the victim in our relationship with others, when we feel we have suffered abuse and cannot forgive those who we perceive to have abused us. Gorse helps us to recognize our part in the story. Withholding love from ourselves and others because of our judgement. Healing communities where there has been a history of conflict, violence, retaliation and retribution. (Use whilst meditating for peace, reconciliation and healing in these areas. Can also be sprinkled in areas which need healing from past events.) For prison rehabilitation work.

Physical: Heart and mind. May aid the healing process for conditions arising from heat and intense sunlight: dehydration, heat exhaustion, sunstroke, burns and fevers. May help plants cope with drought and heat: use when watering and transplanting.

L.H.F.E.

GREAT MARSH THISTLE *Carduus personata*

Nobility, spiritual value. Develops the crown chakra. Trust in the spirit. Maintaining one's spirituality in spite of undermining company. Strength, protection, unhindered growth. Allows true beauty and gentleness of the soul, without fear.   *H.F.E.*

GREAT SALLOW (GOAT WILLOW, PUSSY WILLOW) *Salix caprea*

"Soul". Allows the mind to expand and link with the soul. Understanding of life purpose.

Energising. Links to earth energy.   *G.M.T.E.*

Balancing inner masculine energy and masculine sexuality. Helps in working with dreams.   *L.L.F.E.*

GROUND IVY *Glechoma hederacea*

Stem, leaves, flowers. For understanding and encompassing the earth role. For self-perception.

For self-confidence. For determination to do.   *E.E.*

GROUNDSEL *Senecio*

Integrates ideas into the physical.   *C.H.*

GUELDER ROSE *Viburnum opulus*

Berries. To 'see'. For clarity. For processing the 'idea'.   *E.E.*

Balances higher chakras above crown. Brings awareness to emotional problems. *C.H.*

HAIRY NIGHTSHADE *Solanum luteum*

Encourages one to go forward with sensitivity and awareness, to truly progress on one's real path. Is particularly good for creative visualisations, manifestation work and inner journeying.

(Helps those who feel they have lost direction in their lives.)   *H.F.E.*

HAIRY SEDGE *Carex hirta*

For poor memory caused by mental attitudes. In such people there is a chronic lack of attention to the present moment.   *B.E.*

HAREBELL (SCOTTISH BLUEBELL) *Campanula rotundifolia*

To stay with your wildness. Harebell is both delicate and strong, clear as a bell, yet subtle, almost ethereal. Qualities that come to you when you live close to nature.

'I am part of the natural world. I am gentle and wild and free'.   *H.R.*

Keynote: Prosperity

Harebell is for realigning to the spirit of abundance and releasing material concerns following fear of lack.

Indications: Fear of lack, possessiveness, lack of faith, attachment, poverty consciousness, out of alignment with oneself and one's environment.

Attributes: Manifesting abundance, re-alignment, affirmation, balance, self-reliance, equilibrium. *F.F.E.*

For the shy and nervous, unable to express themselves, especially in groups. *C.H.*

Calming, sedatory.

For peace of mind. Calms on all levels so excellent for insomnia, for hyper-active children (ideal for long distance travellers, passengers NOT drivers!). May stop twitching/jumping legs especially at night. Eliminates irrational fears and is excellent for emotional stress or shock.

Useful for computer and TV addicts as it can shield from electro-magnetic stress. Harebell is a very gentle essence so it is suitable for children, it is also recommended for the terminally ill, for grief and for bereavement. It reduces the trauma to plants when transplanting or pruning.

Contra-indicated for ME or Post Viral Syndrome because of its strong sedatory effect.

Associations include the colour blue, direction South, planets Moon, Neptune and Chiron, Tarot 3 of Cups. *A.F.E.*

HARESFOOT CLOVER *Trilolium arvense*

Loosens up the body joints if taken over one month or more. *C.H.*

HAWKSBEARD (LUNAR)

This remedy can be used to heal the wounds that have occurred on the collective level of consciousness in previous incarnations. Whole communities or nations have greatly suffered at certain times and many souls reincarnate still bearing the wounds of a life that was injured through the suffering of the community or nation. Hawksbeard heals the wounding that has occurred when whole communities are subjected to suffering because of racial characteristics, religious practice, war, famine and many other reasons. Souls who in previous lives have become caught up in a major national disaster would benefit from this remedy. *A.F.R.*

HAWKWEED

Keyword – 'Temperance'.

Negative aspects – Social pariah. Completely sapped of energy. Children with speech problems. Fear of the new.

Positive aspects – Return to the community (prodigal child). Revitalised. For childless couples who want children. Fruitful times.

Physical attributes – Gripping in stomach. *B.F.E.*

HAWTHORN *Crataegus*

Hawthorn brings balance at times of precancerous emotional stress such as grieving for a loved one or the pain of a broken relationship. PHYSICAL USE: eases spread of cancer, especially tumours. *A.F.R.*

Tumours, stress. *R.D.*

Keywords – 'The path finder'.

Negative aspects – Stress related to house moving. Mental congestion. Abuse of friendship.

Child within cries for help.

Positive aspects – Enhances meditative states. Cease being a victim. Helps to find a partner (on any level). Love thyself.

Physical attributes – Post operative on the heart/circulation. Varicose veins. Thyroid.

B.F.E.

Pink and white hawthorn.

Body spray with essential oil.

Supports self love.

Negative focus – Blocked heart energy – turmoil, confusion, anger, grief etc.

When the heart energy is blocked the result can be distressing inner turmoil. This flower essence spray can create an opening which can restore balance and inner stillness. From this space comes the courage to act appropriately and with self love. Spray directly on skin around heart area and work in with a circular motion. Use twice a day, morning and night. *S.E.*

Helps eliminate cancer cells. *C.H.*

Balancing inner feminine energy and feminine sexuality. *L.L.F.E.*

This essence can be used for treating precancerous emotional states and can help to check the spread of tumours. It is very useful when there is a feeling of broken heartedness, or extreme stress after the passing of a loved one. It is useful in connection with a raw food diet used as a cancer therapy.

Planets – All planets are affected

Chakras – All *M.E.F.E.*

Change is an essential part of the rhythm and evolution of life. For change to occur all aspects of our lives must grow be they thoughts, beliefs, relationships or life styles and sometimes this can involve letting go of deeply held patterns of behaviour, ideas, people or objects.

Hawthorn helps one to understand the patterns of clinginess, or why one might 'hang on' to things. It brings patience which is necessary in the process of letting go as there may be set-backs. But in the letting go of the old Hawthorn also reveals the gifts which become available. *U.F.E.*

HAWTHORN (MAY TREE) *Crataegus monogyna*

'Brings hope' calmly protecting body, mind and spirit in times of deep grief or sadness. To know that our sorrows are not endless, not damaging, but a natural part of life.

'My spirit is free. My body is a wise healer. My heart can bear this'. *H.R.*

Mars, Saturn. Heart centre. Activates spiritual properties. Lets go of negativities. Good for grief and stress. Clears the etheric and emotional bodies. Eases cancer distribution. For heartbreaks. Balances the physical to the subtle bodies. *J.J.*

Leaf. To balance the body, mind and spirit. To bring awareness of the 'lone' self, the 'true' self.

To bring awareness of oneness. Powerfully grounding and cleansing. *E.E.*

Flower. To bring awareness of spirit. For understanding 'being'. For self-love. *E.E.*

Berry. To bring awareness of one's true source of nourishment. To bring awareness of the free flow of giving and receiving. *E.E.*

"Love". Stimulates the healing power of love. Trust. Forgiveness. Helps to cleanse the heart of negativity. *G.M.T.E.*

HAWTHORN (LUNAR)

Lunar hawthorn is for those souls who have been unable to shake off the doctrines of previous lives which are proving unhelpful in the present incarnation. Use this remedy when the soul's own wisdom has been at odds with the collective consensus and the soul has had to accept religious and cultural "truths" unsympathetic to its own spiritual development. *A.F.R.*

HAZEL *Corylus*

Access to trance states. Balanced integration of male and female energies within self. *L.L.F.E.*

Corylus avellana

For wisdom, for healing, for understanding and encompassing masculinity, for joyous fertility. *E.E.*

"Skills". The flowering of skills. Ability to receive and communicate wisdom. Helps all forms of study. Clears away unwanted debris. Brings more stability and focus in order to integrate useful information. *G.M.T.E.*

HAZEL (LUNAR)

Hazel can be given to heal wounds inflicted upon the physical body by sharp or heavy weapons in previous lives. Also use when there has been a large display of greed or possessiveness in a previous life which is colouring the present incarnation. Hazel is also indicated where there is a sense of powerful energies and patterns from previous lives, which are now outworn and inappropriate , being retained by the soul and informing the present incarnation inappropriately, pulling the soul down into the depths rather than lifting it up. *A.F.R.*

HEARTSEASE (WILD PANSY) *Viola tricolor*

Eases and 'brings comforting thoughts' to broken or damaged hearts. Letting go of mistaken love.

'I acknowledge my feelings of loneliness. I forgive and let go'. *H.R.*

Saturn. Used for colds and viruses, protection against radiation. Mental body and right brain.

Balances resistance. Heartsease – which helps to lighten a sorrowful heart. *J.J.*

Combats viral infections. Increases intuitive faculties and strengthens mental functioning. *G.M.F.E.*

Developing a strong, loving, warm heart. Bringing out the beauty of the soul. Purification of the heart and soul and of the desires. *H.F.E.*

Viruses, tiredness after meditation. *R.D.*

Strengthens physically.

Pansy has a predominantly physical application. Helps strengthen the body's defence mechanisms against viral attack. Excellent topically in creams and oils. Useful alongside Ramsons and Jack by the Hedge.   *L.F.H.*   *S.E.*

As the name suggests there is a quality of easing the centre of our being with this remedy.

More specifically, Heartsease helps in situations where one is over-indulging, be that with food or drink, self-pity, self-criticism or worry. Heartsease brings an ability to see situations more objectively and to facilitate self-nurturing.   *U.F.E.*

HEATHER *Calluna vulgaris*

For fears of being alone, of the dark and empty spaces in your life. Finding the courage to face shadows.

'I accept all aspects of myself'.   *H.R.*

HEDGE WOUNDWORT *Stachys sylvatica*

For healing deep hurts and tapping a source of inner strength. Helps connect with power animals and guardian angels.   *H.F.E.*

HELIANTHUS *Helianthus multiflorus*

Like sunflower, works on heart chakra, carries the strength of the sun aspect, brings balance to masculine/feminine energies at heart chakra.   *C.H.*

HELLEBORUS *Helleborus*

Brings spiritual awareness to the ageing process.   *C.H.*

Helleborus corsicus

Colon spasm, obesity, spinal degeneration, spinal inflammation, weight control. Anti depressant, anxiety, grief, pre-cancerous emotional states, schizophrenia, too introverted.

Cleansing – colon, intestinal tract, spine and spleen. Works on eighth and shoulder chakras, stomach meridian, syphilitic maism. For psycho-spiritual balance.   *B.F.R.*

HEMP-NETTLE *Galeopsis*

Particularly for strengthening the eyes. May also be used in water as a swab for relieving tired eyes.   *C.H.*

HENBANE *Hyoscyamus niger*

For understanding death and exploring its realms. Preparing for death initiations. Connecting with spirits who have passed on.   *H.F.E.*

HERB ROBERT *Geranium robertianum*

For inflammation of the gums, toothache, has antiseptic qualifies; good for bruises, cuts, boils if used in a cream base. Also has diuretic qualities. For being positive in thought and action.   *S.C.E.*

HIBISCUS *Hibiscus*

Hibiscus helps women to reclaim the dignity and warmth of their sexuality after traumatic or degrading experiences, including the exploitation and commercialisation of female sexuality.   *A.F.R.*

Disorientation after psychic or spiritual shock, brings balance.   *C.H.*

Hibiscus syriacus 'Blue Bird'

This is very grounding. It clears and balances the emotional body, so is helpful after emotional cleansing. It works on the feet, base, sacral and solar plexus chakras and has some effect on the heart energy. Made with the love of St Germain. Good for people who are 'running away', helping them to realise that there can be no escape, but only transformation in whatever form this takes. *S.M.*

HIMALAYAN POPPY

Brings strength and healing to continue on one's spiritual path, opens up to easier meditation and spiritual ideas to come through. *C.H.*

HOLLY *Ilex aquifolium*

"Power of peace". Agitated states, balance of mind. Loss of control, panic, lack of self-worth, unhappiness, loneliness. Active expression of love. Non-aggression, peace-loving yet assertive. *G.M.T.E.*

HOLLY BUDS *Ilex*

Diffusion of confusion. Allows negativity to be acknowledged, passed through and released. *A.T.*

HOLM OAK *Quercus ilex*

"Negative emotions". Relieves emotions and restlessness related to thwarted expression: guilt, jealousy, anger etc. Activates personal creativity and balances emotional and mental energy. *G.M.T.E.*

HOLY-THORN *Crataegus*

Keynote: Rebirth

This essence opens our hearts to love and the acceptance of ourselves and others, allowing intimacy and the expression of our truth and creativity.

Indications: Blocked self expression and creativity, withholding oneself, lack of involvement, creating barriers to friendship, fear of rejection, repression of the true self.

Attributes: Birthing and expressing creative activity on all levels, opening to others, intimacy and nurturing, radiant compassion, warm and loving acceptance of all, universal Christ-like love, transformation through the power of love. *F.F.E.*

Deep contact with subconscious. Releases deep rooted patterns and memories. Attunes to higher soul energies and purpose of incarnation. *L.L.F.E.*

Negative – For extreme suffering and feeling cut off from the source of Love and Light – from God. Feelings of great despair and betrayal – "Why hast thou forsaken me?" Dark night of the soul. For those angelic beings who want to return home, as they can bear it no longer – feeling of abandonment.

Positive – Connecting back to the source and knowing there is no separateness – we are all one! A rebirth and transformation, at one with the Christ energy. A huge weight is lifted off one's shoulders. Enables one to continue to serve mankind, but from a different perspective, coming from a deeper place of compassion. Opens up the heart to greater loving!

Affinity with heart, third eye and crown chakra. Opens up the heart and heals deep wounds.

Stimulates third eye – clairvoyance and channelling. Stimulates crown chakra – connection to the divine. Gentle cleansing action on reproductive organs, purifying and healing any ancient sexual wounds. *G.H.T.E.*

HOLY-THORN BUD

To be taken after using the *G.H.T.E.* flower essence.

For those souls who choose to come and make a great sacrifice, to be reborn and assist in the transformation of this planet. For the new beginnings and great shifts in consciousness occurring on the planet at this moment in time. To bring humour, love and creativity into our lives so that we can serve humanity in the true light of understanding and compassion and to give us the courage to complete and manifest our life's mission. To walk with Grace upon this planet, surrounded by the Christ Light, with reverence for every living thing in this most beautiful creation. *G.H.T.E.*

HONESTY *Lunaria*

Lifts the veil of illusion between the third, fourth and fifth dimensions. *C.H.*

Lunaria redivia

Moon. Pituitary. For right brain – feminine – negative attributes. Often secretive in order to assert. Helps one to become more open and honest. *J.J.*

Lunaria annua

For confusion or lapses in consciousness. Fosters openness with others and honesty with oneself. Reclaiming memory blanks.

'I honour the truth. I am clear about what is real'. *H.R.*

Brings the energy necessary to find knowledge of the Self, clarity of one's personal needs and how to relate to others at an energetic/subtle level. Increases willingness to accept change and flexibility in persona or self-image. Clarity and direction in relationships with others. Helps to clear negative emotions from the heart. Healing negative emotional blocks. *G.M.F.E.*

Maintains peace and beauty amongst stressful surroundings. Simplicity and faith in who you really are. *H.F.E.*

Honesty aligns the mind to the abundance of the universe, thereby lifting consciousness above the negative thought patterns centred around poverty and lack. *A.F.R.*

Positive: Honesty without judgement. For allowing ourselves to experience the full depth and range of our feelings, with love and without judgement. For giving ourselves and our inner child the unconditional love, compassion, approval and recognition that we would seek from others.

For releasing judgement of ourselves and others and showing our true face. For understanding that truth is love and recognising that the greatest gift we can give ourselves and others is the unadorned expression of our human-ness. Being happy to be who we truly are.

Indications: Hiding one's true feelings from oneself, or others, for fear of judgement, fear of exposure. Suppressed emotion, suppressed grief. Sensitivity to criticism or judgement from others. Self-judgement, self-criticism, low self esteem, poor body image. For co-dependency in relationships, helps us to recognise when our actions are motivated by our yearning for love, recognition and approval. For when we feel misunderstood – helps us to understand ourself.

For those who experienced a deep lack of love, recognition and approval during childhood and those who deny their own feelings and who feel threatened and are judgmental, when those around them express their feelings and their human-ness. For when we are denying our truth and are attempting to live according to the (mis)perceived standards of others or of society and for those who work hard to maintain an image of perfection in order to hide their vulnerability. Stage fright.

Physical: For the heart, solar plexus, thymus, lymphatic system, spine. Cleansing, energy releasing. For loving one's body, one's physical expression. To help heal the patterns of anorexia, addictions, alcoholism, drug addiction (combine with Pussy Willow). *L.H.F.E.*

This remedy is for help with bringing openness and receptivity where previously there were subversive negative characteristics. *B.E.*

HONEYSUCKLE *Lonicera periclymenum*

Balancing.

Gives protection from other peoples emotions, releases anger, irrational fears and mental stress.

Helps to achieve inner peace and to improve the memory making this an excellent remedy for teachers as well as students. It helps with the absorption of vitamins and minerals, increases the oxygen levels in the blood and is believed to maintain the cellular structure of bone tissue.

Honeysuckle is indicated for poor circulation, high/low blood pressure, chilblains, pulmonary congestion, diarrhoea and osteoporosis. Associations include the colour red, direction West, planets Venus and Jupiter, Tarot The Chariot. *A.F.E.*

Used for the lungs and bowel. To energise your femininity and the inability to love for clinging to emotions of the past. *S.C.E.*

HOPS *Humulus lupulus*

Mars. Pituitary. Activates the etheric. Good in groups. Relaxes and calms. Stimulates spiritual growth. *J.J.*

For growth on all levels, including physical and spiritual. *C.H.*

HORNBEAM *Carpinus betulus*

"Right action". Deep energising on many levels clearing blocked or stagnant energies. Clarity of purpose. Standing up for personal experience. Increased security in working with others. *G.M.T.E.*

HORSE CHESTNUT (WHITE CHESTNUT) *Aesculus hippocastanum*

"Agitation". Harmonising flows of energy to and from the individual, eases agitation caused by contrast and difference. Clarity of mind. Flow of intuition. Peace. Ability to ground and dissipate excess energy. *G.M.T.E.*

HOYA *Hoya*

Alignment of seven major chakras, only temporarily but if taken over a long period will bring total and more permanent alignment, also helps grounding. *C.H.*

HYACINTH *Hyacinthus*

Integrates spiritual and earthly qualities. Inner hearing.   *C.H.*

Blue hyacinth. Grounding.   *A.T.*

HYDRANGEA *Hydrangea*

For scatteredness, brings mental alignment.   *C.H.*

HYPERICUM *Hypericum 'Hidcote'*

Helps release worrying thoughts to bring more calmness, especially helps calm the stomach area which often suffers from excess worry via ulcers etc.   *C.H.*

HYSSOP *Hyssop officinalis*

'Purge me with Hyssop'. A tonic which can lessen feelings of anxiety and help the acknowledgement and release of guilt.

'I honestly 'own' the true cause of my thoughts and actions. I release all blame'. *H.R.*

Moon, Mars, Jupiter. Releases guilt feelings and being judgmental. Good for groups. Base chakra. 2nd and 3rd chakras and etheric body are balanced. Helps with sleep when astral travel makes one tired on waking. Helps to assimilate gold.   *J.J.*

Hyssop alleviates guilt, thereby allowing a deeper understanding of thoughts and actions to emerge.   *A.F.R.*

Acknowledging and releasing guilt feelings. Tension.   *C.H.*

IRIS *Iris*

Purple iris. Crown chakra. For spiritual, psychic or visionary artists.   *C.H.*

Blue iris. Unblocking of hidden talents.   *A.T.*

Brown/gold iris. This is a connection with the Lord Maitreya and helps all working with this energy.   *C.H.*

Iris 'Amethyst'

Strengthens the connection of those working with the amethyst ray and angels thereof, whether for healing or visionary purposes.   *C.H.*

Iris 'Bluebeard'

Works through all dimensions to clear blockages in throat area, thus helping to spiritualise speech.   *C.H.*

Iris sibirica

Venus moon. For creativity especially through art. Links to the colour of the soul of nature. The triangle of faith, wisdom and valour, Iris means rainbow – the bridge between spirit and matter, light and dark. Recharges the soul to create beauty.   *J.J.*

IRIS (BLUE FLAG) *Iris germanica*

'Symbol of power'. Coming into one's own personal power. Releasing blockages to living to our full potential.

'I am my own authority'.   *H.R.*

IRIS/DIOPTASE *Iris ziphium + dioptase*

Yellow dutch iris plus dioptase crystal – combined in one bowl when made. This works on all chakras up to the 12th, aligning and opening them all at whatever level is needed at the time. It helps to access all the levels of love within you. Relieves guilt.

'Open to receive the light within you'.   *S.M.*

ITALIAN ALDER *Alnus cordata*

"Protected peace". Brings peace, love and protection for delicate energies. Helps with shyness or over-aggression. Courage for new starts.   *G.M.T.E.*

IVY *Hedera*

Grounding and stabilising. Brings out intuition.   *L.L.F.E.*

Hedera helix

Patience, strength, stability, rooting. Gradually growing towards union. Links one to the Earth Mother.   *H.F.E.*

"Fear". Eases hidden fears and anxieties. Helps to release true feelings and identify needs.

Balances the heart chakra and its nadis. Strengthens the immune system.   *G.M.T.E.*

IVY (LUNAR)

Lunar ivy is for past life poisoning and poisoned emotions such as envy, jealousy, hatred and anger. It is used to release the toxicity which is produced through the constant denial, repression or inability to face such powerful emotions. The healing action of ivy is dramatic; a powerful cathartic release of past life toxins can be expected.   *A.F.R.*

JACK BY THE HEDGE *Allaria petiolata*

Supports a delicate immune system.

For sensitive, fragile and delicate constitutions, prone to infection. This essence can help support the heart connection to the body's defence system, so is ideal when emotional pain, e.g. grief, has weakened the constitution. Appropriate with Ramsons in any infection. *L.F.H.*   *S.E.*

JACOB'S LADDER *Polemonium caeraleum*

For being open to receiving or actively seeking help. For those of us who feel we must resolve all our problems alone.

'The help that I desire is on it's way.'   *H.R.*

JAPANESE QUINCE *Chaenomeles japonica*

Strengthens red blood cells and helps them to expand, reproduce.   *C.H.*

JASMINE *Jasminum*

Nasal passages, sinuses, throat and lungs. *R.D.*

Jasmine stimulates the God spark or permanent atom that resides in the heart chakra. Jasmine is given to those suffering from low self-esteem.

Physical use: mucus in the system is regulated. The nasal passages, the sinuses, the throat and the lungs are cleared. Jasmine helps diseases associated with mucous problems such as pneumonia or the common cold.

Viruses are dissolved and discharged. Diseases associated with protein deficiency such as hypoglycemia can be treated. *A.F.R.*

Stimulates Divine spark in heart chakra, self worth. Viruses, excess mucus in system, sinuses, related diseases. *C.H.*

Jasminum officinale

A general stimulant. Helps to process, absorb or eliminate. Good for congestion, low self esteem and practicality★★.

'All that comes to me I either use or let go'. *H.R.*

Moon, Jupiter. For spiritual love. Stimulates the God spark. It has two devas, male and female and a very high vibration. It transmutes physical love to higher levels of spiritual love. Head centre. Universal love awakens the fragrance of jasmine. Strengthens the etheric with the physical. Perfume reaches the angels who deal with colour. *J.J.*

Jasminum ordoratissmum

Empowers.

Stimulates the immune system, heals physical and emotional scars and balances the body fluids. Indicated for colds (not flu), asthma, hay fever and sinus problems, also for post natal depression, candida, IBS, oedema and soft tissue damage. It is a useful bacteria buster and can be used to discourage head lice, nits and fleas. Jasmine can be utilised to tune astrologers into all the planetary influences before they do readings. Jasmine cleans, opens and balances all the chakras and resolves karmic patterns at an emotional level. Associations include the colours orange and gold, direction North, planets All, Tarot Hanged Man. *A.F.E.*

JONQUIL *Narcissus*

Brings higher chakras i.e. throat, brow, crown and higher, into alignment. *C.H.*

JUDAS TREE *Cercus*

Denial and suppression of guilt at duality, original or spiritual guilt. *C.H.*

Cercis siliquastrum

"Channelling". Access to completely new thought patterns and ideas. Openness and acceptance of very subtle levels of energy and the ability to communicate it to others. The ability to discriminate and discern the validity of given information. *G.M.T.E.*

KERRIA *Kerria*

Balance for emotional extremes, violence. *C.H.*

KIDNEY VETCH *Anthyllis vulneraria*

Helps cleanse kidneys and process all energies moving through, on all levels i.e. physical – water, emotional – fears. *C.H.*

For circulation problems, kidney disease. A transformational essence, will help you to understand spiritual matters, will allow the user to connect with their soul. *S.C.E.*

KNAPWEED *Centaurea nigra*

For the bladder and kidneys, it is a tonic and diuretic. For using your intuitive faculties and insights as a resource for aiding others. *S.C.E.*

LABURNUM *Laburnum x watereri "Vossi"*

"Detoxification". Balanced release of stress and tension. Increases detoxification processes and the growth of creative potential. Optimism, positivity and the expression of personal wisdom. *G.M.T.E.*

LADY OF THE NIGHT *Brassavola nodosa*

Gives connection to the beautiful angels of death. Helps take one onto a new level of existence, passing over to the next dimension. *C.H.*

LADY'S BEDSTRAW *Galium verum*

Works on the pattern of passive resistance, helps one to make a stronger stand. *C.H.*

LADY'S MANTLE *Alchemilla mollis*

For the protection and inspiration of wise woman or Goddess energy. Meditation. Prayer.
Wonder working. Fertility. Birth.
'She has been with me from the beginning and is with me now'. *H.R.*
Venus. For protection. Fertility. Alchemy transmutes lower energies into higher. It blends energies into cosmic consciousness of the planet. *J.J.*

Alchemilla vulgaris

Honours the female side.
This essence can help protect the feeling, sensitive, 'female' side of an individual, especially men struggling to be comfortable with their vulnerabilities and holding back emotions through fear. Whatever one's sexual inclination, Lady's Mantle helps give more understanding and acceptance of the feminine aspect. *L.F.H.* *S.E.*

LADY'S SMOCK *Cardamine pratensis*

Attunement with personal guides and higher soul self. Connection with personal power in balanced way. *L.L.F.E.*
Keywords – 'I go forth and multiply'.
Negative aspects – 'I forget details because I am in such a hurry'. 'I hate you'. To help children through learning difficulties. Worried about being close to insanity. For people who are suffering from post child abuse trauma later in their lives.
Positive aspects – Cleansing. Centred and peaceful. Return of personal power. Regain control.
Physical attributes – Helps uterine contractions. For anxiety. *B.B.F.E.*

LAMB'S TONGUE *Stachys byzantina*

Helps to de-fur the body system especially arteries and blood.   *C.H.*

LARCH (EUROPEAN) *Larix decidua*

'Will to express". Helps the communication of personal wisdom from new levels of peace and healing. Inspiration. Physical and sexual energy. Creativity. Balances heart and mind, Will and Desire. Releases suppressed trauma.   *G.M.T.E.*

LARKSPUR *Consolida*

Helps open the channels to kundalini energy.   *C.H.*

LAUREL *Prunus lusitanica*

Keynote: Resourcefulness

This essence represents the abundance of the universe. It enables those wise in heart to empower themselves to find the resources to bring their ideas and ideals into form.

Indications: Inability to 'hold the vision', withholding of talents, initiative and resources of the self, procrastination, giving up easily, failure to act for fear of risk-taking, failure to evoke the will to choose and then follow the way that has been determined upon, overwhelm through inability to integrate many facets of a project, disorganisation.

Attributes: Unfolding the power to manifest, bringing ideas into being and putting them into action, working with the 7th Ray of organisation, order and expression of spirit through form; ability to choose opportunities which serve life purpose, synthesising different facets or energies into a unified whole, evoking the power to hold and maintain silence when necessary, commitment and strength to realise our vision.   *F.F.E.*

LAVENDER *Lavandula*

Helps connection with the higher self and for feeling inner guidance more clearly. Helps to integrate spirituality into daily life, which is often an area of difficulty. Eases emotional tension and brings in a state of calm and peace. Good for those who are physically tense and tend to overstimulate themselves physically, mentally or spiritually (or all of these).   *S.M.*

Lavender activates the crown chakra, connecting us with the higher self. This essence works to clear the karmic blockages that prevent spiritual progress. Lavender also gives balance to those who absorb too much spiritual energy, often resulting in afflictions to the head, neck and shoulders. It teaches the soul how to moderate and regulate spiritual-psychic energy.   *A.F.R.*

Connection to higher self for karmic releases.   *C.H.*

This essence connects people to their higher selves, to remove karmic blockages that are hindering progress. It increases visionary states and can be used to bring emotional balance, as it brings harmony to the feelings. It is also good for people who suffer from nervous oversensitivity.

Planets – Uranus, Neptune

Chakra – 7th   *M.E.F.E.*

Lavandula augustifolia

Antidepressant, for migraines and neurological headaches. Aids contact with own true self and the soul's purpose, will bring enlightenment. *S.C.E.*

Lavandula spica

Soothes and cleanses. Creates a feeling of space and stimulates a clear overview. Good for meditation, balancing the emotions, easing conflict and releasing blocks. Apply to the brow★★.

'My thoughts are calm and clear. l am at peace'. *H.R.*
Emotional support.

Use it to improve sense of smell, to regulate sleeping patterns and for general pain relief. It is indicated for ME, for childbirth, as an aid to digestion – it improves peristalsis of the digestive tract – and can help to regulate menses. It works on the heart centre to promote 'self-love' and 'self-worth'. May also be useful for skin/mouth ulcers and cold sores. Possible aphrodisiac tendencies! Grounds and centres, strengthens all the chakras and balances the subtle bodies.

A useful aid for psychic development. Associations include the colour blue, direction North, planets Mercury, Jupiter and Neptune, Tarot 4 of Disks. *A.F.E.*

Lavandula officinalis

Mercury, Jupiter. Calms and balances. Crown. Opens 1st, 4th, 7th, 8th and 9th chakras and energises 10th chakra. Gives clear insight and understanding. Helps to hear the music of the spheres. Blends the physical, etheric and astral. Removes karmic blocks. For overstimulated nerves – helpful when some spiritual practices and too much meditation can lead to nervous disorders and insomnia. *J.J.*

Spiritual sensitivity, highly refined awareness. For those who are nervous and who have over-stimulation of spiritual forces which deplete the physical body. Keen awareness and alertness.

Cleanses meridians, stimulates visionary states, connections to Higher Self. Karmic and past life conflicts eased. Useful for spiritual practices, especially where there are emotional conflicts blocking spiritual growth. *G.M.F.E.*

LAWSON CYPRESS *Chamaecyparis lawsoniana*

"The Path". Helps identify correct action and one's true needs. Initiates change in the right direction. Increased communication between mind and body. Discipline to attain one's goals and spiritual direction. *G.M.T.E.*

LEMON *Citrus limon*

Balancer.

Lemon is said to stimulate cell regeneration so it is indicated for psoriasis★, eczema★, acne★, stretch marks, scars etc. It reduces blood acidity and balances the digestive juices so it could be useful for stomach ulcers and dyspepsia. Use it to release mental stress, balance right/left brain function and so enhance mental clarity. It is also indicated for hypoglycaemia and may be useful to reduce cholesterol. Lemon gives psychic protection from negative thought forms but not from deliberate attack, it deals with karmic issues on a purely spiritual level. It opens all the chakras and balances all the meridians. Associations include the colour blue, direction North, planets Moon, Mars and Neptune, Tarot Lust.

*Lemon heals the skin but not the cause of the problem so it would also be necessary to find a means to release emotional stress. *A.F.E.*

LEMON BALM *Melissa officinalis*
Sun, Jupiter. Good for concentration. Aligns the chakras. Helps open 3rd and 4th chakras – helps the mental body. For those allergic to cats and dogs. Great healer. Remembering past lives. Comfort to the dying. For groups and spiritual unity. *J.J.*

LEOPARDSBANE *Doronicum pardalianches*
For those who are at a point of major change, but feel as though they are living on a knife-edge. *B.E.*

LESSER CELANDINE *Ranunculus ficaria*
Increasing mental faculties, concentration and memory. *L.L.F.E.*

LESSER STITCHWORT *Stellaria graminea*
For "possession", i.e. for those whose behaviour is dominated by others or by strongly held ideas. *B.E.*

LEWISIA *Lewisia*
Strengthens the immune system, helpful over long term use in all immune system illnesses and diseases. *C.H.*

LEYLAND CYPRESS *Cupressocyparis leylandii*
"Freedom". Helps ease hidden fears and anxieties, increases positive attitudes and sense of humour allowing a sense of freedom to grow and feel comfortable in. For those who dislike being by themselves. *G.M.T.E.*

LIGULARIA *Ligularia*
Far, eardrum infections, perforations, balance. *C.H.*

LILAC *Syringa*
PHYSICAL USE: produces antibodies for spinal inflammation, cleanses and replaces spinal fluid, eases pinched nerves in the spine, disperses solidification of the vertebrae thereby increasing flexibility of the spine. *A.F.R.*
Spine. *R.D.*
Christ consciousness, unconditional love *C.H.*
White lilac. This essence mainly influences the spinal column, working on many things associated with the spine. It also improves posture and gives increased flexibility to the spine. Lilac opens up all the chakras and activates the kundalini energy which travels up the spine.
Planets – Mercury, Jupiter
Chakras – All *M.E.F.E.*

Syringa vulgaris
For ease and grace of movement. Opens and connects the chakras. Helps to lessen rigidity in the body (especially spine) and mind.★★
'I yield, bend, sway and surrender softly to life's changes. *H.R.*

Venus. Flexibility. Aligns the etheric, mental and spiritual bodies. Associated with the fairy kingdom. Good for cleansing and all problems connected with the spine. For rigid attitudes.   *J.J.*

"Spine". Eases all aspects of the spine. Activates all chakras. Helps posture and tension in the back. Lilac is closely aligned with many different types of nature spirit.
G.M. T.E.

Syringa vulgaris 'Massena'

For those whose personal development has been stunted, often caused by a dominant parent.   *B.E.*

LILY *Lilium*

Viruses, builds up immune system for protection.   *C.H.*

Pink lily. Strengthens the veins (and arteries to a lesser extent).   *C.H.*

Lilium 'Apollo'

The Lily essence is for the spiritually insecure, bringing peace, serenity and comfort. These souls are finally reaching their destination or life's purpose, bringing recognition of their whole spiritual being. This realisation can bring great feelings of insecurity and until they can actually become at one with their spirit, they can easily have their faith and security shaken, sometimes rocking their very foundations. This remedy will bring back emotional and spiritual balance so that these souls can carry on, safe in the knowledge that God, creator of all things, is guiding them and their foundations will, once again, become as solid as a rock.   *C.H.*

Lilium 'Enchantment'

This opens up the base and sacral chakras, to release anger and frustration, then allowing the kundalini to rise up the spine in a natural way.   *S.M.*

Lilium 'Star Gazer'

Ability to use power and spiritual talents wisely and with discretion.   *A.T.*

Helps link with the planetary energy of Venus, unconditional love.   *C.H.*

LILY OF THE VALLEY *Convallaria majalis*

Safety, by enshrouding the negative tendencies of the subconscious mind that can draw in trouble.   *H.F.E.*

Menstrual and associated problems, ovaries etc.   *C.H.*

For yearning. For those who have become blocked by desiring the unattainable. *B.E.*

LIME *Tilia platyphyllos*

Keynote: Oneness

Lime helps us open our hearts to the light and love of our universal being. From this awareness we experience our interrelatedness on earth and create harmonious relationships in our lives.

Indications: Introspective or too focussed on self, over-identification with lower self/personality, feelings of powerlessness, over-dependency, fear of domination, intolerance, prejudice or nationalism, lack of awareness of the whole, separativeness.

Attributes: Knowing and experiencing the self as universe, transfer from identification with lower to Higher Self, unification of individual consciousness with collective consciousness and environment, transmuting self-preservation into detached world service, humanitarian activity through recognition of need, service, relationship and sense of responsibility; group consciousness.　　　　*F.F.E.*

LIME (EUROPEAN LIME, LINDEN) *Tilea x europaea*

"Development". Shifting levels of consciousness without disorientation. Calms anxiety where related to practical use of one's psychic and healing potential. Doubts and fears ease. Past programming is lessened.　　　　*G.M.T.E.*

LOBELIA *Lobelia*

Spiritual qualities, peace.　　　　*R.D.*

'Wakes up" the eyes, good in the morning or as a swab (7 drops in a cup of water) over eyelids.　　　　*C.H.*

LOOSESTRIFE *Lythrum salicaria*

For feeling spaced out, too open, brings grounding. Aligns lower chakras bringing balance and spiritual integration.　　　　*C.H.*

Channelling and connection to higher levels. Helps to release grief, good with bereavement and separation.　　　　*L.L.F.E.*

Effect of taking essence: focuses energy to where it is needed. Improves circulation. Balances the energy of the body so the life force flows throughout, from Crown to soles of feet. Grounds in reality. Lifts the veil of our day dreams and returns us to reality to create the world of day dreams.

Presenting condition: Being in your head feeling detached from reality and the rest of humanity. Seeming to be in a dream. Withdrawing or escaping from the reality of what being human is about. Off with the fairies (or leprechauns). Especially when being used as an escape or distraction from the day to day problems of being human.　　　　*L.N.E.*

LORDS AND LADIES *Arum*

Balances inner masculine and feminine energies. Good for couples, people working together to take at same time to harmonise energies.　　　　*L.L.F.E.*

LOVE-IN-A-MIST *Nigella damascena*

Openness to loving and being loved. Increased clarity about one's motivations emotionally. Clarity for spiritual direction by easing frustrations and allowing clearer choices to be made. For getting back to oneself after setbacks. Calms and releases old emotional trauma. Increases energy and blood flow in the circulatory system, especially in the legs.　　　　*G.M.F.E.*

LUCOMBE OAK *Quercus hispanica "lucombeana"*

"Creative energy". Life-supporting creativity, inspiration, ideas. Increased mental focus. Commitment to act and bring change. Wisdom and compassion.　　　　*G.M.T.E.*

LUFFA

Skin disorders.　　　　*R.D.*

LUNGWORT *Pulmonaria*

Good cleanser of the lungs, also good for any associated diseases.   *C.H.*

Assimilation of vital force (chi, prana etc.). Ideal for use with breathing techniques. Releases blockages and deep feelings within lower centres to be consciously worked on.   *L.L.F.E.*

In the process of change we learn new ideas and have experiences which bring new understandings. Sometimes when the old patterns are deeply ingrained it is easy to forget these insights. Lungwort helps to reaffirm lessons and new beliefs. It also supports situations where teamwork is required, helping people to work together and share pleasures.   *U.F.E.*

Pulmonaria officinalis

Cleansing, clearing and protecting air space. Also opening psychic airways. 'Through breathing and meditation I create a clear space to inhabit'.   *H.R.*

Pulmonaria longifolia

Energises auric field.

Lungwort connects one with the lifeforce through the breath which can help re-energise the auric field. This process is gentle as it is in tune with the rhythms of the body and ideal for those of a delicate constitution. Useful in a spray. *L.F.H.*   *S.E.*

LUPIN *Lupinus*

Mental confusion. Integration and calmness.   *C.H.*

LYCHNIS *Lychnis*

Good for physical energy when energies have been used up in the healing process or energy is needed to be moved up from one chakra to another.   *C.H.*

MAGNOLIA *Magnolia*

Digestion.   *R.D.*

Recognition of Divine origins and soul memories. Crown chakra.   *C.H.*

Magnolia x soulangeana

"Restlessness". Eases restlessness and lack of clarity. Helps to maintain balance when difficult changes have to be made. Increases sense of freedom and relaxation. Learning from past experiences, a clearer idea of one's true identity.   *G.M.T.E.*

MAHONIA *Mahonia*

Brings balance to emotions through integration with thoughts. Solar plexus.   *C.H.*

MALLOW

Mallow helps us overcome fear of ageing. The menopause years are made easier. This essence is also indicated for those who experience shyness, finding it hard to reach out to others. It encourages openness, friendliness and warmth.

Physical use: reinforces skin regeneration, treats most diseases associated with the ageing processes.   *A.F.R.*

Mental stability.   *R.D.*

Fears of ageing, phobias relating to physical appearance. Diseases related to ageing.

C.H.

Malva sylvestris

Moon. Used for ageing, any stresses or tensions associated with the elderly. Tonic for the endocrine system. Pituitary. Invigorates the skin tissue, connections and veins to the brain. Helps to find the warmth of a loving relationship for it attracts love.   *J.J.*

For coughs, throat infections, stomach and intestinal conditions, can be used in the bath for abscesses, boils, burns, also used for bronchitis, catarrh and eczema. For loving yourself and accepting love as you love others.   *S.C.E.*

Malva neglecta

For understanding and encompassing the feminine aspects. For 'mother'/self-less' love   *E.E.*

MALTESE CROSS *Lychnis chalcedonica*

Cleansing bloodstream, for blood disorders.   *C.H.*

MANNA ASH *Fraxinus ornus*

"Happy with oneself". Heals the heart and emotions. Being honest with oneself about how one feels. Unresolved emotional issues. Increases understanding and access to creative levels of consciousness.   *G.M.T.E.*

MAPLE *Acer palmatum*

Jupiter. Balances yin and yang. Realigns the meridians. Good with acupuncture.   *J.J.*

MARIGOLD *Calendula*

Communication, joy.   *R.D.*

For energy depletion due to healing process or consciousness raising.   *C.H.*

For deep, unresolved anger that continues to surface. The constant blaming of others and the 'not fair, why me?' attitude.   *G.E.*

Calendula officinalis

Sun. When there is too much materiality, denial of spiritual purpose. Strengthening and comforting. Often connected with psychic matters. Great protection.   *J.J.*

Kind communication.

Marigold is indicated for those aggressive and argumentative types who enjoy provoking a reaction in their contacts with others. This essence helps develop assertive communication, but in a clear and compassionate way. *L.F.H.*   *S.E.*

For stomach disorders, duodenal ulcers, for eczema if used in a cream. For sore skin. When uncertain of your direction in life, for changes and those not motivated. *S.C.E.*

For where there is a rigid materialistic approach to life, often with a total denial of the psychic and spiritual dimensions.   *B.E.*

MARJORAM *Origanum vulgare*

Calms and soothes. Comforts and protects from harm. Supporting life in times of danger. Helps emotional release especially fear.

'I trust in the creative strength of the life preserving force'. *H.R.*

Restores power and will, deep memory and the knowledge of who you truly are. Strengthens the heart chakra. Marjoram is sacred to the Goddess Venus. *H.F.E.*

MARSH CAMPION *Silene*

Where capillaries are broken, helps to restore their link and reduce the effects physically. *C.H.*

MARSH GENTIAN *Gentiana pneumonathe*

Communication with the deepest and most healing levels of the self. The brow chakra is brought to a clearer perception of reality, purified of doubts and enabled to find quieter, deeper levels during meditation. A very deep healing of the spiritual nature allows development of fuller potential, while the mind is able to go beyond apparent darkness to see the underlying unity and love of creation. *G.M.T.E.*

MARSH MARIGOLD *Caltha palustris*

Attunement to the Golden Ray. Spiritualises solar plexus chakra. *C.H.*

Calmness and relaxation, helps with meditation. *L.L.F.E.*

MARSH ORCHID *Dactylorhiza*

Overcoming mental restrictions. Releasing negative thought forms and belief patterns. Overcoming worry. *L.L.F.E.*

MARSH THISTLE *Cirsium palustre*

The remedy for those locked in the past. For those who cling to old outmoded patterns of thought and behaviour. *B.E.*

MARSH WOUNDWORT *Stachys palustris*

For fretfulness. Letting go of old worry and distress. Releasing bitterness and discontent.

'I let go of old feelings from the past. I am open to healing and to the present'. *H.R.*

MAYWEED

This herb has one of those smells that is verging on offensive and its healing quality is about opening to what at first glance (or smell) may not seem acceptable. All life is one, all aspects of life are part of the cycle of life. Decay is as much a part of the magic of life as blossoming. Mayweed helps those who feel tormented because they think they are unacceptable, or they are being subjected to unacceptable behaviour by others. It helps to bring a sense of trust. *U.F.E.*

Matricaria perforata

Integration of different energies. Rising above conflict and stress. *H.F.E.*

Chamomilla recutita

Can be used for stomach conditions, can also soothe eczema, for lack of flora in the intestines. For feeling unloved, lonely, separated, emotionally detached. *S.C.E.*

MEADOWSWEET *Filipendula ulmaris*

Jupiter. Relaxes tension especially in the head. Can uplift. Good in groups. Throat chakra. Perfume expands the possibility to receive love. *J.J.*

False Persona.

Meadowsweet is for those who are concerned about their public image and may put on a false, superficial front. They are usually popular, but their sweet and flattering ways are often a guise for control and an insurance that others will continue to like them. Keeping up a false persona can be so stressful that they often 'take it out' on those close to them. This essence helps balance out such extremes of personality. *L.F.H.* *S.E.*

Keyword – 'Companionship'.

Negative aspects – Boredom in children. To be accepted in an unwelcomed space.

Positive aspects – For children and adults who are studying for exams. Concentration. To help young psyches to realise their potential. To keep one earthed. To aid and strengthen interpretation of omens and symbols.

Physical attributes – Aches in the left shoulder. *B.F.E.*

MELILOT *Melilotus*

Brings clarity of mind in children. *C.H.*

MICHAELMAS DAISY (LUNAR)

Use this remedy when there have been power struggles in past life relationships. Such struggles are usually centred around sex, money or authority. Many souls have a series of incarnations within a particular family: this flower essence works well with the negative karma of family power struggles which inevitably result from such close contacts over several incarnations. Jealousy over money, inheritance or family rifts that have occurred in previous lives can be resolved with this remedy. *A.F.R.*

MILK THISTLE *Sonchus oleraceus*

This remedy is for those who do not love themselves. Often they try to make up for this by trying to please others. *B.E.*

MIMOSA (SILVER WATTLE) *Acacia dealbata*

"Sensitivity". Increased awareness of what is going on inside self. Intuition is better understood. Ability to stand up and express oneself. A sense of peace. *G.M.T.E.*

MISTLETOE *Viscum album*

Balances sexual energy with love. Helps one to be an individual within groups. *L.L.F.E.*

MOCK ORANGE *Philadelphus*

Ability to make use of powerful energy and the material world in a sensible, balanced way. Helps those who are afraid of strong feelings and of losing control. Solar plexus energised, boosting immune system and sense of self. Increased ability to express oneself and one's power in a direct, creative manner. Base chakra strengthened to enhance creativity in mental processes and communication of ideas. Strengthens and protects uniqueness of every being. *G.M.F.E.*

MONKS HOOD *Aconitum napellus*

'Expels poisons'. For protecting spirituality. The ability to recognise and banish bad influences from one's life.

'My true identity and purpose cannot be harmed'. *H.R.*

Understanding the need for illusion, to protect one's spirit when vulnerable. Gives some protection to the 'psychic gate' when opening. For turning people away from what you wish to keep hidden. For those who feel too 'open', helps to draw strength from spirit. *H.F.E.*

For difficulties of long standing that have their roots in the distant past. Helps to bring one up-to-date. *B.E.*

MONTEREY PINE *Pinus radiata*

"Connectedness". Helps remove very deep trauma. Artistic blocks eased. Balances emotions, calms anxieties. Deep peace and connectedness to everything. At ease in one's body, physical well-being. Past life information. *G.M.T.E.*

MORNING GLORY *Ipomoea*

This is useful when we have a hard time waking up in the morning, are lacking in life energy or rely on addictive substances to pull us through. Morning Glory promotes a sparkling life force in tune with one's natural state of being. PHYSICAL USE: removes opiates from sympathetic nervous system and stimulates production of the endorphins. *A.FR.*

Nervous system. *R.D.*

Nervous system. Helps all signs of nervousness, gives morning energy. *C.H.*

Ipomoea purpura

Body rhythms.

This essence can be useful when one is leading an erratic lifestyle often requiring stimulants to stay alert. Morning Glory can gently regulate the body clock so the need for such habits is released. It becomes easier to wake up and feel refreshed. *L.FH.* *S.E.*

Ipomoea violacea

Helps people who don't feel good about themselves or who have low self esteem. These people tend to develop nervous afflictions such as stuttering, insomnia, or habits such as smoking or drug abuse. This essence can help in the breaking of such habits by addressing the root cause and offering support at that level. *J.W.*

MOSS

Acceptance, non-judgement, transmuting karma by living through it without judgement. *H.FE.*

Discranella heteromalla

Whole plant. This is to help those who fear freedom and lightness in their lives. Often a fear of dark spaces within the being. *B.E.*

MOSS ROSE

This essence is good for linking with the animal kingdom, thus enabling us to contact
our instinctual feelings. It can help us to contact our power animals allowing us to
manifest their energies. It can bring clarity in relationships by linking our conscious
to the subconscious, giving a deeper understanding of our two needs and allowing
them expression.

Planets – Sun, Moon

Chakras – 3rd, 4th *M.E.R.E.*

MUGWORT *Artemisia*

Muscular system, IQ. *R.D.*

Artemisia vulgaris

Psychic energiser.

Indicated for low blood pressure, contra-indicated for high blood pressure. Mugwort
stimulates the digestive tract giving a better assimilation of vitamins and minerals. Its
main use however, is for psychic work. Mugwort is spiritually cleansing and
protective, it pulls the subtle bodies together but weakens their boundaries, this
opens up all the psychic abilities especially mediumship and channelling. Ideal for
any meditation, shamanic or ritual work and well known for its use with lucid
dreaming and astral projection. Mugwort strengthens the silver cord but not as much
so as bindweed. It should be used with caution and respect! Associations include the
colours purple and black, planets Venus, Neptune, Uranus, Pluto and Chiron, Tarot
Ace of Disks. *A.F.E.*

MULBERRY *Morus nigra*

"Wrath". Powerful emotions released constructively. Freedom from remorse and
past pain. For those hurt by the world and who react with anger and cynicism.

G.M.T.E.

MULLEIN *Verbascum thapsus*

Inner truthfulness.

This essence can bring the courage and strength to be true to the higher self and
embrace one's rightful path in life. Mullein can be supportive as one explores a sense
of individuality in the face of possible opposition. *F.H.* *S.E.*

For group attunement and purpose. *C.H.*

Verbascum densiflorum

This essence is used for male fertility, also for gastritis, neuralgia and rheumatic pain.
For when you feel you are not living up to your own and others' expectations, trying
to change. *S.C.E.*

MUSHROOM *Boletus edulis*

High level astral protection from psychic attack. *A.T.*

NASTURTIUM *Tropaeolum*

Nasturtium invigorates. It draws in light through the crown chakra, opening locked

doors and allowing fear to lift or subside. For doing what is needed in the moment, removing fatigue and grounding the light. Works also on sacral and brow chakras.
S.M.

Joy.
R.D.

Rigid, narrow obsessive thought patterns. Colour awareness. Good for tiredness after spiritual work/channelling.
C.H.

Brow chakra essence. For lack of awareness, boredom, mental tension and over-activity, delusion, fantasies etc. Encourages intuition, clairvoyance, conscious awareness, creative visualisation and thought, inspiration and insight. Treats dis-ease of the ears, eyes, sinuses and nose, cataracts, headaches behind eyes, endocrine imbalances.
A.F.R.

Tropaeolum majus

Mars. For energy. Good against negativity. For when changes need to be made. To let go of fear. Pituitary gland, endocrine system. For the over-intellectual who causes depletion. For loose earthly alignment. For depletion of the life force. Good for animals when dying. Useful in colour therapy.
J.J.

Balancing energy.

This essence is helpful for the dry, intellectual types who tend to drift into the realms of thought and detach from feelings. Nasturtium can also help to revitalise the mind after periods of excessive mental work. Useful during study.   *L.F.H.*   *S.E.*

Nasturtium leaf. To be able to dream the dreams of all things that are possible to me that I didn't even realise were available – seeing the dream that I know I understand.
A.T.

For those who know that they need to make changes in their life but seem to be unable to make the first move.
B.E.

NETTLE *Urtica dioica*

To provoke warmth and heat in the body and the temperament. For cold angry states and those who feel apart because of frequent hurt.★★

'I am protected by the fire within me'.
H.R.

Mars. Cleansing tonic. For those who blow hot and cold. Emotional states from a broken home, useful in divorce. For those who feel stung in life.
J.J.

Eases all stress associated with a broken home. Useful for asthma, inflammations of the nerves and damage to inner lung tissue. For problems with sibling relationships. Assimilation of nutrients and vitamins. Creates calm in emotional and etheric bodies.
G.M.T.E.

Heals the emotional stress which is associated with a broken home. Stinging nettle is useful for adopted children, those parents who have adopted children and divorced people. Sibling rivalries can also be eased with this essence.

Physical use: tonic to the kidneys and lungs. Asthma, neural inflammations and scarring of the inner lung tissue respond to this remedy.
A.F.R.

Relationships, emotions.
R.D.

For stress and trauma related to divorce, broken home. For all the family, adoptions.
C.H.

Increases willpower and resilience. Helps to develop patience. Overcoming unwanted
habits.   *L.L.F.E.*

There is a feeling of having been attacked when stung by a nettle and in the
homeopathic tradition of like curing like so the Nettle remedy comes to the rescue in
situations where a similar feeling of having been attacked is present. This feeling is
often accompanied by feelings of having been knocked off one's feet – 'unearthed' –
and of having one's energy 'scattered'. Nettle helps to restore a sense of balance,
enabling restorative action to be taken if necessary.   *U.F.E.*

NEW ZEALAND FLAX *Phormium*

Enhances the ability to divide in order to produce unity and growth. Strengthens the
separate aspects of the personality and therefore the whole. For those of proud
nature who have overstretched themselves. The 'networkers' essence'.   *I.C.*

Communication with spirit/higher self. Receiving and transmitting. Stimulates sixth
and seventh chakras.   *J.W.*

NORWAY MAPLE *Acer platanoides*

"Healing love". Love and acceptance, healing, nurturing energy for emotional shock
and trauma. Lightness, happiness, relaxation. Taking back control of life and power
for oneself.   *G.M.T.E.*

OAK *Quercus robur*

Acorn. For understanding the life-cycle. For strength.   *E.E.*

"Manifestation". Absorption and integration of very deep, hidden energy underlying
this Reality, the desire for stability whilst experiencing the polarities of existence.
Ability to manifest one's goals. Channelling energy.   *G.M.T.E.*

OIL SEED RAPE

For those with allergic reactions to oil seed rape.   *C.H.*

ONION *Allium*

Onion is a useful essence in counselling. It aids the counsellor in peeling away the
barriers or protection that surround the root problem. Onion encourages release of
emotions layer by layer in a safe way.

Physical use: opens the pores of the skin to receive more of the life force.   *A.F.R.*

Emotional stress.   *R.D.*

ONION FLOWER

Fulfillment of cycles, to allow change to happen.   *C.H.*

OPIUM POPPY

This essence is mainly useful in dealing with emotional states that can lead towards
drug dependency. Also the states caused by drug dependency, particularly by opium
based substances. It helps to break the dependency and will help to clear the residual
effects both in the etheric and on the physical level. It is good for waking you up
from any unreal dream state that you may create to avoid emotional issues.

Planets – Neptune, Moon, Mercury, Sun

Chakras – 5th, 6th   *M.E.F.E.*

ORANGE HAWKWEED *Pilosella aurantiacum*

Releasing blockages.

This essence is indicated when negative emotional energy starts to affect the physical body. This can be the final result of long-term stressful issues or the immediate effects of shock, operations, accidents, illness, birth for mother and baby etc. Orange Hawkweed can also help clear the effects of negative psychic pollution as this can have a detrimental effect on the physical body. If you feel stuck and don't know why, treatment with this essence might clear the body of old unconscious blocks. It can release the life force which brings an expansion of consciousness, clarity and a renewed growth.

N.B. Used alone the effects can be strong, for sensitive individuals use along with other essences particularly blue flowers. Partners well with Lungwort. *L.F.H.*   *S.E.*

ORCHID *Equestris*

Works on heart at many levels, but most importantly helps to regulate the heartbeat.
C.H.

ORCHID *Oncidium*

Enhances other remedies specifically working on strengthening and repairing the etheric body. *C.H.*

ORIENTAL HELLEBORE *Helleborus orientalis*

Major healing in the endocrine system. Reduces tension and over-excitability in glandular functioning and the emotions. Increases self-assurance and reduces shyness. Helps to establish one's goals and directions in life. Self-awareness, poise, clarity and balance. *G.M.T.E.*

ORIENTAL POPPY *Papaver orientalis*

Tendencies toward oblivion. Making the choice to live, to fully be here without escaping, numbing or pretending.

'I have the capacity to enjoy my life as it is'. *H.R.*

OSIER *Salix viminalis*

"Spiritual void". To contact Higher Self. Energy to adapt, change and grow. Useful when everything seems empty and useless. Energy and understanding. *G.M.T.E.*

OSTEOSPERMUM *Osteospermum*

Helps one to receive, to open up to others and the universal energy. *C.H.*

OX EYE DAISY *Leucanthemum vulgare*

This essence will relax, ease tension and stress, a tonic. For patience, increases one's own individuality. *S.C.E.*

PALE PINK ROSE

This essence helps us to reconnect with the faery realms. Working with the higher chakras it acts as a bridge to help us to cross to subtler realms where we can perceive and feel the workings of the elementals and devas. It is useful for those people who have grown too 'adult' and need to connect with their magical child within.

Planets – Chiron, Neptune, Pan

Chakras – 7th and higher *M.E.R.E.*

PANSY *Viola*

PHYSICAL USE: works against most forms of virus from common cold to AIDS.

A.F.R.

For all forms of viruses including AIDS and colds. *C.H.*

Viola wittrokiana

For hardy strength, builds up resistance when feeling low, vulnerable and susceptible to frequent illness.★★

'I am hardy and strong. I resist and overcome'. *H.R.*

PARSLEY *Anthriscus sylvestris*

Used for kidney disease, water retention, flatulence. For over response to emotional stresses, for a little more openness to yourself and to new ways of living. *S.C.E.*

PASSION FLOWER *Passiflora*

Christ Consciousness. *R.D.*

For Christ Consciousness. Helps sleep, dreamwork. Heart, throat, feet chakras. *C.H.*

Heart chakra essence. For those who are overly protective, withholding love – a closed heart, lack of sympathy, loneliness, depression etc. Promotes unconditional love, nurturing and compassion. Treats diseases in e.g. bronchial tubes, lungs, breast, heart and circulatory system. *A.F.R.*

Passiflora incarnata

Attunement to Christ Consciousness. Stabilises spiritual focus. Opens heart and throat chakras and eases tensions in the dream state. Works upon the spiritual body and brings sharper visionary states. Easier access to higher states of consciousness while remaining stable. *G.M.F.E.*

Passiflora caerulea

Creativity.

Apart from encouraging creativity it is also useful for reducing lethargy, anger and fear. Regular use releases resentments, past life issues and may bring inner child problems to the surface. It gives a good gentle de-tox, improves circulation, balances blood pressure and increases the metabolic rate by boosting the adrenals. Passion flower is also indicated for general pain relief, tooth decay, warts, constipation and sinus problems. It empowers all the psychic abilities especially channelling, giving some psychic protection by strengthening boundaries, grounding and centering. This essence works on the solar plexus chakra to reduce stress. Associations include the colour red, direction East, planets Mercury, Venus and Neptune, sign Aquarius, Tarot 2 of Swords. *A.F.E.*

PEACE LILY *Spathiphyllum wallisii*

Works at expanding consciousness via the belief system *C.H.*

PEACH *Prunus persica*

Helps bring the mind into order and calmness where there is chaos (possibly caused by trauma). *C.H.*

PEAR *Pyrus*

Brings balance to spiritual groupwork. *C.H.*

The pear flower helps to bring harmony to groups involved with spiritual endeavours. It integrates the mental, emotional and spiritual bodies putting things in proper perspective. It is also connected with music, amplifying the creative process for musicians.

Planets – Pluto, Chiron

Chakras – 2nd, 3rd, 5th *M.E.F.E.*

Pyrus communis

Venus. To ground and strengthen. Used with crystals, harmonics will activate the creativity of musicians. Harmonious in groups. Aligns mental, emotional and spiritual bodies. Increases elasticity. Balances the spine in conjunction with therapies. Strengthens 3rd/4th chakras. *J.J.*

"Serenity". Happy to be who you are. Clarity, simplicity, confidence. Reduction of stress in the nervous system. Increased enthusiasm, drive and energy. Deep peace. *G.M.T.E.*

PENNYROYAL *Hedeoma pulegioides*

Strength and clarity of thought, mental integrity and positivity. When there are negative thoughts absorbed from others, when there is psychic contamination. Protection from psychic attack by strengthening the etheric body so that thought forms cannot penetrate. Pennyroyal also expels negative thought forms from out of the subtle bodies. Eases mental confusion and can be of use with addictions. Schizophrenia and possessions. *G.M.F.E.*

Psychic protection. *R.D.*

For protection from negative thought forms. Solar plexus. *C.H.*

PENNYROYAL *Mentha pulegium*

A powerful purifier. Activates the crown chakra. Earths spiritual energies and unconditional love. Encompassing all life without judgement. *H.F.E.*

For displacement of negative thought forms. Feels like a fresh spring breeze after you've spent the night in a well used public toilet! *J.W.*

PENSTEMON *Penstemon*

Helps to keep attunement to spiritual path. *C.H.*

Penstemon barbatus

Encouraging.

For indecisive people. Releases hatred and anger constructively. Aids concentration by synchronising left/right brain function and eases depression. Penstemon is indicated for tinnitus, arthritis and eye strain. Long term use may encourage hair growth and reduce premature greying. It energises the spleen and stomach meridians, balances and closes the major chakras and repairs damage to the aura. Associations include the colour pale green, direction North, planet Saturn, sign Capricorn, Tarot Ace of Cups. *A.F.E.*

PEPPERMINT *Mentha*

Jupiter, Venus, Mercury. Clarity of vision. Struggle between upper and lower selves. Metabolic digestive complaints. A regulator – when craving for food which makes one sluggish, so the metabolism is unbalanced. Third chakra. Links to the higher nature. Lessens the etheric blocking of the soul. A balancer. *J.J.*

Mentha piperita

Clearing.

This flower can help to clear and cool down the thinking processes in times of great emotional strain or extreme mental activity e.g. muzzy or foggy head. *L.F.H.* *S.E.*

PERIWINKLE *Vinca*

Spiritualises those whose consciousness is at base/sacral chakra level. *C.H.*

Vinca major

Earths, empowers and protects the astral body. Prevents energy leakage. Adds impetus to one's intentions and life expression, by focusing energies and preventing dissipation. Good for recentering after astral experiences. *H.F.E.*

Vinca minor

For mouth ulcers, sore throats, eye conditions. A transitional essence, cleanses the bio energy field, so that you may connect with past lives. Also for those in the transition called death. *S.C.E.*

PERSIAN IRONWOOD *Parrotia persica*

"Alienation". Energy, emotional strength, drive, enthusiasm. Grounds spiritual energy into the physical body. Activates deep-level healing. Connectedness to the highest level of planetary consciousness. Strong sense of connectedness, belonging and joy. For feelings of alienation and weakness. *G.M.T.*

PETUNIA *Petunia*

Crown. Links to the higher self. Anti-depressant. For young children or elderly. Works on mental body, left brain. Good for stuttering and in meditation and visualisation. Can be put on bruises. For public speakers. Etheric and emotional links. *J.J.*

Petunia is an anti-depressant, encouraging us to go within and face the blocks or denials that are at the root of our depression. It also re-establishes proper psychological behavioural patterns and is especially good for hyperactive children, the aged and overly logical individuals. PHYSICAL USE: apply over external bruising and scar tissue. *A.F.R.*

Hyperactive children, meditation. *R.D.*

Enables one to see one's actions from a higher point of consciousness and thus to direct them in a more constructive manner. Would be helpful to young people going through adolescence or to old people in a state of senility. *J.W.*

Depression, tension. Childlike behaviour in the elderly. Impish children. Speech and left brain problems. *C.H.*

PHEASANT'S EYE *Narcissus poeticus var. recurvus*

For retinitis and other eye problems caused by friction, soreness from contact lenses etc.   *C.H.*

PHILADELPHUS *Philadelphus*

Crown and higher chakras, more contact with angels and archangels.   *C.H.*

PHLOX *Phlox paniculata 'Fujiyama'*

This essence embodies the idea of purity and what that means to us individually and collectively. Many ideas of personal purity in this day and age are misconceived; phlox helps with the change in perception that is needed to help us to love ourselves and to realise that we cannot be perfect in this life but that with love we can accomplish much and accept and understand the need for change. When we accept that we are all pure within, the need for self-abuse arising from a feeling of being unclean falls away and we are able to nurture ourselves with what we truly need within the physical. May be helpful with eating disorders and to remove toxins from the physical body.   *S.M.*

PINEAPPLE WEED *Chamomilla suaveolens*

Has sedative qualities, used for pineal gland. Deepens your spiritual connections with nature and to release inner knowledge.   *S.C.E.*

PINE CONES *Pinus sylvestris*

This is for those who are trapped by the authoritarian powers of others and feel unable to escape from them.   *B.E.*

PINK *Dianthus 'Mrs Sinkins'*

Jupiter, Sun. The flower of Zeus. Great healing powers of Sun energy. Gives strength. Grounding.   *J.J.*

PINK CAMPION

This essence has a very spiritual effect on the consciousness, giving a clear lucid state of mind that allows one to receive spiritual guidance and help from spirit guides and other great souls who are operating on this level. It operates on levels above the main seven chakras.

Planets – Venus, Jupiter, Chiron, Pan

Chakras – 6th, 7th and higher   *M.E.F.E.*

PINK CHERRY

This essence embodies the qualities of love. It specifically addresses problems some people have with perfection – often they are unable to let go totally into the experience of love because they perceive that they are not perfect. This remedy aids with seeing/accepting blemishes with love (not dismissing the whole for the sake of some damaged parts).

Pink Cherry facilitates the experience of 'oneness' where everything is equal and perfect and a manifestation of love.   *U.F.E.*

PINK PHLOX

This essence is for connecting the child to the adult, allowing the child within to manifest more in the adult world. It helps us to balance our inner child needs with our responsibilities, so that we can achieve a balance of work and play.

Planets – Moon, Jupiter, Saturn

Chakras – 3rd, 6th   *M.E.F.E.*

PINK FOXGLOVE *Digitalis purpurea*

This essence regulates cardiac function, also for sore throats, laryngitis. For feeling dependent on others or feeling over burdened by outside dependencies.   *S.C.E.*

PINK OXALIS *Oxalis articulata*

Flower and leaf. For the ability to communicate in truth, simplicity and gentleness.

E.E.

PINK PURSLANE *Montia sibirica*

This is the remedy for the self-opinionated, for those who go about with "blinkers" on.   *B.E.*

PINK RAMBLING ROSE

To help the heart chakra develop love in young souls, (not necessarily children). *C.H.*

PINK ROSE *Rosa 'Queen Elizabeth'*

An extremely powerful essence to help release and neutralise karmic fear. People in need of this essence will have been much troubled by fear, whether conscious or subconscious. When one has been treated with other 'fear' essences for a considerable time and they have barely scratched the surface Pink Rose is indicated. Very often people suffer from nervous diseases; they may be agoraphobic or asthmatic. It may be more subtle, fears of persecution, burning, water etc.   *C.H.*

PINK ROSE H.F.

For transmuting group energy and Karma related to the heart.   *C.H.*

PITTESPORA *Pittesporium tenuifolium*

"In two minds". Helps to clarify how one truly feels. Useful when loyalties are divided. Helps find solutions to mental worries and conflicts. Increases perspective and sense of humour.   *G.M.T.E.*

PLANE (LONDON) *Platanus x acerifolia*

"Fine judgement". Ability to discriminate subtle levels of the truth. Helps prevent introspection, melancholy and over-analysis. Broadens viewpoints and gives a peaceful space to meditate.   *G.M.T.E.*

PLANTAIN (RIBWORT) *Plantago lanceolata*

For turning resignation or a heavy heart into acceptance. Finding strength and joy in being grounded.

'By accepting my situation I renew my capacity for happiness'.   *H.R.*

Effect of taking essence: A wonderful confidence building essence. Helps give a sense of our uniqueness and divinity, there is a feeling of being surrounded in a halo of light. Accepting your own divine qualities and that everyone is at a different level.

Presenting condition: Feels inferior, feelings of deep hurt especially when you perceive you are being rejected. Can't make the grade, not good enough, seen but not seen therefore feelings of hurt and rejection.

Helps external wounds heal, as without so within healing the wounded child.   *L.N.E.*

Plantago major

An anti-inflammatory, good for the urinary system, cardiovascular system and for toothache and coughs. To be emotionally secure and accepted by other people, for fear and guilt   *S.C.E.*

PLUM *Prunus*

Colon cleansing and associated diseases.   *C.H.*

PLUM (LUNAR)

Plum is for the stresses and tensions created by past life sexual promiscuity. It brings wisdom, understanding and compassion to bear upon the incorrect use of sexual energy in the past, dispelling the emotions of guilt and self-disgust which can so easily attach to this type of karma.   *A.F.R.*

PLUM (VICTORIA) *Prunus domestica*

"Empowerment". Helps the highest spiritual energy enter into the material world. Practical solution to problems. Increased awareness of surroundings and effective use of personal power. Self-worth, self-motivation.   *G.M.T.E.*

POLICEMAN'S HELMET *Impatiens glandulifera*

For inflammation of the throat, lungs and for the female sexual organs. Will support you in the process of your spiritual development, will help you to be focused in meditation.   *S.C.E.*

POPPY

Energy and grounding, cleanses. Activates blockages in base chakra.   *C.H.*

POPPY *Papaver*

Helps overcome addictive tendencies, particularly opium.   *C.H.*

POPPY (LUNAR)

Lunar poppy is for those souls who have in previous lives stood on a battlefield and seen their comrades killed. Poppy is for the souls who have witnessed the most inhuman and barbaric scenes within the theatre of war. It also addresses the tensions created by losing loved ones during war.   *A.F.R.*

POTATO *Solanum tuberosum*

For coming down to earth. Feeling safe and centred. Calming down over excited states.

'It feels good to be calm. I enjoy being ordinary'.   *H.R.*

For depression caused by the inability to grasp new concepts.   *C.H.*

POTENTILLA *Potentilla*

Releases tension in joints.   *C.H.*

PRIMROSE *Primula vulgaris*

For lightness and cleansing, opening and relief. Help for tight held back feelings, toxic ailments and depression.★★

'I can let go now. I can release what is held. All is well'.   *H.R.*

Venus. Cleansing. Renewal after depressions. Raises the vital force. Five petals represent cosmic man. Clears toxins and mental blockages. Good for the liver. Leaves are used for sleep. A remedy for sensitives.   *J.J.*

Lightness to one's inner child.

Primrose is indicated when emotional childhood traumas inhibit personal growth. Melancholy and a deep unexplained sadness may be hidden away. This essence can gently nurture the inner child, give what is needed and open up a crushed spirit bringing comfort, hope and release. It's as if one can start anew, pure, unblemished and refreshed to life. *L.F.H.*   *S.E.*

Like coming home to a soft embrace, the softest touch. Can provide a feeling of non-judgmental support, the kind you get from stroking a pet after you have had a bad day. This essence is all about touch, the hands and possibly the tear ducts. Would be good for intuitive massage and for people who feel displaced to help them cultivate a sense of home. Like a hug from someone who knows and loves you.   *J.W.*

To help studying, mental growth, learning difficulties.   *C.H.*

Balancing the energy centres.   *L.L.F.E.*

Primrose is useful in situations where one feels out of one's natural environment. This can bring up feelings of confusion, paranoia and fear and a sense of being in a very confused and disordered environment. Culture shock would be a good example.

Primrose helps to provide a sense of inner stability and therefore, aids decision making. It also helps with electrical disturbances in the mouth caused by amalgam fillings which are not part of the mouth's natural environment.   *U.F.E.*

For stomach complaints, rheumatism, insomnia. Will help to develop spiritual compassion. Brings forward wisdom from past lives.   *S.C.E.*

For artists, writers and those involved with the creative arts, grounds the creativity bringing it into everyday life. For right-brain imbalance, helps concentration, memory and studying.   *G.E.*

PRIMROSE (LUNAR)

Primrose is the remedy for past life relationships. It is common for souls who have been very close in past lives to make pacts to meet up again at some point in the future: love, the emotional bonding between individual souls survives death. However there are other emotional bonds which are carried across, some of which are not particularly pleasant, life affirming or constructive to the relationship and it is these that primrose will bring to the surface and help the individuals to transcend.   *A.F.R.*

PRIMULA *Primula*

Understanding life's lessons and growing from that knowledge.   *C.H.*

PRIVET *Ligustrum*

Connecting with the Tao by understanding the cycle of uniting and dividing, opening and closing. Linked with the Dark Mother and the owl, Silence and Darkness. *H.F.E.*

Ligustrum vulgare

"Old wounds". Works with subtle bodies to repair physical shock and trauma. Creates harmonious vibration that helps to heal on fine levels. Increases life force to allow letting go of old wounds. *G.M.T.E.*

PULSATILLA *Pulsatilla*

Inability to focus on one thing. Unbalanced emotions, PMT. *C.H.*

PURPLE COMFREY

This remedy helps people who acknowledge that they have self-abusive behaviour. This abuse may take any form from smoking, to self-denial to self-mutilation.

Comfrey plays a fundamental role in herbal medicine and as a flower remedy it plays a fundamental role in self-acceptance and accepting mistakes. There are so many negative messages attached to self-abuse; Purple Comfrey helps to readdress the balance and allow some positivity and creativity to shine through. *U.F.E.*

PURPLE LOOSESTRIFE

Keyword – 'Wisdom'.

Negative aspects – Failure in exams. Last chance. Despair – lost in a maelstrom. Tension.

Holding on to negative thought processes. Moodiness especially in men.

Positive aspects – Relaxes. Reflection. Composure.

Physical attributes – When thoughts of disease bring fear and shame. *B.F.E.*

PURPLE TOADFLAX *Linaria purpurea*

For chest infections, coughs, the bronchia. For being aware of your sensitivities and believing in your own inner guidance, expression of feelings. *S.C.E.*

PUSSY WILLOW *Salix daphnoides*

Positive: For deeply loving and nurturing ourselves and our inner child, for knowing we are supported by life, for flexibility born out of responding to the real Flow of life, for self approval, relaxation, abundance, peace, joy and fun. New beginnings, renewal, cherishing and following inner dreams and talents. To comfort, soothe and nurture the newborn and children.

Indications: For anger, resentment, depression, rigidity, self-denial, self-defence, victim mentality, powerlessness, not honouring one's integrity. For too much doing and never Being, for when we have created difficult stressful situations and bleak lifestyles. For not allowing love, relaxation, abundance, beauty, fun and joy in our lives and patterns arising from a lack of love and support in childhood or from past lives of poverty and self denial.

Physical: To restore physical flexibility, for arthritis, depression, exhaustion, for spinal problems caused by lack of self-nurturing, feeling unsupported by life, driving oneself too hard and lack of flexibility. For eating disorders, anorexia/bulimia and weight problems: helps us to give ourselves the deep love and nurturing that we need and to let go of the need for control. Infertility in women, where there is a pattern of tension, overwork and denial of inner needs – to love and nurture and listen to the inner child. Rapid healing of wounds, cell regeneration, youthfulness and vigour.

L.H.F.E.

PYRAMID ORCHID *Anacomptis pyramidalis*

To be used for the pineal gland and all renal conditions. For trusting in others and recognising your own sensitivities.

S.C.E.

QUEEN ANNE'S LACE *Anthriscus sylvestris*

Helps with inner sight, seeing auras. For over intellectualizing and those who are confused. Pineal gland and crown chakra. For mental calm. Bridges the gap between physical and spiritual. Strengthens the rods of the eyes.

J.J.

Inner vision, eye problems, crown chakra.

C.H.

Cydonia oblonga

Loving strength, active femininity balanced with inner masculine. For those unable to catalyse or reconcile feelings of strength and power with essential qualities of the feminine self, or who have a distorted connection with the inner masculine self or animus.

G.M.F.E.

RAGGED ROBIN *Lychnis flos-cuculi*

Keynote: Purity

This aids in releasing, on all levels, congestion, obstruction and toxicity and facilitates the free flow of life force and energies.

Indications: Congestion, toxicity, obstruction, blockages, unclean living, hindrance of spirit.

Attributes: Inner purification, promotes circulation, facilitates free flow of life force, purgation, wholesomeness.

F.F.E.

Brings soul qualities into the physical.

C.H.

For nerve cells, bronchia, cardiovascular problems, arteries, capillaries, brain and spinal cord. 'I like to love, be loved and care for others'.

S.C.E.

Keywords – 'I love life'.

Negative aspects – Unable to celebrate life. When one is let down by a co-worker. Life is at 'boiling point'.

Positive aspects – To reunite – individuals, families, friends and communities. Helps you to avoid conflict. Sensuous. Be blessed.

Physical attributes – Pre-menstrual oedema.

B.F.E.

RAGWORT *Senecio*

Forgiveness of self and others.

L.L.F.E.

Senecio jacobaea

For trusting the body. Letting go of over active mental states. Centering all our separate selves. 'I love and respect my body and surrender all thoughts which are not in the service of my wise intuitive self'.   *H.R.*

RAMSONS *Allium ursinum*

Supports body's defences.

By bringing white light into a sluggish, toxic system, this essence can help cleanse the body, which if not corrected, can be debilitating and may deplete the immune system. This treatment can raise vitality levels and resistance to infection. Excellent as a spring cleanser, but also as a boost to the body's defences at the beginning of winter. *L.F.H.*   *S.E.*

This remedy comes up for people who are having 'problems' with other people, perceiving that it is the other person who has the problems. In these situations it is useful for the person being treated to see how the external situations can be mirrored internally and provide information about the sense of separation within.

Ramsons, therefore, aids in a growing sense of self-acceptance and self-responsibility.
                                                        U.F.E

RASPBERRY *Rubus idaeus*

Venus. Base and 2nd chakras. Cleanses the etheric. Used for bonding especially with children and the newly born. Releases a sense of fun which children know.   *J.J.*

RED CAMPION

There are times when we know that in order to move through a particular problem we must talk to someone else. Other times we may know that we are being affected by emotional problems but can't put a finger on exactly what the problem is.

Red Campion helps in sharing problems and in the release of emotional problems at a subtle level (not necessarily verbalised or consciously recognised). It is also useful in coming to terms with what we might perceive as failure, i.e. accepting that we don't always achieve what we aim for – the prize may be in the path rather than the goal.   *U.F.E.*

RED CAMPION (LUNAR)

This remedy is for those who have suffered in previous lives for being a wise woman. Give this essence to those who have been tortured, burnt at the stake or persecuted in other barbaric ways for possessing female wisdom. Red campion also has the ability to work with the whole range of emotional issues that arise out of such abusive past life treatment, so what is an extremely complicated karmic wound is simple to treat with this one remedy.   *A.F.R.*

RED CHESTNUT *Aesculus x carnea*

"Fear for others". A feeling of serenity and protection at a deep level of being, both for oneself and others. This reduces fear and anxieties and brings a peace and detachment from the worries of what may, (but probably won't), be. Helps create a clear, positive, unselfish link with others. Fears and phobias ease.   *G.M.T.E.*

RED CLOVER *Trifolium pratense*

Well known 'for shock'. Calms and soothes any person, child or animal who has had a fright. Lessens the tendency to panic or react in an unharmonious way. Helps the release of fear and encourages concentration on our own needs.★★

'I trust that the world will care for itself, if I care for myself'. *H.R.*

Mercury. For shock. For those in a panic. To help lose identity with the negative forces. Helps to lead in a crisis. Throat and base chakras. For all emotional issues which cause blockages. Balances right/left brain. Helps oneness with animals. *J.J.*

A powerful cleanser and balancer. It can be used when there is a need to be strong, aware, calm and balanced in an emergency situation, when all around are succumbing to panic and hysteria. PHYSICAL USE: strengthens the blood vessels.

A.F.R.

Calm, peace. *R.D.*

Brings a calm mind to situations of panic. *C.H.*

Lack of focus, confusion, indecisiveness. *L.L.F.E.*

Has a dermatological key. It is used for psoriasis, eczema and as a sedative for the lungs. For intolerance of others and for feelings of rejection. *S.C.E.*

This is for those who are blocked off by fear of their own emotional nature. *B.E.*

Positive: For letting go of fear, breaking the pattern of habitual fear, recognising that we are never alone and never have been, that we are powerful, not powerless and that we separate ourselves from our birthright of love and healing and everpresent good, by our fear. Red Clover helps us to disengage from fear, to let it be and let it go and to allow ourselves to experience a new reality of the complete safety, invulnerability, wholeness and union of our divine expression. For the understanding that we are constantly supported by life, if only we will allow and recognise this in our lives.

Indications: Panic, trauma, terror, accidents and emergencies, mass fear, crowd fear, panic attacks, habitual fears and phobias, fear – both conscious and unconscious, nightmares, faintheartedness, for when we are influenced by fearful images from the media or received fears from society, i.e. fear of the outcome of illness or accident, fear of cancer/Aids, fear of being alone, fear of annihilation, fear of abandonment, fear of violent attack, fear of food poisoning etc.

Physical: Kidneys, adrenals, heart, mind. All chakras, but especially the base, sacral, solar plexus and heart. Panic attacks. Any condition accompanied by fear and feelings of powerlessness. For accident and rescue workers, hospital and psychiatric staff, soldiers, police, aid workers, healers and all those who work in traumatic and stressful conditions. *L.H.F.E.*

RED DEAD NETTLE *Lamium purpureum*

Releasing and understanding suppressed anger. *L.L.F.E.*

Sacral chakra essence. Treats creative blocks, overly dry or serious personality, internalised anger, obsession with sex, confusion over sexual orientation, blocked or suppressed emotions. Encourages passion for life, increases creativity and libido, expression of sensual emotions and sexuality, detoxification. Eases diseases of e.g. reproductive organs, bladder, large and small intestines, stiffness in the body including arthritis. *A.F.R.*

RED OAK *Quercus rubra*

"Practical support". Bones and skeletal system energised. Growing conviction of one's place and purpose in the world. Clearing of self-doubt and false views. Very practical searching for the Spirit.   *G.M.T.E.*

RED/ORANGE ROSE

This essence enables one to tune into the heart's vision/wish. It stimulates the pineal gland enabling one to visualise the heart's ideals in a clear way. It helps to deal with wounds stemming from the parents, which impair the vision; by bringing the mother/father inside into a state of harmony. Freeing oneself to follow one's vision.

Planets – Mercury, Venus, Chiron, Neptune

Chakras – 3rd, 7th   *M.E.R.E.*

RED PHEASANT'S EYE *Adonis*

For angina and for heart conditions. For lack of physical energy and for anger. *S.C.E.*

RED POPPY *Papavar rhoeas*

For energy and vitality, both physical and mental. An uplifting essence, stimulating the base chakra, this could be used for people of low vitality, either physically or mentally, people convalescing though not after heart attacks as it may be too stimulating. Athletes and those in training could benefit; helpful for those who need to manifest their thoughts into action. May improve circulation.   *J.W.*

RED ROSE *Rosa floribunda*

For boldness and passion. Being true to your desires and against shame.
'I am proud of my passionate nature. I live a life of enthusiasm and delight'.   *H.R.*

RED ROSE-BUD *Rosa floribunda*

Opening up to love and sexual feelings. Puberty. New relationships.
'It is safe to give and to receive gentle tender love'.   *H.R.*

REDSHANK *Polygonum persicaria*

Anti-inflammatory, for piles, heart problems. Will connect you with the Christos energy and open the user to love, compassion and initiation.   *S.C.E.*

Effect of taking essence: Helps to see the inherent good in oneself. Allows one to take responsibility for one's own health and well-being. You ARE important. Realisation that it is not selfish to look after yourself.

Presenting condition: There is a sense of bitterness towards self, low self-worth. Being subservient and self sacrificing only adds to the feeling of bitterness. Putting others before self, feelings of I don't count. On a physical level may have circulation problems, diabetes or gallbladder problems, due to internalising the bitterness. *L.N.E.*

RED STRAWBERRY

This essence helps to calm emotional turmoil that threatens to engulf one. It allows you to look at the root of the problem and communicate it rather than be caught up in the surface turbulence. Also allowing the release of blocked emotions in a controlled way.

Planets – Moon, Mercury, Jupiter

Chakras – 2nd, 3rd, 7th   *M.E.F.E.*

RED TULIP *Tulipa 'darwinii'*

To overcome shyness. Not trusting one's fire (can be daring, vibrant and outgoing but tend to lose our centre).

'I am strong and centred. I can be outrageous. I give birth to myself'.   *H.R.*

REDWOOD *Sequoiadendron giganteum*

Body spray with essential oil.

Resilience.

Negative focus – Vulnerability, easily hurt by others, hooked into abusive situations, fear. Where extreme patterns of self-defeating behaviour create painful vulnerability. There is an inability to take care of oneself and feel supported in life. This flower essence spray can bring feelings of resilience and the ability to stay detached from others and in your own power. Helpful in relationships and supports commitment. Spray directly on skin around lower back and feet, two to three times a day.   *S.E.*

REST HARROW *Ononis repens*

Cleanses the urinary system, also the gall bladder. Supports the process of reawakening and will encourage spiritual strength.   *S.C.E.*

RHODODENDRON *Rhododendron*

Helps one towards following the will of the spirit.   *C.H.*

Rhododendron ponticum

This is for those who lack flexibility and keep trying to push through blind alleyways.
                B.E.

RHUBARB *Rheum nobile*

Exhibitionism. For the insecurity of being way off centre. Extrusive behaviour (talking too much etc.). Unaware of boundaries.

'I am good enough as I am. It is all right to feel my feelings. I let go of the need to show off'.   *H.R.*

RIBES *Ribes*

Diseases of the pituitary gland.   *C.H.*

ROCK ROSE *Helianthemum*

Stress buster, emergency use only.

For relaxation, physical stress and feeling 'burnt out', also releases guilt feelings. It helps tone muscle, reduce fat, balance blood sugar levels and acts as a diuretic. Unfortunately it uses up precious (Jing) life force energy to do all this, so use it in emergencies but use it sparingly. Rock rose is contra-indicated for thrombosis and varicose veins because it increases the risk of blood clotting. Associations include the colours purple and white, direction North, planet Mars, Tarot 4 of Disks.   *A.F.E.*

ROSE BAY WILLOW HERB *Epilobium angustifoliumn*

Numbness or 'cut off' toward others. Old defensive patterns that are hard to change.★★

'I release old injury and injustice. I can respond without fear'. *H.R.*

Connections to the etheric can become blocked causing one to feel alienated. Removes blockages in the subtle bodies so that energy can move freely. *J.J.*

Keynote: Power

Willowherb helps to balance the personality expressing self-seeking, authoritarian or overbearing behaviour, bringing about the responsible integration of will and power issues.

Indications: Self-aggrandisement, self-importance, judgmental, self-will, attached to power and position, authoritarian, eruptive temperament, oppression, anger.

Attributes: Integrity, self-empowerment, congruence, adept use of will, authority, self-tempering, humility, diplomacy, synergy. *F.F.E.*

Another remedy for letting go – letting go of the past, of old perceptions. A useful remedy for people who find themselves living in the past through reminiscing. Rose Bay Willowherb helps to move on – to see something familiar in a new way.

U.F.E.

Heart, circulation. For grief, renewed hope, relax your mind and listen to your heart. *S.C.E.*

ROSE *Rosa 'Alba Maxima'*

Mother.

The remedial qualities are to do with mothering and the bond between mother and child. A good remedy for those who have been denied this or to help with the bonding process during pregnancy and the infant years. Beyond this it also creates a bonding to earth helping those who find it difficult to concern themselves with earthly things. Physically it relates to the womb and is good for problems related to the reproductive system. Emotionally it brings a sense of being loved and nurtured. Spiritually it links to the Divine Mother. *C.F.R.*

Rosa 'Alexander'

Breath.

Alexander is a remedy related to the breathing system, excellent as a combination with Louise Odier to help the functioning of the heart and lung systems. Physically it relates to the lungs, throat and sinuses. Emotionally it helps to strengthen the will to live and to be alive. Spiritually it vitalises the centres in the lungs and those around the nape of the neck and shoulders enabling a better assimilation of the life force that enters at those points. *C.F.R.*

Rosa 'Arthur Bell'

Balance.

Arthur Bell is to do with balancing one's earthly life with one's spiritual quest. It is related to the fathering aspect of parenthood. Combined with Alba Maxima it makes an excellent remedy for all children who are experiencing the lack of some aspect of parenting and are going through a difficult time. Physically it is a remedy for the head and mind. Emotionally it brings balance and stability. Spiritually it is the harmoniser balancing the energies between mind, body and spirit *C.F.R.*

Rosa 'Blue Moon'

Clears shadow side from heart chakra. *C.H.*

Rosa 'Cadfael'

Peace.

Cadfael helps to bring calmness to those who find difficulty in resting. Physically it is for the nervous system where it helps to soothe a hyperactive system and to uplift the nervously tired. Emotionally it helps to steady the nerves to allow recovery from shocks. Spiritually it dispels fear of the unknown. *C.F.R.*

Rosa centifolia

Joy.

Raises the spirit. Moves beyond human grief, whether personal or collective. Enables one to see beyond tragedy to the reflection of joy. Restores balance after trauma, grief and destruction. Good for those involved in war situations, unrest and disruption. Links to the star Sirius, the Atlantean energies and the Sun or star within. Physically it works with the nervous system and emotionally the heart. *C.F.R.*

Church Farm Rose

Wisdom.

This remedy connects very much to wisdom and to the stars, a wisdom beyond earthly perception. It is a remedy for those who are seeking the truth and wish to expand their consciousness, to open the heart and mind to the wisdom of the divine source. Beneficial to those wanting to work on the higher levels of communication. It is very much connected to the spiritual aspects of mankind. Physically it helps to calm and clarify stress and trauma, confusion and instability. Spiritually it is an awakener. *C.F.R.*

Rosa 'Claire'

Clarity.

Claire helps promote clarity of mind and thought, helping to free us from negative thought processes, especially those who only see the darker side of life. Emotionally it helps those who are possessive and those who are possessed to release and be released. Physically it relates to all the senses helping to clean and clear them. Spiritually the clearer. *C.F.R.*

Rosa 'de la Hay'

Aligns heart chakra with crown, helping transform belief into inner knowing. *C.H.*

Rosa 'Evelyn'

Abundance.

Evelyn is a remedy relating to the generative organs. Physically the kidneys, bladder and reproductive systems. Emotionally it is for those who have suffered or are suffering abuse. Spiritually it connects with creativity and abundance. *C.F.R.*

Rosa 'Fisherman's Friend'

Purity.

Fisherman helps clean and purify the system. Physically it relates to the blood and bone systems. Emotionally it helps those who find life exhausting and burdens too heavy to bear. Spiritually it brings strength and enlightenment   *C.F.R.*

Rosa 'Gallica'

Humility.

A remedy for the over sensitive, fragile, weepy. The old and the new born that are delicate. Helps recovery from ill health. Brings purity to heart and mind. Links to the angelic realms and helps attain communication from these realms. Helps the spiritually ambitious to come back to a point of humility. Befriends the ego and prepares for integration of the ego and soul to reach the Christ light within. Relates to the brow and alta major chakras and the bloodstream. Its quality is peaceful strength. Helpful for those who work with lunar cycles and energies.   *C.F.R.*

Rosa 'Handel'

For strength, courage and the release of lack of self worth when stuck at heart chakra.   *C.H.*

Rosa 'Ispahan'

Gratitude.

To do with gratitude and graciousness. Useful for those who find it hard to receive and to say thankyou, to be loved by the world. Those who are disillusioned by life. Helps attune to the love aspect of the Divine Source, works very much with the higher aspects of the heart energy. Opens the heart to the Christ Light within, to Divine Love and prepares for the connection to Divine Love. Physically it relates to the heart working on the higher emotional aspects to open to Love Divine.   *C.F.R.*

Rosa 'Louise Odier'

Heart.

Louise Odier is a remedy relating to the heart centre covering all aspects of the heart. Physically the heart itself including stress related problems. Emotionally it is to do with all affairs of the heart including grief and heartache in its many forms. Spiritually it opens the heart centre and awakens a sense of beauty, creativity and spirituality.   *C.F.R.*

Rosa 'Maidens Blush'

Heart chakra, gentle loving energy, good for the sensitive and children.   *C.H.*

Rosa 'Mary Rose'

Protector.

This remedy is the protector, on all levels. Good for the worried, the nervous, the afraid. it has a calming influence which helps to restore a feeling of order back into uncomfortable or distressing situations. It gives Love to those who feel unloved. It helps those who can not seem to give or receive Love. Physically it relates to the immune system. Emotionally to the nervous system. Spiritually it brings protection.   *C.F.R.*

Rosa 'Peace'

For deep inner peace, transmuting any fear vibrations stuck in heart chakra.   *C.H.*

Rosa 'Pilgrim'

Light.

Pilgrim essence is for those souls who have lost hope, related to sight, vision and light. Physically it relates to the eyes and liver. Emotionally it is useful for anger and those who despair. Spiritually it helps to promote a greater acceptance and awareness of the Light.   *C.F.R.*

Rosa 'Regensberg'

Aligns all higher chakras.   *C.H.*

Rosa 'Spontanea'

Canary Bird Rose.

Aids, Alzheimer's, arteriosclerosis, arthritis, asthma, M.S., muscular diseases, toxaemia, dryness of body. Guilt, identity crisis, unbending rigid people, cleanses subconscious mind. Increases physical flexibility and vitality, sense of physical relaxation. General strengthener, oxygenates the body. Works on all chakras especially twelfth and wrists, all miasms.   *B.F.R.*

Rosa 'Superstar'

Brings energy to the heart chakra and helps to align it with the throat chakra.   *C.H.*

Rosa 'Swan'

Grace.

The Swan essence is related to the digestive system. Physically it is for the lower gut and intestines. Emotionally it helps resolve and release jealousy and peevish ness. Spiritually it brings an awareness of Grace.   *C.F.R.*

Rosa 'Sweet Juliet'

Twins.

Sweet Juliet is related to twins and twin energy. It helps those who feel alienated and not at home on earth to adjust to life on earth. A good remedy for the dreamer, the loner and the fear of earthly things. It has a strong link with the nature energies and is useful for those who need to link more closely with nature. It is the connector between heaven and earth, body and soul. Physically it is good for headaches, migraines, insomnia and the spine, particularly the lower back. Emotionally it is a good remedy for feelings of isolation, disorientation and problems arising from being a twin or a part of a multiple birth, especially if there has been a loss. Spiritually it has a balancing influence harmonising body and soul.   *C.F.R.*

Rosa tormentosa

Venus, Jupiter, Mars. Heart chakra. Spiritual love. Strengthens the etheric, opens 8th chakra. Best used alone. Brings peace and comfort. Links with the higher spiritual forces uniting human and spiritual love. A very high vibration connected to the monad. Gladdens the heart linked to Christ Consciousness.   *J.J.*

ROSE (LUNAR)

Lunar rose is for past life bereavement. It is not uncommon for the grieving process to take more than one life time to complete, particularly if the initial bereavement was so deeply wounding. Rose will ease the emotional burden of such bereavement. This type of past life loss can colour present life relationships detrimentally: over-possessiveness and deeply rooted fear of losing a loved one are common manifestations of this karmic condition.

A.F.R.

ROSEMARY *Rosmarinus officinalis*

'For remembrance'. This essence strengthens the heart and mind. Helps trust in friendship, strong bonds and common purpose. Especially good for fear of loss of love and for the freedom and autonomy of the sexes.

'I receive strength from friendship. I will always be loved'.

H.R.

Sun. When absent minded and forgetful, often when the incarnation is not well earthed. For psychic protection. When extremities are cold because of lack of warmth from poorly connected etheric/spiritual bodies. Stimulates the pineal gland and crown chakra to draw down the warmth of the sun to gladden the heart. Transforms, brings joy and light. A stimulator.

J.J.

Brings clarity when there is great emotional or mental stress, loss of trust, or confusion. Restores harmony by shifting the focus to the underlying perfection in all things. Helps with memorising and remembrance.

H.F.E.

Promotes trust by healing early traumatic experiences which have left us feeling vulnerable and insecure. Classic indicators for this essence are forgetfulness and spending a lot of time out of the physical body. Rosemary increases vitality within our incarnated being.

A.F.R.

Helps creativity. Brings joy to the unhappy and withdrawn personality. Crown chakra. Sharpens all five senses.

C.H.

Releasing stuck emotions. Cleanses and purifies energy system.

L.L.F.E.

For self-nurturing. Works on thymus, spleen, all chakras especially ninth, throat nadis. For white corpuscle imbalance and SV40 virus.

B.F. R.

ROSE OF SHARON *Hypericum calicynum*

Helps transmute vibrations of anger. Solar plexus.

C.H.

This essence gives access to past life information and teachings. It is particularly useful when there is a blockage towards manifesting this knowledge, as it involves a release of power which the individual may find difficult to handle. It enables us to manifest this power in a safe way. This remedy can help to develop or retrieve knowledge of healing through the hands.

Planets – Sun, Mercury, Venus, Pluto, Chiron

Chakras – 4th, 5th

M.E.F.E.

ROWAN *Sorbus aucuparia*

Keynote: Forgiveness

Rowan helps us to let go of resentments and to heal old wounds. As we learn to forgive ourselves and others, we can heal the past.

Indications: Clinging to old behaviour patterns, judgmental, avoidance, self-pity, shame, defensiveness, self-destructive patterns, unwillingness to give in and let go, resentment.

Attributes: Ability to forgive oneself and others, learning from past experiences, resolving karma, harmony through conflict, releasing stored tension and pain, facing deep repressed emotions.   *F.F.E.*

"Nature". Attunement to the energies of nature, particularly wood and earth. Enlarges perspectives to a cosmic level, allowing deep understanding of the universe.
G.M.T.E.

Evoking soulfulness. To draw on the rich experience of personal attachment to people, places, nature and culture. Embracing the familiar, the unexpected and the paradoxical. Refining the raw materials of life into something valuable.
'My experience is grounded by the deep threads of soul'.   *H.R.*

RUBY RED ROSE

For transmuting pain and sorrow from heart chakra into love and compassion. Attunement to the Christ Consciousness and the new ruby red ray of forgiveness.
C.H.

RUDBECKIA *Rudbeckia*

Raises lower emotional energies to the heart chakra.   *C.H.*

RUE *Ruta graveolens*

Energises and strengthens emotions and sensitivity, even to the extent of being an aphrodisiac. Gives energy to one's true desires and acceptance of oneself. Enhances appreciation of the body, improves self-image. Self expression as an aspect of one's spiritual nature.   *G.M.F.E.*

For water retention, can be used as a tumour inhibitor. For high ideals and compassionate thoughts.   *S.C.E.*

RUNNER BEAN

Removes spikiness and rigidity.   *A.T.*

RUSSIAN LETTUCE *Lactuta tartarica*

For sinuses, bronchia, throat infections. Encourages the user to find their true philosophy of life and to go with the flow.   *S.C.E.*

SAGE *Salvia officinalis*

For the wisdom of not taking oneself too seriously (essential secret of longevity). Awakens the higher self.
'I can relax and enjoy life. I affirm my essential foolishness'.   *H.R.*

Jupiter. Connects the mental/spiritual bodies. 2nd and 4th chakras. For unconditional love, wisdom in that we accept that we do not know everything. For not taking life too seriously, so it promotes long life. A balancer, for when too much mental energy makes one agnostic and too much spiritual energy makes one a religious fanatic. Great cleanser of negative psychic energy. Important in rituals.   *J.J.*

Ability to draw wisdom from life experience. To review and survey life processes from a higher perspective. Reduces the tendency to see life experience as ill-fated or undeserved. For those unable to perceive higher purpose and meaning in life's events. Aligns mental and spiritual bodies thus preventing religious fanaticism or atheism. Laughter, psychic faculties, philosophical interests. Strengthens etheric body, augments digestive system, cleanses meridians. Heart and solar plexus chakras.

G.M.F.E.

Wisdom.

When looking for a positive aspect on a difficult situation, past or present, sage can bring a detached viewpoint. This essence can help distil wisdom from life's various experiences and encourage one to see a new angle on the problem. *L.F.H.*   *S.E.*

Sage enhances the ability to see things as they are, in a grounded way and enhances the strength to accept that truth. Used to treat lack of acceptance of reality; shock, from bad news, sudden change; the feeling that you can't carry on in the face of the truth.

I.C.

Understanding of the Book of Revelation. Psycho-spiritual aspects activated. Jet lag.

C.H.

Solar Plexus chakra essence. For wisdom. Enables the soul to view life events from a wise or higher perspective. Treats victim consciousness, lack of control, stress, domination or abuse of others, anger, aggression, fatigue. Encourages the taking back of personal power, assertiveness, confidence, outward vitality. Treats diseases in the organs of digestion and purification – stomach, pancreas, liver, gallbladder, spleen, ulcers, diabetes.

A.F.R.

This essence aligns the mental and spiritual bodies bringing a balance between the two. It awakens interest in spiritual matters, psychic and mediumistic abilities. It also stimulates laughter. Sage helps the digestive system by producing enzymes and it is a good essence to take whilst fasting.

Planet – Jupiter

Chakras – 3rd, 4th

M.E.F.E.

ST JOHN'S WORT *Hypericum perforatum*

For protection, guidance and containment. Seals the aura and promotes sound sleep. Helps any frightened, anxious or paranoid state. Especially good with children or with psychotherapy.★★

'I can trust All is well. I am held and protected'.

H.R.

Sun. Releases fear from the past. Clears nightmares. Links with the Divine. For sensitive people who are prone to stress and negative elemental forces. Gives light through the darkness. Crown chakra.

J.J.

Illuminated consciousness, light-filled awareness and strength. For those who are too open or over-exposed leading to psychic and physical vulnerability. Eases deep fears and disturbed dreams. Releases hidden fears or obvious fears, including those from past lives. Ability to separate thought from emotion. Useful for skin complaints.

G.M.F.E.

Fear.

R.D.

Gives divine protection and guidance when in an overly-expanded, dream-like or 'spaced-out' state of consciousness; for vulnerability to harmful influences when spiritually open. For fears related to out-of-body experiences, fearful dreams, bed-wetting and other night-time childhood traumas; helpful for feelings of inadequacy and doubt. Chiefly affects solar plexus chakra.

C.G.

Karmic and hidden fears released. Nightmares. *C.H.*

For hyperactive children, PMT. It is also a sedative. For better communication, more self awareness. *S.C.E.*

Hypericum elatum

Energises and calms.

Provides motivation and inspiration. Calms and helps to release guilt feelings. Balances right/left brain function improving memory and concentration. Use it to help with general pain relief, amenorrhea, eye strain and poor circulation. It is indicated for angina, high blood pressure and varicose veins, it may also reduce cholesterol. Energises the meridians and the nadis. Very useful for reducing the shock caused to plants by pruning. Associations include the colour red, direction South, planet Sun, Tarot Queen of Swords. *A.F.E.*

SALPIGLOSSIS *Salpiglossis*

Emotional stabiliser for the over-sensitive. *C.H.*

SALVIA *Salvia*

Cleanser for bloodstream. *C.H.*

SAXIFRAGE *Saxifraga*

Balances mind, intellect and imagination. Peace, calm and detachment that allows space for new ideas and concepts to be carefully considered. Encourages the practical use of all spiritual experience. *G.M.F.E.*

SCABIOUS *Scabiosa*

Help to become more sensitive to and to feel energies. *C.H.*

Scabiosa caucasica

Enthusiasm to reach for new possibilities. Communication from and on subtle levels. Opening to higher learning. Finding other ways of doing things, exploring other worlds. Heals indifference and over-cool detachment from the roots of existence. *G.M.F.E.*

Succisa pratensis

For respiratory complaints, coughs, asthma and skin conditions. Helps to find self love and inner peace. Will help you to understand the laws of karma. *S.C.E.*

SCARLET PIMPERNEL *Anagallis arvensis*

Gives strength to those who feel taken over by others. Breaks psychic bonds. Helps the kundalini power. Aligns mental/emotional/spiritual bodies. Crown chakra. Assists the loving nature when kundalini awakens. *J.J.*

Eases the passage of kundalini when it has been awakened. Harmony in dream state: recurring nightmares and other dreams can be understood and assimilated. Vitalises pineal, pituitary and heart energies. Release of stored spiritual information and subtle emotions. *G.M.*

Strengthens and nourishes the navel chakra and etheric body. Strengthens against psychic contamination. Aids one to be recharged and nourished through meditation.

Replenishes creative and sexual energies. Good to use in meditation. Also helps to bring resentments into the consciousness, particularly linked with sexual issues.

H.F.E.

Stem, leaves and flowers. For understanding and encompassing raw earth/sexual energy. For vitality. For joy.

E.E.

This essence works mainly on the etheric levels. It is useful for people working with releasing kundalini energies, as it helps to activate the chakras and increases understanding of what is going on. It also helps people who have trouble with their father image and men who have trouble relating to women.

Planets – Mercury, Uranus, Pluto

Chakras – 4th, 6th, 7th

M.E.F.E.

Anaemia, disorders of the liver and gall bladder, skin infections, has a cleansing action. It also aids the intestines to absorb nutrients. Restores your physical endurance; for vague fears and feelings of rejection.

S.C.E.

For those who are emotionally trapped by others, often with a psychic dependence.

B.E.

Keywords – 'I breathe new life'.

Negative aspects – Inertia threatens. Expectations too high. Isolated in grief. Lack of communication.

Positive aspects – Breathes new life and love where previously life was barren. Allows one's tears to flow. Helps to understand loss. Support in time of crisis.

Physical attributes – For tough dry skin. Fear of snow. Liverish people. *B.F.E.*

SCILLA *Scilla verna*

Balancing energy levels.

This essence is useful when undertaking work activities that create an imbalance e.g. too much head work, driving, etc. Helps one to be calm, steadfast and clear about what is needed to re-balance the energy levels. Useful in a spray around head area. F.H.

S.E.

SCOTS PINE *Pinus sylvestris*

Keynote: Wisdom

Scots Pine helps us in finding directions in our search for answers. In being open to listening, we can be guided from within by the all-knowing self and the inner teachers.

Indications: Barriers to trusting inner knowing and intuition, blocks to inner and outer listening, resistance to hearing the truth, overly dependent on outside validation, indecision.

Attributes: True listening, trusting one's inner knowing and intuition, hearing inner spiritual guidance, openness to the Ancient Wisdom within oneself and nature, learning and teaching.

F.F.E.

"Insight". Helps activate third eye and development of subtle awareness in a balanced way. Brings penetrating insight and increases tenacity and patience. Broadens one's outlook.

G.M.T.E.

SCOTTISH PRIMROSE *Primula scotica*

Keynote: Peace

Scottish Primrose brings inner peace and stillness to the heart when confronted by fear, anxiety, conflict or crisis.

Indications: Fear, constriction, panic, shock, paralysis, anxiety, hysteria, inner struggle, conflict in relationships, disheartenment.

Attributes: Inner peace and stillness, coming back to earth, inner harmony, relaxation, purity of feeling, experience of love, compassion. *F.F.E.*

SEA CAMPION *Silene maritima*

For separation in early childhood and its consequent insecurity and fears. Stimulates loving protective energies. *B.E.*

SEA LAVENDER *Limonium vulgare*

For coughs, nerves, to ease throat infections, indigestion. A transformational essence, a spiritual cleanser. *S.C.E.*

SEA PINK *Armeria maritima*

Keynote: Harmony

This essence aligns and infuses our being with Spirit. Blending and melding our life force with Divine Will, it helps to balance the energy flow between all energy centres.

Indications: Burn-out or blocks in energy systems of the bodies, overload, stuckness, vacillation between the opposites, following desires of the lower self, craving stimulating experiences, untimely kundalini situation, split personality, the fundamental problem of the relationship between Spirit and Matter.

Attributes: Healing the split between higher and lower selves, soul and personality; achievement of stability and balance between the opposites, harmonisation of crown and root chakras and soul and form; surrendering the lower to the higher, will-to-be, kundalini awakening, magnetic potency which binds the soul and personality in functioning relationship. *F.F.E.*

SEDUM *Sedum*

Clears surplus bile from the system. *C.H.*

SELF HEAL *Prunella vulgaris*

Looking within for healing and nourishment. Releasing self doubt and confusion, developing self love and acceptance.

'I let go of suffering, take control and trust in my healing process'. *H.R.*

For taking control of ourselves, trusting in our own inner strength. Crown chakra. For assimilation of spiritual energy. Used with mineral waters when fasting. Strengthens the thermal body. Powerful cleanser of the etheric when this is weakened. Useful when one has lost confidence in one's own capacity for healing.

J.J.

Taking responsibility.

Self-heal can be used in all healing situations. It re-energises the life force from within, reducing the need to seek support from others. One can then take greater responsibility for healing the self through very difficult life challenges. *L.F.H.*   *S.E.*

Helps people who see others' problems better than their own to re-focus and get 'the beam out of their own eye'.   *J.H.*

Self-heal is appropriate for people who have 'their fingers in a lot of different pies' – giving their attention to many different tasks simultaneously. It feels a bit like juggling with a lot of balls and there is a sense that it is a bit too precarious and may all collapse.

Self-heal facilitates a sense of ease with the situation so that there is an experience of smoothness and competence with lightness and fun.   *U.F.E.*

Used for the throat and mouth, external wounds and arthritis. For sensitivity to one's personal and spiritual needs. Contacting one's intuition.   *S.C.E.*

Effect of taking essence: Cleanses the systems both physical, mental and spiritual, on all levels.

Part of a convalescence after a dis-ease.

Will give a really good spring clean. It will balance the feeling of 'phew – there's a lot going on for me'. Helps neutralise unqualified energies. A good tonic restoring spirit as well as body to bring back a sense of well-being and reconnection with our divinity. Revitalises. Works well in combinations.

Presenting condition: When the body feels under pressure from illness. Also the body is in need of a tonic, because of wrong diet etc. When convalescing, feeling lethargic or a lack of connection to higher self or divine source.   *L.N.E.*

SERBIAN SPRUCE *Picea omorica*

This remedy is for those whose "male" energy is lacking, producing frustration and a lack of clarity.   *B.E.*

SIDALCEA *Sidalcea*

Helps bring to consciousness past associations with Greece.   *C.H.*

SILVER BIRCH *Betula pendula*

This essence is about balance, but not a static balance, balance in motion, in time. This is tied with the tree's natural grace and beauty – grace is perfect rhythm. This is the natural pattern of movement in time. The essence rebalances systems that are out of sync and acts as a regulator. Also good for skin conditions, especially peeling ones and for people with problems caused by unbalanced subtle energy rhythms which ultimately result in physical ailments.   *J.W.*

Gives flexibility to thoughts, ideas flow. Arthritis.   *C.H.*

"Beauty". Ability to experience beauty and calmness. Tolerance of self and others. For those who find it difficult to express themselves.   *G.M.T.E.*

SILVER MAPLE *Acer saccarinum*

"Moods". Helps balance the flow of energy through the body and regulates mood swings.

Realigns the meridians, so useful for acupuncture.   *G.M.T.E.*

SILVERWEED *Potentilla anserina*

Keynote: Simplicity

Silverweed helps us to detach ourselves from material concerns and over-indulgence, by promoting moderation and self-awareness.

Indications: Overindulgence, fussiness, pernickety, narrowmindedness, disconnection from spirit, self-centredness, greed, pretentiousness.

Attributes: Awakening to spirituality, breakthrough of self-awareness, integrity, self-discipline, enjoyment of simple pleasures of life, getting back to grass roots, moderation, frugality, humbleness. *F.F.E.*

For bladder and kidney complaints, throat infections and painful menstruation. For poor self image, feelings of frustration or limitation. *S.C.E.*

SINGLE SNOWDROP *Galanthus nivalis*

For those experiencing difficulty in breaking through to new levels of awareness and consciousness. *B.E.*

SINGLE WHITE CHERRY *Prunus shirotae*

Promotes antibodies, balances right and left brain. Breathing trouble and bronchial conditions, colds, fevers, laryngitis, mucous colitis, sinus congestion, hay fever, throat diseases, typhoid fever, viral inflammations. Emotional cleansing, frustration, grief, guilt, immaturity, past life problems, self-righteousness, stuttering, lack of discipline. Cleanses subconscious mind. Works on all miasms, all chakras especially 10th, lung meridians; finger, hand, heart and throat nadis. *B.F.R.*

SKULLCAP *Scutelleria gallericulata*

Facilitates contact with the Divine/the Higher Self. Clears the head and calms the system, can help clear head pain where it originates from congestion; clears blocks in the crown chakra and helps where the spiritual connection has been lost and a person feels isolated and alone.

Helpful for childbirth. Chakras chiefly affected are crown and sacral. *C.G.*

SLOE

Keywords – 'I am fragile yet I can live through a storm'.

Negative aspects – Fragility. Things are falling apart. Bad judgement. Fickleness. Forgetfulness. Frustration. Fear of success.

Positive aspects – Rebirth of creativity and knowledge.

Physical attributes – Inner knee pain. Lassitude in shoulders and arms. Headaches. *B.F.E.*

SNAKE'S HEAD FRITILLARY *Fritillaria meleagris*

Smoothness to the skin, skin complaints. Throat. *C.H.*

SNAPDRAGON *Antirrhinum*

Larynx. *R.D.*

Speech difficulties, throat problems, helps express emotions. *C.H.*

This essence is for treating the vocal cords, lips, jaw, facial tissues and muscles. It also treats allergies that manifest as spots on the skin. It is primarily physical in its effects, but also helps one to express feelings when there is difficulty, such as in the case of stuttering. It can help one to release anger that has been held back.

Planets – Mercury, Venus, Mars, Jupiter

Chakra – 7th   *M.E.F.E.*

Antirrhinum majus

Allowing expression of so called 'negative' emotions. Irritation in the throat or voice. Tightness in the face (lips and jaw). Frustration and speech problems.★★

'I express myself clearly and boldly. All my feelings and valid'.   *H.R.*

Lively dynamic energy; healthy libido; verbal communication that is emotionally balanced. Counters verbal aggression and hostility, repressed or misdirected libido. Eases tension around jaw. Aligns cranial plates, tempero/mandibular joint disorders (TMJ) and throat disorders. Speech disorders, self-expression and communication.

G.M.F.E.

SNOWDROP *Galanthus nivalis*

Simplicity, innocence and trust. Sexual cleansing. Protecting your inner child.

'I affirm my essential innocence. I am open and trusting and safe'.   *H.R.*

Spiritual confidence. A clearer direction in life. Increases the ability to plan practically – energises the thought processes. Brings insight, imagination, discernment and healing wisdom.   *G.M.F.E.*

Keynote: Surrender

Snowdrop allows us to surrender to the end of past events and attachments in life. In the death of the old we find the seed of our eternal inner light and behold new vistas.

Indications: Personal darkness and suffering, negative or destructive attitudes, fear of death and dying, depression related to seasonal darkness (S.A.D. Syndrome), dark night of the soul, grief.

Attributes: inner radiance in times of darkness, resilience, inner strength, ability to yield, letting go as a prelude to spiritual rebirth or initiation, acceptance of the processes of death leading to liberation, knowing of the Eternal Self, detachment, transcendence of the form side of life, optimism and hope for the future.   *F.F.E.*

Energy blocks, cleansing.   *R.D.*

Bereavement. Allows hope and joy to return.   *C.H.*

This is the essence of inner awakening at the end of a long period of darkness or dormancy. It helps to awaken the energies and prepares for new things, like the light at the end of the tunnel, it offers new hope and a new way forward.

Planets – Sun, Saturn, Pluto

Chakras – 1st, 7th   *M.E.F.E.*

Snowdrops are the first flowers associated with the beginning of a New Year and this essence was the first made in the Unitive range. It represents aspects of the underlying qualities of the remedies as a whole.

Snowdrop facilitates group consciousness, supporting the fundamental aim of the Unitive range to promote Unity within and between individuals, be they cells, organs, people or groups. One of the main contributing factors to distress of any sort is the inability to see beyond the personal and/or individual. Illness, traumas, parts of the body, home, work, play, environment, family etc, tend to be seen in isolation of each other whereas every aspect of our lives and environment are interrelated and can be seen as a whole. A movement of perception from the individual to a wider understanding of the Universe requires trust and an inner peace – Snowdrop brings courage and tranquillity. *U.F.E.*

Enlightenment.

Body spray.

Negative – Frozen and numbed out feelings, blocked creative expression. Heart and sacral energies closed, particularly when situations are perceived as threatening. When someone has taken on much negativity. Little free exchange of energy.

Positive – Cleansing and purification of emotions. Moving you to a place where you can start again. Gives new light on situations and initiates forgiveness and trust. Frees up energies, learning to hang loose and be more enlightened, open and creative. Beginning to hold personal power but being able to let go and connect in loving situations in a different way. *S.E.*

SNOWDROP (LUNAR)

Snowdrop is given to heal the deepest wounds society has inflicted upon the soul in previous incarnations, or the soul has inflicted upon society; it is for the abused and the abuser. It brings a greater sense of true self or individuality which was lacking in previous lives. The sense of self may well have been lost or distorted in a previous incarnation whilst functioning within the bounds of social convention; snowdrop helps to deal with the imbalances in the present incarnation which are a result of the self being denied in previous lives. *A.F.R.*

SNOWFLAKE *Leucojum vernum*

A positive space within which the Self can flourish. Clarity of purpose, one-pointedness and confidence. Calms and quietens the emotions to experience deep silence and the flow of universal energy and information. Helps protect from unwanted external thoughts and feelings that would interrupt the correct Path for the individual. *G.M.F.E.*

SOAPWORT *Saporania officinalis*

Mental cleansing. Heart chakra. *C.H.*

Saponaria ocymoides

For use where there is bewilderment and lack of vision. For the "What the Hell am I doing here?" type of feeling. *B.E.*

SOLOMONS SEAL *Polygonatum*

Mental relaxation. *R.D.*

Polygonatum verticillatum

For the busy mind. This remedy helps bring quietness and detachment. *B.E.*

SORREL

Sorrel grows in many forms depending on the conditions in which it grows. The energy of the remedy can match many characteristics; it is useful for those who recognise that their state of being has a tendency to be dependent on their external circumstances. They may feel out of control of their feelings – depending on who they're with or what arrived in the post they can experience wildly varying emotional states from day to day; for example adventurous, anger, vulnerable, worthiness, tenderness.

Sorrel helps with the understanding that we are a product of our environment but that we are also self-determining. *U.F.E.*

Rumex acetosa

For kidney and liver complaints and acute muscular weakness. For feeling consumed by worry or fear, uncertain about the future. *S.C.E.*

SPEEDWELL *Veronica*

Stem, leaf and flower. For understanding and encompassing change. For renewal.
E.E.

For children in times of change and mental growth. *C.H.*

This essence is the traveller's remedy as it enables you to go from one place to another with a sensation of effortless ease. No sooner than you have set off it appears that you are arriving. It is useful if you have a lot of small journeys to undertake e.g. delivering messages or a long journey.

Planets – Sun, Mercury, Jupiter

Chakras – 3rd, 4th *M.E.F.E.*

Most people experience at some time a feeling of not wanting to return to ordinary life – maybe after a good holiday or course of study. There is a perception that doing the same daily routine for the foreseeable future will be dull and that nothing exciting will ever happen again. Speedwell lightens this perception bringing an understanding that by living in the moment we can carry a sense of anticipation and newness into daily routines. This is not a one off change in perception; it requires a resolution to change – Speedwell supports this. It is also a useful remedy for those who dislike the cold, which is a related issue in that part of the change in perception which comes with Speedwell is an acknowledgment of the rhythmic nature of life of which the seasonal changes are the most obvious. *U.F.E.*

Veronica officinalis

Safe travel, moving with ease, changes, crisis periods, 'more-haste-less-speed' situations.

'I see clearly my new direction and therefore travel with ease'. *H.R.*

Has diuretic qualities, a tonic after illness or operation. Will help tissues to repair. For mental exhaustion, problems with decision making. *S.C.E.*

Veronica persica

Jupiter. More haste less speed. For safe travel and movement. For seeing the way clear. *J.J.*

SPINACH

Develops the higher octave of the heart chakra. Shifts the focus from giving on a

personal level to a universal level. For growing out of a repeated pattern. Strengthens
one's spiritual integrity. Oneness.   *H.F.E.*

SPINDLE
Overcoming frustration and aggressive tendencies.   *L.L.F.E.*

Euonymus europaeus
"Self-integration". Understanding one's true nature and needs. Increased sense of
security, reducing the need to compare oneself to others. For feelings of
superiority/inferiority. Energises soul, accesses energies of the shadow-self in an
integrated, positive way.   *G.M.T.E.*

SPOTTED ORCHID *Dactylorhiza fuchsii*
Keynote: Perfection
Spotted Orchid enables us to go beyond pessimism and self-interest to seeing the
best in everyone and everything.
Indications: Cynicism, self-centredness, pessimism, inability to see beyond oneself
and personal circumstances, nostalgia, stuckness.
Attributes: Self-expression, nurturing and creativity, positive outlook, inspiration,
seeing the best in everyone and everything.   *F.F.E.*

Dactylorhiza maculata
For skin disease, also for the lungs, infection and catarrh. For fear of being unloved,
emotional traumas.   *S.C.E.*

SPRING SQUILL *Scilla verna*
For major change points in a person's life when they are prepared to open up to new
views of reality.   *B.E.*

SQUARE-STALKED WILLOW HERB *Epliobium tetragonum*
Overwhelmed when bombarded with mental activity or ideas. Unable to function
properly, "can't see the wood for the trees". Square-stalked willow-herb helps one to
focus and unscramble the mental activity, producing clarity of thought. Profoundly
calming, good for meditation, stillness of the mind and insomnia.   *G.E.*

SQUASH
Hormonal balance.   *R.D.*

STAGS HORN SUMACH *Rhus typhina*
"Meditation". Brow chakra energised. Flow of information. Balances energies for.
meditation. Stills mental and emotional processes while allowing clear intuition and
communication at deep levels.   *G.M.T.E.*

STAR OF BETHLEHEM *Ornithogalum*
Trauma.   *R.D.*

STINKING HELLEBORE *Helleborus foetida*
Balances love and power. Helps break out of conditioning and outer influences which

seek to 'mould' you, while maintaining a state of love. Protects the heart chakra.

H.F.E.

Releasing negative energies from aura. Helps with flow of energy through meridians. Brings flow to life, overcoming rigidity.

L.L.F.E.

STITCHWORT *Stellaria holostea*

Brings a joy and lightness to the emotions and releases cares and worries. Once this process is underway there is an increase of calming, quiet energy where one can rest in relaxed alertness. Releases excess energy wherever it may be in the system. *G.M.F.E.*

As an essence it will boost your immune system after trauma, operation, also for skin conditions. To be open minded and ready for new pathways in life, new ideas, new insights.

S.C.E.

STONECROP *Sedum*

This essence is connected to the wounded child that needs to feel part of a family. It is the child within us that wants to feel warmth and protection with a group of people that feel like a family. Stonecrop can help us to find our own healing family where we feel secure and loved. It also helps to promote group healing and can be used by a group to focus healing energy, to someone either in the group or absent.

Planets – Moon, Chiron

Chakras – 3rd, 4th

M.E.F.E.

Sedum anglicum

Keynote: Transition

Stonecrop helps us to maintain inner stillness whilst in the process of breaking through inertia and resistance to change in the face of imminent transformation.

Indications: Resistance to change, stuck in the past, loneliness, isolation, inertia, stagnation, stubbornness.

Attributes: Profound self-transformation, revelation, incarnation, breakthrough, self-reliance, patience, inner stillness, state of grace.

F.F.E.

STRAWBERRY *Fragaria vesca*

This will increase the blood flow; for stomach upsets and various inflammatory disorders. For being open to new ideas, to counteract negative thinking; releases over burdening.

S.C.E.

STRAWBERRY TREE *Arbutus unedo*

"Quietude". Quietens and clears the mind of all unnecessary thought. Brings stillness and silence, which allows change to occur on deep levels. Energises crown chakra. Good for healers and meditation.

G.M.T.E.

STRELITZIA *Strelitzia*

Renewal, rejuvenation. For feelings of vulnerability, not knowing which way to go. For times of crisis and for inner strength. Helpful for the terminally ill, or those in bereavement, for loss, separation, alienation.

G.E.

STREPTOCARPUS *Streptocarpus*

To help regulate stools, diarrhoea. *C.H.*

SUMACH *Rhus typhina*

For those who ignore their own potentials due to fear of loss of their old identities.

B.E.

SUNDEW *Drosera rotundifolia*

Effect of taking the essence: Helps with awareness of possible opportunities for growth. Some opportunities are taken and others are passed by. Often when opportunities are not taken we can live in regret of that "missed opportunity". This essence helps to release these feelings of regret and therefore allows us to be alert to all future opportunities as they present themselves.

Sundew can also help with discerning the most appropriate opportunity at this particular time. It will increase our sensitivity within our discernment and increases the potential for one's synchronistic development.

On a physical level, it helps with glandular problems, especially in early teens and at the start of adulthood. At this time we are unsure of ourselves, our independent life is just beginning. If we have not had the appropriate support in childhood we can feel emotionally insecure to go out into the world. We may be unequipped for the opportunities that will present themselves. These feelings of being overwhelmed by having to make our own decisions lead to a real feeling of lack of "support" which can be turned inwards.

Presenting condition: Nothing seems to work for me, insecurity because of living in regret of missed opportunities, can dwell in the past. Lack of childhood support resulting in a lack of confidence and an indecisive nature. *L.N.E.*

SUNFLOWER *Helianthus annus*

Aligns all chakras from throat to feet, connecting to the earth guardians. A balancing essence for those who have too much 'father' energy. Helps to remove sun toxicity. Good to take when meditating to connect father sun to mother earth for healing.

S.M.

True enthusiasm and balanced masculinity. Softens the ego. For disconnectedness to the feelings, stress and deprivation. *H.F.E.*

Empowerment.

When the male aspects of the personality are under-developed sunflower can bring greater empowerment. Like the sun, one feels able to radiate outwards and reach for the peaks of personal achievement. It can balance an overdeveloped ego. Also useful where there are problems with the father figure. *L.F.H.* *S.E.*

Balances the ego. It helps us to shine and show our true self. Sunflower is also associated with the masculine aspect of self; it is useful for a poor relationship with one's male self or father.

Physical use: improves posture, strains in the spinal column and heart disease. Eases sunburn and heat exhaustion. *A.F.R.*

Spine. *R.D.*

Father problems, male ego, spiritualising, heart chakra. *C.H.*

SWEET CHESTNUT *Castenea sativa*

"The Now". Focussing and centering in the present moment. Release of guilt, particularly alienation with physical world. Creates detachment and understanding to regain wider perspective. Finding ways out of difficult situations.　　*G.M.T.E.*

SWEET PEA *Lathyrus*

Helps you to live in the now, grounding, overcrowded families.　　*C.H.*

Lathyrus odoratus

Libra. For relationships. Helps those who do not know where they belong and are always searching, never becoming involved, always moving around. When one needs bonding to the community. When there is little sense of belonging to the earth. Those lonely and seeking. For those who are antisocial or escape into fantasy. Good in overcrowded situations.　　*J.J.*

Sweet Pea is given for antisocial behaviour and the need to develop a sense of social responsibility. It helps us to form a connection with the community, home and Mother Earth. Sweet Pea is also useful for those who live in overcrowded or urban situations.　　*A.F.R.*

Lathyrus latifolius

To help people to come to terms with living in crowded conditions. Stimulates the pancreas. Just as the flower seems to be throwing a hood from over its head, this essence can help individuals to do this for themselves or their own situations.　　*J.W.*

SWEET VIOLET *Viola odorata*

For loving. Believing in and practising unconditional love with oneself and others. Allowing oneself to be more loving and most of all to let in the love that is around us. 'I surrender to love'.　　*H.R.*

Venus, Moon. Links to the 7th ray. For the very sensitive. Yin energy – calming. Strengthens the immune system. Purifies the lymphatics. For those who are poor mixers. For those who have a highly refined soul force, who do want to shine, yet hold back for fear of losing their identity. Often feeling lonely. Appear cool, yet have inner strength. The subtle perfume flows and helps to shift the fears to open and flow with the warmth of others. Very much a new age essence. Protection from radon.　　*J.J.*

Acceptance of one's spiritual self.

This essence is indicated when one has a strong awareness of the spiritual side of life but through a fear of rejection, denies this aspect of the self. White violet brings feelings of self acceptance, truth and trust, so it becomes safer to be open with others. Useful in spray around crown. *F.H.*　　*S.E.*

Opens crown chakra. For forgiveness of others.　　*C.H.*

For lack of self-worth, love and forgiveness of yourself, releasing past negative patterning and traumatic events from this life and allowing you to let go and move on.　　*G.E.*

SYCAMORE *Acer pseudoplatanus*
Keynote: Softness

Sycamore recharges and uplifts body and soul when we are stressed allowing the emergence of a soft yet powerful new energy supply.

Indications: Profound fatigue and exhaustion, worn down over time by effort or over-exertion, depletion of energies, stretched to the limit, at breaking point, spiritually testing times, negative influences, bad environmental effects, heavy hearted, stress.

Attributes: Ability to tap inner reserves of strength, patience, constancy, endurance and persistence, continuity of effort, catalysing energy, restoring gentleness and smoothness in our energy flow, surrendering strain, conflict or anxiety, setting boundaries, encouraging when facing challenges, tests or trials; enthusiasm, softness and openness, ability to be flexible and resilient under stress. *F.F.E.*

"Lightening up". Energy levels increase, so helps with lethargy. Awareness of the sweetness of life, harmony and relaxation. Lifts heavy moods. *G.M.T.E.*

TAMARISK *Tamarix gallica*

"Fire of transformation". Finding spiritual direction, freeing up energies for personal expansion and growth. Deeply cleansing and uplifting, cleanses age-old dross for the true self to emerge. *G.M.T.E.*

TANSY *Tanacetum vulgare*

Causes one to look at oneself and examine one's motives, while providing some protection against outside influences. *H.F.E.*

Drive.

When there is lack of motivation, procrastination and a poor sense of self, it becomes difficult to see a way forward. Tansy can help one to connect to a solid centre within, bringing an instinctive sense of the right direction, which propels one forward into action. *L.F.H.* *S.E.*

For the deeply ingrained pattern of opting out of life and withdrawing energy when faced with emotional trauma of any kind. Those of us in need of Tansy may appear withdrawn, indifferent, lazy or indecisive. This essence helps us to reconnect with life. *A.F.R.*

Strengthening and sedatory.

Ideal for couch potatoes and computer buffs or anyone who has been mentally overstimulated because it brings peace and quiet to the brain. Excellent for insomnia for the same reason as it encourages deep, restful sleep. Can be used to reduce the pain of mental stress. Contra-indicated during pregnancy. Tansy strengthens all the subtle bodies and closes all the major chakras. Associations include the colour pale blue, planets Moon, Mercury, Venus and Mars, relates to Gemini, Cancer and Libra, Tarot Lovers. *A.F.E.*

For varicose veins, rheumatics. Transforms spiritual ideas into matter. Will help you to connect with inner guidance. *S.C.E.*

TENBY DAFFODIL *Narcissus obvallaris*

For muscular weakness, tetany, osteoporosis and as a nervine laxative, asthma, eczema and for rheumatoid arthritis. To attain deep inner wisdom, use this as a light tool, which gives guidance on which spiritual path to take. *S.C.E.*

THISTLE

To release defence mechanisms built up around aura by ego, i.e. spikes, armour. *C.H.*

Cirsium vulgare

Keeping integrity and self respect. Staying faithful to our own views. Loyal to and supportive of those who share them.

'I respect myself, my own beliefs and personal truths'. *H.R.*

Keynote: Courage

Thistle helps us to find true courage in times of adversity and to respond with positive action.

Indications: Fear, dread, threat, immobility to act, powerlessness, frightening situations, fight/flight syndrome.

Attributes: Courage in the face of adversity, empowerment when facing great challenge, strengthening, facilitates confident action, fortitude. *F.F.E.*

Buds. Enables you to unfold your mysteries by being your own true self. *A.T.*

Buds. Made overnight. Joining in the higher spirituality into being here. *A.T.*

The purple Spear Thistle has a beautifully lush and delicate flower head atop and surrounded by a formidable construction of thorns. Some people construct an energetically similar barrier around themselves to protect their inner being but this barrier usually causes a deep sense of separation between themselves and others. The barrier may manifest physically as an overweight body, or mentally as a very defensive attitude. The sense of separation can result in a deep unhappiness and lack of self-confidence.

Spear Thistle works gently to bring a sense of trust and openness – that I can open my heart and still feel protected. As with Speedwell this issue is deeply rooted and will not be resolved overnight. Spear Thistle supports the intention and brings the experience of ecstasy which comes when the heart is open. *U.F.E.*

THISTLE (LUNAR)

This is the remedy for past life imprisonment. Incarceration for long periods of time causes deep wounding to the soul and may well have to be healed in future lives. Often there is deep frustration and anger still felt as a result of having lost the freedom of a past life; this can be projected onto almost anything. This remedy also treats the loneliness and isolation of the past life detention and the psychological effects of being separated from loved ones which can manifest in the present life relationships. *A.F.R.*

THORN-APPLE *Datura stramonium*

'Soulvine'. Aids movement between different planes of existence. Breaking conditioning and limitations of the mind. Seeing the oneness of life and death. Taken after using the Henbane essence, it can take one deeper into the death initiation. This is a very initiatory essence and should be taken with the utmost respect and with clarity of motivation. *H.F.E.*

Helps people unlock their creative potential which may have been protected by psychological barriers put up in childhood or past harsh experiences. *J.W.*

Cleanser and stimulant.

Works on the pituitary to stimulate the mental process. Could be useful long term for dyslexia and has indications for ME and MS. Thorn apple assists the repair of all physical tissue damage, it helps to clean the blood, lower blood pressure and encourages the lymph system to de-tox. Use when dealing with food and drink – but not drug – addictions. It can cause a slight increase in the metabolic rate and could be used for some types of pain relief. Thorn apple is especially recommended for tension headaches caused by constricting blood vessels, brilliant for hangover headaches. It stimulates all the psychic abilities, energises the meridians, cleans, realigns and heals all the subtle bodies. Associations include the colours brown and green, direction East, planets Moon, Saturn and Neptune, Tarot Hanged Man. *A.F.E.*

THRIFT *Armeria*

Helps bring art, spiritual, scientific concepts into consciousness. *C.H.*

Armeria maritima

For skin blemishes, skin cancer, blood. For emotional support for oneself and others. Lack of self acceptance. 'Yes, you can love yourself'. *S.C.E.*

For helping to open up the psychic sensitivity but keeping the person firmly grounded at the same time. *B.E.*

THYME *Thymus*

Thyme is used when there is not enough time. It has the ability to alter our perception of the flow of time, thereby allowing it to speed up or slow down. It can be used for past life work. It is also an amplifier of other essences, speeding the healing process. *A.F.R.*

Strength, augments other essences. *R.D.*

Amplifies other flower essences. Past and future lives. *C.H.*

Attunement with devas. Helps to connect to inner joy. Brings back a sense of humour to serious people. *L.L.F.E.*

Thymus vulgaris

Venus. Etheric/mental bodies. 3rd, 4th and 9th chakras. Left brain. Alters the time flow of love to the heart. Will speed up remedies being taken. Used in far memory trips. Can travel from the past to the future – our cells carry the blueprints, thyme helps release the information. Gives a sense of direction. Linked to the animal kingdom. *J.J.*

Used as a sedative, for coughs, bronchitis and whooping cough. This essence can be used with all essences. A healing protection essence. *S.C.E.*

TOADFLAX *Lunaria*

Inner ear, perforated eardrum, hearing and balance. *C.H.*

Lunaria vulgaris

Mars. Deals with connections to the throat or voice. Aligns emotional/mental/causal bodies. For any inability to speak or express. Verbal aggression. For when the lower centres are unbalanced and creative expression is not communicated. *J.J.*

TOBACCO *Nicotiana*

Clears the body of nicotine. Helps people deal with dependency on all levels.   *J.W.*

Helpful for nicotine addiction.   *C.H.*

TORMENTIL *Potentilla erecta*

To resist being crushed. Refusing to be dispirited or overpowered. Springing back
with renewed confidence and hope.

'I have the faith to overcome whatever tries to put me down'.   *H.R.*

This essence helps to ease the tormented mind. If you are experiencing a lot of
mental pain and are needing a rest from it for a while, tormentil will shut things
down allowing you to rest. It won't necessarily deal with the problems but will give
respite. It could be very useful if someone is on a 'bad trip' and would like to close
down the mind for a while.

Planets – Moon, Mercury, Neptune

Chakras – 3rd, 7th   *M.E.F.E.*

There are times when a fundamental aspect of one's being rises to the surface and
begins to assert itself – it can be seen as the child within asserting itself. This
assertion can herald a change in one's being – a gathering of energies to create a new
pattern, a new way of being. Tormentil brings a quality of strength and an ability to
handle the shift which is being undergone.

Keywords – 'Go forth and multiply'.

Negative aspects – For women who have lost their partner. For children who do not
'hear'. Pure anger. Hopes for survival.

Positive aspects – Feeling of 'eternal life'. Reclaiming one's creativity.

Physical attributes – Dehydrated. Migraines.   *B.F.E.*

TRADESCANTIA *Tradescantia*

Helps repair torn muscles and heal muscular system.   *C.H.*

TREE LICHEN *Usnea subfloridana*

'Wisdom". Accesses past knowledge and ancient wisdom. Brings a sense of
independence and detachment without isolation. Letting go of things no longer
needed, in order to grow.   *G.M.T.E.*

TREE MALLOW *Lavatera arborea*

Develops the spiritual heart. Soothes pain, gives strength and allows rapid growth
through adversity.   *H.F.E.*

Enhances the ability to connect with the inner, ancient knowledge. For those who
feel the weight of ignorance a burden; for those who feel worthless because of lack of
perceived or learned knowledge.   *I.C.*

Developing visualisation enhancing the ability to manifest on earth plane.   *L.L.F.E.*

TREE OF HEAVEN *Ailanthus altissima*

"Heaven on earth". Dynamic, energising, spiritual energies. Maintains integrity of
self whilst removing barriers and allowing growth of new levels of awareness.
Practical spirituality, practical wisdom.   *G.M.T.E.*

TREFOIL *Trifolium dubium*
Used for the lungs. To help one express new ideas and oneself. *S.C.E.*

TRILLIUM *Trillium*
Spiritual understanding and love for Mother Earth, appreciation of its beauty. *C.H.*

TRINE TREE *Carpinus betulus quercifolia*
Synthesis.
A rare form of Hornbeam bearing 'leaves like the Oak' hence its latin name. This tree can bring strength and endurance when struggling to harmonise opposing aspects of life i.e. giving equal importance to the diverging needs of the body, mind and spirit. Supports health as it regulates all body systems during times of personal growth, crisis or stress. *H.B.* *S.E.*

TUFTED VETCH *Vicia cracca*
For circulation problems and chilblains if used in a cream. To trust in your feelings, use your intuition, for protection from over involvements. *S.C.E.*
Sexual difficulties caused by an incorrect sexual self-image – usually due to childhood conditioning. *B.E.*

TULIP *Tulipa*
Brings pride in one's work and self worth in a dignified way. *C.H.*
Clears blocks in heart center. Brings an open and loving energy to all aspects of life. *L.L.F.E.*

TULIP TREE *Liriodendron tulupifera*
"Spiritual nourishment". Nourishing on spiritual levels, particularly for those feeling restless and dissatisfied or those with addictive tendencies. Finding positive outlets for energy and expression. Artistic. Balance for meditation. *G.M.T.E.*

TUTSAN
This essence opens us up to the flower kingdom allowing us to tune into these subtle energies, making us aware of any flowers that may be needed. By bridging the gap between the human and the plant kingdom we can heal the wounds wreaked upon nature by man and at the same time heal our own personal wounds.
Planets – Sun, Mars, Pan
Chakras – All are involved *M.E.F.E.*

VALERIAN *Valeriana officinalis*
Keynote: Humour
Valerian lifts our spirits and helps us to rediscover delight and happiness in living. It helps us to be at peace by taking ourselves lightly.
Indications: Weighed down by sense of responsibility, over-seriousness, the glamour of being busy and hard-working, hurry and worry, over-striving, stress and tension, too focussed on one's own problems, sombreness, lack of sense of fun or humour.
Attributes: Experiencing life wholeheartedly, contentment, sensibility, sensitivity to impression, ability to laugh at oneself, pleasure, delight and happiness in being, joyful thanksgiving, true appreciation, spontaneity. *F.F.E.*

A karmic essence for lack of interest in present circumstances. Perhaps this person is subconsciously locked into past incarnations, possibly to happier times in the soul memory to which it would like to escape, therefore unable to focus on the present. Valerian is the key to unlock that door so that we may realise the importance for our soul to learn this life's lessons thoroughly and to let go of the past. Also for those continually needing 'grounding' to help stay in the body. *C.H.*

For those who have not had their need for love fulfilled during their childhood. *B.E.*

VALERIAN *Centranthus*
White valerian. Calming, soothing. Brings peace and light and enables one to rest. Good for shock and stress. *H.F.E.*

Centhranthus augustifolium
Venus. For the pathetic. Those who are lost, never having received true love, so they find it difficult to love themselves. *J.J.*

Centranthus ruber
For emergency use. Dealing with specific shocks. For when one is feeling overwhelmed, by any intense emotion or experience. It is good to follow with white valerian. *H.F.E.*

VETCH
Spiritual independence. To go away from guru needs. *C.H.*

Vicia cracca
To balance yin/yang. When sexual identity is confused. *J.J.*

VIBURNUM (LAURUSTINUS) *Viburnum tinus*
"Reassurance". Support and reassurance. For those who feel unsettled, vulnerable or unhappy. Helps to establish identity and direction, particularly after life-threatening situations. *G.M.T.E.*

VIOLET
White. Forgiveness of self. Soul aspects of purity. *C.H.*

Releasing depression. Connection to inner inspiration. *L.L.F.E.*

Sometimes life can seem like an abstract painting; a collection of random events seemingly unconnected, a disconnectedness with the environment, meaningless sensual impressions. Nothing makes sense, has meaning or a flow of continuity.

Violet makes connections, it transcends boundaries including time. With Violet there is a sense of connectedness with past, present and future, possibly an experience of communion with ancient beings and definitely seeing patterns in the Universe. *U.F.E.*

Viola rivinana
For earache, catarrh, coughs, has anti tumour quality, muscle fibres, pancreas. For those restricted by authority, who have difficulty in trusting others completely. *S.C.E.*

VIPERS BUGLOSS *Echium vulgare*
Understanding primordial powers. Linked with the spider and snake. Very useful for resolving emotional tensions and conflicts which are due to the emergence of

subconscious forces. (N.B. This flower will initiate one through these forces, but will not suppress them.) *H.F.E.*

Balances the love energies.

Vipers bugloss helps to re-align the love energies. When these are extremely out of balance people may become the perpetrator or victim of manipulative patterns in an effort to meet their needs. This flower can help dissolve the distorted patterns, which have become ingrained, thus helping the life force to flow more freely. *L.F.H.*   *S.E.*

For physical problems between ears, nose, throat. *C.H.*

Used for the blood, epilepsy, throat problems, fertility. To enhance your wisdom and discernment. *S.C.E.*

WALLFLOWER *Erysimum/Cheiranthus*

Digestion. *R.D.*

Erysimum x allionii

For the homeless, helps find inner security. *C.H.*

WATER FORGET ME NOT *Myosotis scorpioides*

Balancing of water and air. Brings air qualities to watery types and vice versa. Tempers the ego and allows one to express themselves gently. Helps bring subconscious fears and repressed feelings to the surface and supports peacefully and gently. Aids connection with the angelic realms. *H.F.E.*

WATER LILY

Yellow. Strengthens emotional/mental body links. *C.H.*

Nymphaea odorata

Provides an inner sense of space, for detachment, stability and safety. Inner nourishment and connectedness to the source of life. *H.F.E.*

Nuphar lutea

The karmic problem of persons needing Water Lily is a loneliness brought into this lifetime by the soul, a residue from past incarnations where perhaps much time was spent alone or unable to communicate with our fellow man. This loneliness will feel soul deep and will bring with it an acute sadness. The sadness and the loneliness will be gently eased away in the shortest possible time. *C.H.*

WEIGELA *Weigela*

Unconditional love. Heart chakra becomes more expressive. *C.H.*

WEEPING WILLOW *Salix chrysocoma*

"Ego". Proper use of personal power and energy. Useful for those who get annoyed by others' views and attitudes. Tolerance of others and acceptance of one's own shortcomings. Energising, motivating in a wise, balanced way. *G.M.T.E.*

WELD *Reseda luteola*

To be used for the spinal column and for the vertebrae. For balance, strength, harmony, lack of insight. *S.C.E.*

WELSH POPPY *Meconopsis cambrica*

Nervine laxative, constipation, liver complaints. Loneliness, communication of feelings.   *S.C.E.*

For those who have lost their fire and inspiration and become day-dreamers.   *B.E.*

WHITE BLUEBELL *Endymion non-scriptus*

This essence is indicated for those souls that are extremely over-sensitive. Those who are so influenced by negative vibrations around them that they are unable to concentrate on their own individuality/work. Useful for those choosing a spiritual path or perhaps spending much time in meditation. Many healers often need this essence especially if using psychic faculties in their work.   *C.H.*

WHITE CHESTNUT *Aesculus hippocastanum*

Worry.   *R.D.*

WHITE CLOVER *Trifolium repens*

Balance.   *R.D.*

Whole plant. For consideration. For patience. For 'inaction'.   *E.E.*

WHITE FOXGLOVE *Digitalis purpurea alba*

To deepen meditation. Once used 'to induce trance'.★★

'I surrender to a deeper consciousness. My spirit is free'.   *H.R.*

Developing sensitivity. Helps in getting in touch with feelings. Helps to release blockages to communication. Sensitivity to others' feelings.   *L.L.F.E.*

Digitalis lutea

For heart conditions. For unity, need for spiritual protection, insight, perception.
                                        S.C.E.

WHITE LEAVED OAK *Quercus robur variegata*

Very centering and grounding. Brings the balance of roots firmly anchored in the earth and connecting with the Divine Source in the Heavens. Gets to the heart of the matter. Giving strength, confidence, courage and resilience to bounce back in times of adversity. Gives meaning to life's journey.

Cleansing and purifying both soul and body (particularly skin conditions).

Doorway to the inner realms, encouraging psychic intuition and visionary experiences.   *G.H.T.E.*

WHITE NARCISSUS *Narcissus actaea*

Letting go of being overly self conscious. Moving from thinking too much to being more aware of your feelings and in touch with the spontaneous child within.

'I trust myself to be guided by my heart'   *H.R.*

WHITE POPLAR *Populus alba*

"Starting again". Increase of wisdom, joy and contentment. Healing of mind and emotions. Energy and courage to recover from emotional setbacks.   *G.M.T.E.*

WHITE ROSE

Purity of heart. Developing your own soul note, without reacting to distracting influences.   *H.F.E.*

This essence attunes one to the pure white light within. It is good for purifying the mental state and giving receptivity to spiritual guidance from higher realms. There is a pure white angelic form attached to this flower. Good for clarity of vision in meditation, especially when wishing to meditate on the white light.

Planets – Jupiter, Chiron, Mars

Chakras – 6th, 7th, 1st   *M.E.R.E.*

WHITE ROSE BUD *Rosa floribunda alba*

For infants and babies in the womb (children and adults too) to help us grow and keep our sense of heaven on earth.★★

'I rest and grow safely in the light of grace'.   *H.R.*

WHITEBEAM *Sorbus aria*

"Otherworld". Stimulates fine levels of perception. Understanding of the animal and plant kingdoms. Opens heart and mind to finer levels of creation.   *G.M.T.E.*

WHITE WILLOW *Salix alba*

"True Self". The perception of the self is put in the context of its universal existence. This clarity brings a truer balance within oneself. Ego is cleansed and filled with a sense of bliss and love welling up. Spiritual cleansing.   *G.M.T.E.*

WILD CLARY *Salvia verbenaca*

Good for digestive problems, useful for psychotherapy, also kidney disease. Reduces outside pressures, to see clearly.   *S.C.E.*

WILD GARLIC *Allium triquetrum*

Saturn, Mars, Moon. Great protection against negative forces. Helps transition at death. Heart chakra. Good for animals. Effects are short-lived. For low vitality, poor immune system. Eases radiation. Rids fears and wards off possessing entities.   *J.J.*

WILD IRIS *Iris pseudacorus*

Iris is the essence for the person who possibly in past lives has held positions of great authority, or responsibility, either for others or greater things. Hence, brought into this lifetime are very often deep feelings of worry or concern. These feelings may be difficult to pin down; possibly a deep anguish and concern for the planet, which many are suffering at present, or possibly concern for one's fellow man or a need to take on their pain. As used, the person will be able to look at global, cosmic or mankind's problems in the right perspective.   *C.H.*

WILD ORCHID *Dactylorhlza praetermissa*

This beautiful purple flower brings a degree of consciousness raising, for as our uncertainties and indecision become positive vibrations within us so we become more aware of our spiritual being. This awareness that we are a part of our Creator, all as one and not different to our fellow man is a very necessary step along our soul's path and evolution. Only with this realisation comes our spiritual security, enlightenment, strength and courage, giving us a solid foundation from which to work. *C.H.*

WILD ROSE *Rosa canina*

Bringing out the beauty in your wildness. Overcoming limited conditioned beliefs and finding your true self. Love and appreciation of all things, including self. Acceptance of all Life.

Strength through opening the heart to the oneness of nature. *H.F.E.*

Helps to develop love. Brings understanding of one's own and others loving needs. Helps to discover where in life one is lacking in love. *L.L.F.E.*

WILD THYME *Thymus serpyllum*

Helps to open clairvoyant vision. Enhances feminine power and the feminine will, creative energy and subtle wisdom of the heart. Regenerates the female base chakra. Initiation into feminine power. *H.F.E.*

Thymus praecox

Strengthening by purification. Especially of thought, motivation and intention. Can be used to enhance or potentise other essence mixes, also to cleanse crystals or other objects used in healing or divination.

'I cleanse mind and affirm my good intention. I am strengthened by clear and appropriate motivation. *H.R.*

WILD VIOLET *Viola riviniana*

Acceptance and understanding of' one's needs and energy to fulfil one's goals. Courage to the timid. Reduction of negative, aggressive tendencies in favour of life-supporting activity. The ability to perceive and live one's own life for personal fulfilment (rather than society's expectations and stereotypes). Adaptation of beliefs to one's own standpoint. Poised self-expression. Passionate expression of true potential. Brings love and healing to feelings of confusion and emptiness. Heart chakra. *G.M.F.E.*

WILLOW *Salix caprea*

Clarity of focus and discernment. *A.T.*

WINTER ACONITE (LUNAR)

This remedy is for those who have in a previous life suffered from narrow-mindedness or blinkered vision because of strict and dogmatic religious beliefs, denying spontaneity, joy, material comfort and happiness. It will also treat the karma which has resulted from being part of a community which has been too inwardly focussed at the expense of shunning the rest of society. *A.F.R.*

WINTERSWEET *Acokanthera oblongifolia*

Hope, mental understanding of barrenness. Inspiration. *C.H.*

WISTERIA *Wisteria*

Subtle body imbalances. *R.D.*

Strengthens meridians, useful tool for acupuncturists. *C.H.*

WITCH HAZEL

Keywords – 'Bring forth light'.

Negative aspects – Addictions, fragility, fear of unknown, panic attacks, clumsiness, greed, moving house, work.

Positive aspects – Fruitful work. Accepts life's limitations, recuperation after an addiction. Coping in adverse conditions, clarity of thought, the light has been turned on.

Physical attributes – Oedema in hands. Heals deep tissue injuries/trauma. *B.F.E.*

Hamamelis virginica

Mentally stimulating.

Recommended for creative writers, authors and students. Witch hazel balances right/left brain function and appears to regulate brain patterns. It is indicated for epilepsy and Parkinsons disease. Suggested use is as a nerve tonic for shingles, for muscle spasms, tics and twitches. It does not improve memory or concentration but does encourage lateral thinking and the acceptance of radical new concepts or ideas. Witch hazel clears the negativity from all the subtle bodies, it stimulates the meridians especially the central vessel and opens and balances the ninth chakra. Associations include the colour red, direction West, planets Sun, Mars and Chiron, Tarot 6 of Cups. *A.F.E.*

Hamamelis mollis

For those who sacrifice themselves in trying to live up to the expectations of others. *B.E.*

WOOD ANEMONE

Wood Anemone is concerned with the workings of the mind. It is suited to people who along with a difficulty in concentrating and absentmindedness are able to spot small but vital details. They may perceive the first two traits as being culturally undesirable (although not creating problems in their own lives) and this may bring feelings of insecurity. However, they often fail to recognise their minds are acutely alert in other ways enabling access to avenues not normally explored by everyone else.

Wood Anemone supports these uniquely creative individuals. *U.F.E.*

Anemone nemorosa

For arteriosclerosis, urinary problems, fevers. For those who suffer with loneliness, or those who isolate themselves from others. *S.C.E.*

For use where there are very old difficulties – genetic or Karmic. *B.E.*

WOODRUFF

Brings a calm, natural sleep pattern to babies. *C.H.*

WOOD SORREL

This essence is suited to people who undervalue themselves, comparing their lack of beauty, strength, character, intelligence or connectedness to that of others. But look a little deeper and they reveal a great strength of character when tested, a settled energy as in meditation and an innate trust in the Universe.

Wood Sorrel brings a quiet confidence and self-acceptance. *U.F.E.*

WOUNDWORT (LUNAR)

This remedy is for those who have suffered at the hands of another, who in a previous life have been robbed or cheated of something which has been of great value, such as material possessions, trust or even life. Present life lack of trust is often the result of past life robbery. *A.F.R.*

YARROW *Achillea millefolium*

Offers protection against negative influences in the environment and in the thoughts and emotions of others. Enhances and strengthens the aura (energy field surrounding your body).

'I am surrounded by a strong white light. I am protected from harm'. *H.R.*

Venus. Special protection against radiation and psychic attack. Pink yarrow protects against negative emotions. Gives radiance to the aura. As the spiritual path becomes more open, so there is a need to protect against vulnerable forces which can cause depletion. Yarrow gives a shield of shining light. Very necessary new age essence. One of the oldest plants on earth. *J.J.*

Enhances the aura. Protection. Over identification with other peoples' energies and outside influences. *H.F.E.*

Counselling, psychotherapy etc. help to release the memories, experiences and trauma associated with oppression and violation, but they cannot obliterate or wipe out what has happened. At some point the experience must be integrated into the whole life experience. Yarrow helps with this integration bringing an acceptance of and a release or transcendence from the 'negative' states which initiated the process. *U.F.E.*

Pink yarrow. Protection.

This essence is for those who are empathic and may absorb the negative feelings of others. This can cause confusion and a drain of energy. Pink yarrow can strengthen and protect the aura so it is also of great help to therapists working with clients. Useful in a spray. *L.F.H.* *S.E.*

Pink yarrow. This essence gives emotional strength and balance, helping to overcome emotional oversensitivity and reactiveness. It is useful if you act like a psychic sponge absorbing negative or draining energies that happen to be around. This remedy is also a useful defence against psychic attack as it strengthens the aura, acting like a shield so you don't get caught up in the negative energies.

Planet – Moon

Chakra – 1st *M.E.F.E.*

White yarrow. Environmental protection.

This essence can help to protect the aura from negative environmental influences e.g. noise, fumes, pollution, radiation, computers etc and the resultant energy drain.

Useful in a spray. *L.F.H.*   *S.E.*

White yarrow. This is a remedy that strengthens the aura. It creates a shield of white light around you, giving protection from negative environmental things, such as background radiation or pollutants. This essence is really good if you are over sensitive or feeling vulnerable.

Planet – Moon

Chakra – 3rd   *M.E.F.E.*

Yarrow is recommended for those who are involved in healing or whose openness and sensitivity require protection from environmental and psychic toxicity. Yarrow is a protector of light. PHYSICAL USE: protects against radioactivity.   *A.F.R.*

Protection.   *R.D.*

Pink. Protection from psychic attack. White. Protection from radioactivity. Available as a mixed extra strong potency.   *C.H.*

Protecting and strengthening auras.   *L.L.F.E.*

Pink Yarrow. Used as a shield against negative energy, particularly of an emotional nature.   *J.W.*

YARROW IN SEA WATER *Achillea millefolium*

Exposure to and protection from radiation.

'I release my vulnerability to radiation. I let the sea wash me clean'.   *H.R.*

YELLOW ARCHANGEL *Lamiastrum galeobdolon*

Aids in contacting and understanding the hidden realms. Helps attune with the angelic intelligences and develop an attitude of acceptance and non-judgement towards all that one may have to face on the path of these planes. Understanding the need for balance of light and dark, all having a divine role and place.   *H.F.E.*

Inner Peace.

A living essence.

Negative – Loss of spiritual direction, arrogance. In trying to be other than what you really are, may have unreasonable expectations of the self and even display extremes of behaviour. A possible scattering of energies, rushing to get somewhere and an urge to keep up with everyone else. Unable to take care of personal spiritual needs as have completely lost sight of them.

Positive – At peace with the self, happy to be where you are on your spiritual path. Great inner stillness and poise. Everything in perspective and priorities clear. Content to move at your own pace and able to take care of one's needs.   *S.E.*

YELLOW BUCKEYE (SWEET BUCKEYE) *Aesculus flava*

"Devas". A way to link to devas, elementals and nature spirits in all environments. Modifies personal energy patterns in order to understand different sorts of communication.   *G.M.T.E.*

YELLOW DOCK *Rumex crispus*

Soothing to the joints, for rheumatics. For being optimistic, smiling, for those who have been hurt.   *S.C.E.*

YELLOW FLAG
For stress and bad nerves. *L.L.F.E.*

YELLOW IRIS *Iris pseudacorus*
General tonic, also used for jaundice. To enhance your communication abilities and for tolerance. *S.C.E.*

YELLOW LOOSESTRIFE *Lysimachia vulgaris*
This essence brings up problems which are stored in the subconscious. The dis-ease associated with these problems is brought into focus in the mental body. Spiritual help is then received and the issue is brought to rest, working through the levels until it is discharged into the earth. As the name implies it is for letting loose strife.

Planets – Moon, Mercury, Pluto

Chakras – 1st, 6th, 7th *M.E.F.E.*

Digestive disorders, liver complaints and for the blood. For too many thoughts, sharing with others. *S.C.E.*

YELLOW POPPY *Glaucium flavum*
Calms emotions and activates the mind. Helps to memorize, synthesize and adapt. Ideas, inspiration, clarity of mind. *H.F.E.*

YELLOW RATTLE *Rhinanthus minor*
Souls in need of this remedy carry a weight, an innate sadness, which in all likelihood they will be unable to express. A melancholy which echoes from previous lives in a similar way to the dried seed pods in the flower. When winds cast upon a meadow of Yellow Rattle the rattling sound will echo; the vibrations reverberating over surrounding fields in a similar way to the echoes of past hopelessness and despair.
C.H.

YELLOW ROSE
Brings feeling of security and courage to the heart. *C.H.*

This essence is concerned with cleansing as preparation for opening channels to the higher self, for the receiving of inspirational creativity to give out to the world. It also helps in opening oneself to trusting in the nourishing and sustaining energies of the universe. When this process has taken place one is able to communicate love and beauty from the heart.

Planets – Mercury, Venus, Chiron, Neptune

Chakra – 3rd *M.E.R.E.*

YELLOW WOUNDWORT *Stachys recta*
Used for gout, cramps, jaundice. For despair or depression, expressing yourself.
S.C.E.

YEW *Taxus baccata*
Connecting with the void through the understanding of opposites. Putting the mind aside and listening to the hidden wisdom of matter. *H.F.E.*

Develops wisdom, helps one to see the grander scheme of things. *C.H.*

"Protection". Protects from harm by activating the highest spiritual values of survival and protection. Aids the memory and discrimination, helps the immune system and increases energy.

G.M.T.E.

Deep healing. Letting go of what is no longer needed. Brings soul back to body.

L.L.F.E.

For resilience where previously the person has been too brittle – not bowing to the inevitable.

B.E.

YUCCA *Yucca*

Helps remove the veil of doom and gloom – for mild or long-term depression. Gives lightness, joy, a zest for life, providing energy and vitality. For mental and chronic fatigue.

G.E.

ZINNIA *Zinnia*

Laughter, humour.

R.D.

Laughter, restores humour. To get in touch with child-like properties within, helpful for unfulfilled parental or maternal instincts. Festivity.

C.H.

ZUCCHINI

Male sexuality, fertility problems. Sexual diseases. Hormonal imbalances. Base and sacral chakras.

C.H.

Chapter 8

Individual sets of essences

❀ ARTEMIS FLOWER ESSENCES ❀

This is a small selection from the Artemis range of Flower and Crystal Essences made in Devon by Kay Harrison. Kay's original intention was to explore Crystal Essences as part of her own spiritual development, but the flowers intruded and soon became too important to be ignored. Both organic garden and wild varieties are used as both have something valuable to offer. As many of these essences do similar things in slightly different ways they can be tailored very specifically for differing requirements. Combinations can be prepared to order. All the Artemis Essences assist the body to heal itself by restoring balance, releasing stress and stimulating change while offering support during the process.

Much of the information on the Essences has been acquired while on Shamanic journeys and from 'channelling' and this is reflected in the emphasis on spiritual and psychic uses.

BINDWEED

Connecting, binds ideas/people together.

Use to resolve karmic and inner child issues. It is indicated for people who stifle their emotions – helps them to recognise and come to terms with their deepest emotions. Bindweed encourages the resolution of karmic patterns by forming the connection between current stresses and past life issues. It is also useful for connecting therapist/clairvoyant and client together for more effective work (both would need to use the essence at least a half hour before the session). Protects by strengthening the silver cord for astral travel. Bindweed strengthens all the subtle bodies and meridians and gives all round protection at all levels. It's associations include colours gold and yellow, direction North, planets Earth, Moon and Saturn.

BLACKBERRY

Strengthening. Use for poor circulation and mental clarity.

It is suggested for: cleaning the blood, improving circulation, balancing blood pressure and increasing the absorption of oxygen throughout the body. It stimulates the adrenals to increase stamina, encourages kidneys and lymph to throw out toxins and the muscles to throw off lactic acid. It is also useful for spleen, liver and urinary problems. Use for mental fatigue, depression and lethargy. It calms the mind for meditation and channelling. Blackberry energises and balances all the meridians and nadis, it opens all the chakras but does not balance them. Blackberry amplifies other essences in combinations and assists their assimilation. Its associations include the colour red, direction South, planets Venus and Mars, Tarot Emperor.

BUTTERCUP

Comforting, use if feeling overwhelmed.

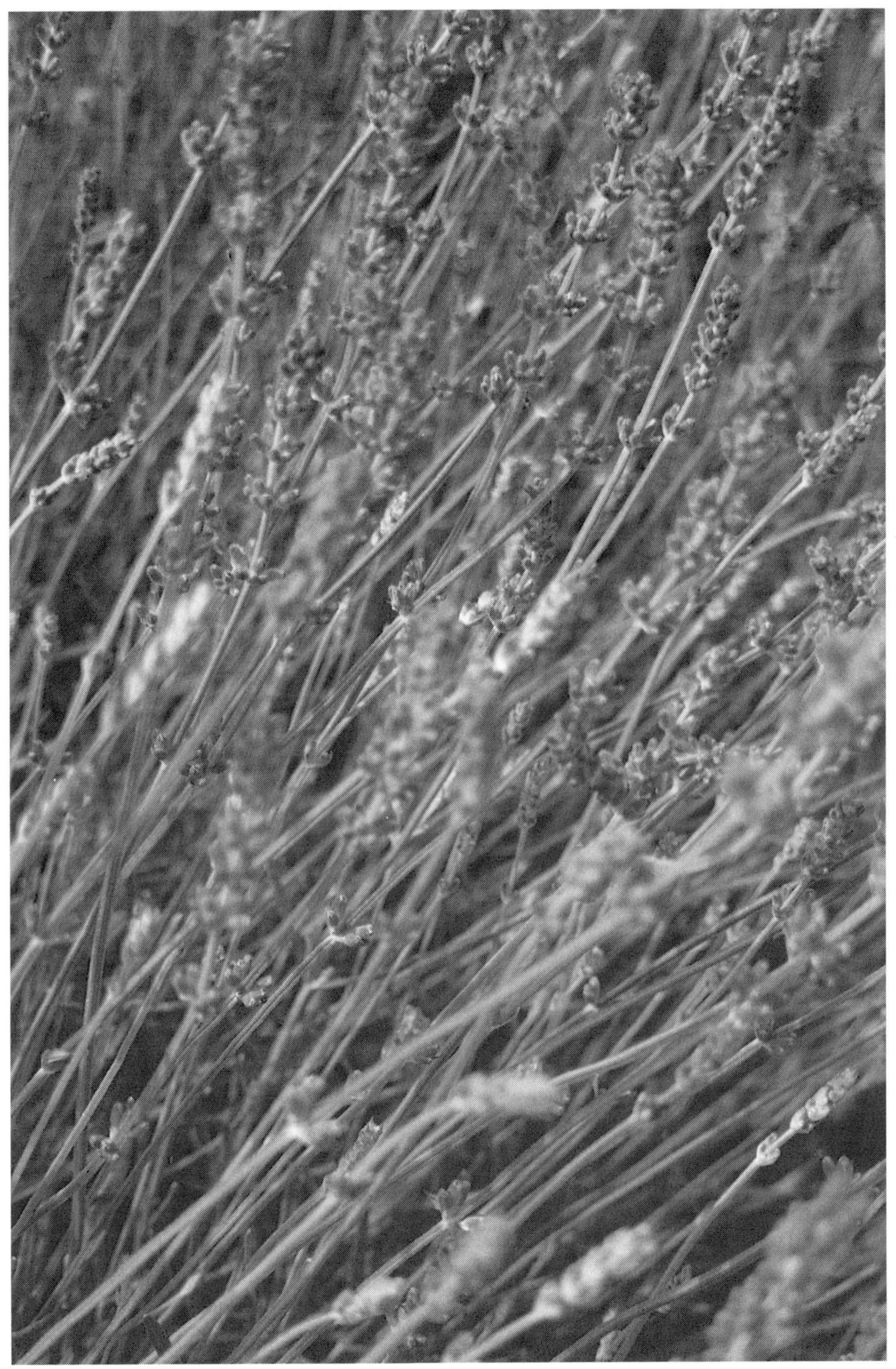

It is useful for all types of stress as it opens and strengthens the solar plexus chakra. It could be used to encourage a gentle de-tox and for general pain relief. It is recommended for removing stress from the site of an injury and is indicated for teenagers to bring some stability to their rioting hormones. Gives psychic protection by re-establishing boundaries, realigns the subtle bodies bringing them back into balance. Associations include the colour gold, direction East, planets Sun and Moon, Tarot 5 of Cups.

EVENING PRIMROSE

Sedatory, balancing.

Helps to promote emotional stability and is especially useful for relationship traumas, divorce, bereavement etc. Assists you to become emotionally self sufficient. Used regularly it releases tension in the uterus easing pre-menstrual syndrome and period pain, this may also eventually help to reduce the size of fibroids. Evening primrose also stimulates the nervous system and so may well be of long term benefit for Multiple Sclerosis. It is also indicted for an over-active thyroid, but it is definitely contra-indicated for ME and Post Viral Syndrome because of its strong calming effects. It does not combine well with other essences. Associations include the colours gold and yellow, direction West, planet Sun, sign Libra and Tarot Art.

GOLDEN SAGE

Motivating.

Reduces mental clutter so use before meditation. Provides motivation and a sense of purpose. Ideal for the stress of exams/interviews etc. Encourages self forgiveness and improves self esteem. Golden sage is recommended for nervous, introverted, shy people. It is indicated for: flatulence and digestive disturbances, shingles and chickenpox, tension or sick headaches, neuralgia, balancing blood pressure and as a gentle de-tox. Golden sage is very grounding, it balances the meridians, opens the solar plexus chakra and strengthens the subtle bodies. Associations include the colour pink, direction East, planets Venus and Mars, Tarot 3 of Swords

HAREBELL

Calming, sedatory.

For peace of mind. Calms on all levels so excellent for insomnia, for hyperactive children (ideal for long distance travellers, passengers NOT drivers!). May stop twitching/jumping legs especially at night. Eliminates irrational fears and is excellent for emotional stress or shock. Useful for computer and TV addicts as it can shield from electro-magnetic stress. Harebell is a very gentle essence so it is suitable for children, it is also recommended for the terminally ill, for grief and for bereavement. It reduces the trauma to plants when transplanting or pruning. Contra-indicated for ME or Post Viral Syndrome because of its strong sedatory effect. Associations include the colour blue, direction South, planets Moon, Neptune and Chiron, Tarot 3 of Cups.

HONEYSUCKLE

Balancing.

Gives protection from other peoples emotions, releases anger, irrational fears and mental stress. Helps to achieve inner peace and to improve the memory making this an excellent remedy for teachers as well as students. It helps with the absorption of vitamins and minerals, increases the oxygen levels in the blood and is believed to maintain the cellular structure of bone tissue. Honeysuckle is indicated for poor circulation, high/low blood pressure, chilblains, pulmonary congestion, diarrhoea and osteoporosis. Associations include the colour red, direction West, planets Venus and Jupiter, Tarot The Chariot.

JASMINE

Empowers.

Stimulates the immune system, heals physical and emotional scars and balances the body fluids. Indicated for colds (not flu), asthma, hay fever and sinus problems, also for post natal depression, candida, IBS, oedema and soft tissue damage. It is a useful bacteria buster and can be used to discourage head lice, nits and fleas. Jasmine can be utilised to tune astrologers in to all the planetary influences before they do readings. Jasmine cleans, opens and balances all the chakras and resolves karmic patterns at an emotional level. Associations include the colours orange and gold, direction North, planets All, Tarot Hanged Man.

LAVENDER

Emotional support.

Use to improve sense of smell, to regulate sleeping patterns and for general pain relief. It is indicated for ME, for childbirth, as an aid to digestion – it improves peristalsis of the digestive tract – and can help to regulate menses. It works on the heart centre to promote 'self-love' and 'self-worth'. May also be useful for skin/mouth ulcers and cold sores. Possible aphrodisiac tendencies! Grounds and centres, strengthens all the chakras and balances the subtle bodies. A useful aid for psychic development. Associations include the colour blue, direction North, planets Mercury, Jupiter and Neptune, Tarot 4 of Disks.

LEMON

Balancer.

Lemon is said to stimulate cell regeneration so it is indicated for psoriasis★, eczema★, acne★, stretch marks, scars etc. It reduces blood acidity and balances the digestive juices so it could be useful for stomach ulcers and dyspepsia. Use it to release mental stress, balance right/left brain function and so enhance mental clarity. It is also indicated for hypoglycaemia and may be useful to reduce cholesterol. Lemon gives psychic protection from negative thought forms but not from deliberate attack, it deals with karmic issues on a purely spiritual level. It opens and balances all the chakras and balances all the meridians. Associations include the colour blue, direction North, planets Moon, Mars and Neptune, Tarot Lust.

★Lemon heals the skin but not the cause of the problem so it would also be necessary to find a means to release emotional stress.

MUGWORT

Psychic energiser.

Indicated for low blood pressure, contra-indicated for high blood pressure. Mugwort stimulates the digestive tract giving a better assimilation of vitamins and minerals. Its main use however, is for psychic work. Mugwort is spiritually cleansing and protective, it pulls the subtle bodies together but weakens their boundaries, this opens up all the psychic abilities especially mediumship and channelling. Ideal for any meditation, shamanic or ritual work and well known for its use with lucid dreaming and astral projection. Mugwort strengthens the silver cord but not as much so as bindweed. It should be used with caution and respect. Associations include the colours purple and black, planets Venus, Neptune, Uranus, Pluto and Chiron, Tarot Ace of Disks.

PASSION FLOWER

Creativity.

Apart from encouraging creativity it is also useful for reducing lethargy, anger and fear. Regular use releases resentments, past life issues and may bring inner child problems to the surface. It gives a good gentle de-tox, improves circulation, balances blood pressure and increases the metabolic rate by boosting the adrenals. Passion flower is also indicated for general pain relief, tooth decay, warts, constipation and sinus problems. It empowers all the psychic abilities especially channelling, giving some psychic protection by strengthening boundaries, grounding and centering. This essence works on the solar plexus chakra to reduce stress. Associations include the colour red, direction East, planets Mercury, Venus and Neptune, the sign Aquarius and Tarot 2 of Swords.

PENSTEMON

Encouraging.

For indecisive people. Releases hatred and anger constructively. Aids concentration by synchronising left/right brain function and eases depression. Penstemon is indicated for tinnitus, arthritis and eye strain. Long term use may encourage hair growth and reduce premature greying. It energises the spleen and stomach meridians, balances and closes the major chakras and repairs damage to the aura. Associations include the colour pale green, direction North, planet Saturn, the sign Capricorn and Tarot Ace of Cups.

ROCK ROSE

Stress buster, emergency use only!

For relaxation, physical stress and feeling 'burnt out', also releases guilt feelings. It helps tone muscle, reduce fat, balance blood sugar levels and acts as a diuretic. Unfortunately it uses up precious (Jing) life force energy to do all this, so use it in emergencies but use it sparingly. Rock rose is contra-indicated for thrombosis and varicose veins because it increases the risk of blood clotting. Associations include the colours purple and white, direction North, the planet Mars and Tarot 4 of Disks.

ST JOHN'S WORT

Energises and calms.

Provides motivation and inspiration. Calms and helps to release guilt feelings. Balances right/left brain function improving memory and concentration. Use it to help with general pain relief, amenorrhea, eye strain and poor circulation. It is indicated for angina, high blood pressure and varicose veins, it may also reduce cholesterol. Energises the meridians and the nadis. Very useful for reducing the shock caused to plants by pruning. Associations include the colour red, direction South, planet Sun, Tarot Queen of Swords.

TANSY

Strengthening and sedatory.

Ideal for couch potatoes and computer buffs or anyone who has been mentally overstimulated because it brings peace and quiet to the brain. Excellent for insomnia for the same reason as it encourages deep, restful sleep. Can be used to reduce the pain of mental stress. Contra-indicated during pregnancy. Tansy strengthens all the subtle bodies and closes all the major chakras. Associations include the colour pale blue, planets Moon, Mercury, Venus and Mars, relates to Gemini, Cancer and Libra and Tarot Lovers.

THORN APPLE

Cleanser and stimulant.

Works on the pituitary to stimulate the mental process. Could be useful long term for dyslexia and has indications for ME and MS. Thorn apple assists the repair of all physical tissue damage, it helps to clean the blood, lower blood pressure and encourages the lymph system to de-tox. Used when dealing with food and drink – but not drug – addictions. It can cause a slight increase in the metabolic rate and could be used for some types of pain relief. Thorn apple is especially re-commended for tension headaches caused by constricting blood vessels, brilliant for hangover headaches! It stimulates all the psychic abilities, energises the meridians, cleans, realigns and heals all the subtle bodies. Associations include the colours brown and green, direction East, planets Moon, Saturn and Neptune and Tarot Hanged Man.

WITCH HAZEL

Mentally stimulating.

Recommended for creative writers, authors and students. Witch hazel balances right/left brain function and appears to regulate brain patterns. It is indicated for epilepsy and Parkinsons disease. Suggested use is as a nerve tonic for shingles, for muscle spasms, tics and twitches. It does not improve memory or concentration but does encourage lateral thinking and the acceptance of radical new concepts or ideas. Witch hazel clears the negativity from all the subtle bodies, it stimulates the meridians especially the central vessel and opens and balances the ninth chakra. Associations include the colour red, direction West, planets Sun, Mars and Chiron and Tarot 6 of Cups.

❁ AQUARIUS NEW GENERATION FLOWER ❁ REMEDIES

This is a set of forty popular flower essences which are made mostly in Northumberland by Aquarius Flower Remedies to promote health and healing on all levels. The set ranges from Angelica to Yarrow and the essences have all been documented elsewhere. We have found that all of the essences in this set have come up time and time again in readings and consultations with clients.

ANGELICA

Angelica allows us to feel a greater degree of protection, guidance and love from the angelic kingdom. It is particularly important at major life passages. PHYSICAL USES: treats epilepsy and many other neurological disturbances, skin ulceration and eczema.

BABY BLUE EYES

Baby Blue Eyes is for those of us who feel unsafe and insecure in this world due to a lack of emotional support during childhood. Taking this essence helps to restore the soul's original innocence and child-like trust.

BASIL

Basil is used when there is a sense of shame, guilt or disgust around sex. It heals the separation experienced between sexuality and spirituality.

BLACKBERRY

Blackberry aligns the mind with the will, making it easier to ground goals and ideals in the physical world. It is also given to those who fear death. PHYSICAL USE: helps the blood absorb food throughout the body and purifies the entire endocrine system.

BLEEDING HEART

Bleeding heart is a very powerful heart cleanser and strengthener for those who must learn the deeper spiritual lessons of love and freedom. This essence promotes the ability to love unconditionally. PHYSICAL USE: alleviates heart disease, regulates blood pressure and is a tonic for muscle tissue.

BORAGE

Borage is for courage. It can be used for any situation that is difficult to face. Borage stimulates love and compassion, bringing joy, optimism and light into life. PHYSICAL USE: stimulates adrenals, circulatory system, skeletal structure and thyroid.

BUTTERCUP

Buttercup is for when we feel low self-worth. This essence shows the soul the radiant light shining from within.

CALIFORNIAN POPPY

Californian poppy encourages a balanced psychic opening, aligning heart with spirit, giving a strong sense of inner knowing. PHYSICAL USE: treats multiple sclerosis and other nerve diseases, strengthens the eyes and the middle ear.

CHAMOMILE

Chamomile brings the gifts of serenity, emotional balance and a sun-like disposition. PHYSICAL USE: augments the entire nervous system and strengthens the ductless glands.

CHRYSANTHEMUM

Chrysanthemum is for when we identify too strongly with the material world and lose touch with our spiritual self. Chrysanthemum is also given for fear of death.

COSMOS

Cosmos gives clear articulation of thoughts, especially when speaking. Cosmos can be given to shy, introverted or procrastinating individuals, such people could express themselves more clearly.

DAISY

Daisy helps when we feel intellectually scattered; it brings clarity and understanding to what is trying to be learnt. Daisy is a good essence for students of any kind. It increases humility by opening the high heart chakra, located where the breast bones meet below the throat.

DANDELION

Dandelion is a wonderful essence for stress. It is for when we overdo it and are unable to sit still and reflect. Dandelion helps us listen to the body and emotions. PHYSICAL USE: many uses including alleviation of muscular degeneration, fevers and leukemia.

EVENING PRIMROSE

Evening primrose can be given to anyone who has experienced, whilst in utero or early infancy, lack of emotional support, rejection, neglect or abuse by the mother. Fear of commitment, coldness or emptiness within are classic symptoms of this early pain. Evening primrose literally rebirths the soul, providing all emotional nutrients that were lacking at incarnation.

FORGET ME NOT

Forget me not helps us remember those in other realms, those who have died and those who are incarnating. This essence makes us aware of karmic relationships and so widens consciousness and self-responsibility. PHYSICAL USE: increases communication between the cells in the brain, which in turn allows the brain's electrical messages to reach different parts of the body faster and more effectively.

FRENCH MARIGOLD

French marigold develops psychic abilities. It is further used for hearing difficulties or understanding what others are trying to say. It is useful for schizophrenia and autism. PHYSICAL USES: eases inflammation in the inner ear and pancreas, treats muscles which are attached to the bones, such as tendons and eases genetic deterioration of the spine and viral inflammations.

FUCHSIA

Fuchsia helps the soul to encounter and transform deep, hidden and painful emotions which are often covered up by a hyperactive emotional front. Powerful remedy to aid deep cathartic release.

GARLIC

Garlic is used to alleviate fear. It is useful for periods of low vitality when there is openness to disease and attack on all levels.

GOLDEN ROD

Golden rod is given when we are too easily influenced by social pressure and family ties in our desire for love and acceptance. This essence strengthens the sense of individuality.

GORSE

Gorse is given to those who experience deep depression, despair, hopelessness and resignation. Gorse brings the qualities of faith, hope and joy back into life.

HAWTHORN

Hawthorn brings balance at times of pre-cancerous emotional stress such as grieving for a loved one or the pain of a broken relationship. PHYSICAL USE: eases spread of cancer, especially tumours.

HIBISCUS

Hibiscus helps women to reclaim the dignity and warmth of their sexuality after traumatic or degrading experiences, including the exploitation and commercialization of female sexuality.

HONESTY

Honesty aligns the mind to the abundance of the universe, thereby lifting consciousness above the negative thought patterns centred around poverty and lack.

HYSSOP

Hyssop alleviates guilt, thereby allowing a deeper understanding of thoughts and actions to emerge.

JASMINE

Jasmine stimulates the God spark or permanent atom that resides in the heart chakra. Jasmine is given to those suffering from low self esteem. PHYSICAL USES: mucous in the system is regulated. The nasal passages, the sinuses, the throat and the lungs are cleared. Jasmine eases diseases associated with mucous problems such as pneumonia or the common cold. Viruses are dissolved and discharged. Diseases associated with protein deficiency such as hypoglycaemia can be treated.

LAVENDER

Lavender activates the crown chakra, connecting us with the higher self. This essence works to clear the karmic blockages that prevent spiritual progress. Lavender also gives balance to those who absorb too much spiritual energy, often resulting in afflictions to the head, neck and shoulders. It teaches the soul how to moderate and regulate spiritual-psychic energy.

LILAC

PHYSICAL USE: produces antibodies for spinal inflammation, cleanses and replaces spinal fluid, eases pinched nerves in the spine, disperses solidification of the vertebrae thereby increasing flexibility of the spine.

MALLOW

Mallow helps us overcome fear of ageing. The menopause years are made easier. This essence is also indicated for those who experience shyness, finding it hard to reach out to others. It encourages openness, friendliness and warmth. PHYSICAL USE: reinforces skin regeneration, treats most diseases associated with the ageing processes.

MORNING GLORY

Morning glory is used when we have a hard time waking up in the morning, are lacking in life energy or rely on addictive substances to pull us through. Morning Glory promotes a sparkling life force in tune with one's natural state of being. PHYSICAL USE: removes opiates from sympathetic nervous system and stimulates production of the endorphins.

ONION

Onion is a useful essence in counselling. It aids the counsellor in peeling away the barriers or protection that surround the root problem. Onion encourages release of emotions layer by layer in a safe way. PHYSICAL USE: opens the pores of the skin to receive more of the life force.

PANSY

PHYSICAL USE: works against most forms of virus from common cold to AIDS.

PETUNIA

Petunia is an anti-depressant, encouraging us to go within and face the blocks or denials that are at the root of our depression. It also re-establishes proper psychological behavioural patterns and is especially good for hyperactive children, the aged and overly logical individuals. PHYSICAL USE: apply over external bruising and scar tissue.

RED CLOVER

Red clover is a powerful cleanser and balancer. It can be used when there is a need to be strong, aware, calm and balanced in an emergency situation, when all around are succumbing to panic and hysteria. PHYSICAL USE: strengthens the blood vessels.

ROSEMARY

Rosemary promotes trust by healing early traumatic experiences which have left us feeling vulnerable and insecure. Classic indicators for this essence are forgetfulness and spending a lot of time out of the physical body. Rosemary increases vitality within our incarnated being.

STINGING NETTLE

Stinging nettle heals the emotional stress which is associated with a broken home. It is useful for adopted children, those parents who have adopted children and divorced people. Sibling rivalries can also be eased with this essence. PHYSICAL USE: tonic to the kidneys and lungs. Asthma, neural inflammations and scarring on the inner lung tissue respond to this remedy.

SUNFLOWER

Sunflower balances the ego. It helps us to shine and show our true self. Sunflower is also associated with the masculine aspect of self; it is useful for a poor relationship with one's male self or father. PHYSICAL USE: improves posture, strains in the spinal column and heart disease. Eases sunburn and heat exhaustion.

SWEET PEA

Sweet pea is given for antisocial behaviour and the need to develop a sense of social responsibility. It helps us to form a connection with the community, home and Mother Earth. Sweet pea is also useful for those who live in overcrowded or urban situations.

TANSY

Tansy is given for the deeply ingrained pattern of opting out of life and withdrawing energy when faced with emotional trauma of any kind. Those of us in need of Tansy may appear withdrawn, indifferent, lazy or indecisive. This essence helps us to reconnect with life.

THYME

Thyme is used when there is not enough time. It has the ability to alter our perception of the flow of time, thereby allowing it to speed up or slow down. It can be used for past life work. It is also an amplifier of other essences, speeding the healing process.

YARROW

Yarrow is recommended for those who are involved in healing or whose openness and sensitivity requires protection from environmental and psychic toxicity. Yarrow is a protector of light. PHYSICAL USE: protects against radioactivity.

AQUARIUS MOON FLOWERS

Made by the process of lunarisation, these essences heal the karmic patterns carried across from previous lives.

LUNAR ALDER

Alder is the remedy to heal sexual problems that have occurred in past lives. It is particularly applicable to those souls who have experienced sexual servitude of some form and are still suffering. Past life cases where disempowerment has occurred through such actions as rape, abuse or prostitution can be healed by this flower remedy. Alder is useful where there has been incest for it has a strong therapeutic impact upon sexual abuse committed in the family. Alder treats the guilt and self-disgust of those souls who are aware that they themselves have sexually abused in a previous life.

The karma of the water element is retention; this element stores all past life experiences in the memory. Alder can be given to souls who have a great deal of karma to release. Some souls are "walking karma", their whole lives seem to be reliving old karma, paying off karmic debts, continuing work on karma which was not completed and looking increasingly unlikely to be finished this time. There may be a sense of always being pulled back into the past with little opportunity to develop or move forward towards future lives to meet new karma. Alder has the ability to draw excessive water from the soul, dry out the ground, so to speak, so that the new seeds can be raised on well-drained soil.

The Deva of Alder came to Earth during the time of the first attempts at hierarchical structure on the continent of Atlantis. For the first time human souls were subjected to servitude and the loss of free will. An empathetic link was created between Alder and those who found themselves in positions of subordination. This pattern is carried through to the present use of Alder. Lunar Alder resonates with the water element.

LUNAR CAT'S EAR

Cat's Ear is the remedy for past life deceits or misunderstandings.

This remedy is useful for those who have in a previous life uttered falsehoods. Certain roles in society require one to be economical with the truth or twist facts to suit one's own position. Karma inevitably has to be encountered from such actions and Cat's Ear is the essence to help untie such past life actions. Those who have been politicians, barristers or who have had to use the power of words to persuade others may benefit from this remedy. Those who have used words to undermine or intentionally hurt another in a previous life will find healing from Cat's Ear.

Cat's Ear can also be used in past life relationship therapy. Frequently positions of misunderstanding remain unresolved to return in future lives. Lack of understanding of the others point of view, not being able to hear the truth of another and judging them wrong are common enough dynamics within human relationships. Cat's Ear may be able to dissolve the boundaries between two individuals, allowing greater understanding of the other's point of view, if the problem is rooted in a previous life relationship. Cat's Ear is an excellent remedy to bring clarity and understanding when past life regression is proving confusing. Conversely, Cat's Ear may well cause confusion if taken by someone who has clarity.

During the earliest stages of the Atlantean colonisation this Deva acted as a messenger between the newly formed colony and the mother-shores of Lemuria. The Deva presently associated with Cat's Ear has taken on different material forms in the past. This level of consciousness comes through in the flower essence. Cat's Ear is able to bring so much clarity to past life confusion and mis-representation because it has itself gone through many changes.

LUNAR COLTSFOOT

Coltsfoot aids the process of deep karmic release where there is a sense of something forcing its way to the surface.

Give Coltsfoot when deep past life patterns or habits are attempting to emerge onto the conscious level. Such patterns have been held down in the lower levels of the subconscious in order to be denied or repressed; consequently they find it difficult and painful to be released. When they rise it can be as if something large is pushing or welling up inside, stretching or pulling apart the tightness or rigidity that has for so long held it all down and there can be a sense of disgust, regret, guilt, shame or other negative emotions around the patterns as they force their way out. Coltsfoot relaxes that tightness or rigidity, which is most likely fear and thereby affords a greater ease of passage for the release into consciousness of the deep karma.

The Deva of Coltsfoot helped bring compassion, empathy and understanding to humanity towards the end of the Atlantean civilisation. A great many mistakes had been made by this time and it became necessary for humanity to reflect, take stock, so to speak, before the final demise of Atlantis.

Lunar Coltsfoot resonates strongly with passive Jupiter/Pluto contacts.

LUNAR FEVERFEW

Feverfew is the remedy for past life confusion.

At certain points during its evolution the soul seeks greater clarity in a particular incarnation. One is able to discern past karma of confusion, uncertainty about meaning, direction, purpose or identity. Such souls have spent lifetimes lost in a maze, unable to release themselves from muddled thinking, tying themselves in knots. They may well have been mentally ill in a previous life.

Now they are seeking to transform this karma into clarity; they are moving out of the dark maze into the simplicity and truth of light. However their karmic habit is to turn around and return to the maze for it is very hard for them to accept that life can be sharp, focussed, single pointed. For these souls to hold a vision, to be committed, to know their path is one of the greatest challenges of the life. To step out of the maze is the most exciting and frightening action to take, bringing intensity, polarization and crisis. Their past confusion is the safety net, the escape hatch in case living in the reality of light and truth is too difficult.

Feverfew aligns these souls with their true destiny, allowing them to contact their own personal power which has been unused in previous lives. It also brings them into contact with their ability to believe, trust in the future, have hope and faith. The souls in need of feverfew have learnt a great deal from previous incarnations wandering the endless avenues of possibility, now they are being asked to get in touch with the seat of their power which is the direction they have to take.

Certain types of karma require more than one life time's experience to deal with so each soul, during a series of incarnations, works through specific karmic patterns, resulting in similar life experiences being encountered through several life times. Feverfew is also used for those souls who, for whatever reason, have strayed or been led astray from working with their karmic destiny.

Lunar feverfew resonates with the mutable cross.

LUNAR HAWKSBEARD

This remedy can be used to heal the wounds that have occurred on the collective level of consciousness in previous incarnations. Whole communities or nations have greatly suffered at certain times and many souls reincarnate still bearing the wounds of a life that was injured through the suffering of the community or nation. Hawksbeard heals the wounding that has occurred when whole communities are subjected to suffering because of racial characteristics, religious practice, war, famine and many other reasons. Souls who in previous lives have become caught up in a major national disaster would benefit from this remedy.

Lunar Hawksbeard resonates particularly strongly with any of the trans-Saturn planets in the twelfth house.

LUNAR HAWTHORN

This is the remedy for past life indoctrination.

All societies, no matter how liberal they claim to be, have religious, moral or philosophical doctrines that have to be adhered to. Lunar Hawthorn is for those souls who have been unable to shake off the doctrines of previous lives which are proving unhelpful in the present incarnation.

Many souls have, in a previous life, been deeply wounded by strict, petty and narrow cultural belief systems, frequently perpetuated by the establishment. Lunar hawthorn can be used to heal such wounds, often resurfacing during present incarnation childhood experiences of moral teaching and indoctrination. Use this remedy when the soul's own wisdom has been at odds with the collective consensus and the soul has had to accept religious and cultural "truths" unsympathetic to its own spiritual development. Hawthorn can also be used for those who have in a previous life been severely judged by society for transgressing the moral/religious principles of the time. Those who have had the courage, to challenge the "accepted wisdom" will almost certainly fall in this category. The angel of hawthorn offers protection and this comes through the process of lunarisation. Lunar Hawthorn protects the soul from the powerful invasive "shoulds and shall nots" dictated by society, giving its own wisdom the opportunity to flourish.

LUNAR HAZEL

Hazel can be given to heal wounds inflicted upon the physical body by sharp or heavy weapons in previous lives.

Deep or fatal wounding in a previous life can resurface in the physical vehicle of the present life. Intensely traumatic injuries have an impact upon the soul, causing the wound to reoccur in successive incarnations; such karmic scarring is not uncommon.

Use hazel to bring healing to the wounds that have been inflicted by sharp or heavy weapons still existing on the soul level: these frequently manifest as complaints in the area of the body which had in a previous incarnation been injured. Use hazel when there has been a large display of greed or possessiveness in a previous life which is colouring the present incarnation.

Old and outworn patterns which were important, profound or intense in a previous incarnation can be retained by the soul and inform the present incarnation inappropriately. The soul is clinging to something which was of great value to its spiritual evolution in a past life yet is completely unnecessary this time. The "gold" of a previous life, stored for future use, turns out to be a handful of dust needing to be released. This previous life experience, prized by the soul, may have manifested on the conscious level as a positive, beautiful, helpful quality or the reverse, negative and painful; in either case hazel can be used to release the soul. Hazel is indicated when there is the sense that these powerful energies from the previous life are pulling the soul down into the depths rather than lifting it up.

The Deva of Hazel has an extremely old relationship with humanity for it agreed to help in the very earliest stages of the colonisation of Atlantis – this implies there was already a well established relationship between the two. The Deva of Hazel helped prepare the ground of the newly formed continent for human migration from Lemuria and also eased the psychological problems which accompany migration. This Deva, therefore, had an important role to play in the establishment of Atlantis.

Lunar Hazel resonates with the Taurus/Scorpio axis and the second/eighth house polarity of the horoscope.

LUNAR IVY

Lunar Ivy is for past life poisoning and poisoned emotions such as envy, jealousy, hatred and anger.

Deep seated anger and other dark or poisoned emotions can be carried through to future lives; they reside in the aura, often close to the physical. Ivy is used to release the toxicity they produce through the constant denial, repression or inability to face such powerful emotions. Such dark, one might say evil, sentiments leave a deep wound on the soul which may require healing in a future life. The healing action of ivy is dramatic, rather like taking a knife to an infected wound or lancing a boil. A powerful cathartic release of past life toxins can be expected.

Ivy can also be used when the individual has ben poisoned in a previous life or suffered through septicemia or other infections that have entered through the skin.

Lunar Ivy resonates with Scorpio, Pluto and Mars in opposition or square to the Sun.

LUNAR MICHAELMAS DAISY

Use Michaelmas Daisy when there have been power struggles in past life relationships.

This remedy is able to address the tensions which continually surface in relationships from time to time, transforming repeated patterns that have their roots in power struggles from previous lives. Power is one of the most highly magnetic qualities and consequently returns with as much force as it delivered in past lives. Michaelmas Daisy is asking to heal, through transformation, the battles that have raged between individuals in their past incarnations. Such struggles are usually centred around sex, money or authority.

Many souls have a series of incarnations within a particular family: this flower essence works well with the negative karma of family power struggles which inevitably result from such close contacts over several incarnations. Jealousy over money, inheritance or family rifts that have occurred in previous lives can be resolved with this remedy.

The consciousness of the great angel Michael has always been close to humanity. He played an important role in our initial descent from spirit onto the Earth, helping in the process of separation. Michaelmas Daisy was first used to heal the traumas of our separation from loved ones in spirit. At a later period in Atlantis the flower was used to assist the process of the emergence of the hierarchical social structure and heal the painful rifts that occurred when certain individuals were seen as being more important or more blessed than others. This remedy resonates with Scorpio/Pluto in the seventh house as well as Mars in the fourth.

LUNAR PLUM

Plum is for the stresses and tensions created by past life sexual promiscuity.

Over or unwise use of sexual energy in a previous life can result in patterns of pain and suffering emerging in the present incarnation. Plum is a remedy which brings wisdom, understanding and compassion to bear upon the incorrect use of sexual energy in the past, dispelling the emotions of guilt and self-disgust which can so easily attach to this type of karma.

Sexual activity is vulnerable to attack from a wide range of negative and judgmental thoughts. The sexual promiscuity of a former life may well have incurred little or no negative karma; sexual openness can be natural, creative and joyful. However, profound stresses and tensions may have been created in the present incarnation due to current cultural and socially acceptable standards of behaviour in this area being so different from those of the previous life. Whatever the suffering, plum will tease the knot open if it has been formed by previous life sexual promiscuity.

LUNAR POPPY

Poppy is for the psychological dis-ease created by involvement in warfare in previous lives.

Lunar Poppy is for those souls who have in previous lives stood on a battlefield and seen their comrades killed. It is the remedy to address the profound wounding the soul carries from such lifetimes. Poppy is for the souls who have witnessed the most inhuman and barbaric scenes within the theatre of war. Such visions remained with them for the rest of that life and were carried through into subsequent incarnations to be healed. Lunar poppy is the remedy to give for this type of karma, a type of haunting from the past which will not go away. The use of this flower remedy may awaken the memory in order to relive and release the tensions. Poppy does not address the physical injuries that may have occurred during the heat of battle, see Lunar Hazel for this particular condition.

This remedy is also for those who in a previous life have lost loved ones through war. It addresses the tensions manifesting in the present incarnation which are a direct result of this deepest of losses. Our souls are all born out of the same cosmic womb; at this level of being we are all brothers and sisters. Taking sides with the intent to kill an enemy creates a wounding at the deepest of soul levels. Lunar Poppy has much healing to offer in reconciliation between old enemies.

LUNAR PRIMROSE

Primrose is the remedy for past life relationships.

Each soul will, during the course of a particular incarnation, meet with souls it has known from previous lives. It is common for souls who have been very close in past lives to make pacts to meet up again at some point in the future: love, the emotional bonding between individual souls survives death. However there are other emotional bonds which are carried across, some of which are not particularly pleasant, life affirming or constructive to the relationship and it is with these that primrose is concerned.

Primrose will bring to the surface, make a couple conscious of the dysfunctional aspects of their relationship which have been carried across from previous incarnations. At first primrose will highlight or amplify these inharmonious patterns so that the individuals concerned can become fully aware of the karmic patterns and make conscious decisions about what needs to be changed. Primrose is able to awaken the deep memory, revealing the nature of past life relationships.

Deeply ingrained patterns of behaviour, carried across from previous relationships, are rather like a rutted road; once the car slips into the ruts it becomes impossible to get out. Primrose works with individuals to transcend this unhelpful relationship karma by helping to fill in the ruts, so to speak. Slowly and gently the patterns become less deep and those concerned become less inclined in the continuation of the karmic patterns.

Lunar primrose resonates with Libra and the seventh house.

LUNAR RED CAMPION

Wisdom is an important soul quality to be learnt over many incarnations, yet there are a great many souls who, whilst in the body of women, have severely suffered in the pursuit of knowledge and wisdom. This remedy is for those who have suffered in previous lives for being a wise woman. Give this essence to those who have been tortured, burnt at the stake or persecuted in other barbaric ways for possessing female wisdom. Furthermore Red Campion has the ability to work with the whole range of emotional issues that arise out of such abusive past life treatment so that what is an extremely complicated karmic wound is simple to treat with this one remedy.

Lunar Red Campion resonates with the Moon, Venus or Jupiter in Sagittarius.

LUNAR ROSE

Lunar Rose is for past life bereavement.

If the etheric cord linking us to loved ones has, in a past life, been cut in a violent or unexpected way, the trauma can be carried through to future lives. Use this remedy for any shocking separation from loved ones. The sudden death of a partner or a child and becoming orphaned are just a few instances which suggest the use of rose. It is not uncommon for the grieving process to take more than one life time to complete, particularly if the initial bereavement was so deeply wounding. Rose will ease the emotional burden of such bereavement. This type of past life loss can colour present life relationships detrimentally: over-possessiveness and deeply rooted fear of losing a loved one are common manifestations of this karmic condition.

During the later times on the continent of Lemuria, as part of the preparation for the exodus to the newly forming continent of Atlantis, there was a conscious drive to loosen the bonds with the spiritual realms, particularly the links with spiritual companions. The Angel of Rose appeared on Earth at this time to help this process by strengthening the bonds of love between souls residing on the physical plane.

LUNAR SNOWDROP

Snowdrop is given to heal the deepest wounds society has inflicted upon the soul in previous incarnations, or the soul has inflicted upon society.

Give snowdrop when the soul has been alienated from society, spurned or rejected in some fashion. Snowdrop treats any form of abuse meted out by society. Any negative karma resulting from actions carried out to fulfil a role in society can also be treated with snowdrop. The most vicious, inhuman deeds perpetrated can be cleansed by this flower essence: such karma inevitably creates profound stress for the soul in the present life. Snowdrop flower essence is for the abused and the abuser in society. It brings a greater sense of true self or individuality which was lacking in previous lives. The sense of self may well have been lost or destroyed in a previous incarnation whilst functioning within the bounds of social convention: Snowdrop helps to deal with the imbalances in the present incarnation which are a result of the self being denied in previous lives.

Snowdrop's current destiny is to serve humanity as an extremely powerful, cathartic healer. The Snowdrop Deva suffered at the hands of science during the last era of Atlantis, when many scientific abuses occurred. It is these wounds which make it such a powerful healer, helping us to release the wounds that have occurred through communal living.

Snowdrop resonates with Aquarius and the eleventh house.

LUNAR THISTLE

This is the remedy for past life imprisonment. Incarceration for long periods of time causes deep wounding to the soul and may well have to be healed in future lives. Often there is deep frustration and anger still felt as a result of having lost the freedom of a past life; this can be projected onto almost anything. This remedy also treats the loneliness and isolation of the past life detention. Being separated from loved ones has profound psychological effects which can manifest in the present life relationships.

The experience of being locked away can cause the individual to see the whole of life as a prison. Confinement forces the inner life to develop at the expense of the outer so the individual may well be introverted, quiet, shy and retiring and find it difficult to express the extrovert side of their personality. There may also be a strongly developed psychic life as a result of the past life imprisonment which needs to be integrated into the whole being. There may well be within the individual a yearning to escape, leave the physical body and return to the loved ones in the spiritual realms.

Thistle assists in the balancing process that needs to occur for the individual to find harmony within and without. The Deva of Thistle has an extremely ancient relationship with humanity. From the very earliest times in Lemuria some human souls were finding it difficult to bond with the collective consciousness. Thistle made contact with such souls to offer healing and help in their rediscovery of their own sense of individuality.

Lunar Thistle resonates with Saturn and Uranus in Pisces or the twelfth house.

LUNAR WINTER ACONITE

This remedy is for those who have in a previous life suffered from narrow-mindedness or blinkered vision because of strict and dogmatic religious beliefs.

This is the remedy to use for those souls who have in the past been members of strict religious sects that have practised austere regimes and denied spontaneity, joy, material comfort and happiness. Winter Aconite will also treat the karma which has resulted from being part of a community which has been too inwardly focused at the expense of shunning the rest of society. Winter Aconite also addresses the karma of spiritual elitism, living a previous life in the belief of being one of the chosen few.

LUNAR WOUNDWORT

This remedy is for those who suffered at the hands of another. It is the remedy for those who, in a previous life, have been robbed or cheated of something which has been of great value. This may well have been material possessions, trust or even life.

Woundwort is useful to heal karma from past life relationships where one party experienced the other taking something of value away from the relationship. It is not what has been taken away which is of importance but the accompanying feeling; the shape of that emotional wound is what returns in future incarnations to be healed. Therefore Woundwort can be used to heal any form of past life robbery, be it physical, emotional, mental or spiritual. Present life lack of trust is often the result of past life robbery.

The initial relationship between Woundwort and humanity was established when the first dwellings were built on the continent of Atlantis: Woundwort was taken inside to bless and protect the properties. Woundwort played a similar yet more complicated role in the royal palaces during the height of the Atlantean nobility. Woundwort's present name is an empathetic link to a later Atlantean period: because of the already well-established relationship between this plant consciousness and humanity it was universally used to treat many physical ailments that arose out of the use of nuclear energy.

Lunar Woundwort resonates with the Taurus/Scorpio polarity.

AQUARIUS CHAKRA FLOWER ESSENCES

Seven essences to unblock and balance each of the seven major chakras, bringing well being to the physical, emotional, mental and spiritual levels.

COMFREY – THE ROOT CHAKRA

Indicators – not properly grounded, difficulty with day to day living, disorientation, overly aggressive, restlessness, anxiety, stress, getting stuck, lack of concentration, fear of injury, inability to release the past or assimilate the present.

Attributes – the initiation of spiritual practice or any project, developing strength of character, stability, releasing past-life talents, will to live, creativity.

Physical complaints – dis-ease of bowels, rectum, anus, urethra, adrenals, difficulty with any of the eliminative processes.

RED DEAD NETTLE – THE SACRAL CHAKRA

Indicators – creative block, overly dry or serious personality, internalised anger, confusion over sexual orientation, obsession with sex, blocked or suppressed emotions.

Attributes – passion for life, increasing creativity and libido, expression of sensual emotions and sexuality, detoxification.

Physical complaints – dis-ease of reproductive organs, bladder, large and small intestines, appendix, lumbar vertebrae, infertility, stiffness in body including arthritis.

There is a long and powerful history between humanity and the angel of Red Dead Nettle which started on the ancient continent of Lemuria. Lemuria is better known as the Garden of Eden, the place of innocence we inhabited prior to colonising the continent of Atlantis. The angel made itself known to humanity at this time to help in the assimilation of knowledge as we became more awake and wise to the ways of the world. There are parallels with the episode of tasting the forbidden fruit, perhaps a rather negative interpretation of our need to know.

The angel of Red Dead Nettle made further contact at the height of the golden age of Atlantis. During this Atlantean era there were souls for the first time in positions of great power and control over people, similar to the pharaohs of Ancient Egypt. Red Dead Nettle helped both the souls who exercised power and the souls who were subject to it come to terms with their roles. It was later used as a powerful healer during the great epidemics which swept over the continent of Atlantis.

SAGE – THE SOLAR PLEXUS CHAKRA

Indicators – victim consciousness, lack of control, stress, domination or abuse of others, anger, aggression, fatigue.

Attributes – taking personal power, control in life, assertiveness, outward vitality, confidence, feeling the world is a safe place to live.

Physical complaints – dis-ease in the organs of digestion and purification – stomach, pancreas, liver, gallbladder, spleen, ulcers, diabetes.

Sage means wisdom and the angel of this flower brings this attribute Sage flower essence bestows the ability to draw wisdom from life experiences, to review and survey the processes of life from a higher perspective. Sage can be taken when we need to draw a spiritual dimension into our being. This essence also brings the quality of laughter.

PASSION FLOWER – THE HEART CHAKRA

Indicators – overly protective, withholding love – a closed heart, lack of sympathy, loneliness, depression, grief, self-blame, guilt.

Attributes – unconditional love, ability to love oneself, compassion, nurturing, empathy, open-heartedness.

Physical complaints – dis-ease in bronchial tubes, lungs, breast, heart, entire circulatory system, strokes, blood clots, thymic atrophy, weak immune system.

The vine acquired its current name from the Jesuit priests who sailed to the New World. They discovered in its signature the whole passion of their saviour god. The three stamen resemble the nails used for the crucifixion, the petals are like the crown of thorns placed on Christ's head and the ten sepals represent the disciples minus the two, Judas and Peter, who betrayed and denied. Christ is the universal principle associated with the heart and Christ Consciousness is heightened when this flower essence is used. It is the essence to use if there is long-term emotional pain that has not yet been released. The passion, the suffering of Christ flows through the angel of this flower, bringing universal healing and peace directly into the area it is needed, the heart chakra. Any individual who is opening up spiritually will benefit from the use of this essence as it helps assimilate and stabilise the experience. One further use for Passion Flower Essence is as an aid to sleep; it promotes deep sleep, eases nightmares and helps in the remembering of dreams.

CELANDINE – THE THROAT CHAKRA

Indicators – difficulty in self-expression, unaware of own needs and desires, suppression of self, introversion, sullen.

Attributes – greater and clearer communication, speaking one's truth, diplomacy.

Physical complaints – dis-ease of thyroid glands, mouth, vocal cords, trachea, cervical vertebrae, nervous system, speech impediments.

NASTURTIUM – THE BROW CHAKRA

Indicators – lack of awareness, narrow-mindedness, blinkered vision, sluggish mind, boredom, mental tension and over-activity, delusion, hallucinations, fantasies.

Attributes – intuition, clairvoyance, conscious awareness, creative visualisation and thought, inspiration, insight.

Physical complaints – dis-ease of the ears, eyes, sinuses and nose, cataracts, headaches behind eyes, endocrine imbalances.

Nasturtium also opens the pituitary chakra, acts as a mild tonic for the entire endocrine system, enhances the assimilation of B vitamins and finally increases sensitivity to colour, making it a good essence to us alongside colour therapy.

DAFFODIL – THE CROWN CHAKRA

Indicators – searching for meaning, crisis of belief or faith, psychosis, perfectionist, elitism, frustration, low intellectual capacities, manic depression, psycho-spiritual imbalances.

Attributes – enlightenment, knowing, acceptance, fulfilment, completion, alignment with higher forces.

Physical complaints – dis-ease of the nervous system, synchronisation between the left and right hemispheres of the brain, ulcerous conditions.

Daffodil can be used to gain a greater degree of contact with spirit guides or other non-physical beings whose consciousness is reached through the crown. It is an excellent remedy to use when a higher perspective is required for it extends the consciousness through the mental into the spiritual bodies. Its connection with the crown gives Daffodil the ability to make us more sensitive to intuitive work. Any form of self-condemnation affects the crown chakra, so Daffodil is a remedy which dispels negative attitudes about the self. There is great joy about the angel of Daffodil, reflected in the vibrant yellow of the flower and this quality is transmitted through the essence.

❀ THE BAILEY FLOWER ESSENCES ❀

The Bailey Flower Essences were created over 30 years ago by Dr. Arthur Bailey. Arthur Bailey has a rigorous scientific background, but has always had a love of nature and felt particularly drawn towards flowers. He has been involved in healing and meditation for the last 30 years and it was from that background that the essences were developed.

Mind and body interact with each other. When the mind is not at ease, neither is the body. It is this unease of the mind that often is the origin of our illnesses. Out of date attitudes and conditionings can disempower us and make us very unhappy. They stand in the way of positive personal change. The Bailey Essences act as catalysts for this needed change. They are concerned with helping us to come up to date.

The Bailey Essences are compatible with and complementary to many other flower essences. They are gentle in their action, non-addictive and totally non-toxic. They can be safely used on small children.

Most of the Essences are made by the Sun method. Those made instead by alcohol extraction have an asterisk (*) after the botanical name. Not all the essences are made from flowers. A few are produced from the fruit or the leaves of a plant or from the whole plant. These are indicated by the initial (F) for fruit, (L) for leaf, OR (P) for whole plant after the plant name.

PLEASE NOTE WHEN ORDERING ESSENCES: The single essences below are all included in the current, recently updated, Bailey Essence Set, with the exception of those at the end after the title 'Extra Essences'. These were included in the original set but have now been incorporated into composite remedies listed in Chapter 9, after considerable research and testing to find which essences have affinities with others. The 'Extra Essences' will still be available as there may be practitioners who wish to continue using these as well as the composites which include them, but those persons ordering a 'Bailey Essence Set' will not receive these essences.

ARIZONA FIR

In many religions it is assumed that any enjoyment of life is "not spiritual", that life should be a hard process. Indeed any enjoyment of life is seen as a severe stumbling block on one's path. I feel that such ascetic teachings are distortions of the Truth. Clinging to a path of suffering and mortification can be just as disastrous to one's personal growth as living the life of a hedonist. It is the clinging that is the problem, not what one is clinging to. What is needed is balance.

Many people do not enjoy their life. For them, it is full of woe and suffering. Yet from a different viewpoint, life can be seen as an amazing and wonderful experience – something to be enjoyed. The essence of Spruce can help us to celebrate our life and existence. It can stimulate a sense of freedom and joy. It is only when we can really open up and rejoice that the Heart Chakra (which represents love) can be fully energised. We need to be able to love life and to love our own self, "warts and all", celebrating life as a spiritual being, on this earth. There is nothing wrong about enjoying ourselves, it is the attachment to such enjoyment which is the difficulty.

When we can dance in celebration and we, the dancer, no longer exist, then there is only the dance. That is true celebration. In such timelessness there is no ego, just a unity with all creation. Spruce softens our rigidity and opens the door to the mysteries of true celebration.

BLUEBELL

This is the essence to promote openness, vitality and "upliftment" beyond the restrictions of the past. Like the bluebells in the woods in Spring, there is now colour and fragrance after the dark winter. The typical "Bluebell" person will be someone who has lost most, if not all, of their self-esteem. There is usually a feeling of self-dislike, often coupled with a sensation of somehow being rotten inside, rather like the guilty "sinner" who feels that they are beyond redemption. Such a person will most likely feel that everything they have worked for is somehow dying. They have become locked into negative ways of looking at themselves. Nearly always their distorted self-image has arisen from childhood conditionings where little that they did was met with approval. Bluebell helps to bring openness and joy where previously there was darkness and fear. We can become locked in that "winter of discontent". Bluebell releases the spirit from old conditioned beliefs and attitudes relating to feelings of being sinful or unworthy and encourages the regrowth of self-love and self-respect. Outgrowing old negative conditionings brings us into a new and much more vital period of growth. Bluebell is about unlocking our hidden potential and bringing us into a period of personal blossoming.

BOG ASPHODEL

Bog Asphodel is for the willing servant or slave, whose driving ambition is to help other people, whilst ignoring their own needs. What is not understood is that help for others can only come from a natural overflowing of their own strengths and wisdom. Enthusiasm and powerful opinions are not a substitute for this and may indeed hinder rather than help. The "Bog Asphodel person" often finds it difficult to see that sometimes a suffering person may need to work out their own salvation. Imposed "help" can block the true healing process especially where the helper is influenced by their own prejudices and beliefs. Bog Asphodel people tend to be trapped by their emotional reactions to the suffering of others. They need to spend more time gently looking to their own personal growth and developing their true sense of humour. A lightness of touch and a slightly whimsical approach is essential to all "healers" if they are to fully help others and not become trapped by their work. Bog Asphodel encourages people to take their "mission in life" more lightly and to avoid entanglements with the suffering of others. The irony is that many of the people whom they try to help may well be suffering from the same problem – that of living their life at too great an intensity!

BRACKEN (Aqueous extract) (L)

This essence relates to the blocking of psychic sensitivity in childhood. This particular difficulty is not covered by the "Childhood" combination included in chapter 9. Children are naturally psychically aware from the moment of birth. However, this sensitivity often becomes blocked due to the influence of others (usually adults). They may call it "childish imagination" and something that needs to be grown out of. Children having imaginary playmates is just such psychic sensitivity in action. If this sensitivity is blocked by the attitudes of others, it can lead to a deep-rooted fear of the intuitive mind. It may show as a feeling that there is something wrong or unreliable about intuition. It is this fear of coming "up-front" and accepting these suppressed abilities that causes the problem. If the conditioning has gone very deep, then the person can react violently against any suggestion that these faculties exist. This denial may be extremely vehement, even leading to accusations of such faculties being of the devil. A Bracken person usually appears to be very "left-brain" or logical-mind dominated, yet in fact they have great sensitivity that is well hidden. Often there is a tendency to put higher values on "things" rather than people. Things, being predictable, fit much more comfortably into their adopted logical view of the world. Attempts to fit people into this logical view can cause many problems, as people inconveniently refuse to fit into a steady predictable pattern. Bracken helps to gently unblock the intuitive mind. Communication can then take place at levels other than the "logical", bringing much joy as a result. Being involved in artistic pursuits may well help a suppressed intuitive and creative side to awaken. This in turn will encourage the left and right hemispheres of the brain to 'talk to each other', promoting increased personal harmony and ease. The 'Yang" composite essence included in Chapter 9 may also be helpful in maintaining stability in the logical side, whilst forging links with the intuitive.

BUTTERBUR

This essence relates to self-esteem and personal power. Many people who are working on their own personal growth suddenly block-off at a particular point along their path. This can be caused by getting a glimpse of the awesome power that is beginning to open up within themselves. Blocking of this sort can result in the person becoming very negative about their personal growth. They may well criticise the methods they have been using or perhaps the teacher they have been working with. If the person concerned has always shied away from power – refusing to accept their rightful place in the world – then they may become very fearful about their power becoming destructive. In the Butterbur personality there is a failure to recognise their own innate "goodness" – the Kingdom of God within. Instead, there is a feeling that if they go on developing their powers they could end up inflicting damage on other people. It is a lack of self-esteem and trust in themselves that lies at the back of such difficulties. Perhaps there are childhood memories of being labelled "wicked" or "naughty". Perhaps they were not truly loved as a child and so lack the self-confidence that such love brings. Perhaps they believed that they were "Born in Sin" or that they were a "miserable sinner" (both corrupt interpretations of the original biblical texts). All of these can have a very negative effect on one's self-esteem. Butterbur helps to dissolve these feelings of self-distrust, so revealing our innate power and spiritual birthright. Opening up to a much greater vision of the world and one's rightful place in it, is the message of this essence.

BUTTERCUP

This is for those who need to open up and let the "sunshine" into their life. Often they have a sunny nature that has been suppressed. Due to their experiences however, they may well have developed a negative "jaundiced" view of things. Indeed they might have become the habitual cynic, always ascribing negative motives to any good deed performed by others. These are people who have been badly treated in the past and their confidence in others severely shaken. Perhaps they put their trust in someone and then had it betrayed. This flower can therefore be very helpful for the sceptic or cynic; the person who looks for ulterior motives (real or imaginary) in the actions of other people. Signs of this tendency sometimes show in such things as telling jokes that have a hidden cutting "edge" to them. It is for the person who has lost their trust in others and who needs to let more light and warmth into their own life. From that point of ease they can then open up to others without prejudice. The lovely Buttercup is the flower that puts us in touch with the flame of loving-kindness that lies within each of us. We can then see people as they really are, "warts and all", but with love and compassion and without judgement. It is one of the flowers for the "Heart Centre" of the body.

COMPACT RUSH

The remedy for sadness, for those who feel that life is passing them by. As people become older they often become sad as they begin to dwell on what might have been. They feel that somehow they have missed out on life, that they have not and are not being fulfilled. They begin to dwell on wasted opportunities, or opportunities that were denied them. This sadness is suppressed anger, anger that things were not different. Yet there now seems to be little that can be done. They feel disempowered and resentful. They may resent the actions of others in the past, or they may blame themselves.

Flowering Rush is about new beginnings, fresh starts; about wiping the slate clean. It helps us to look on the past with compassion; that things were as they were because of the surrounding circumstances at that time. It helps to pull the sting from those past memories and so to understand with compassion just why things happened. Looking back is then like seeing an old movie with one's self as one of the actors. The old emotional ties are now no longer present, neither are the sadness and angers that were involved. What lies ahead is then seen as a great number of new possibilities, possibilities that are no longer inhibited by all the old resentments. Flowering Rush helps us to break free of the past and so embrace the present moment with new energies and insights.

DOUBLE SNOWDROP

This is for those who have become too set in their ways. Often they have become, in some way, frozen in their attitudes to life and the world around them. They may have become "experts" – where nothing new is allowed to challenge their established views. Should that happen, they will often react in a very hostile way. In extreme cases the person will become very autocratic, totally believing that they are right. In addition they may well feel that they have a duty to correct the erring ways of others! Luckily most Double Snowdrop people are not so extreme; they are much more likely to have become stuck in a rut and feel unable to get out of it. Feeling "old before one's time" is a classical symptom of this. What is needed is the insight to see that in reality everything is changing and that change, however uncomfortable it may feel at times, is a fact of life.

It is fear of change that is the main Double Snowdrop characteristic. Often this fear results in heavy serious feelings. This essence encourages a lightness of touch and a rejoicing in the newness of life. One can then see that, not only is nothing the same moment-to-moment, but that one can rejoice that it is so. Double Snowdrop helps to break up the crusts of rigid attitudes that are preventing joy and freedom from entering one's life. It also helps to build trust and a feeling of safety as one eases out of the shell of old, rigid patterns. There is then the discovery that the old rigidity was actually very uncomfortable.

EARLY PURPLE ORCHID

This essence is concerned with helping us to get in touch with our own true nature. It can be particularly helpful when old patterns are falling away and the new ways of being have not become firmly established. At these times we can feel weakened by the loss of personal identity that is taking place. It is then that we are vulnerable and can easily fall back into the negativity of old outmoded ways, just because they are familiar. Often we may prefer to polish the bars of our cage rather than fly away through the open cage door! Early Purple Orchid begins to dissolve the blocks which are impeding our progress, whilst bringing harmony to the mind-body-spirit. It helps to open the channels of communication within us, including "blocked chakras".

Because these blocked areas distort our main energy flows, they can and do manipulate our lives. Often we may be totally unaware of these patterns asserting themselves. Sometimes this essence can greatly assist the action of another, more specific, essence. For example, Milk Thistle, for a blocked off ability to really love, will be enhanced by Early Purple Orchid. Similarly, it can be very helpful to use it with the "Transition" composite (included in chapter 9) when the person is having difficulty in allowing new energies into their life.

FIRETHORN (F*)

This is the essence for helping to balance energies. Many people with unstable energies have problems due to suppressed emotions. A typical Firethorn pattern is where suppressed emotions (often caused by old conditionings) stay hidden until they finally "blow their top". After seeing the resulting violent release of energy that has taken place, panic often occurs and the person retreats within themselves. This can lead to a blow-hot/blow-cold alternating energy pattern. Energy or mood swings of this nature can make life very difficult for anyone else involved. Additionally,

"Firethorn" people may have difficulties due to an over-emotional involvement in what they do. They may become very possessive about their own work or expect everyone else to live up to excessively high standards. What is required is that the energy is appropriate for the matter in hand, not too little and not too much. Firethorn helps to bring balance and a more mature attitude in handling one's life so that the energies can ebb and flow as they are needed. The result is a much more tranquil and easy way of living. Once the energies have stabilised, the underlying cause or causes of the instability can usually be seen.

From here it is much easier to see how to deal with the original root causes of the problem, or often, by then, there is the realisation that they have already been dealt with!

FLOWERING CURRANT

This is for those who feel that they are facing inevitable defeat in some part of their life. They have largely lost heart but are still courageously trying to keep on going. The emotional pressure will have made them feel twisted and collapsed, yet they still try to protect the spark that keeps them going. Indeed their physical body may have twisted in response to the mental pressures.

The real problem with people in this state is that they do not recognise their own strengths. They find it difficult to look directly at what opposes them. Often they are so frightened or intimidated, that, like children, they try to hide their faces, hoping it will all go away. Flowering Currant helps with the discovery of one's inner strengths and thereby brings confidence when facing up to opposition. It is only by fearlessly looking directly at opposing forces that we can see how to deflect or overcome them. The truth is always less frightening than the fears that arise from not being able to look things straight in the face. Even when things are not so extreme Flowering Currant can be very helpful. It encourages us to let go of fears and open up to seeing what is actually present in our life.

FOXGLOVE

This is the essence for those who are confused and bewildered. Due to a variety of circumstances, including over-work, people can lose their bearings and their sense of direction. They can become very despondent and lose all their drive. They know that somewhere there is a way out of their difficulties, but somehow they just cannot find it. This can result in trying to push through ways that are blocked to them, with all the consequent frustration. Often there is a clear way out of their difficulties but they are too emotionally blocked to see it. Someone who is continually seeking new therapies for their ailments may well fall into this category. They are often too intellectual about their difficulty trying to think their way out of their problems. The resulting mental exertion makes things even more confused and woolly. Foxglove lessens the emotional entanglement with difficulties, thereby creating distance from the "problem". With the resulting quieter mind, new ways of looking at things will emerge, the confusion and bewilderment naturally falling away. The answers that the person needs will then reveal themselves with such clarity that there will be little doubt as to their accuracy.

HAIRY-SEDGE

This essence is for those who find difficulty in living in the present. There is a tendency to dwell either in the past or in possible futures. This lack of present-moment awareness often causes difficulty with their short-term memory. Some things will bring the person into the present moment; perhaps something that has an impact on their personal well-being, or something that brings them pleasure. These things will normally be remembered. However, things that seem to be of less importance will most likely be forgotten as the person is not then putting their whole attention into what is happening around them. Sometimes poor memory can be due to fear. There may be a reluctance to see what is really there due to the threat that such awareness could bring to established ideas. Awareness therefore becomes restricted, dealing mainly with possible futures and things of the past. This causes memory to be selective, reinforcing personal attitudes and opinions. Anything which would be threatening to those beliefs would then be ignored and forgotten. If a person is too entrenched in their beliefs, it might be better to start with Double Snowdrop. Alternatively both essences could be given together. The amount of progress that can be made with such a client will largely depend upon their willingness to take part in the whole healing process.

LEOPARDSBANE

This is the essence for those who are awakening to their true self, whether consciously or not. They may feel that they are living on a knife-edge and indeed may begin to believe that they are going mad. Such feelings can be very distressing. Yet they may be a very positive sign, showing that the person is beginning to see through the veils of conditioned thought. The negative aspect of the Leopardsbane characteristic is that it can lead to serious depression and even to suicidal thoughts. because of the powerful emotions generated in such states, there is often a real problem with addiction to the feelings of negativity. Leopardsbane helps in two ways. First it helps to lessen the attachment to emotional extremes and secondly it helps the perceptions to broaden. The people who suffer in this way are often very perceptive and may be seeing something of the nature of the "madness" of mankind – the madness of clinging to beliefs or situations that can only cause pain and suffering. They need to see beyond that pain and suffering. Hopefully they will then reach a point where they can understand that this "madness" is an inevitable part of life; at least until people begin to awaken and change. Leopardsbane helps one to see one's own sufferings, as well as those of others, with understanding and compassion.

LILAC

This is for those who have failed to fully develop and blossom in their life and whose personal growth has therefore been stunted. There may be a feeling of being shrivelled-up and sometimes this may show in a shrivelled or stunted physical appearance. This may have been caused by the domination of someone else, for example a parent, partner or teacher. The result of such domination is an inability to freely express what is felt. Lilac encourages an opening up and a restart into growth. It helps one to realise that all is not lost, it is just that one has been hibernating. Unblocking locked-in energies can give remarkably rapid personal growth, rather like plant growth in the spring. Often "Lilac" people have difficulty in accepting their own worth and potential. Indeed they may have become addicted to being a "victim", feeling safe in their prison. Opening the door of the cage and looking out into a much greater world can feel pretty threatening. Love and support is needed to help them through such a major change. We are talking here about true love, not sentimentality – support, not indulgence.

It is often advisable to give the "Transition" composite at the same time as this will give the added support needed through such a period of major change. A description of this is given in chapter 9.

LILY OF THE VALLEY

This is the essence for yearning. It is the essence for those emotionally involved with desiring things that are beyond their grasp. Perhaps they are in love with someone and those feelings are not returned. Perhaps they yearn to experience contact with the "spiritual" planes and the search has proved fruitless. It is like searching for the Holy Grail and never finding it, however hard one tries. Behind the yearning there is a desperate longing. There is a feeling of being incomplete until the object of desire is achieved. It is like a heart-burn that will not go away. The answer lies in giving up the search! Things will then begin to resolve themselves. Emotional searching only blocks the process. In effect, things have been seen back-to-front. It has been likened to playing hide-and-seek with Truth. After desperately searching we find nothing. It is only when we give up and sit quietly that we feel a tap on the shoulder and find that Truth has found us. It is easy to try too hard in our quests in life. Lily of the Valley helps to create "the empty cup" so that what we truly need can find the space within us and enter in. It is about learning to trust the forces that created us in the first place.

MARSH THISTLE

This essence is for those who are locked in the past. At some time in their life many people will have experienced this state. It is where the familiar and routine are depended upon for support and anything new is looked upon with fear and suspicion. When this attitude becomes chronic, it is a difficult one to break. Marsh Thistle helps the fear of newness to fall away but allows the change to take place gently. This gentle approach is necessary when the views have been very entrenched and without it one of two possibilities may occur. Fear could lead to a rebound back into the original state. Alternatively, the personality may go headlong into the opposite state of welcoming everything new, however inappropriate it may be. Once the person has moved away from their fixed viewpoints, then what was previously seen as a haven from the threats of the world will be seen as it really was – a cage – a prison where the door was locked. Marsh Thistle helps to unlock that door so that the person is free to come and go as they please. It is the remedy for all those who are trapped in routine attitudes and situations. Marsh Thistle is about being joyous and free in the world – instead of the old cage there is now a whole new fascinating world to explore. It is about being open to newness and change and welcoming those changes as they occur. Like the down of the Marsh Thistle, one can now float effortlessly with the currents of the lifeforce itself.

MILK THISTLE

This essence relates to the chest area of the body – in eastern terms the Heart Centre (Heart Chakra). For many people this is a place of great vulnerability because it is where they experience fear as well as love. In many ways love and fear are opposite. Fear can suppress love, yet love can overcome fear. Difficulties in this part of the body are often due to blocked-off love of the self and of other people. Typical physical symptoms are a "caved-in" look where the shoulders are pulled forwards and downwards and the breathing is restricted due to a pinched-in chest. In this case it can be very helpful to encourage working with suitable exercises. These need to be designed to ease the shoulders back and help the chest-box to expand forwards, outwards and upwards. The "defeated" posture in someone is a fairly sure sign that they have a poor opinion of themselves – self-love and self-esteem being at a very low level. Milk Thistle encourages the person to open to love and let go of the fears that are restricting them. In opening at this level, there may be temporary feelings of pain or increased vulnerability. This is due to positive change taking place. Reassurance and loving help may be needed until sufficient courage has been gained to enable the person to look the world straight in the face. They will then begin to understand that the world itself is, in reality, a loving environment. A very useful and powerful essence, Milk Thistle is about helping people to bring more light and love into their lives. Early Purple Orchid assists the process when given at the same time.

MONK'S HOOD

This is for long-standing difficulties, the roots of which lie in the past – very often childhood. Such chronic difficulties show that problems have been carried forward rather than being resolved at the time when they originally occurred. Very often the Monk's Hood person has not updated their views of the world and tends to see things with old attitudes and beliefs. In childhood they could well have been heavily indoctrinated with ideals and dogmas of religion, politics or nationalism. As a result there is often a dogmatic stance in these areas of belief. What is needed is the ability to understand just how they were indoctrinated in those early years. Monk's Hood gently helps one to see things of the past as they really were – with all the old attitudes and emotions stripped away. It enables us to see our past with the wisdom of our present status, bringing with it a compassionate understanding. This encourages the person to see parents and other dominant influences in far less "black and white" terms. It is only through such insight that we are freed from the past. When attitudes of the past let go, then the problems that are energised by those old tensions usually let go at the same time.

MOSS (P★)

This is the essence for those who fear the dark spaces within themselves. Like the childhood fears of darkness, many people fear the uncharted areas within their own being. For some, there may be fears instilled by childhood teachings, such as that of being inherently sinful. For others it may be the feeling of having dark secrets hidden within the subconscious mind. There are many people who struggle on, dogged with these deep fears. Sometimes they feel compelled to help others in a desperate attempt to atone for the "evil" that they feel within themselves. Moss helps to show that fears about the subconscious are only "Paper Tigers" – shadows that disappear when light is shed on them. It is fear that prevents the light of insight from entering the mind and fear is therefore responsible for the dark spaces. Moss lessens these addictive fears and loosens up the constrictions. The dark spaces are then transformed into places of light and illumination. This remedy relates to Butterbur, but operates more on the level of the subconscious mind. As we are released from our fears, we will then discover that our subconscious mind is a treasure-house. It is not the "Freudian" dark place of repressed sexual feelings. It is the residence of our intuition and our essential link with the infinite and loving essence of the universe.

PINE CONES (F*)

This is for those who feel trapped by the authoritarian power of others and are totally unable to escape. The source of these feelings of inadequacy and the need for the approval of others, can usually be traced back to childhood. There is such a lack of self-confidence that the ability to express one's own personal authority may well be impossible. In adolescence, the inhibiting forces may have been so great that the normal changeover from parental authority to self-authority will not have taken place. Often there will have been a dominant parent who was over-protective, thus preventing the child from making its own decisions and learning from its own mistakes. If the dominant authoritarian power came from a priesthood then there may well be fears of evil, of the Devil, or of losing one's own soul, unless one does exactly as one is told. To those who have been heavily dominated, the world can seem to be a frightening place, resulting in a need to turn to to others for help and reassurance. This essence helps to free one from worrying about pleasing others, so bringing the understanding that "authorities" are simply people, people who may well know less about the truth of things than you do. The opinions of others are then seen in their true perspective. Pine Cones opens one to the realisation that in breaking free from the authoritarian control of others, all one has to lose are one's own chains.

PINK PURSLANE

Many people have illusions about what really goes on in the outside world. In some, this tendency can become very deep-rooted and they may become quite obsessive about what they consider to be reality. This can show up as religious or political dogmatism. Very often these ideas will have been implanted within the person at an early age. In other words their views are a reflection of those held by their parents or teachers. Pink Purslane is about helping people to gain a quiet detached viewpoint where they can begin to see the limitations of their previous view of the world. To protect their conditioned opinions of "reality" such people can become very defensive and opinionated. Indeed they may have become revered teachers as they will have spent much time getting their beliefs into a coherent and ordered form. They usually have a plausible answer to any question, yet their arguments often have hidden flaws. This blinkered approach means that there will be large areas of reality not encompassed by their doctrines. Pink Purslane is concerned with expanding one's awareness and bringing the realisation that there is no end to learning or to enlarging one's view of reality.

RHODODENDRON

For those who always seem to be "pushing the river". They try to find ways out of
blind alleys, or try to force ready-made solutions onto problems. Often there is a
degree of desperation behind their actions as they become more and more frustrated
in their efforts. When things refuse to work for them, then an ever increasing effort is
expended in trying to make them work, rather than taking a quiet overall look at the
whole situation. When things either break under the pressure, or refuse to budge,
then other factors may well be found to take the blame for the situation (often other
people). This essence helps to bring a detachment from and a lessening of, our
dependence on particular beliefs or theories. It enables us to stand back from
situations and feel into just what is happening. With humour we may then see how
we became trapped in the situation. The fixed ideas at the back of these states often
relate to childhood conditionings and the expectations of others. We may have
become fixated by the idea that to any particular problem, there must be a solution.
The patterns characterised by Rhododendron may also have developed in
adolescence. One example would be a teenager trying to live up to a parents
expectations regarding academic work. The "workaholic" who is locked into his work
is also a typical Rhododendron personality. What is needed in all these cases is an
increasingly relaxed, less frenetic, approach to life. For this, Rhododendron is the
essence of first choice.

SCARLET PIMPERNEL

A useful essence for those who are emotionally entangled with another person. There
are two states – either being obsessed or being "possessed" by someone else. In
either case they are unable to break free, even though they may realise that the
relationship is unsatisfactory and probably very bad for them. There may well be
strong psychic bonds originating from the dominant person. These can be difficult
to break as the other person usually has a lot to gain from the relationship on a
possessive level. Often there is a deep-rooted fear in the "victim" so far as breaking
free from this connection is concerned. The affected person fears that breaking the
connection will leave them void and desolate. In addition they know that they will
have to face the anger of the dominant person. Domination by others saps our willpower and subverts our energies. The process frequently starts by someone seeming
to offer us something that we want or feel we need – for example, love, sex, money
or spiritual growth. We fail to see that sometimes the person offering us these things
is, in some way, a predator and that we may well become a victim if we fall under
their spell. Scarlet Pimpernel works at a hidden level, enabling us to disconnect the
ties that bind us and helping us to gain sufficient power to finally break free. To
lessen the chance of the other person seeing the process of change and therefore
"upping the stakes", Early Purple Orchid can, with advantage, be given at the same
time.

SEA CAMPION

This essence is for those who suffered separation early on in their life. Whilst this is
most frequently due to a separation from the mother, equally a separation from the
protective male energy of the father can cause trauma. All human babies and many
animal ones, need a close bond with their mother during the early stages of their life.

This builds up a sense of security and one of being cared-for and loved. That in turn gives a strong firm basis for the youngster to grow up feeling secure in the world in which it finds itself. As well as the loving maternal background, babies also need the feeling of firm protective energy around them. Ideally this comes from the father, but can be provided by some equally supportive Yang energy.

If a loving stable background is weak or missing, then the youngster will feel insecure and fearful. This can lead to nightmares and bed-wetting in childhood. When older they may have deep-rooted feelings of insecurity and be dogged by fears. Such fears can greatly disempower that person, preventing them from properly expressing themselves in the world.

Sea Campion is a flower that relates to the Earth Element. If we are properly "earthed", then we are in harmony with nature. We have a strongly rooted quality that enables us to withstand "The slings and arrows of outrageous fortune", as Shakespeare would put it. The element Earth is to do with nurturing, with "being at home" with situations, with belonging to this Earth that is our present home.

Sea Campion is therefore a flower that helps us return to our roots, to find contentment and peace in the world. It grows on bleak windswept cliffs that are battered with the winter storms, yet it still blossoms in the Spring. Sea Campion is a "Return to Earth" flower, helping to bring ease to the insecure heart.

SOAPWORT

This is the essence that is needed when there is great bewilderment and confusion. There may well be that "What the hell am I doing here?" feeling, which is usually followed by the mental question "How do I get out of here?" This state is often encountered during personal development as the older identities lose their grip and fall away. The loss of personal self-image at such times can be quite devastating. It can be a time of distress and trauma, the old having fallen away and the new not yet fully emerged. It is in this personal "void" that many deep positive changes can take place, so what is needed is encouragement. A "Better the devil you know rather than the one you don't" feeling can so often take over at this time. Soapwort prevents one from falling back into these old ways. It can be viewed as helping to wash away the past negative influences and providing love and encouragement for the new. Often it is best complemented with the "Breakthrough" composite (see chapter 9) to stabilise the psyche as the new states of being emerge.

SOLOMON'S SEAL

This is the essence for the busy mind; for the person who has things that need doing, but somehow cannot get round to completing them. All too often, the person gets bogged down with trivia, unable to settle to the more essential jobs in a clear and competent manner. What is usually not perceived is that it is the act of being busy that is the real problem. By becoming quiet and apparently doing less, we actually become much more efficient, spending far less time and energy doing things in the "wrong" way. Indeed hopefully we will question the need for doing some things at all! This "busy-ness" is often exploited by other people who see us as a "soft-touch", using us to do what they want, irrespective of our own needs. As we quieten, we increasingly discover what we need to be doing for our own fulfilment. Less and less will we be automatically carried away by the requests of others. This essence can also be very helpful to those who practice meditation but who have problems with a constantly chattering mind. This is a very common complaint – having a mind that just will not shut up. Our mind should be our servant, not the master. Solomon's Seal helps us to reassert our rightful control over our wayward mind. It is rather like training an unruly dog, so it may take an appreciable time. However, the end result is well worth the time taken.

SUMACH (L★)

The essence for those who steadfastly refuse to accept their own potentials. Many gifted people "hide their light under a bushel" and try to pretend that they do not have those gifts. There are many different reasons. It could be that much dedicated work or a considerable financial input is needed. Perhaps their partner is deeply opposed to it. Maybe there is a problem of self-image such as "People like me can't do things like that", or "Others do these things far better than I ever could". These are usually just excuses put up by their conscious mind. The reality is that they are frightened of owning up to their full powers and potentials. In accepting their true role in life they would have to accept a new self-image – that of a powerful adult. They would then have to come out into the open, which could well cause great feelings of vulnerability. Sumach shows us that there is no hiding place and that it takes far less energy to accept what one is rather than waste energy in trying to oppose it. When one finally accepts one's true status the reaction is always the same – "Why did I put up so many barriers to change, when life is so much easier this way?" Sumach helps to reveal our true self.

THRIFT

This essence is indicated where stabilisation of the psychic areas of insight is needed. It is the essence for those whose psychic gifts are developing, but who need this development to be strongly "earthed". A tree cannot grow to maturity without firm roots. In just the same way, we must be strongly rooted in ordinary everyday life before it is safe to open up to other aspects of reality. Some people tend to go "over the top" in the psychic areas and become very emotionally involved in beliefs and concepts. Thrift helps to stabilise the being so that the psychic gifts can develop in balance with other aspects of the personality. These gifts will then be seen as neither more, nor less, "spiritual" than those in any other area. For many, this "earthing" is very necessary. Opening up to psychic areas without sufficient grounding can easily give rise to "psychic attack" or other forms of vulnerability. Thrift helps to establish a strong safe base for our inner development. This essence can be very helpful to those who work as healers or teachers and who find that they tend to take on the symptoms of their clients. In Chakra terms, this essence relates to stabilising the energy flows between the Brow and Root centres.

TUFTED VETCH

The key remedy for many sexual difficulties. People frequently have a fairly mixed-up sexual self-image. This is hardly surprising considering the number of manipulative power games that are played out with sex as a basis. A wholesome human characteristic has variously been portrayed as "dirty", obscene, something to lust for, manipulate others through, etc. With all the heavy conditioning from childhood onwards, many people have difficulties in this area. Sex, like money and power, has traditionally been used to manipulate people and we grow up in an environment where such manipulations are widespread. Tufted Vetch helps us to rebalance our own sexual self-image in both male and female aspects. At the same time it is worth looking to see if either the "Yin" or "Yang" composite (see chapter 9) is needed, to bring the "male" and "female" characteristics into closer balance. As we become more balanced between our own male and female sides, then we will find that much of the sting is taken out of our relationships with other people at a sexual level. Only when we are really at ease with our own sexuality will we find the ease in sexually relating to other people. Only then can we truly honour our own sexuality and then, by reflection, honour the sexuality of others.

WELSH POPPY

This is for those who have lost their fire and inspiration and have become day-dreamers. It is for those who have previously been energised and active, but somehow their usual driving energies have been dissipated. Previous goals have lost their meaning. There is a day-dreaming, bewitched feeling. Sometimes this daydreaming state is like following a path into a sunny field full of beautiful flowers. We get so carried away with lying in the sun and looking at the flowers, that we forget there is a path that goes on beyond that field. People in this state frequently feel that their problems are due to the negative influence of others. In fact the problem relates to changing perceptions; old goals, now being seen in a new light, have lost their allure. Welsh Poppy helps to bring energy and inspiration back into one's life. It helps to liberate blocked creative energies and points us towards our true path.

WITCH HAZEL

This is for those who are for ever trying to live up to the expectations of others – the "willing horses" who are constantly trying to please their parents, teachers, partners, children, or whoever. You may find them on committees; the "eager-beavers" who are always busy and always helpful. They feel that to "let the other side down" is to fail, so they drive themselves relentlessly. This state often relates to childhood, when the person felt that to keep their parents' approval they had to live up to their parents' expectations of them. This in turn gave rise to a conditioned response of always trying to gain the approval of others. What they now need is a wider view of the world where they take their "mission" in life rather less seriously, ceasing to give themselves such a hard time. Witch Hazel helps the mind to drop its dependence on this continual stimulation and thus breaks the vicious circle. With progressive quietening and ease, a completely new evaluation of one's life then becomes possible. Solomon's Seal can be very helpful when used at the same time.

WOOD ANEMONE

For problems where the roots are very old, often before birth. Some of these may well be karmic. "Acting completely out of character" can be an indication of this state. Where there are deep-rooted psychic problems, this is often the best remedy to start with. Sometimes there can be a blaming of others for "psychic attack" with an unconscious refusal to accept the part that they themselves may have played in the process. There can be deep feelings of guilt and fear in such people, even though they have no idea why they are feeling fearful or guilty. Wood Anemone helps to clear these old blocked areas, illuminate them and so resolve the old tension patterns. Because of their very old origins, karmic problems have gained the reputation of being difficult to eradicate. In fact if the person deals with problems as they arise in this lifetime, the past difficulties will also be resolved. It is in the present time, not in the past, that we rebalance our life. Monk's Hood can often be helpful when used at the same time.

EXTRA ESSENCES

BISTORT (*) (Incorporated in Transition composite)

Bistort helps those who are at a major change-point in their life. They are at a point where old ways of relating to the world are under pressure from new and more relevant ones. In many ways it mirrors the needs of people at the present time. At times of severe personal crisis people may arrive at the point where they begin to suffer from "Nervous Breakdown". Their old ways of being are no longer working for them. Bistort can help to convert this possible breakdown into a "breakthrough". It also helps to awaken the person's own love and self-protection at times of major emotional upheaval. For many people, these times of personal crisis are very traumatic – often giving rise to much negativity and depression. "Why should this happen to me?" is the cry that is often expressed. This negativity can produce a "self-destruct" outlook where people may progressively withdraw from sources of possible help, even becoming suicidal. Bistort helps to provide an "inner scaffolding" to maintain the basic structure of the personality and it also provides loving support during the change processes. It is important to give positive encouragement to people undergoing traumatic changes in their lives. These times are like the pain of giving birth – in this case it is the possible birth of a new and more positive way of living one's life.

BLACKTHORN (Incorporated in Despair composite)

Blackthorn is for those who are in the depths of despair, when all seems lost, with life having no meaning and death having no meaning. Often there is a feeling of being in a deep black pit with no way out. Sometimes the person may feel that they are travelling through the "Valley of the Shadow of Death". This is the ultimate point of the "self-destruct" of the personality. It is the point where all our illusions have been shattered by the force of outside circumstances. Blackthorn mirrors this feeling with its sharp black thorns everywhere. Yet from these depths a completely new growth into a much lighter way of living is possible – leaving the old restricting ways behind. There is a dawn beyond the darkest night; it is only our fears that block us from seeing the light. Many "Blackthorn people" find themselves in that deep pit because of their strong Ego, their own powerful personal approach to life. Facing the fact that those personal opinions may be fatally flawed is not easy when there has been a strong personal investment in them. It is the conflict between strongly held personal opinions and Truth, (as it is experienced in the person's life) that finally precipitates the collapse into despair. The basic problem is that the Ego can be so powerful that, rather than accept that the strongly held beliefs were incorrect, it can produce in the person despairing or even suicidal thoughts. There is however, always a way out of this despair if the person will accept the challenge and acknowledge that a new way of living is possible. Blackthorn can help to ease the trauma of this change and also illuminate the way forward.

BRACKEN (L*) (Incorporated in Childhood composite)

This is for those who have habitually played the "child" role in life. Such people often have a chronic inability to express their inner feelings and insights. Perhaps due to parental or other domination, the person was never encouraged to take increasing responsibility for their life. As a result, there can be a tendency to try to get their own way by acting the "child" role. Such people may fill with tears when spoken to harshly. The problem with playing the subservient role is that it becomes difficult to express ones own true self in the world. When things have been bottled up for many years there will inevitably be deep resentments. These resentments, when not expressed openly, can lead to feelings of frustration, depression, toxic dejection and defeat. When feelings are hidden or suppressed it is rather like a volcano that never blows its top. This suppressed energy often gives rise to chronic sadness. A failure to fully grow-up mirrors in life as an insistence on playing the role of the child – being submissive yet often subversive. This subversion is how many children get back at their parents to whom they cannot face up to directly. The alcoholic extract of bracken helps to dissolve the influence of these old childish states. However some people may find the positive changes quite threatening. It is rather like coming out into the light, after living your previous life in a dark cave. In these cases Transition composite should also be given, for vital support and comfort.

CHARLOCK (Incorporated in Childhood composite)

For the "Peter Pans" of this world – the essence for those who have never fully grown up and moreover do not want to grow up. They want to live in a world where everything is good and things are predictable. "Charlock people" tend to have a naive and trusting approach to life. They believe that if you are nice to other people, then they will be nice to you. They can become prime targets of the world's "con-men" and are often genuinely puzzled that they are so frequently hurt by others. What is needed is for them to leave being their attachment to childish ways, but without losing the openness of the child-like way of approaching anything new. This remedy helps to show that an adult approach to life can be infinitely more rewarding than the restrictions of childhood. It also helps the person to see that responsibility does not have to mean a heavy way of dealing with things. Charlock helps to open the door to being a confident, competent, joyful adult.

HONESTY (Incorporated in Yin composite)

This is for a lack of openness and receptivity. This can occur when the Yin (right brain) aspect of the person has been used, but in a negative way. If the assertive Yang side has been suppressed, perhaps due to a dominant parent, then that person may misuse the "female" Yin side of their nature in an attempt to assert themselves. The difficulty is that the Yin aspect of one's personality cannot be used to mimic the Yang. The result is that the person then attempts to control situations by subversion. This "negative female" shows in being secretive, in not telling the whole story about things, thus maintaining a hold on the situation. This characteristic is due to not having really grown up – the "deceitful child" who resorts to deceitfulness because that is the only way they can assert themselves. Honesty helps one to overcome these subterfuges. Reducing emotional dependency on negative female ways encourages openness and honesty. At the same time a calm Yang "male" energy will develop to protect the otherwise vulnerable new state of being.

LESSER STITCHWORT (Incorporated in Possession composite)

The essence for those who need to escape from the thought patterns and influences that "possess" them. Such possession may even feel as if someone else is controlling their actions. The things that possess us can be many and various. It may be attitudes and opinions that we have come to believe in. It may be that someone is trying to obtain a dominant position so that they can control our life. Or perhaps we have become so involved with our own possessions that in reality they now possess us, as we endeavour to hold on to them. What we need in our life is to reduce our dependency on things and relationships. When that happens, what we truly need will naturally stay with us and the rest will fall away. Lesser Stitchwort works in two ways. First, it helps to dissolve our emotional entanglement with objects, events and people. These greatly restrict our freedom of action in the world. Second, it acts, like a guiding star, to illuminate the path ahead. It also gives us the insight and encouragement to follow that path as it opens up before us.

MARIGOLD (Incorporated in Yin composite)

This is the essence for the person who has totally blocked their Yin sensitivity. Whereas the Aqueous Bracken personality is merely suppressing their sensitivity, the Marigold personality has gone one stage further. They may well vehemently deny and attack any suggestion that there is anything in this universe but that which can be "scientifically" detected and explained. The extreme of this is the professional sceptic who seeks to expose "fake" healers, mediums, dowsers, etc. Often these people are inherently sensitive but are afraid to admit it. As Shakespeare put it "Methinks they protesteth too much". They could well find it too threatening to embrace the "feminine" Yin side of their nature. Marigold is therefore particularly useful for all those who have blocked the light from their feminine side. It helps to dissipate the fear of the feminine aspects and gently encourages the growth of positive insight.

NASTURTIUM (Incorporated in Yang composite)

This is for those who know that they need to make changes in their life. They may wish to do so, yet they feel unable to make the first move to start the change process. Somehow there always seems to be something that prevents them from getting started. There are two factors needed for the process to start and Nasturtium helps with both of them. The first is that of having sufficient energy to initiate the change. The second is a recognition of the need to let go of the attitudes and fears that will otherwise inhibit the change process. In fact it is usually this latter factor that is the key problem. For some people, guilt feelings or fears about the changes in personal status will almost certainly occur. For others there will be fears of having to come up-front and accept a more responsible role in life. Nasturtium helps us to accept different future roles in life. It helps us to accept the challenge of change and to view such change with lightness and positivity rather than fear or dread. Nasturtium encourages change, growth and a whole new future.

RED CLOVER (Incorporated in Yang composite)

This is for those who are emotionally blocked off. This blocking off is the result of a deep-rooted fear of the emotional side of one's nature. There is a real fear of the serious damage that unbridled emotions can bring. Red Clover helps the emotional side to gently emerge. It is important that this change is gradual so that the person can integrate the changes without stress. The usual indications are when someone has the tendency to appear hard, cold and calculating and everything is equated to utilitarian ends. To this "machine" type of person "art for art's sake", just "watching the world go by", doing "useless" things, may appear incomprehensible. Here the problem is usually due to a largely blocked-off right (intuitive) brain function. Red Clover encourages communication between the two sides of the personality. The left (logical) brain will then begin to allow and trust the activities of the right brain and finally rejoice that it has such an amazing partner to work with.

SERBIAN SPRUCE (Incorporated in Yang composite)

This is for those whose Yang "male" energy is low. It is the essence to choose for a lack of assertiveness. Many people prefer to take a low profile rather than come up-front and accept personal responsibility for their actions. Sensitive people, whose Yin "feminine" aspect is dominant, often have difficulties in dealing with the Yang side of their nature. It is the opposite aspect to the Red Clover personality. Both are equally unbalanced but in opposite directions. Here it is a fear of being exposed to the "hard light of reality" that is the problem. Often there is an exaggerated emotional response to life. What is needed is a gentle but firm "earthed" energy and Serbian Spruce points the way to this. Many people have the mistaken belief that the "Rambos" of this world represent the "true" male aspect, whereas in fact they represent the negative aspects of the male. The positive male aspects of uprightness, openness and "outgoingness" are the qualities needed and encouraged by this essence. Serbian Spruce helps to lift the Yang energies up to the level of the Yin.

SINGLE SNOWDROP (Incorporated in Transition composite)

This is for those who are experiencing difficulties in breaking through to new levels of consciousness and awareness. It is the essence for the person who seems to have met a barrier on their path towards personal freedom. The usual problem is that of being open to "corruption" by old habit patterns. It is as if these old patterns realise that their future existence is under threat and so they react in an attempt to remove that threat. The net result is that one's efforts are continually being subverted, in spite of having the best of intentions. There can also be difficulties due to increasing insight. Seeing things more clearly can, at first, give the impression that it is rather a bleak world that surrounds one (rather like the world that the snowdrop sees as it emerges). Single Snowdrop helps to reveal the joyful potential of a true and wider vision. Old identities can then be seen for what they really are – apparently comfortable strait-jackets!

SPRING SQUILL (Incorporated in Transition composite)

For those who are breaking through to new freedoms, the "Jonathan Livingstone Seagulls"† of this world. These are the ones who are finding joy in realising that they really can be free, where previously they had been limited by their own ideas and concepts, rather than anything else. Sometimes this transition is difficult. There may be pressure from family, peer groups, "friends", etc. who find these new ways very threatening and who may try nearly anything to prevent or reverse the change. Those breaking through into these new freedoms often need support for their vulnerable self-confidence. It can seem quite lonely, flying in freedom, apparently alone. Spring Squill, relating as it does to the Crown Chakra, can assist in this. From the viewpoint of freedom, the world is then seen as it is; an amazing workshop for emerging souls. Without that insight, our fears and attitudes may well paint it as a dark and fearsome place, to endure or to escape from; Spring Squill helps us to see more widely and more deeply into the true nature of reality. This remedy is most effective when other major blockages (particularly at the Heart centre) have been eased. Only when all the groundwork has been done can a person truly begin to fly free.   †*Jonathan Livingstone Seagull by Richard Bach.*

VALERIAN (Incorporated in Childhood composite)

The essence for the "lost child". This person may even look rather like a pathetic lost child that is in need of help and support. Instinctively one feels one's heart go out to them – they seem so alone and helpless. However they can easily become very manipulative – always getting others to provide help and support. This manipulation is not normally at a conscious level and they may be totally unaware of its existence. Many people feel sorry for the lost child and may try to bring them out of their loneliness and misery. In reality, help in this form is most likely not needed at all. Often the original cause of the problem is that the Valerian personality has had a childhood deprived of true love. Although they may put a brave face on things, deep down they feel bereft and unable to love other people. They also know that something within them needs the love, support and encouragement that was previously denied them. Valerian encourages the development of self-love and self-esteem, lessening the need for external support and so reducing the demands placed on others. Ironically, as this happens, it is far more likely that the person will then gain the support that is really needed.

YEW(*L & F) (Incorporated in Yang composite)

For resilience and for escaping from rigid patterns of thought and behaviour. Due to tensions in their life, many people become brittle and although they may appear to be strong, they may suddenly crack under pressure. They are like cast iron which, although very strong, can fracture easily under a sudden shock. They may have developed strong principles about which they are very protective. This can result in them reacting fiercely against what they see as opposing forces. Yew helps people to see that there is no sin in being both resilient and flexible, or indeed bowing before the storm. It also helps to bring the discernment needed to accurately assess just what forces are involved in any particular situation. After all, only a fool will stand in the path of an express train. Yew helps people to become less proud of their own ideas and concepts and more open to new approaches and ideas. It helps to break up the rigidity of outmoded patterns of thought and behaviour. A very useful essence for people who have become trapped by their own beliefs and opinions.

❀ BALLYBANE FLOWER ESSENCES ❀

Back in 1992, spring time to be exact, I was out in the garden looking at the season unfolding. Inside myself it was chaos. As a herbalist I always look to what is growing. On a bank, beside a stream a beautiful carpet of sweet violets grew. I sat and looked at them, admiring their beauty and wishing I was like them, content with life. At this point they began to sing to me and show me things, telling me I could be beautiful if

I just allowed them into my life. That was the start. The flower essences are dedicated to St. Brigid.

BLUEBELL

Keywords – 'No one is more powerful than thou'.

Negative aspects – Always weepy. Over eager. Scattered thoughts. Recovery from bad judgement. Lacking vitality.

Positive aspects – Quality time with your children. Feeling happy and content. Recognising a reincarnation.

Physical attributes – Lassitude. P.M.S.

COMFREY

Keyword – 'Transformation'

Negative aspects – Environmental chaos. Wintery feeling inside. When words are inadequate. Fear of giving self time out.

Positive aspects – 'I understand the Great Unknown'. Preparation for a winter hibernation. Helps lift the Spirit. Regaining faith.

Physical attributes – Pains in the joints. Profuse menstruation.

CREEPING BUTTERCUP

Keywords – 'Secrets, Binding'

Negative aspects – When life is disintegrating. Perplexed. Unsure. Pensive parents. Attention seeking in children.

Positive aspects – Brings lovers together. Transmutation. Feminine principle. Getting to the mountain. Remembrances.

Physical attributes – A rescue remedy for children specifically.

DOG VIOLET

Keywords – 'Down Trodden'

Negative aspects – For despair and violence especially toward children. Reluctance. Overload.

Positive aspects – Oneness; Joy enters one's life like a beam of sunlight.

Physical attributes – Some cancer conditions, head problems, congestion in chest, sore feet.

EARLY PURPLE ORCHID

Keywords – 'Shape Shifter'

Negative aspects – Temper tantrums in children. For children who tell tales. For children who bully. Misrepresentation. Self obsessed. Overload. Bad spellers. Do not want to be alone.

Positive aspects – Clinging to Life. Feeling of unconditional love. Helps physically disabled people to respect themselves. Surprise out of the blue.

Physical attributes – Insomnia. Serous back injury. Trauma. Pain in the right pelvis in women.

EUPHRASIA

Keyword – 'Intuition'

Negative aspects – For children who cry wolf. When one feels like a servant. "On the verge of murdering someone feeling". Let down by one's best friend.

Positive aspects – Sheer joy. Intuition working well. Encourages psychic signals. Good for single parents. For parents who feel they are neglecting their children. For children who are going through a 'rite of passage'.

Physical attributes – Itchy eyes and sinus problems/hay fever.

FIELD SCABIOUS

Keyword – 'Balance'

Negative aspects – Depression when life feels incomplete. Illusion. Fear of growing old. Fear of life.

Positive aspects – Raised consciousness. Regaining intelligence. Communal healing. Spellbinding.

Physical attributes – Delayed menstruation. Good for the onset of clinical depression.

FLOWERING RED CURRANT

Keyword – 'Survival'

Negative aspects – Mood swings. Overly arrogant. Restlessness. Worries on money matters.

Positive aspects – One's presence is felt from afar. Empathy to new surroundings. Nine lives like a cat. Reconciliation. First Spring Day feeling. 'Sweet success comes my way.

Physical attributes – Diarrhoea, shakes, blows to the extremities.

FORGET ME NOT

Keywords – 'Forget me not'

Negative aspects – Nervous about life, remorse with tears, inadequacy.

Positive aspects – 'I can deal with delicate situations'. 'This phase of my life is complete'. Revitalises. Quenches spiritual thirst.

Physical attributes – Pain in lower back.

FUCHSIA

Keywords – 'I have no regrets'

Negative aspects – 'I don't like myself'. Coming to terms with loss either physically or emotionally. Flighty unreal ideas. Fear comes easily. Disobedience in children.

Positive aspects – Co-operation in children. Set one's personal boundaries. Allows one's truth to blossom. 'I need to give to me'. Vision to go on.

Physical attributes – For infertility. Music therapy.

HAWKWEED

Keyword – 'Temperance'

Negative aspects – Social pariah. Completely sapped of energy. Children with speech problems. Fear of the new.

Positive aspects – Return to the community (prodigal child). Revitalised. For childless couples who want children. Fruitful times.

Physical attributes – Gripping in stomach.

HAWTHORN

Keywords – 'The path finder'

Negative aspects – Stress related to house moving. Mental congestion. Abuse of friendship. Child within cries for help.

Positive aspects – Enhances meditative states. Cease being a victim. Helps to find a partner (on any level). Love thyself.

Physical attributes – Post operative on the heart/circulation. Varicose veins. Thyroid.

LADY'S SMOCK

Keywords – 'I go forth and multiply'

Negative aspects – 'I forget details because I am in such a hurry'.' 'I hate you'. To help children through learning difficulties. Worried about being close to insanity. For people who are suffering from post child abuse trauma later in their lives.

Positive aspects – Cleansing. Centred and peaceful. Return of personal power. Regain control.

Physical attributes – Helps uterine contractions. For anxiety.

MEADOWSWEET

Keyword – 'Companionship'

Negative aspects – Boredom in children. To be accepted in an unwelcomed space.

Positive aspects – For children and adults who are studying for exams. Concentration. To help young psyches to realise their potential. To keep one earthed. To aid and strengthen interpretation of omens and symbols.

Physical attributes – Aches in the left shoulder.

PURPLE LOOSESTRIFE

Keyword – 'Wisdom'

Negative aspects – Failure in exams. Last chance. Despair – lost in a maelstrom. Tension. Holding on to negative thought processes. Moodiness especially in men.

Positive aspects – Relaxes. Reflection. Composure.

Physical attributes – When thoughts of disease bring fear and shame.

RAGGED ROBIN

Keywords – 'I love life'

Negative aspects – Unable to celebrate life. When one is let down by a co-worker. Life is at 'boiling point'.

Positive aspects – To reunite – individuals, families, friends and communities. Helps you to avoid conflict. Sensuous. Be blessed.

Physical attributes – Pre-menstrual oedema.

SCARLET PIMPERNEL

Keywords – 'I breathe new life'

Negative aspects – Inertia threatens. Expectations too high. Isolated in grief. Lack of communication.

Positive aspects – Breathes new life and love where previously life was barren. Allows one's tears to flow. Helps to understand loss. Support in time of crisis.

Physical attributes – For tough dry skin. Fear of snow. Liverish people.

SLOE

Keywords – 'I am fragile yet I can live through a storm'

Negative aspects – Fragility. Things are falling apart. Bad judgement. Fickleness. Forgetfulness. Frustration. Fear of success.

Positive aspects – Re-birth of creativity and knowledge.

Physical attributes – Inner knee pain, lassitude in shoulders and arms. Headaches.

TORMENTIL

Keywords – 'Go forth and multiply'

Negative aspects – For women who have lost their partner. For children who do not 'hear'. Pure anger. Hopes for survival.

Positive aspects – Feeling of 'eternal life'. Reclaiming one's creativity.

Physical attributes – Dehydrated. Migraines.

WITCH HAZEL

Keywords – 'Bring forth Light'

Negative aspects – Addictions, fragility, fear of unknown, panic attacks, clumsiness, greed, moving house, work.

Positive aspects – Fruitful work, accepts life's limitations, recuperation after an addiction. Coping in adverse conditions, clarity of thought, the light has been turned on.

Physical attributes – Oedema in hands. Heals deep tissue injuries/trauma.

❀ BRIDGET'S FLOWER REMEDIES ❀

Bridget and Alf Craig's flower remedy system may only be purchased after consultation, diagnosis and instructions as to it's use. Phone: 01580 – 763334.

COWSLIP

Common wild flower, small yellow flowers in bunches, on stems 6" high. Blooms May.

Physical – Nervous system, liver, solar plexus, stomach.

Psychological states – Anorexia nervosa, cannot make decisions, confusion, inability to cope with life, over analytical mind, self critical.

Professions – Psychic abilities, spiritual healing.

Diseases – Anorexia nervosa, bacterial inflammation, eczema, liver imbalance, psychosomatic illnesses, solar plexus imbalance.

Cellular level – Liver.

Major chakras – Eleventh chakra, all chakras.

Minor chakras – Breast bone, liver.

Subtle bodies – Spiritual body, Permanent Atom.

Nutrients – Vitamin A, Zinc.

Psycho-spiritual – Wisdom.

Miasms – All miasms.

Twelve Rays – Eleventh Ray.

THE BRIDE (Exochorda macrantha 'The Bride')
Small shrub, with small white flowers the size of 5p pieces, very pretty. Flowers May.
Physical – Breasts, pelvis, stomach.
Psychological states – Confusion, joy, mental clarity, self nurturing.
Professions – Yoga teachers.
Diseases – Circulatory system, fatigue, motion sickness.
Cellular level – Nerve tissue
Major chakras – Sixth chakra, all chakras.
Minor chakras – Shoulders, wrists.
Subtle bodies – Soul body, Permanent Atom.
Nutrients – Vitamin B.
Psycho-spiritual – Spiritual quest.
Meridians & nadis – Throat nadis.
Twelve Rays – Sixth Ray.

AMELANCHIER
Medium sized tree. White star shaped flowers, blooms in April. Wonderful autumn colours.
Physical – Control of glands improved, lymphs, pancreas, strengthening.
Psychological states – Clarity of thought, compulsive gamblers, courage, drug addiction symptoms, selfishness, will power balanced, will power weak, stopping smoking.
Professions – Spiritual healers.
Diseases – Smoking, torn tissue rejuvenated, varicose veins.
Cellular level – Tissue regeneration.
Major chakras – Fifth chakra, all chakras, Permanent Atom.
Nutrients – Vitamin C, zinc.
Meridians & nadis – Throat nadis.
Twelve Rays – Fifth ray, twelfth ray.

CHRISTMAS ROSE
Cup-shaped yellow/green flowers 2" blooms, March/April. Evergreen.
Physical – Cleansing, colon, intestinal tract, lower intestinal tract, small intestines, spine, spleen.
Psychological states – Anti-depressant, anxiety, grief – death of beloved, pre-cancerous emotional state, schizophrenia, too introverted.
Diseases – Colon spasm, obesity, spinal degeneration, spinal inflammation, weight control.
Cellular level – Fatty tissue removed.
Major chakras – Eighth chakra.
Minor chakras – Shoulders.
Subtle bodies – Causal body.
Nutrients – Fatty tissue, potassium, Vitamin D.
Psycho-spiritual – Psycho-spiritual balance.

Meridians & nadis – Stomach meridian.

Miasms – Syphilitic.

Twelve Rays – Eighth Ray.

ROSEMARY

A herb, deep blue flowers borne on dark green leaves. Flowers March/April.

Physical – Spleen.

Psychological – Self nurturing.

Professions – Travellers.

Diseases – Sun's ultra violet rays blocked, SV40 virus, white corpuscle imbalance.

Cellular – Thymus.

Major chakras – 9th chakra, all chakras.

Minor chakras – Spleen.

Subtle bodies – All subtle bodies, aura, odic force, thermal body, Permanent Atom.

Nutrients – Vitamin E

Psycho-spiritual – Superconscious and subconscious minds

Meridians & nadis – Throat nadis.

Twelve Rays – Ninth Ray.

SINGLE WHITE CHERRY

An elegant tree, large white flowers borne in clusters. Flowers have pretty maroon tipped stamens.

Physical – Antibodies, balances left and right brain, brain, cleansing, conscious mind immune system, kundalini, larynx, left brain, lungs, lymphs, mucus regulated, nasal passages cleared, nature morphines, nerve ganglion in throat, nose, respiratory system, sense of smell, sinuses (hay fever), sweat glands, throat, thyroid, vocal cords.

Psychological states – Emotional cleansing, frustrated, grief, guilt, immaturity, past life problems, self-righteousness, stuttering, subconscious mind cleansed, undisciplined.

Professions – Enhances flower essences, past life therapy, psychic abilities.

Diseases – Breathing trouble, bronchial conditions, common cold, fevers, laryngitis, lung imbalance, mucous colitis, sinus congestion, throat disease, sore throat, tonsillitis, typhoid fever, viral inflammation.

Cellular – Cell communication, circulatory system, DNA, immune system, larynx, liver, lungs, sweat glands.

Major chakras – Tenth chakra, all chakras.

Minor chakras – Tip of index finger.

Subtle bodies – Astral body, emotional body, spiritual body.

Nutrients – All vitamins, manganese, vitamin K.

Psycho-spiritual – Karmic problems, spiritual quest.

Meridians & nadis – Lung meridians, finger nadis, hand nadis, heart nadis, throat nadis.

Miasms – Tuberculosis, all miasms.

Twelve Rays – Tenth Ray.

CANARY BIRD ROSE

A beautiful single flat bright yellow rose, about 1³/₄" across, borne in profusion close to the stem. Flowers in May.

Physical – Cleansing, physical flexibility increases, sense of physical relaxation, strengthening, vitality increased, vocal cords.

Psychological states – Guilt, identity crisis, subconscious mind cleansed, unbending rigid people.

Professions – Crystal ball cleansed.

Diseases – Aids, Alzheimer's, arteriosclerosis, arthritis, asthma, dryness (entire body), M.S., toxaemia.

Cellular – General strengthening, oxygenates the body.

Major chakras – Twelfth chakra, all chakras.

Minor chakras – Wrists.

Subtle bodies – Emotional body, soul body.

Nutrients – Sulphur.

Psycho-spiritual – None.

Meridians & nadis – None.

Miasms – All miasms.

Twelve Rays – Twelfth Ray.

DOG TOOTH VIOLET

Small yellow/green upturned lily shaped flower with nodding head. The name derived from the tooth shaped bulb.

Physical – Capillaries, ears, face, hormones, lips, coccyx, eyes, hair, jaw, nose, retina, scalp, sinuses, skin, teeth, sense of hearing.

Psychological states – Claustrophobia, fear from past lives, needs love, past life problems, self righteousness, universal emotionalism.

Professions – Past life therapy, vegetarians.

Diseases – Eczema, eye problems, hair loss, hearing loss, inner ear problems, motion sickness, periodontal diseases, scalp problems (psoriasis), skin conditions, skin ulcers, smallpox, ulcers (internal).

Cellular – Ovaries, skin, teeth enamel.

Major chakras – All chakras.

Minor chakras – None.

Subtle bodies – Spiritual bodies.

Nutrients – Iron.

Psycho-spiritual – Spiritual quest.

Twelve Rays – None.

❀ CAROLE GUYETT ❀

These essences were made in Berkshire, England.

SKULLCAP

Facilitates contact with the Divine/the Higher Self.

Clears the head and calms the system, can help clear head pain where it originates from congestion.

Clears blocks in the crown chakra and helps where the spiritual connection has been lost and a person feels isolated and alone.

Helpful for childbirth.

Chakras chiefly affected: Crown and sacral.

ST. JOHN'S WORT

Gives divine protection and guidance when in an overly-expanded, dream-like or 'spaced out' state of consciousness.

For vulnerability to harmful influences when spiritually open.

For fears related to out-of-body experiences, fearful dreams, bed-wetting and other night-time childhood traumas.

Helpful for feelings of inadequacy and doubt.

Chakra chiefly affected: Solar Plexus.

❀ CHURCH FARM ROSE ESSENCES ❀

"The rose, where in the world 'Divine' makes itself flesh"

Dante, (Italian poet 1265-1321)

Church Farm Roses are a set of so far 17 essences prepared solely from roses. Because the rose has a unique mystical association with the Divine, the rose carries within its essence a very strong vibration to do with 'Love'. This may be why these rose essences tend to be more subtle and gentle in their effect.

Originally prepared for the newborn they were later also found to be very helpful for the dying, in fact for every situation both physically and emotionally that is more sensitive, vulnerable and fragile. Church Farm Roses, unlike most other flower essences were prepared by moonlight. This is to do with the rose's affinity with the mother, the feminine principle of the Divine source.

Church Farm Roses are also prepared in 7 different combinations, see chapter 9. These combinations cover all the life movements we can expect to encounter, as well as the major body systems.

Church Farm Roses are carried in a vegan base cream which is scented with organic rose oil. This makes them simple and pleasant to use.

ALBA MAXIMA – MOTHER

The remedial qualities are to do with mothering and the bond between mother and child. A good remedy for those who have been denied this or to help with the bonding process during pregnancy and the infant years. Beyond this it also creates a bonding to earth helping those who find it difficult to concern themselves with earthly things. Physically it relates to the womb and is good for problems related to the reproductive system. Emotionally it brings a sense of being loved and nurtured. Spiritually it links to the Divine Mother.

SWEET JULIET-TWINS

Sweet Juliet is related to twins and twin energy. It helps those who feel alienated and not at home on earth to adjust to life on earth. A good remedy for the dreamer, the loner and the fear of earthly things. It has a strong link with the nature energies and is useful for those who need to link more closely with nature. It is the connector between heaven and earth, body and soul. Physically it is good for headaches, migraines, insomnia and the spine, particularly the lower back. Emotionally it is a good remedy for feelings of isolation, disorientation and problems arising from being a twin or a part of a multiple birth, especially if there has been a loss. Spiritually it has a balancing influence harmonising body and soul.

MARY ROSE – PROTECTOR

This remedy is the protector, on all levels. Good for the worried, the nervous, the afraid, it has a calming influence which helps to restore a feeling of order back into uncomfortable or distressing situations. It gives Love to those who feel unloved. It helps those who can not seem to give or receive Love. Physically it relates to the immune system. Emotionally to the nervous system. Spiritually it brings protection.

CHURCH FARM ROSE – WISDOM

This remedy connects very much to wisdom and to the stars, a wisdom beyond earthly perception. It is a remedy for those who are seeking the truth and wish to expand their consciousness, to open the heart and mind to the wisdom of the divine source. Beneficial to those wanting to work on the higher levels of communication. It is very much connected to the spiritual aspects of mankind. Physically it helps to calm and clarify stress and trauma, confusion and instability. Spiritually it is an awakener.

ARTHUR BELL – BALANCE

Arthur Bell is to do with balancing one's earthly life with one's spiritual quest. It is related to the fathering aspect of parenthood. Combined with Alba Maxima it makes an excellent remedy for all children who are experiencing the lack of some aspect of parenting and are going through a difficult time. Physically it is a remedy for the head and mind. Emotionally it brings balance and stability. Spiritually it is the harmoniser balancing the energies between mind, body and soul.

EVELYN – ABUNDANCE

Evelyn is a remedy relating to the generative organs. Physically the kidneys, bladder and reproductive systems. Emotionally it is for those who have suffered or are suffering abuse. Spiritually it connects with creativity and abundance.

LOUISE ODIER – HEART

Louise Odier is a remedy relating to the heart centre covering all aspects of the heart. Physically the heart itself including stress related problems. Emotionally it is to do with all affairs of the heart including grief and heartache in its many forms. Spiritually it opens the heart centre and awakens a sense of beauty, creativity and spirituality.

ALEXANDER – BREATH

Alexander is a remedy related to the breathing system, excellent as a combination with Louise Odier to help the functioning of the heart and lung systems. Physically it relates to the lungs, throat and sinuses. Emotionally it helps to strengthen the will to live and to be alive. Spiritually it vitalises the centres in the lungs and those around the nape of the neck and shoulders enabling a better assimilation of the life force that enters at those points.

SWAN – GRACE

The Swan essence is related to the digestive system. Physically it is for the lower gut and intestines. Emotionally it helps resolve and release jealousy and peevishness. Spiritually it brings an awareness of Grace.

PILGRIM – LIGHT

Pilgrim essence is for those souls who have lost hope, related to sight, vision and light. Physically it relates to the eyes and liver. Emotionally it is useful for anger and those who despair. Spiritually it helps to promote a greater acceptance and awareness of the Light.

FISHERMAN'S FRIEND – PURITY

Fisherman helps clean and purify the system. Physically it relates to the blood and bone systems. Emotionally it helps those who find life exhausting and burdens too heavy to bear. Spiritually it brings strength and enlightenment.

CADFAEL – PEACE

Cadfael helps to bring calmness to those who find difficulty in resting. Physically it is for the nervous system where it helps to soothe a hyperactive system and to uplift the nervously tired. Emotionally it helps to steady the nerves to allow recovery from shocks. Spiritually it dispels fear of the unknown.

CLAIRE – CLARITY

Claire helps promote clarity of mind and thought, helping to free us from negative thought processes, especially those who only see the darker side of life. Emotionally it helps those who are possessive and those who are possessed to release and be released. Physically it relates to all the senses helping to clean and clear them. Spiritually the clearer.

GALLICA – HUMILITY

A remedy for the over sensitive, fragile, weepy. The old and the new born that are delicate. Helps recovery from ill health. Brings purity to heart and mind. Links to the angelic realms and helps attain communication from these realms. Helps the spiritually ambitious to come back to a point of humility. Befriends the ego and prepares for integration of the ego and soul to reach the Christ light within. Relates to the brow and alta major chakras and the blood stream. Its quality is peaceful strength. Helpful for those who work with lunar cycles and energies.

CENTIFOLIA – JOY

Raises the spirit. Moves beyond human grief, whether personal or collective. Enables one to see beyond tragedy to the reflection of joy. Restores balance after trauma, grief and destruction. Good for those involved in war situations, unrest and disruption. Links to the star Sirius, the Atlantean energies and the Sun or star within. Physically it works with the nervous system and emotionally the heart.

ISPAHAN – GRATITUDE

To do with gratitude and graciousness. Useful for those who find it hard to receive and to say thank you, to be loved by the world. Those who are disillusioned by life. Helps attune to the love aspect of the Divine Source, works very much with the higher aspects of the heart energy. Opens the heart to the Christ Light within, to Divine Love and prepares for the connection to Divine Love. Physically it relates to the heart working on the higher emotional aspects to open to Love Divine.

COMFORT CREAM

A combination of Mary Rose, Arthur Bell and Louise Odier in one cream for protection, balance and strength. Useful when someone has suffered a shock at any level to help them feel comforted and secure.

❀ CRYSTAL HERBS – FLOWER ESSENCES ❀

All of the essences listed have been made with love, wonderful help and guidance from spiritual guides and Masters, devas and the angelic kingdom. By using the natural power of the four elements, the pure water into which the flowers are placed becomes potentised. The water then contains the life force or energy of the plant and carries its own unique healing vibration. This vibration is then preserved in brandy, forming a mother tincture, which is then amplified using crystals, pyramids and natural elements, under guidance. All are then hand bottled and labelled with loving care.

AGAPANTHUS

Brings courage and strength to higher purposes.

AGERATUM

Brings the soul qualities into the physical, grounding.

ALMOND

Mental maturity, fears of ageing.

AMARYLLIS

Can be used to perfect the art of meditation, brings calm and stillness, helping to go within.

ANEMONE

Balancing all chakras.

ANGELICA

Affinity with angelic forces.

ARTEMISIA

Helps develop telepathy, for left brain hemisphere damage.

AUBERGINE

Lifts the base chakra energy, shifts blockages. Sexually related problems.

AURICULA

Balances the emotions, solar plexus.

BABY BLUE EYES

Childhood emotional issues, any age.

BASIL

Heart and throat chakras, brings clearance to grief, allowing it expression.

BEGONIA

To move to the next stage of development from a healing plateau.

BELLFLOWER

New borns' adjustment to sound. Children's creative expression. Throat chakra.

BELLS OF IRELAND

Links to Divinity of nature, stress and anxiety.

BERGAMOT

For cleansing and disinfecting wounds and infections. Use internally and externally as a swab with 7 drops in a small cup of water.

BLACKBERRY

Dreams stimulated. Death/dying fears and bereavement depression.

BLACK EYED SUSAN

Will help draw to you that which is needed for your growth and change.

BLACKTHORN

Brings spiritual understanding to fear. Use at night after taking karmic fear essence during the day for release during sleep.

BLEEDING HEART

For those too emotionally attached. Heart chakra, heart diseases.

BLUEBELL

Creative expression, singing, music, chanting, sound therapy. Throat chakra.

BORAGE

Opens the heart chakra, bringing joy.

BROMPTON STOCK

To help those new to spiritual ideas, insight and initiation. Crown and ajna chakras.

BUDDLElA

Helps one to feel spiritual contact in the darkest of situations.

BUTTERCUP

Recognition of self worth from within, not from others' perceptions.

CALENDULA

For energy depletion due to healing process or consciousness raising. Adjustment to new ideas during this period. Base and sacral chakras.

CALIFORNIAN POPPY

Spiritual and psychic balance. Helps assimilation of gold therefore good for nervous diseases and M.S.

CALLA

After physical abuse or cruelty this essence helps restore dignity and self worth.

CAMELLIA

To open, develop and balance heart chakra.

CAMPANULA

Frankness and honesty in expression. Eliminates need for secrecy.

CAMPION

Most pregnancy and birth problems.

CANNA 'PRESIDENT'

Energy. To build stamina and strength.

CANTERBURY BELL

Throat chakra. Inner hearing, in combination with other essences for clairaudience.

CARNATION

Attunement with devic orders and fairies. Crown chakra.

CASTOR OIL PLANT

Helps repair brain neurones, brain disorders. Motor neurone and Alzheimers disease.

CATMINT

Brings alignment between the throat and heart chakras.

CEANOTHUS

Throat chakra, related problems, thyroid. Unconditional love.

CEDAR

Stimulates hair growth, scalp disorders. Colon, intestinal tract.

CELANDINE

Vocal cords, throat chakra, thyroid. Helps access information including contact with spiritual guides.

CENTAUREA

For cleansing of the higher chakras i.e. throat and above.

CHAMOMILE

For calmness, serenity, releasing anxiety. Solar plexus.

CHEIRANTHUS

For strengthening/cleansing of the spleen.

CHICORY

White. Victims of sexual abuse, purity.

CHIONODOXA

Hope, joy and upliftment.

CHRYSANTHEMUM
Helps to bring those of differing ideas more together into harmony. Liver and kidneys cleansed and strengthened.

CINQUEFOIL
Solar plexus. Good for stubbornness.

CISTUS
Cleanses pancreas, useful in a fast.

CLEAVER
For releasing the need for emotional control, possessiveness and taking advantage of others.

CLEMATIS
('Nellie Moser'). Cleanses and opens the 8th chakra, just above the crown.

CLOVER
(Haresfoot). Loosens up the body joints if taken over one month or more.

COLUMBINE
Helps activate brow and crown chakras. Attunement to angelic kingdom.

COMFREY
Nerve endings, nervous system diseases. Memory, left-right brain balance.

CONE FLOWER (ECHINACEA)
Powerful flower, created in Lemuria to symbolise the descent of man into matter. Works powerfully on the physical body, helps strengthen heart, lungs, kidneys and abdomen. Helps purify the blood and helps cells to better communicate with each other.

CONVOLVULUS
Brings alignment to the crown and higher chakras.

CORAL BELLS
Spiritualising sacral/sexual energy.

COREOPSIS
Helps spiritualise the intellect.

CORN
Allergies to corn. Detachment and rationality to emotions.

CORN COCKLE
Helps draw in energy through 9th and 10th chakras.

COWSLIP
Helps children understand relationship and environment problems, helps parents understand children.

CRANESBILL
Helps one become single minded, spiritually and mentally.

CYCLAMEN
Helps the individual to absorb higher energies, especially the new rays currently being directed to earth, consciousness raising transformation of DNA pattern. 1990's essence.

DAFFODIL
Increased sensitivity, inner hearing, higher self attunement.

DAHLIA
Transmutes sexual energy to higher expression. Base and sacral chakras.

DAISY
Brings clarity to thoughts, inner knowing.

DANDELION
Releases muscle tension caused by mental stress.

DAY LILY
Symbolising rebirth, it helps give an understanding of external life.

DEADNETTLE
Helps activate chakras above the crown, especially the 13th. Spiritual energy.

DELPHINIUM
Brings awareness of the need to be a channel for expression of one's individual spirit. Throat chakra.

DEUTZIA
Angels of perfume ray operate with this flower, helps attunement to them.

DIASCIA
Helps those striving towards unconditional love. For distant and earth healers.

DIGITALIS
Helps soften those who are hard hearted. Heart disorders. N.B. This essence does not contain any sap from the plant or flower.

DILL
Brings light to problems. Depression. Obsession with death.

DIPLADENIA
Yellow. Attunement to angelic realms.
White. Grounding spiritual ideas and visions.

ELDERFLOWER
Helps the individual to trust that all their needs will be provided for. Inner security.

ERTHRINA
Liver cleanser. Tonic for nervous system.

EVENING PRIMROSE
For tension at the time of full moon, P.M.T., rebalances hormones.

FEVERFEW

Helps disturbed sleep caused by insecurity.

FIG

Releases hidden blocks and fears in the subconscious, memory and psychic development.

FLAX

Throat problems, throat chakra, for speaking up in group situations.

FORGET-ME-NOT

Anxiety, sleep disturbances, memory, clarity of mind.

FORSYTHIA

Bereavement. Helps us to see higher aspects.

FREDONTODENDRON

Specifically for skin rashes caused by allergies and also for shingles, especially when it is around the solar plexus area.

FRENCH MARIGOLD

Inner hearing, psychic abilities. Inflammation, viruses.

FUCHSIA

White. Gentle emotional release.

Red, white/blue, pink or combination. All work to bring attention to underlying emotions.

GALTONIA

Brings to a head unresolved issues in relationships, especially when having a sexual base.

GARLIC

Cleanser and purifier at many levels. Anger and fear.

GAZANIA

Helps open and cleanse crown chakra. Good to help visualisations with white light.

GENISTA (BROOM)

Heals differences in relationships, particularly parent/child. Helps sinus symptoms.

GEUM

Energy. For those whose confidence was damaged in childhood.

GLADIOLUS

Helps to become stabilised in spiritual intent, when drawn back into ego dimensions. Crown chakra.

GOLDEN ROD

Spiritual guidance through increased connection with higher self.

GROUNDSEL

Integrates ideas into the physical.

GUELDER ROSE
Balances higher chakras above crown. Brings awareness to emotional problems.

HAREBELL
For the shy and nervous, unable to express themselves, especially in groups.

HAWTHORN
Helps eliminate cancer cells.

HEMP NETTLE
Particularly for strengthening the eyes. May also be used in water as a swab for relieving tired eyes.

HELIANTHUS
Like sunflower, works on heart chakra, carries the strength of the sun aspect, brings balance to masculine/feminine energies at heart chakra.

HELLEBORUS
Brings spiritual awareness to the ageing process.

HIBISCUS
Disorientation after psychic or spiritual shock, brings balance.

HIMALAYAN POPPY
Brings strength and healing to continue on one's spiritual path, opens up to easier meditation and spiritual ideas to come through.

HONESTY
Lifts the veil of illusion between the third, fourth and fifth dimensions.

HOPS
For growth on all levels, including physical and spiritual.

HOYA
Alignment of the seven major chakras, only temporarily but if taken over a long period will bring total and more permanent alignment, also helps grounding.

HYACINTH
Integrates spiritual and earthly qualities. Inner hearing.

HYDRANGEA
Scatteredness, brings mental alignment.

HYPERICUM 'HIDCOTE'
Helps release worrying thoughts to bring more calmness, especially helps calm the stomach area which often suffers from excess worry via ulcers etc.

HYSSOP
Acknowledging and releasing guilt feelings. Tension.

IRIS 'AMETHYST'
Strengthens the connection of those working with the amethyst ray and angels thereof, whether for healing or visionary purposes.

IRIS 'BLUEBEARD'

Works through all dimensions to clear blockages in throat area, thus helping to spiritualise speech.

IRIS

Brown/gold. This is a connection with the Lord Maitreya and helps all working with this energy.

Purple. Crown chakra. For spiritual, psychic or visionary artists.

JAPANESE QUINCE

Strengthens red blood cells and helps them to expand, reproduce.

JASMINE

Stimulates Divine spark in heart chakra, self worth. Viruses, excess mucus, sinuses, related diseases.

JONQUIL

Brings higher chakras into alignment, throat, brow, crown and higher.

JUDAS TREE

Denial and suppression of guilt at duality, original or spiritual guilt.

KERRIA

Balance for emotional extremes, violence.

KIDNEY VETCH

Helps cleanse kidneys and process all energies moving through, on all levels i.e. physical – water, emotional – fears.

LADIES BEDSTRAW

Works on the pattern of passive resistance, helps one make a stronger stand.

LADY OF THE NIGHT

Gives connection to the beautiful angels of death. Helps take one onto a new level of existence, passing over to next dimension.

LAMBS TONGUE

Helps to de-fur the body system especially arteries and blood.

LARKSPUR

Helps open the channels to Kundalini energy.

LAVENDER

Connection to higher self for karmic releases.

LEWISIA

Strengthens the immune system, helpful over long term use in all immune system illnesses and diseases.

LIGULARIA

Ear, eardrum infections, perforations, balance.

LILAC

Christ Consciousness, unconditional love.

LILY

Viruses, builds up immune system for protection.

LILY 'STARGAZER'

Helps link with the planetary energy of Venus, unconditional love.

LILY PINK

Strengthens the veins (and arteries to a lesser extent).

LILY OF THE VALLEY

Menstrual and associated problems, ovaries etc.

LOBELIA

'Wakes up" the eyes, good in the morning or as a swab (7 drops in a cup of water) over eyelids.

LOOSESTRIFE

For feeling spaced out, too open, brings grounding. Aligns lower chakras bringing balance and spiritual integration.

LUNGWORT

Good cleanser of the lungs, also good for any associated diseases.

LUPIN

Mental confusion. Integration and calmness.

LYCHNIS

Good for physical energy when energies have been used up in the healing process or energy is needed to be moved up from one chakra to another.

MAGNOLIA

Recognition of Divine origins and soul memories. Crown chakra.

MAHONIA

Brings balance to emotions through integration with thoughts. Solar plexus.

MALLOW

Fears of ageing, phobias relating to physical appearance. Diseases related to ageing.

MALTESE CROSS

Cleansing bloodstream, for blood disorders.

MARSH CAMPION

Where capillaries are broken, helps to restore their link and reduce the effects physically.

MARSH MARIGOLD

Attunement to the Golden Ray. Spiritualises solar plexus chakra.

MELILOT

Brings clarity of mind in children.

MORNING GLORY

Nervous system. Helps all signs of nervousness, gives morning energy.

MULLEIN

For group attunement and purpose.

NASTURTIUM

Rigid, narrow, obsessive thought patterns. Colour awareness. Good for tiredness after spiritual work/channelling.

NETTLE

For stress and trauma related to divorce, broken home. For all the family, adoptions.

OIL SEED RAPE

For those with allergic reactions to oil seed rape.

ONION FLOWER

Fulfillment of cycles, to allow change to happen.

ORCHID 'ONCIDIUM'

Enhances other remedies specifically working on strengthening and repairing the etheric body.

ORCHID 'EQUESTRIS'

Works on the heart at many levels, but most importantly helps to regulate the heartbeat.

OSTEOSPERMUM

Helps one to receive, to open up to others and the universal energy.

PANSY

For all forms of viruses including AIDS and colds.

PASSIONFLOWER

For Christ Consciousness. Helps sleep, dreamwork. Heart, throat, feet chakras.

PEACH

Helps bring the mind into order and calmness where there is chaos (possibly caused by trauma).

PEAR

Brings balance to spiritual groupwork.

PENNYROYAL

For protection from negative thought forms. Solar plexus.

PENSTEMON

Helps to keep attunement to spiritual path.

PERIWINKLE

Spiritualises those whose consciousness is at base/sacral chakra level.

PETUNIA

Depression, tension. Childlike behaviour in the elderly. Impish children. Speech and left brain problems.

PHEASANTS EYE

For retinitis and other eye problems caused by friction, soreness from contact lenses etc.

PHILADELPHUS

Crown and higher chakras, more contact with angels and archangels.

PLUM

Colon cleansing and associated diseases.

POPPY

Energy and grounding, cleanses. Activates blockages in base chakra.

POPPY 'PAPAVER'

Helps overcome addictive tendencies, particularly opium.

POTATO

For depression caused by the inability to grasp new concepts.

POTENTILLA

Releases tension in joints.

PRIMROSE

To help studying, mental growth, learning difficulties.

PRIMULA

Understanding life lessons and growing from that knowledge.

PULSATILLA

Inability to focus on one thing. Unbalanced emotions, PMT.

QUEEN ANNE'S LACE

Inner vision, eye problems, crown chakra.

RAGGED ROBIN

Brings soul qualities into the physical.

RED CLOVER

Brings a calm mind to situations of panic.

RHODODENDRON

Helps one towards following the will of the spirit.

RIBES

Diseases of the pituitary gland.

ROSE OF SHARON

Helps transmute vibrations of anger. Solar plexus.

ROSEMARY

Helps creativity. Brings joy to the unhappy and withdrawn personality. Crown chakra. Sharpens all five senses.

RUDBECKIA

Raises lower emotional energies to the heart chakra.

SAGE

Understanding of the Book of Revelation. Psycho-spiritual aspects activated. Jet lag.

SALPIGLOSSIS

Emotional stabiliser for the over-sensitive.

SALVIA

Cleanser for bloodstream.

SCABIOUS

Helps become more sensitive to and feel energies.

SEDUM

Clears surplus bile from system.

SIDALCEA

Helps bring to consciousness past associations with Greece.

SNAKESHEAD FRITILLARIA

Smoothness to the skin, skin complaints. Throat.

SNAPDRAGON

Speech difficulties, throat problems, helps express emotions.

SNOWDROP

Bereavement. Allows hope and joy to return.

SOAPWORT

Mental cleansing. Heart chakra.

SPEEDWELL

For children in times of change and mental growth.

ST JOHN'S WORT

Karmic and hidden fears released. Nightmares.

STREPTOCARPUS

To help regulate stools, diarrhoea.

SUNFLOWER

Father problems, male ego, spiritualising, heart chakra.

SWEET PEA

Helps you to live in the now, grounding, overcrowded families.

THISTLE

To release defence mechanisms built up around aura by ego, i.e. spikes, armour.

THRIFT
Helps bring art, spiritual, scientific concepts into consciousness.

THYME
Amplifies other flower essences. Past and future lives.

TOADFLAX
Inner ear, perforated eardrum, hearing and balance.

TOBACCO
Helpful for nicotine addiction.

TRADESCANTIA
Helps repair torn muscles and heal muscular system.

TRILLIUM
Spiritual understanding and love for Mother Earth, appreciation of its beauty.

TULIP
Brings pride in one's work and self worth in a dignified way.

VETCH
Spiritual independence. To go away from guru needs.

VIPERS BUGLOSS
For physical problems between ears, nose/throat.

VIOLET
Sweet. Opens crown chakra. For forgiveness of others.
White. Forgiveness of self. Soul aspects of purity.

WALLFLOWER
For the homeless, helps find inner security.

WATER LILY
Yellow. Strengthens emotional/mental body links.

WEIGELA
Unconditional love. Heart chakra becomes more expressive.

WINTERSWEET
Hope, mental understanding of barrenness, inspiration.

WISTERIA
Strengthens meridians, useful tool for acupuncturists.

WOODRUFF
Brings a calm, natural sleep pattern to babies.

YARROW
Pink. Protection from psychic attack.
White. Protection from radioactivity.
Available as a mixed extra strong potency.

YEW

Develops wisdom, helps one to see the grander scheme of things.

ZINNIA

Restores humour by uplifting a person's outlook on life. For people who need to laugh. Gets people in touch with their child-like qualities.

ZUCCHINI

Male sexuality, fertility problems. Sexual diseases. Hormonal imbalances. Base and sacral chakras.

CRYSTAL HERBS – ROSES

Any 10 can be purchased as a set, as well as individually. All roses work on the heart chakra.

BLUE MOON

Clears shadow side from heart chakra.

REGENSBERG

Aligns all higher chakras.

RUBY RED

For transmuting pain and sorrow from heart chakra into love and compassion. Attunement to the Christ consciousness and the new ruby red ray of forgiveness.

MAIDENS BLUSH

Heart chakra, gentle loving energy, good for the sensitive and children

PINK ROSE H.F.

For transmuting group energy and karma related to the heart.

HANDEL

For strength, courage and the release of lack of self-worth when stuck at heart chakra.

PINK RAMBLING

To help the heart chakra develop love in young souls, (not necessarily children!).

DEEP RED ROSE

Works on lowest section of heart chakra to draw up and transmute negative energy from solar plexus.

SUPERSTAR

Brings energy to the heart chakra and helps to align it with the throat chakra.

ROSA DE LA HAY

Aligns heart chakra with crown, helping to transform belief into inner knowing.

YELLOW

Brings feeling of security and courage to the heart.

PEACE

For deep inner peace, transmuting any fear vibrations stuck in heart chakra.

CRYSTAL HERBS – KARMIC ESSENCES

These seven essences have been developed to follow on from the 'traditional 38' essences rediscovered in the 1930s. They work on a much higher vibrational level than the traditional 38 essences, through the crown chakra which is our centre for receiving spiritual guidance and help.

Many people will recognise that often the more deep rooted mental/emotional states, which can often be the cause of disease, have their origins in past incarnations. These states, not having been eliminated previously, are brought into this life by the soul so that they may be overcome. This enables one to progress both spiritually and mentally, to become clear, whole and balanced, free to perform one's Divine purpose.

The traditional 38 essences were placed in 7 main groups. There is one new karmic essence for each of these main groups; the essence will help to clear karmic lessons and blockages.

N.B. These essences are very powerful and should be used with care. They may only be used at a rate of 4 drops 4 times per day for three days. If further treatment is necessary leave 7 clear days to monitor results before using the same dosage for another 3 days, or take as prescribed, or use intuition.

OVERSENSITIVITY – WHITE BLUEBELL

This essence is indicated for those souls who are extremely over sensitive. Those who are so influenced by negative vibrations around them that they are unable to concentrate on their own individuality/work. Useful for those choosing a spiritual path or perhaps spending much time in meditation. Many healers often need this essence especially if using psychic faculties in their work.

FEAR – PINK ROSE

An extremely powerful essence to help release and neutralise karmic fear. These people will have been much troubled by fear, whether conscious or subconscious and as such will have already used one or probably more of the existing fear essences extensively. When one has been treated with these for a considerable time and they have barely scratched the surface Pink Rose is indicated. Very often people suffer from nervous diseases; they may be agoraphobic or asthmatic. It may be more subtle, fears of persecution, burning, water etc. Most people have a karmic lesson to learn regarding conquering fear.

OVERCARE & CONCERN FOR OTHERS – WILD IRIS

Iris is the essence for the person who possibly in past lives has held positions of great authority, or responsibility, either for others or greater things. Hence, brought into this lifetime are very often deep feelings of worry or concern. These feelings may be difficult to pin down; possibly a deep anguish and concern for the planet, which many are suffering at present, or possibly concern for one's fellow man or a need to take on their pain. This essence is indicated for use after a course of any of the existing essences in this group. As used, the person will be able to look at global, cosmic or mankind's problems in the right perspective.

UNCERTAINTY – WILD ORCHID

This beautiful purple flower brings a degree of consciousness raising, for as our uncertainties and indecision become positive vibrations within us so we become more aware of our spiritual being. This awareness that we are part of our Creator, all as one and not different to our fellow man is a very necessary step along our souls path and evolution. Only with this realisation comes our spiritual security, enlightenment, strength and courage, giving us a solid foundation from which to work.

LONELINESS – WATER LILY

The karmic problem of this group is a loneliness brought into this lifetime by the soul, a residue from past incarnations where perhaps much time was spent alone or unable to communicate with our fellow man. The difference between Water Lily and the existing essences in this group is that this loneliness will feel soul deep and will bring with it an acute sadness whose depth is out of reach of Heather etc. People in need of this essence will have been treated with a loneliness essence, possibly for a long time. However, they should be able to recognise the shift to soul level and may feel extremely sad. The sadness and the loneliness will be gently eased away in the shortest possible time.

DISINTEREST – VALERIAN

A karmic essence for lack of interest in present circumstances. Perhaps this person is subconsciously locked into past incarnations, possibly to happier times in the soul memory to which it would like to escape, therefore unable to focus on the present. Valerian is the key to unlock that door so that we may realise the importance for our soul to learn this life's lessons thoroughly and to let go of the past. Also for those continually needing "grounding" to help stay in the body.

DESPAIR AND DESPONDENCY – YELLOW RATTLE

Souls in need of this remedy carry a weight, an innate sadness, which in all likelihood they will be unable to express. A melancholy which echoes from previous lives in a similar way to the dried seed pods in the flower. When winds cast upon a meadow of Yellow Rattle the rattling sound will echo, the vibrations reverberating over surrounding fields in a similar way to the echoes of past hopelessness and despair.

CRYSTAL HERBS – 'THE TRINITY'

Linking the seven new essences above with the traditional 38 essences are a trio of 'spiritual light' essences. These are often necessary bridges between the two, as experienced practitioners will recognise. Intuition will guide to the correct remedy.

GERANIUM

For those still in the dark, gloom, possibly even despair, but recognising the need to contact their spirituality. Like a person in a darkened room, moving around, bumping into things but unable to find that light switch. This is their essence. Their fingers will find the switch and their whole being will be flooded with light and love, which in turn will illuminate the world.

FUCHSIA

A wonderful essence for dislodging and releasing blocked energy. Fuchsia opens up the heart chakra, bringing out all that which has been locked inside. The floodgates will open releasing any pent-up emotions which are causing blockages preventing spiritual attunement. Once these emotions have been recognised they can be treated and worked through; this is a very important part of the learning process. The resultant emotions can be treated with other flower essences such as the traditional 38 or the seven karmic essences, as it is then that the person can recognise their karmic lessons, duties and obligations, releasing and transmuting them, thus bringing about a complete healing.

LILY

The Lily essence is for the spiritually insecure, bringing peace, serenity and comfort. These souls are finally reaching their destination or life's purpose, bringing recognition of their whole spiritual being. This realisation can bring great feelings of insecurity and until they can actually become at one with their spirit, they can easily have their faith and security shaken, sometimes rocking their very foundations. This remedy will bring back emotional and spiritual balance so that these souls can carry on, safe in the knowledge that God, Creator of all things, is guiding them and their foundations will, once again, become as solid as a rock.

Lily, Fuchsia and Geranium may be taken at a rate of 4 drops 4 times per day until a noticeable improvement is obtained, for as long as necessary. Because these and the karmic essences above vibrate at a very high rate, they lose up to 45% efficiency if diluted, so for best results use from stock level, directly from the bottle.

❀ DAWN CAROL THE LIVING RAINBOW AURA ❀ ESSENCES

The Living Rainbow Aura Essences represent a co-operation between the devic angels and higher spirit, under the watchful eye of Archangel Michael. They are the vibrational representation of colour and have the ability to transform negative patterns in the aura, helping the recipient to change their lives. They are made from flowers and are the vibrational representation of colour.

"The Living Rainbow" appertains mainly to the physical aura. "The Crystal Light Essences" to the spiritual aura and the higher chakras, "The Aura Gems" work on the etheric body, "The New Age Remedies" work on the emotions and the dimensional and lateral essences work on the expansiveness of those involved in spiritual work. All come under the umbrella of "The Living Rainbow". Dawn Carol teaches vibrational medicine; contact her for details.

SET 1

These are made up of the basic colours and shades of these colours. All these are made from basic wild and garden flowers.

1st chakra (around soles of feet) POPPY – for grounding.

2nd chakra (to the ankles) ORANGE – renewal of creative force, energy.

3rd chakra (to the knees) YELLOW – helps those who are too flexible to set boundaries.

4th chakra (the base or kundalini) EMERALD – sexual cleansing. PINK CRIMSON – grounded sexuality, balance.

5th chakra (solar plexus) ALL SHADES OF BLUE – peace and calm. SPRING

GREEN – gentle cleansing and GOLD – dispels rigidity. Relaxes.

6th chakra (the spleen) ORANGE – renews life force, energises.

7th chakra (the heart) ROSE PINK – love and comfort. AMETHYST – gentle understanding and releasing of fears. VIOLET – deep understanding and karmic responsibilities taken. MOTHER OF PEARL RAY – THE CHRIST RAY – gentle healing. Mother of Pearl is the Christ Ray and gives a gentle rainbow of colours which is nevertheless very powerful as a healing tool. Give also to whole aura. LOTUS TREE – deep peace and stillness.

8th chakra (the throat) MAGENTA – removes blocks. BLUE – calms, eases pain. GOLD – flexibility.

9th chakra (the third eye) RUBY ROSE – clears and activates. GOLD – eases tension. BLUE – calms.

10th chakra (the crown) GOLD – raises consciousness, brings new flexibility and inner happiness.

SILVER – raises the vibration and gives clarity.

Whole Aura LIVING RAINBOW – puts back colour and lifts depression.

The throat and solar plexus – BLUEBELLS (Blue of flowers and green of leaves) – calms, soothes, cleanses and clears: relieves pain, is the headache remedy, used for allergic, toxic, inflamed conditions, stomach upsets, digestive problems. Works on the physical symptoms first and then sorts out the underlying emotional problems. Excellent for children.

SET 2

These are meant for the five higher chakras above the crown which opened up for some in early 1989.

11th chakra (the chakra approx. 5" above the crown) EMERALD – cleansing.

12th chakra (5" above 11th) SAPPHIRE – peace and calm.

13th chakra (5" higher again, higher heart) PINK LAVENDER – love and understanding.

14th chakra (5" higher again, through which the higher self may be balanced) CRYSTAL BLUE WHITE LIGHT – centres and balances.

15th chakra (5" higher again and gives us our contact with the Angelic realms) DIVINE WHITE – angelic connection.

16th chakra (5" higher again and activates our highest aspirations and helps us to keep our intent and purpose pure) PUREST WHITE – highest aspiration and purity of intent.

DAWN CAROL – CRYSTAL LIGHT ESSENCES

These are intended for the Crystal Light chakras which began to open in 1990 and form a pyramid of crystal light energy at arms length above the crown. Combinations of flowers seen through purest white.

1. CRYSTAL SUN GOLD Highest spiritual enlightenment.

2. CRYSTAL SUN ROSE PINK Highest spiritual love.

3. SUN SILVER DIAMOND LIGHT Highest possible energy.

4. CRYSTAL MERCURY Highest possible clarity and creativity.

5. CRYSTAL VENUS Highest possible integration.

6. CRYSTAL CELESTIAL Highest possible peace, tranquillity and balance.

7. CRYSTAL GALAXY Highest possible grounding.

8. CRYSTAL EARTH EMERALD Highest possible cleansing.

9. CRYSTAL EARTH VIOLET Highest possible understanding and protection from negative rays.

10.CRYSTAL EARTH INDIGO Highest possible sleep vibration.

11 CRYSTAL LIGHT TURQUOISE Highest transformation.

12.CRYSTAL LIGHT RAINBOW This is a combination of the above 11 crystal light essences.

All aura essences are used as follows: 3 drops on left hand, rub hands together, with right hand put into aura at appropriate chakra point(s). May also be used in the bath.

DAWN CAROL – HOLY ARCHANGEL ESSENCES (DIMENSIONAL)

DIVINE LOVE
DIVINE PEACE
DIVINE STRENGTH
DIVINE BEAUTY
DIVINE DELIGHT
DIVINE LAUGHTER
DIVINE TRUTH
DIVINE UNDERSTANDING
DIVINE WILL
DIVINE HEALTH
DIVINE MUSIC

Use on clothes you are wearing or drop drops in room or leave bottle open.

DAWN CAROL – NEW AGE REMEDIES

These essences are intended primarily for use by practitioners in healing centres who are able to monitor the recipient and give them the right sort of support and counselling. This is because the New Age Remedies work very swiftly bringing results in 24 hours. They are really for those advanced souls who have come to a block in their progress. They also lend themselves strongly to use in group situations.

UNCERTAINTY
OVERCARE FOR OTHERS
OVERSENSITIVITY
DISINTERESTED IN THE PRESENT
LONELINESS

DESPAIR AND DESPONDENCY
FEAR
CONFRONTATION OF TRUTHS
SELF CONFIDENCE
THE FLOW

Dosage – 4 drops on clean tongue every hour for 24 hours or until release is experienced.

❀ DR ANDREW TRESIDDER ❀

The range of essences which Dr Tresidder has been helped to develop concentrate on unlocking right-brain intuitive talents.

'Alcoholic infusion' denotes that the essence has been made with alcohol rather than water. Where a specific number of blooms, berries etc to use in making the essence has been obtained intuitively, this has been noted.

*Essences for sale.

AZALEA 'WAYFORD WOODS'

White and slightly scented. Channelling/inspiration – unleashing creative focus to channel and be inspired.

BARLEY GRAINS

Dissolving the belief of needing to rely on the leadership of others for my own truth.

BAY BUDS

Five buds. Alcoholic infusion. Unblocking the need to be led. Settling into yourself and distributing the energy evenly.

BLACKBERRY

Five blackberries. High level astral protection from psychic attack.

BLUE IRIS*

Alcoholic infusion. Unblocking of hidden talents.

BOLETUS EDULUS

High level astral protection from psychic attack.

BULL THISTLE BUDS

Alcoholic infusion. Three buds. Enables you to unfold your mysteries by being your own true self – raising the mantle so that the light can be lit – the paraffin allows you to don the mantle of your spiritual talents and accept those talents.

Aqueous infusion. Three buds. Overnight. Brings the light down to the mantle – joining in the higher spirituality into being here – (the oxygen).

COTONEASTER BERRY

Alcoholic infusion. Seven berries. Lights a match to spirituality.

FUCHSIA

Aqueous infusion. Pale pink sepals, purple corolla. Opening up of the heart centre to allow unconditional love to flow.

Alcoholic infusion. Seven flowers. Red sepals, double purple corolla. Brings deep peace and a remembering of the secrets of life.

HOLLY BUDS

Diffusion of confusion. Allows negativity to be acknowledged, passed through and released.

HYACINTH*

Alcoholic infusion. Three blue flowers. Grounding.

LILY 'STARGAZER'

Ability to use power and spiritual talents wisely and with discretion.

NASTURTIUM LEAF

Alcoholic infusion. To be able to dream the dreams of all things that are possible to me that I didn't even realise were available – seeing the dream that I know I understand.

ORANGE AZALEA*

Self forgiveness.

ORNAMENTAL CRAB APPLE

Alcoholic infusion. Final piercing of the web of illusion.

PUSSY WILLOW

Seven flowers. Clarity of focus; discernment.

RUNNER BEANS

Alcoholic infusion. Three flowers. Removes spikiness and rigidity.

WILD FUCHSIA

Alcoholic infusion. Seven flowers. Dissolving the weakness of the disbelieving self.

❀ EARTH ESSENCES ❀

It is my belief that there are no definitive bounds attached to any particular essence, merely an understanding that each of us is a unique vibrational being and will so respond to each unique vibrational essence.

In pursuing this theory I have attempted to reduce limitations by providing only broad positive indications and by revealing the chosen essences only when the healing cycle is completed. There are currently 24 Earth Essences (most of which are detailed below) and the Emergency Essence, to which there is the recent addition of Wild Violet. With the exception of Emergency Essence the individual dosage is based in communion wine. It is taken morning and evening only and in conjunction with the lunar cycle.

Earth Essence is an inspiration derived from my own healing process. I thank Douglas Perkins for introducing me to vibrational medicine and communion wine and I thank Susan Fletcher for her encouragement.

BINDWEED
For the ability to face fear.
For inner strength to conquer.
For resilience.

BITTERCRESS
For understanding, encompassing and channelling 'THE LIGHT'.

BLACK MEDICK
To balance the black/white, positive/negative aspects of the self.
For understanding and encompassing power.
For fearlessness.

BUTTERCUP
To bring awareness of one's environment.
For adaptability.
For resilience.

COMMON MOUSE EAR
For scrutiny.
To bring understanding of the 'whole'.

DAISY
For connection (especially to the Earth).
To bring a sense of purpose and belonging.

DANDELION
To balance the male and female aspects of the self.
For acceptance.
For tolerance.
For flexibility.

DWARF MALLOW
For understanding and encompassing the feminine aspects.
For 'mother'/'self-less' love.

FIELD PANSY
To bring awareness of energy fields.
To bring awareness of energy interaction.
To cleanse the aura.

GROUND IVY
For understanding and encompassing the earth role.
For self-perception.
For self-confidence.
For determination to do.

GUELDER ROSE BERRY
To see.

For clarity.

For processing the 'idea'.

HAZEL FLOWERS

For wisdom.

For healing.

For understanding and encompassing masculinity.

For joyous fertility.

HAWTHORN BERRY

To bring awareness of one's true source of nourishment.

To bring awareness of the free-flow of giving and receiving.

HAWTHORN FLOWER

To bring awareness of spirit.

For understanding 'being'.

For self-love.

HAWTHORN LEAF

To balance the body, mind and spirit.

To bring awareness of the 'lone' self, the 'true' self.

To bring awareness of oneness.

OAK ACORN

For understanding the life-cycles.

For strength.

PINK OXALIS

For the ability to communicate in truth, simplicity and gentleness.

SCARLET PIMPERNEL

For understanding and encompassing raw earth/sexual energy.

For vitality.

For joy.

SPEEDWELL

For understanding and encompassing changes.

For renewal.

WHITE CLOVER

For consideration.

For patience.

For 'inaction'.

EMERGENCY ESSENCE

Combination of oak acorn, ground ivy and bindweed.

❀ FINDHORN FLOWER ESSENCES ❀

Findhorn Flower Essences are made using wildflowers from Scotland and pure water collected from sacred healing wells. They are prepared by the sun-infusion method pioneered in the 1930's by Dr. Edward Bach, whose own remedies revived the age-old use and understanding of the natural healing power expressed by flowering plants and trees.

These essences have been created in co-operation with the forces of Nature. The elements of earth, air, fire and water combine to create the physical form of every plant according to the divine blueprint. Our love and thanks must go to the angels, the divine architects and to the nature spirits, who work according to the plan to bring each plant into being. Vis Medicatrix Naturae, the healing power of Nature, is their gift to us in the form of flower essences. Through the love with which the essences are prepared and the intention that those taking them maintain, these natural essences reaffirm our connection with the divine and the oneness of all life.

The description of each essence is followed by an affirmation.

APPLE

Keynote: Higher Purpose

The essence of apple helps us to integrate our desires and our willpower to realise positively our goals and visions. By aligning with Higher or Divine Purpose we channel these powerful energies into right action: will-to-good

Indications: Blocks to realising inherent power and ability, unable to sustain self-discipline, the glamour of power and superiority, lack of the power to act or self-assertion, succumbing to lower desires, unbalanced sexual expression, depletion of sexual creative forces.

Attributes: Development and the right use of the will, removing blockages to positive action, concertedness, inner strength to overcome inertia, self-discipline, humility, obedience to higher will, reforming lower desire into love and selfish will into will-to-serve.

Apple facilitates the contacting of our higher aspirations, freeing our attachment to our personal desires and enabling us to use our will to truly serve for the good of all.

"I align myself with my Higher Purpose and act for the good of all".

BALSAM

Keynotes: Relationship and Intimacy

Balsam essence facilitates love and acceptance of the physical bodies we have chosen to incarnate into as souls. We feel fully present in the world and can express feelings of true love.

Indications: Fear of separation, life or birthing, fear of intimacy, feeling unloved or unwanted, feelings of neglect, abandonment or rejection; feelings of rootlessness or homelessness, lack of bonding, alienation from the mother or the feminine aspect of self, fear of relationships, reduced physical warmth and presence; physical dislike, frigidity, aloofness, permissiveness, exhibitionism, unfulfilled desire.

Attributes: Capacity for intimacy and expression of love, to nurture and nourish oneself and others, feeling at home in one's body and environment, awareness of bodily needs, sensations and feeling; warmth, sensitivity, sensuality, relationship bonding, celebrating sexuality, healing with the mother/feminine aspect, creative feminine power, connecting with mother nature.

When we feel out of place, ill at ease or fail to nourish ourselves, we may have difficulties relating and feel separated from others or unloved. Balsam reminds us of the divinity of our being in physical form. We experience feelings of warmth, sensitivity and tenderness towards ourselves and others and a new joy and harmony in our relationships.

"I am happy and at home in my body and in the world".

BELL HEATHER

Keynote: Stability

Bell Heather helps to access inner strength and resolve to stand one's ground after stress, trauma or conflict: Self-confidence

Indications: Loss of faith in self, lack of confidence, mood swings, easily swayed, apparently victimised by circumstance, loss of direction or purpose, fragile.

Attributes: Tenacity, affirmation, trust inner knowing, faith in oneself, standing up for one's self, resolute in stance and purpose, assertiveness, following one's own path with confidence, resilience, self-recovery.

Bell Heather is stabilising. It allows consolidation: the strength to stand firm while remaining flexible. After setback, disappointment or misfortune, essence of Bell Heather helps to foster trust and faith in the self.

"I stand firmly and securely in my being. I have faith and trust in my self".

BIRCH

Keynote: Perception

Birch essence helps us to broaden our perceptions and transcend limitations of mind. Through expanding our consciousness and seeing our cosmic connections we gain understanding and peace of mind: vision

Indications: Obscured or unclear vision, stuck in thought patterns which hold us back, inability to see beyond ourselves or concerns, worry, introspection, dulled senses, living in the past or future, escapism or day-dreaming, out of body states, 'blind spots', not learning from past mistakes, confusion of mind.

Attributes: Bringing in the light of the mind, expanding one's awareness into the cosmos, contacting Universal Mind, direct experience of the infinite here and now, deep mindfulness, realising the inner wisdom of life experiences, focussed and intuitive attitude and power to see the vision and direct one's course to it, cultivating spiritual vision.

Essence of Birch facilitates breakthrough to understanding the causes of our life circumstances and predicaments. When we identify with our lower self, conflicts or behaviour patterns, it can influence or restrict how we view ourselves and the world and thus impede our highest aspirations. Birch essence frees our imagination and gives us hope for the future.

"I open my mind to new ways and understanding".

BROOM

Keynote: Clarity

Broom stimulates mental clarity and concentration, facilitating ease in communication and creative thought when in a state of bewilderment: illumination

Indications: Memory loss, dullness, feeble-mindedness, bewilderment, confusion, lack of integration, co-ordination or communication.

Attributes: Mental clarity, concentration, communication, integration, decision making, self-expression, guidance, intuition, creative thought, clarity of purpose.

Broom brings light into our minds. When our mental body is clouded or dull or when we are distracted, we are hindered in our expression and communication. Essence of Broom allows the light of the intuition to illuminate our minds, inspiring us with its brilliance and bringing creative thought into outer expression.

"My mind is clear. I express myself, my thoughts and ideas with ease".

DAISY

Keynote: Innocence

Daisy allows us to remain calm and centred amid turbulent surroundings or overwhelming situations, creating a safe space in which to be vulnerable: grace

Indications: Being overwhelmed, fear of losing control, distraction, confusion, easily swayed, inconsistency, indifference, "up in the clouds", fickleness, oversensitiveness.

Attributes: Calm and centred amid intense activity, lightness, presence, being or staying on purpose, protection, ability to enjoy, rediscovering innocence, playfulness.

Daisy allows us to maintain that innocence, vulnerability and sensitivity when in our busy lives we fear losing our calm centre within the storm. The essence of Daisy helps us to stay on purpose and on course and protects us while we do so.

"I am calm and centred and feel safe in my world".

ELDER

Keynote: Beauty

Essence of Elder stimulates the body's natural powers of recuperation and renewal. It helps us to contact and radiate the beauty and joy of our inner eternal youth: rejuvenation

Indications: Feelings of unworthiness or self-consciousness, dislike of oneself or body, feelings of ugliness or heaviness, feeling old, dullness, overidentification with one's image, subdued or held-in personality, masking of the true self, lack of personal vitality or aliveness.

Attributes: Invoking recuperative powers of the body, self-acceptance, enthusiasm, youthfulness, acknowledgement of the process of ageing, lightening-up, new energisation on cellular level through increased inflow of pranic energy; revealing and radiating our true being and beauty, joyful expression of the physical body.

Through Essence of Elder we allow greater penetration into our bodies of the sun forces which regenerate us. Our energy centres or chakras become irradiated, bringing feelings of wellbeing and thus illuminating our inner beauty.

"I am renewed and revitalised. I radiate the beauty and joy of my wellbeing".

GLOBE-THISTLE

Keynotes: At-one-ment and Wholeness

Globe-thistle essence helps us recognise the order of life and our evolutionary process, enabling us to willingly and joyfully make sacrifices which will liberate us on our path.

Indications: Personal handicap, misfortune or discouragement; preoccupation with personal suffering or loss, feeling a victim, martyrdom, self-condemnation, feeling chained to the wheel of life, addictions, self-indulgence, self-gratification, self-pity, waspishness, irritability.

Attributes: Wholeness through balance, centredness, temperance, giving oneself in service to humanity and to the world, self-sacrifice, radiating strength and flexibility, goodwill, Christ/sun/cosmic wholeness, peace and humility, stable, supportive energy; ability to accept the suffering of others, empathy, patience, willingness to moderate, sobriety, restitution.

Often we hold on to the non-essential aspects of our lives rather than risk the pain of letting go. With Globe-thistle we reconnect with the inner strength and flexibility to free ourselves from burden. We discover that surrendering to a higher order for the good of the whole brings us the deepest peace and joy.

"I am strong and whole. I serve joyfully in the spirit of goodwill".

GORSE

Keynote: Joy

Gorse is a light bringer, stimulating vitality, enthusiasm and motivation at times of apathy and low immunity, bringing light-heartedness and enjoyment of life: passion for life

Indications: Apathy, burn-out, low immunity, listlessness, lack of motivation or joy, unable to join in or to share oneself.

Attributes: Renewal of life force, vitality, motivation, enthusiasm, living in the moment, enjoyment and celebration of life.

Gorse is a bringer of light, heralding joy – that soul quality which can heal us. When we run ourselves down, we have no energy left to participate fully in life. We risk withholding our energies in order to conserve them for ourselves but in so doing deny ourselves the very source of replenishment we require. Essence of Gorse brings us back to the enjoyment of living every moment to the full. It gives us hope. This strengthens the will and the body's immunity.

"I live my life with joy and passion".

GRASS OF PARNASSUS

Keynotes: Translucency and Perpetual Serenity

Essence of Grass of Parnassus transforms and diffuses the powerful inflowing universal energies into a gentle and graceful vibration which uplifts our souls and opens the heart to the healing power of love.

Indications: Conflicts between power and love, fear of being in one's power, faint-hearted, delicacy, fragility, protective barriers to feeling deep pain and strong emotion, hardened to pain, deep sadness and sorrow, fear of helplessness or vulnerability well guarded by shields of self-protectiveness, feeling 'out of control', holding back in sharing oneself, elusiveness, coyness.

Attributes: Inner peace and spiritual receptivity, emptying the chalice of one's being to inflow from the spiritual source, power of vulnerability, radiating the pure light of love, purity of heart, transmuting power into love, feminine receptive qualities: gentleness, softness, delicacy, subtlety, openness and gracefulness; impeccability, modesty, innocence, virtuousness, releasing sadness and sorrow.

When we feel weighed down by strong emotions, fear or vulnerability we may create protective barriers which cut us off from our true feelings. Grass of Parnassus opens us to full expression of the Self and to access soul qualities of bliss, peace, joy and serenity.

"I open my heart to let in love. I feel and express my love in the world".

HAZEL

Keynotes: Liberation and Freedom

Hazel essence can help free us to flow with the river of life. Letting go of all that restricts one's growth, advancement and potential unfoldment, we discover the joy and bliss of surrendering as we travel into the unknown.

Indications: Failure to meet one's goals and objectives, lack of power to follow through, procrastination, controlling the flow and direction of one's life, fear or inability to break free of old ties, attachments to the past, keeping within self-imposed limits, fear of failure or making mistakes, not daring to move out of one's depth, discouragement, disappointment, dissatisfaction, frustration, agitation, restlessness without direction

Attributes: Flowing with and trusting the Source, acceptance and trust in the progression of one's life path and destiny, unfoldment and realisation of one's purpose and potential, perseverance to attain one's goals and objectives, motivation to carry through, intentionality, catalyst to stimulate movement and freedom of action, faith to overcome obstacles, joyful liberation and surrender.

We often use considerable effort and energy trying to control the direction and flow of our lives, hanging on to what has ceased to serve us, or through the limitations of our thinking. Hazel essence brings us present in time, helping us to shatter the bonds which bind us to the past. We move forward in the wonder and joy of newness and trust the power of the infinite movement as we let Life flow freely.

"I travel forward in life with wonder and joy".

HOLY-THORN

Keynote: Rebirth

Holy-thorn essence opens our hearts to love and the acceptance of ourselves and others, allowing intimacy and the expression of our truth and creativity: creation

Indications: Blocked self-expression and creativity, withholding oneself, lack of involvement, creating barriers to friendship, fear of rejection, repression of the true self.

Attributes: Birthing and expressing creative activity on all levels, opening to others, intimacy and nurturing, radiant compassion, warm and loving acceptance of all, universal Christ-like love, transformation through the power of love.

Holy-thorn essence is made from the flowers of the Glastonbury Thorn. The original tree is said to have grown from the stave of Joseph of Arimathea where he struck it on Wearyall Hill in Glastonbury. This essence awakens us to the presence of the love of the Christ in ourselves and others.

"I open my heart to feel and express love and acceptance of myself and others".

HAREBELL

Keynote: Prosperity

Harebell is for realigning to the spirit of abundance and releasing material concerns following fear of lack: faith

Indications: Fear of lack, possessiveness, lack of faith, attachment, poverty consciousness, out of alignment with oneself and one's environment.

Attributes: Manifesting abundance, re-alignment, affirmation, balance, self-reliance, equilibrium. Harebell is about realigning with Spirit. When we lose faith in ourselves, we may block the flow of spiritual energies. Fear of lack can produce attachment and possessiveness, hindering our ability to give and receive. Essence of Harebell opens our awareness to all that life has to offer and allows us the grace and gratitude to accept it.

"I align myself with the spirit of abundance and have faith that all my needs are met".

IONA PENNYWORT

Keynotes: Perspicacity and Transparency

Essence of Iona Pennywort brings light into the darkest corners of our souls. Through conscious recognition of the shadow self, we can let go of unfounded fears, understanding that the darkness serves to highlight the essential Truth of our being.

Indications: Glamour of the Path of Light, denial of the shadow side, concealing the darkness within, fear of dark and darkness, nightmares, hiding one's dark thoughts, negative, dark or demonic thoughts or states of mind, psychic fears: possession, supernatural or demonic forces; superstition; fascination for, spellbound or enchantment with the powers of darkness; secretiveness, to distort or veil the truth from oneself or others, suspicion, delusion, torment, paranoia, temptation, pride, transgression or defiance of Law, judgement, guilt, remorse, shame.

Attributes: Bringing in the light of conscious awareness, to face the truth when it comes to light, to master the forms of darkness in the underworld, to acknowledge and integrate all aspects of the self, confronting hidden fears honestly, quest for the Truth, the spirit of renewal, protective Light of the Holy Spirit, obedience to one's higher principles, trial of strength, initiation testing, discipline, observance, to make amends, redemption, salvation, impeccability, to be without judgement.

When we deny or fear the dark aspects of ourselves, or of life, we create illusion and self-deception and judgement of ourselves and others. With Iona Pennywort we realise that the darkness co-exists as part of the whole to reveal the clarity and brilliance of the Light. We move forward with a new awareness and purity of aspiration.

"I acknowledge and respect all aspects of myself. I am light".

LADY'S MANTLE

Keynotes: Awareness and Omniscience

Lady's Mantle essence allows us to access the infinite knowledge and wisdom available to us through the unconscious mind. From this union of unconscious and conscious knowing we realise deeper awareness.

Indications: Limiting one's understanding to the conscious, rational mind; lack of imagination or vision, insensibility to inner world of feeling, low attention span, easily distracted, ignorance, apathy, dyslexic disorders, unthinkingness, unmindfulness, day-dreaming, impassivity, non-responsiveness, guarded, conservatism, scepticism, reactive, projecting out one's problems.

Attributes: Bringing the light of consciousness into the unconscious, embracing all-knowing unlimited wisdom, integrating soul life with ordinary reality, surrender to and trust in the inner knowing of the true self, receptivity to spiritual wisdom through dreams and the realm of archetypes, interpreting symbols from the unconscious, co-ordination of rational and abstract thinking, comprehension, responsiveness, powers of observation, mindfulness, communication.

When we are unable or unwilling to embrace the unconscious sides of ourselves, our awareness and understanding become limited. Lady's Mantle facilitates the reconciliation of our outer and inner paths so that we can experience the union and wholeness which we seek, bringing to light our inherent all-knowing wisdom.

"I bring to light all the wisdom and awareness I need".

LAUREL

Keynote: Resourcefulness

The essence of Laurel represents the abundance of the universe. It enables those wise in heart to empower themselves to find the resources to bring their ideas and ideals into form: manifestation

Indications: Inability to 'hold the vision', withholding of talents, initiative and resources of the self, procrastination, giving-up easily, failure to act for fear of risk-taking, failure to evoke the will to choose and then follow the way that has been determined upon, overwhelm through inability to integrate many facets of a project, disorganisation.

Attributes: Unfolding the power to manifest, bringing ideas into being and putting them into action, working with the 7th Ray of organisation, order and expression of spirit through form; ability to choose opportunities which serve life purpose, synthesising different facets or energies into a unified whole, evoking the power to hold and maintain silence when necessary, commitment and strength to realise our vision.

The essence of Laurel has a harmonising and synthesising effect. When we bring plans to fruition, we need to be bold and to blend our energies of individuality with Higher Will. Laurel essence helps us to trust that we are supported by the spiritual world when we act for the good of the whole.

Note: this essence is not recommended where the consciousness of abundance is lacking. Refer to Harebell essence.

"I manifest all that I need to fulfil the Divine Plan. I work for the good of the whole".

LIME

Keynote: Oneness

Essence of Lime helps us open our hearts to the light and love of our universal being. From this awareness we experience our interrelatedness on earth and create harmonious relationships in our lives: universality

Indications: Introspective or too focussed on self, over-identification with lower self/personality, feelings of powerlessness, over-dependency, fear of domination; intolerance, prejudice or nationalism, lack of awareness of the whole, separativeness.

Attributes: Knowing and experiencing the self as universe, transfer from identification with lower to Higher Self, unification of individual consciousness with collective consciousness and environment, transmuting self-preservation into detached world service, humanitarian activity through recognition of need, service, relationship and sense of responsibility; group consciousness.

Essence of Lime helps us to anchor universal love in our hearts. Supporting us in overcoming feelings of separation from our spiritual self or others, essence of Lime can empower and encourage us to work for peace and spiritual harmony on earth.

"I open my heart to create harmonious relationships in life. I am one with all other beings".

MALLOW

Keynotes: Alignment and Attunement

Mallow essence helps us to experience the unification of the mind and heart and we learn to 'think in our hearts'. When we come in thought and activity from this fusion, we open up to God's Grace.

Indications: Separation or detachment of thought from feeling, relationship conflict, discord, polarisation, 'stuck in the head', over-thinking, repetitive thoughts, loquaciousness, incoherence, tenaciousness, impoliteness, disorderliness, unruliness, intolerance, gaucheness.

Attributes: Harmonising thinking with feeling in the heart, leading to 'love in action'; bringing soul energies into one's thoughts and actions, the power of the unity between heart and mind, intuitive thinking through the heart, letting the heart guide, being and acting with one accord, wholeheartedness, integrity, refinement, graciousness.

When we create separation in our lives between our thinking and feeling, the ability to bring through Higher Will is impeded. With essence of Mallow we glory in the unification of body and soul, mind and heart and live congruently through right relationship.

"I align myself with Divine Will. I am love-in-action".

MONKEY FLOWER

Keynotes: Personal Power and Soul Infusion

Monkey Flower essence helps raise the vibrational energy from the personality level, fusing it with the soul's intention. We are empowered to celebrate and use the uniqueness of our experience and qualities to BE WHO WE TRULY ARE.

Indications: Inability to express and act from one's truth, timidity, nervousness, apprehension, yielding temperament: over-compliancy, over-apologetic; giving one's power away, fear of exploitation or domination by others, patterns of dependency; fear of disapproval: reproach, blame, criticism, ridicule, humiliation, indignation, difficulty in saying 'NO'.

Attributes: Standing in one's power, evoking the soul in personal expression and empowerment, soul and personality fusion, radiating power of the Self, the uniqueness of our personal being, acting from strength of individual purpose and with inner conviction, boldness and force of character, assertiveness, self-assurance, self-realisation, fearlessness in accepting feedback from others, ability to set clear boundaries.

Sometimes we are reluctant to be fully in our power for fear of recrimination, or believing that in our strength or dominance we are acting from the lower self or ego. Monkey Flower essence helps us to know and trust our inner guidance and we find the power and courage to act NOW.

"I celebrate who I am. I stand in my uniqueness and truth to serve all".

RAGGED ROBIN

Keynote: Purity

Ragged Robin aids in releasing, on all levels, congestion, obstruction and toxicity and facilitates the free flow of life force and energies: Inner purification.

Indications: Congestion, toxicity, obstruction, blockages, unclean living, hindrance of spirit.

Attributes: Inner purification, promotes circulation, facilitates free flow of life force, purgation, wholesomeness.

Pollution within ourselves and in our environment creates toxicity, congestion and obstruction to the free flow of life forces and energies. Ragged Robin essence helps us clear the channels and purify on all levels.

"I purify myself and clear my channels. My energies flow free and I am restored to wholeness".

ROSE ALBA

Keynotes: Will-to-love and Omnipotence

Rose Alba is the essence of positive outgoing creative expression. Through aligning higher mind with the Ancient Wisdom, words and action reflect the power of Universal Truth.

Indications: Dictatorial and authoritarian use of will, driving for personal power and control, controlling situations or others, abuse of power, overbearing, using words or excuses to defend, attack or justify oneself or action; hiding behind self-protective shields, emotional insecurity, withholding oneself or one's expression, feelings of inadequacy or impotency in being able to initiate, actuate or perform; inflexibility, rigidity of ideas, strict adherence to convention or tradition, pride, arrogance, criticism, judgement, stubbornness.

Attributes: Enlightened individual power, the creative power of the Word, spiritual will and purpose, will directed consciousness, divine direction and protection, positive action through intuition, ability to be self-responsible and to take initiative, leadership, to speak and act from inner authority, patience, persistence, perseverance, determination, strength, benevolence, honour, the masculine principle: the outgoing creative; healing with the father/father principle, virility, potency.

Without love, power can be misused. Through learned control patterns, feelings of inadequacy or pride, the lower self or ego can undermine the inner authority of the true Self. Rose Alba assists in connecting with the higher self to bring forth deep inner spiritual insight and understanding and with this comes the strength to 'walk our talk'.

"I align my mind with the Ancient Wisdom to stand in my truth. I align my words with love and power to speak my truth".

ROSE WATER LILY

Keynotes: Presence and Ascension

'Here I am, bold and true. Forever I am yours in this Truth of Being. Purity of heart, I bring gladness. Spirit ever moving in the spiral to be – manifest here, now, forever. Courage of heart when despairing of knowing the True Self. I remind you of the Presence'.

Made from a single bloom grown in the final tank of the Living Machine, this lily has emerged from the depths of the purified sewerage, a symbol for the spirit of man, emerging out of the depths of darkest matter to ascend into the Light, radiating from the heart purity, beauty and Presence of Being.

Indications: Sense of loss of connection with Spirit, feeling abandoned or forsaken by God, powerless to penetrate into the depths of one's soul or spirit, losing heart when faced with difficult next steps on the Path of Return, inability to yield but desperate yearning to be delivered into Spirit, death.

Attributes: To feel the intimate closeness and relationship to Spirit, the Beloved; spiritual evolution, spiritual poise, ascension, to penetrate the mystery of Presence through surrender.

When we fervently aspire to move on to higher levels of unfoldment or when in despair we cry out for help essence of Rose Water Lily brings courage of heart. In faith we can descend to the depths and ascend to the heights to uncover the Truth of our Being: indestructible, immutable Spirit, our connection with the Beloved.

"Pure in heart and in truth I stand. I AM".

ROWAN

Keynote: Forgiveness

Rowan helps us to let go of resentments and to heal old wounds. As we learn to forgive ourselves and others, we can heal the past: reconciliation.

Indications: Clinging to old behaviour patterns, judgmental, avoidance, self-pity, shame, defensiveness, self-destructive patterns, unwillingness to give in and let go, resentment.

Attributes: Ability to forgive oneself and others, learning from past experiences, resolving karma, harmony through conflict, releasing stored tension and pain, facing deep repressed emotions.

Rowan essence addresses our attachment to habitual, inherited or karmically acquired emotions and patterns. By accepting the lessons of our past experiences, we can avoid repeating mistakes, reconcile and live congruently with ourselves and the world. Rowan opens us up to a higher level of being; power to surrender to unconditional healing love.

"I experience forgiveness of myself and others and surrender to unconditional healing love".

SCOTS PINE

Keynote: Wisdom

Scots Pine helps us in finding directions in our search for answers. In being open to listening, we can be guided from within by the all-knowing self and the inner teachers: truth.

Indications: Barriers to trusting inner knowing and intuition, blocks to inner and outer listening, resistance to hearing the truth, overly dependent on outside validation, indecision.

Attributes: True listening, trusting one's inner knowing and intuition, hearing inner spiritual guidance, openness to the Ancient Wisdom within oneself and nature, learning and teaching.

The essence of Scots Pine helps us to clear the channels to true inner listening and in the silence, in the seeking and asking, we can tap into our own source of wisdom within. The truth then stands revealed.

"I am receptive to the truth and wisdom within my being".

SCOTTISH PRIMROSE

Keynote: Peace

Scottish Primrose brings inner peace and stillness to the heart when confronted by fear, anxiety, conflict or crisis: unconditional love.

Indications: Fear, constriction, panic, shock, paralysis, anxiety, hysteria, inner struggle, conflict in relationships, disheartenment.

Attributes: Inner peace and stillness, coming back to earth, inner harmony, relaxation, purity of feeling, experience of love, compassion.

Scottish Primrose stands for peace. When we are afraid, anxious or in conflict, essence of Scottish Primrose can help to restore natural rhythms. As we find ourselves at peace, we re-establish harmony, thereby allowing the free flow of life force to all parts of our being, bringing equilibrium.

"I am at peace in my heart and in the world".

SEA PINK

Keynote: Harmony

The Essence of Sea Pink aligns and infuses our being with Spirit. Blending and melding our life force with Divine Will, it helps to balance the energy flow between all energy centres: unification.

Indications: Burn-out or blocks in energy systems of the bodies, overload, stuckness, vacillation between the opposites, following desires of the lower self, craving stimulating experiences, untimely kundalini stimulation, split personality, the fundamental problem of the relationship between Spirit and Matter.

Attributes: Healing the split between higher and lower selves, soul and personality; achievement of stability and balance between the opposites, harmonisation of crown and root chakras and soul and form; surrendering the lower to the higher, will-to-be, kundalini awakening, magnetic potency which binds the soul and personality in functioning relationship.

Sea Pink helps us to release those lower desires or blocks which interfere with the harmonious flow of vital life force. When we feel split-off from our Higher Self, essence of Sea Pink helps to dissolve this barrier and by adjusting the life and consciousness energy streams, seeks to unite the polarities within us, allowing us to follow the 'middle way'.

"I unite all energies within my being and welcome the balance and harmony".

SEA ROCKET

Keynotes: Regeneration and Providence

Sea Rocket essence infuses into our being the experience of abundance in all its forms. We trust in the universal supply to receive and give freely and act from a point of purity of purpose, knowing that all our needs will be met.

Indications: Fear of scarcity, poverty, evaporation or dissipation of one's reserves, feelings of destitution, wasteful or superfluous expenditure of resources, over-materialistic, hoarding with episodic splurging, overprotectiveness, impoverished or depleted, failing to thrive, wasting conditions, lack of absorption from the lifeblood to nourish or replenish the body, dehydration, dryness, barrenness, difficulty giving or receiving, self-absorbed or consumed.

Attributes: Blessed with inner knowing and trust in the abundance of Nature, reverance for and cherishing life through purity of being, tapping into the reservoir of the Self for replenishment and restoration, rehydration, succulence, ability to bring forth and sustain life, conservation of resources, fecundity.

We may experience the feeling that we do not have sufficient resources for our needs, whether materialistically, emotionally, or spiritually and this can create a constant looking outwards for the means to provide. Sea Rocket helps us to reconnect with the Laws of Manifestation and Being.

When we remember that we carry the power to call forth the All out of Nothing, we no longer need to accumulate so much to support our insecurities and we share the abundance with an open heart.

"I give and receive freely knowing that all my needs are met".

SILVERWEED

Keynote: Simplicity

Silverweed helps us to detach ourselves from material concerns and over-indulgence, by promoting moderation and self-awareness: self-realisation.

Indications: Overindulgence, fussiness, pernickety, narrowmindedness, disconnection from spirit, self-centredness, greed, pretentiousness.

Attributes: Awakening to spirituality, breakthrough of self-awareness, integrity, self-discipline, enjoyment of simple pleasures of life, getting back to grass roots, moderation, frugality, humbleness.

Silverweed speaks of the necessity for living lightly on the earth. It is useful in times when we become overly engrossed in material concerns and cut off from our higher purpose or being. It allows us to get back to basics, to grass roots. It can help us lift our awareness through deep contact with the forces of Nature and through earthliness to break through into higher spirituality.

"I live lightly on the earth and treasure all of nature's gifts".

SNOWDROP

Keynote: Surrender

Snowdrop allows us to surrender to the end of past events and attachments in life. In the death of the old we find the seed of our eternal inner light and behold new vistas: Immortality.

Indications: Personal darkness and suffering, negative or destructive attitudes, fear of death and dying, depression related to seasonal darkness (S.A.D. syndrome), dark night of the soul, grief.

Attributes: Inner radiance in times of darkness, resilience, inner strength, ability to yield, letting go as prelude to spiritual rebirth or initiation, acceptance of the processes of death leading to liberation, knowing of the Eternal Self, detachment, transcendence of the form side of life, optimism and hope for the future.

The essence of Snowdrop allows us to access deep, inner stillness and to surrender to the processes whereby we can release the past. Then we can see the light at the end of the tunnel and move towards it and the all-pervading Presence of God, celebrating the death of the old and rejoicing in the coming of the new.

"I surrender and release that which has passed and rejoice in the coming of the new".

SPOTTED ORCHID

Keynote: Perfection

Spotted Orchid enables us to go beyond pessimism and self-interest to seeing the best in everyone and everything: creative expression.

Indications: Cynicism, self-centredness, pessimism, inability to see beyond oneself and personal circumstances, nostalgia, stuckness.

Attributes: Self-expression, nurturing and creativity, positive outlook, inspiration, seeing the best in everyone and everything.

When we become too focussed on ourselves or our work, our vision can become limited and our outlook on life reflects this limitation. If we focus on the negative, or the ugly in life, then disillusionment or pessimism may result. Essence of Spotted Orchid allows us to see the beauty and perfection in everything, thus reflecting the beauty and perfection of our true selves. We are then able to express that creatively.

"I see the very best in everyone and everything".

STONECROP

Keynote: Transition

Stonecrop helps us to maintain inner stillness whilst in the process of breaking through inertia and resistance to change in the face of imminent transformation: transcendence.

Indications: Resistance to change, stuck in the past, loneliness, isolation, inertia, stagnation, stubbornness.

Attributes: Profound self-transformation, revelation, incarnation, breakthrough, self-reliance, patience, inner stillness, state of grace.

Stonecrop aids in times of profound personal transformation. We can sense that change is happening around us and within us at the deepest levels. It corresponds to the pupa stage of a becoming butterfly. This process has its own timing. Stonecrop essence allows us to release our attachments to the past, embrace change and find the point of stillness within.

"I maintain my inner stillness and calm whilst welcoming the change and transformation in my life".

SYCAMORE

Keynote: Softness

Sycamore recharges and uplifts body and soul when we are stressed, allowing the emergence of a soft yet powerful new energy supply: revitalisation.

Indications: Profound fatigue and exhaustion, worn down over time by effort or over-exertion, depletion of energies, stretched to the limit, at breaking point, spiritually testing times, negative influences, bad environmental effects, heavy hearted, stress.

Attributes: ability to tap inner reserves of strength, patience, constancy, endurance and persistence, continuity of effort, catalysing energy, restoring gentleness and smoothness in our energy flow, surrendering strain, conflict or anxiety, setting boundaries, encouraging when facing challenges, tests or trials; enthusiasm, softness and openness, ability to be flexible and resilient under stress.

When we are worn down by time, effort or stress, our energy levels can fall and become depleted. Essence of Sycamore helps us tap into the unlimited energy source of our inner light and life force which radiates, illumines and energises our whole being. We can then experience the smooth flow of our energies in our selves and in life.

"I enjoy the smooth and gentle flow of energies in myself and in life".

THISTLE

Keynote: Courage

Thistle helps us to find true courage in times of adversity and to respond with positive action: self-empowerment.

Indications: Fear, dread, threat, immobility to act, powerlessness, frightening situations, flight/fight syndrome.

Attributes: Courage in the face of adversity, empowerment when facing great challenge, strengthening, facilitates confident action, fortitude.

When we encounter fear, our performance can be crippled. Thistle essence encourages us to access inner strength and to take appropriate action with confidence and certainty.

"I have the courage and strength to stand in my truth. I bring confidence and certainty into all my actions".

VALERIAN

Keynote: Humour

Essence of Valerian lifts our spirits and helps us to rediscover delight and happiness in living. It helps us to be at peace by taking ourselves lightly: jubilation.

Indications: Weighed down by sense of responsibility, over-seriousness, the glamour of being busy and hard-working, hurry and worry, over-striving, stress and tension, too focussed on one's own problems, sombreness, lack of sense of fun or humour.

Attributes: Experiencing life wholeheartedly, contentment, sensibility, sensitivity to impression, ability to laugh at oneself, pleasure, delight and happiness in being, joyful thanksgiving, true appreciation, spontaneity.

The essence of Valerian is uplifting to our mind, body and spirit. When we are weighed down in our busy lives by our responsibilities we can miss the simple or transient joys in life which bring us solace and happiness. Through Valerian essence we may become more responsive in the moment, lighten-up and have fun.

"I delight in the happiness of living and I walk my spiritual path with lightness and humour".

WATERCRESS

Keynotes: Wellbeing and Sanctification

Watercress essence infuses into our bodies a vibrational note of purification. It can act as a powerful cleanser, stimulating our immunity to clear stagnant energies and overcome disease.

Indications: Ill health through unhealthy or unwholesome conditions, lifestyle or environments; exposure to harmful substances or agents, unmindful or negligent of health or wellbeing, contamination through defilement, susceptibility to disease, miasms, low immunity; debilitation, feverish delirium, frenzy, inflamed, inflated, eruptive, carrying the weight of one's transgressions.

Attributes: Purification of self and environment, cleansing and cooling agent, restoring calm, peace and restfulness; cooling fiery desire body, clarification, elimination, purgation, miasmatic clearing, reflecting glowing good health, stimulating and strengthening immune defences, resistance to disease through vigilance, conscientiousness and hygiene; enhancer to transformative processes, extracting usable goodness and nutrients, dissolves, refines, purifies and transforms waste elements; drainage and discharge of dross through flushing out the systems, antisepsis, disinfection, anti-inflammatory.

As we travel through life our bodies absorb excesses and hold toxins from our emotions and lifestyle and pollution from the environment and we may feel heavy, slow down or become ill. Essence of Watercress helps us in refining, purifying and transforming our physical form so that the purity of our bodies reflects the light and truth of the soul.

"I cleanse my body and purify my soul".

WILD PANSY

Keynotes: Resonance and Radiance

Wild Pansy essence illuminates, clarifies and purifies the channels which connect the mind and heart. When we energise and enliven this connection, the Life energies are free to flow into the heart and radiate throughout the whole being.

Indications: Poor circulation of energies through blockage, deviation or dissipation; blocked energy flow to the heart, impeded or non-receptive to higher energies, turbulent, fluctuating or disturbed energy currents; sense of being detached or disconnected, convulsion, spasm, pressure, tension, nervousness, agitation, tremulousness, loss of mental coherence, fogginess, distractedness, abstractedness, absentmindedness, confusion, forgetfulness, disarrangement of one's sense of direction.

Attributes: Receptivity, sensitivity and contact with higher energies; clearing the channels to energy flow, circulation and distribution; infusing mind and body with vital life energies, illumination, vivification, vibrancy, lucidity and luminosity through expansiveness and receptive awareness in the heart, replenishes heart centre and facilitates circulation,co-ordination and synergistic functioning of thinking, feeling and willing processes; sense of aliveness and wellbeing through balance and composure, reassurance of mind/body stability and connectedness.

When the channels linking the head and heart become blocked, the energies flowing through will become diverted, impeded or lost and we may experience lack of clarity, confusion, detachment or disconnection. Wild Pansy helps clear the head and the channels enabling receptivity, sensitivity and contact to be re-established and we register the presence of this infinite flow of energy which is Divine Love.

"My mind and my heart are open. I radiate light and love".

WILLOWHERB

Keynote: Power

Willowherb helps to balance the personality expressing self-seeking authoritarian or overbearing behaviour, bringing about the responsible integration of will and power issues: self-mastery.

Indications: Self-aggrandisement, self-importance, judgmental, self-will, attached to power and position, authoritarian, eruptive temperament, oppression, anger.

Attributes: Integrity, self-empowerment, congruence, adept use of will, authority, self-tempering, humility, diplomacy, synergy.

Willowherb addresses forcefulness and self importance. When we are attached to our positions of power, we are in danger of overinfluencing or manipulating others with our willpower. We need to temper ourselves. Essence of Willowherb helps us to balance force of personality with true power through humility and the correct use of the will.

"I master my personality and power. I bring humility and right use of will into all my actions and deeds".

❀ GAIA ESSENCES ❀

Gaia Essences evolved in reverence to Mother Earth for the healing gifts of nature she has given us – the plant and mineral kingdoms.

The essences are made in rural Suffolk using cultivated flowers and also wild flowers, the preservation and protection of which being paramount.

Gaiai Essences also make many gem and crystal essences and is part of the East Anglian Flower and Vibrational Essence Forum. (See Appendix).

APRICOT

For arrogance, brashness, egocentric people, selfishness, greed, materialism. Brings about a softening, gentleness, sweetness and humility and a compassion for others.

CAMPSIS

Aligns and balances all the chakras. For right/left brain imbalances, dyslexia, learning difficulties, neurological disorders and diseases of the nervous system. Helps with psychic development and intuition.

MARIGOLD

For deep, unresolved anger that continues to surface. The constant blaming of others and the 'not fair, why me?' attitude.

PRIMROSE

For artists, writers and those involved with the creative arts, grounds the creativity bringing it into everyday life. For right-brain imbalance, helps concentration, memory and studying.

SQUARE-STALKED WILLOW-HERB

Overwhelmed when bombarded with mental activity or ideas. Unable to function properly, 'can't see the wood for the trees'. Square-stalked willow-herb helps one to focus and unscramble the mental activity, producing clarity of thought. Profoundly calming, good for meditation, stillness of the mind and insomnia.

STRELITZlA

Renewal, rejuvenation. For feelings of vulnerability, not knowing which way to go. For times of crisis and for inner strength. Helpful for the terminally ill, or those in bereavement, for loss, separation, alienation.

SWEET VIOLET

For lack of self-worth, love and forgiveness of yourself, releasing past negative patterning and traumatic events from this life and allowing you to let go and move on.

YUCCA

Helps remove the veil of doom and gloom – for mild or long-term depression. Gives lightness, joy, a zest for life, providing energy and vitality. For mental and chronic fatigue.

❀ GLASTONBURY HOLY THORN ESSENCES ❀

These two essences, the Flower and the Bud are made from the Holy Thorn Tree which grows in the Chalice Well Gardens in Glastonbury and is one of the descendants of the original tree on Wearyall Hill.

One legend tells how Joseph of Arimathea arrived in Glastonbury and planted his staff, reputed to have belonged to Jesus, on Wearyall Hill. It took root and blossomed and the descendants still flower both at Easter and Christmas time. Another legend links the tree with the crown of thorns which was used at Jesus' crucifixion.

The Essences are prepared with love and reverence in a sacred manner in the peaceful and healing atmosphere of the Chalice Well Gardens, using the Chalice Well Water to make the Mother Tincture. The same love and attention is given throughout the process including the bottling stage after which the Essences are energised further under a copper pyramid before being sent out.

The inspiration for the qualities and properties of the Essences came through during meditation at the time they were being prepared.

It is recommended that the Flower and Bud Essence are used together. First the Flower to assist in clearing and transmuting past and present memories of pain and suffering, both personal and collective, followed by the Bud to help process the new energies as we move towards a higher vibrational rate. Together they are a powerful catalyst for change and rebirth and bring in the light of the Christ Consciousness during this age of transformation.

FLOWER ESSENCE – UNIVERSAL SUFFERING

Negative Aspects:

For extreme suffering and feeling cut off from the source of Love and Light – from God.

Feelings of great despair and betrayal – 'Why hast thou forsaken me?"

Dark night of the soul.

For those angelic beings who want to return home, as they can bear it no longer – feeling of abandonment.

Positive Aspects:

Connecting back to the source and knowing there is no separateness – we are all one! A rebirth and transformation, at one with the Christ energy.

A huge weight is lifted off one's shoulders. Enables one to continue to serve mankind, but from a different perspective, coming from a deeper place of compassion.

Opens up the heart to greater loving

Has an action on the following:

Affinity with heart, third eye and crown chakras:

Opens up the heart and heals deep wounds.

Stimulates the third eye – clairvoyance and channelling.

Stimulates crown chakra – connection to the divine.

Gentle cleansing action on reproductive organs, purifying and healing any ancient sexual wounds.

BUD ESSENCE

To be taken after using the flower essence.

For those souls who choose to come and make a great sacrifice, to be reborn and assist in the transformation of this planet.

For the new beginnings and great shifts in consciousness occurring on the planet at this moment in time.

To bring humour, love and creativity into our lives so that we can serve humanity in the true light of understanding and compassion and to give us the courage to complete and manifest our life's mission.

To walk with Grace upon this planet, surrounded by the Christ light, with reverence for every living thing in this most beautiful creation.

WHITE LEAVED OAK

This is a recent addition, following on from the Glastonbury Holy Thorn essences. The White Leaved Oak is found in the Malvern Hills, one of the oldest geological formations in Britain. This particular species of oak is so called because of the white markings on its leaves. The ancient Druids revered it and would consult the size and shape of the markings as an oracle.

The essence was made on the Summer Solstice in the Vale of the White Leaved Oak, overlooked by Midsummer Hill, an ancient beacon site and hill fort. Water from the nearby 'Holy Well' spring, which is of exceptional purity and gushes from the crystalline rocks of the Malvern Hills was used in the making of the essence.

The Vale of the White Leaved Oak is at the centre of the Circle of Perpetual Choirs where the saints were said to have maintained a ceaseless chant. Three of the known sites are Stonehenge, Glastonbury and Llantwit Major. The Vale is also the meeting point of the three counties of Gloucester, Hereford and Worcester who host the Three Choirs Festival, which echos the same theme.

The oak, an ancient symbol of strength is placed at the Summer Solstice on the Tree Wheel Calendar. It was the traditional fuel for the ancient midsummer beacons. The Druids used oak essence for internal cleansing and the water from the hollow of the tree for their outer cleansing in preparation for the Midsummer Festivals.

Qualities and properties: Very centering and grounding. Brings the balance of roots firmly anchored in the earth and connecting with the Divine Source in the Heavens. Gets to the heart of the matter. Giving strength, confidence, courage and resilience to bounce back in times of adversity. Gives meaning to life's journey. Cleansing and purifying both soul and body (particularly skin conditions). Doorway to the inner realms, encouraging psychic intuition and visionary experiences.

❁ GREEN MAN FLOWER ESSENCES ❁

These essences were the first we made ourselves from our own garden and from the hedgerows in Devon. They consist of those we found useful for our own therapy clients and those that at the time weren't available elsewhere.

BILBERRY

Integration of the Self. Calms and brings peace to thought processes. Communication clarified. Increases equanimity and balance in all situations, especially where there are extremes of emotion that may bring conflict. Clarity, discrimination and wisdom brought to spiritual states.

CAMPHOR

Toxicities removed from subtle bodies allowing vibrational remedies, homoeopathy etc to work more effectively. Camphor and coffee no longer impede life-force through body, but camphor essence won't prevent long term effects of those substances on the physical. Activates meridians.

CHAMOMILE

Serene, sunny disposition, emotional balance. For those easily upset, moody and irritable, unable to release emotion and tension. Meditative states made more easy. Emotional tensions eased. Nervous system, endocrine system enhanced. Mental clarity and logical functioning.

COLUMBINE

Activates higher chakras located above the crown chakra. This greatly enhances the healing and integration of higher faculties and functions. Aids in the rebirth and complete healing of the Self. Inspirational.

DAFFODIL

Aligns mental body with Higher Self. Useful in deep meditation techniques and for listening to guides or the Self. Works with the crown chakra to pass information to the conscious mind. Useful in deepening daily meditation practices.

DAISY

Spiritualises intellect. Scattered information brought into clear focus. Understanding from an intuitive level. Stabilises those who are constantly seeking but not finding. Clarity and understanding, especially in spiritual areas. Relieves hiccups and shallow breathing.

DANDELION

Dynamic, effortless energy, lively activity balanced with inner ease. For those overly tense especially in muscles, overstrung and hard-driving on themselves. Relaxation of stress and muscular tension. Useful for poor posture, highly-strung individuals.

FLOWERING CURRANT

Relaxation of tense muscles. Calms anxious, nervous and fearful states. Cleanses and harmonises the functions of the mental, astral and causal bodies which helps to heal conflicts that have arisen between one's beliefs and ideas and the appropriate life-purpose. Stabilisation of emotions, peace and joy.

FORGET-ME-NOT

Awareness of karmic connections in our personal relationships and with those in the spiritual world. Deep mindfulness of subtle realms. For those with soul isolation, lack of awareness of spiritual connection with others. Blocked communication from other dimensions. Memory, clarity of thought, release of negative thought patterns. Faster reaction time; enhances functions of subconscious and dream state. Integrates crown chakra activities of meditation, dreams and visions.

GOLDEN CROCUS

Self-image improves, forgiveness and tolerance within oneself. Ability to express one's own feelings, if needs be forcefully. Integrity of one's own energy and protection. Healing from past hurts. Fears and anxieties ease. Joy, wisdom and personal power are strengthened. For under-dogs and scaredy-cats!

GOOSEBERRY

Sense of ease and relaxation of cares. Improves attitudes to the world outside. Enjoyment of life and living. For those who wish to save the world single-handedly. For those who fear getting involved. Improves poor circulation in hands and feet.

HONESTY

Brings the energy necessary to find knowledge of the Self, clarity of one's personal needs and how to relate to others at an energetic/subtle level. Increases a willingness to accept change and flexibility in persona or self-image. Clarity and direction in relationships with others. Helps to clear negative emotions from the heart. Healing negative emotional blocks.

LAVENDER

Spiritual sensitivity, highly refined awareness. For those who are nervous and who have over-stimulation of spiritual forces which deplete the physical body. Keen awareness and alertness. Cleanses meridians, stimulates visionary states, connections to Higher Self. Karmic and past life conflicts eased. Useful for spiritual practices, especially where there are emotional conflicts blocking spiritual growth.

LOVE-IN-A-MIST

Openness to loving and being loved. Increased clarity about one's motivations emotionally. Clarity for spiritual direction by easing frustrations and allowing clearer choices to be made. For getting back to oneself after setbacks. Calms and releases old emotional trauma. Increases energy and bloodflow in the circulatory system, especially in the legs.

MARSH GENTIAN

Communication with the deepest and most healing levels of the self. The brow chakra is brought to a clearer perception of reality, purified of doubts and enabled to find quieter, deeper levels during meditation. A very deep healing of the spiritual nature allows development of fuller potential, while the mind is able to go beyond apparent darkness to see the underlying unity and love of creation.

MOCK ORANGE

Ability to make use of powerful energy and the material world in a sensible, balanced way. Helps those who are afraid of strong feelings and of losing control. Solar plexus energised, boosting immune system and sense of self. Increased ability to express oneself and one's power in a direct, creative manner. Base chakra strengthened to enhance creativity in mental processes and communication of ideas. Strengthens and protects uniqueness of every being.

NETTLE

Eases all stress associated with a broken home. Useful for asthma, inflammations of the nerves and damage to inner lung tissue. For problems with sibling relationships. Assimilation of nutrients and vitamins. Creates calm in emotional and etheric bodies.

ORIENTAL HELLEBORE

Major healing in the endocrine system. Reduces tension and over-excitability in glandular functioning and the emotions. Increases self-assurance and reduces shyness. Helps to establish one's goals and directions in life. Self-awareness, poise, clarity and balance.

PANSY

Combats viral infections. Increases intuitive faculties and strengthens mental functioning.

PASSIONFLOWER

Attunement to Christ Consciousness. Stabilises spiritual focus. Opens heart and throat chakras and eases tensions in the dream state. Works upon the spiritual body and brings sharper visionary states. Easier access to higher states of consciousness whilst remaining stable.

PENNYROYAL

Strength and clarity of thought, mental integrity and positivity. When there are negative thoughts absorbed from others, when there is psychic contamination. Protection from psychic attack by strengthening the etheric body so that thought-forms cannot penetrate. Pennyroyal also expels negative thought-forms from out of the subtle bodies. Eases mental confusion and can be of use with addictions, schizophrenia and obsession.

QUINCE

Loving strength, active femininity balanced with inner masculine. For those unable to catalyse or reconcile feelings of strength and power with essential qualities of the feminine self, or who have a distorted connection with the inner masculine self or animus.

RUE

Energises and strengthens emotions and sensitivity, even to the extent of being an aphrodisiac. Gives energy to one's true desires and acceptance of oneself. Enhances appreciation of the body, improves self-image. Self expression as an aspect of one's spiritual nature.

SAGE

Ability to draw wisdom from life experience. To review and survey life processes from a higher perspective. Reduces the tendency to see life experience as ill-fated or undeserved. For those unable to perceive higher purpose and meaning in life's events. Aligns mental and spiritual bodies thus preventing religious fanaticism or atheism. Laughter, psychic faculties, philosophical interests. Strengthens etheric body, augments digestive system, cleanses meridians. Heart and solar plexus chakras.

SAXIFRAGE

Balances mind, intellect and imagination. Peace, calm and detachment that allows space for new ideas and concepts to be carefully considered. Encourages the practical use of all spiritual experience.

SCABIOUS

Enthusiasm to reach for new possibilities. Communication from and on subtle levels. Opening to higher learning. Finding other ways of doing things, exploring other worlds. Heals indifference and over-cool detachment from the roots of existence.

SCARLET PIMPERNEL

Eases the passage of kundalini when it has been awakened. Harmony in dream state: recurring nightmares and other dreams can be understood and assimilated. Vitalises pineal, pituitary and heart energies. Release of stored spiritual information and subtle emotions.

SNAPDRAGON

Lively dynamic energy; healthy libido; verbal communication that is emotionally balanced. Counters verbal aggression and hostility, repressed or misdirected libido. Eases tension around jaw. Aligns cranial plates, tempero-mandibular joint disorders (TMJ) and throat disorders. Speech disorders, self-expression and communication.

SNOWDROP

Spiritual confidence. A clearer direction in life. Increases the ability to plan practically – energises the thought processes. Brings insight, imagination, discernment and healing wisdom.

SNOWFLAKE

A positive space within which the Self can flourish. Clarity of purpose, one-pointedness and confidence. Calms and quietens the emotions to experience deep silence and the flow of universal energy and information. Helps protect from unwanted external thoughts and feelings that would interrupt the correct Path for the individual.

STITCHWORT

Brings a joy and lightness to the emotions and releases cares and worries. Once this process is under way there is an increase of calming, quiet energy where one can rest in relaxed alertness. Releases excess energy wherever it may be in the system.

ST JOHN'S WORT

Illuminated consciousness, light-filled awareness and strength. For those who are too open or over-exposed leading to psychic and physical vulnerability. Eases deep fears and disturbed dreams. Releases hidden fears or obvious fears, including those from past lives. Ability to separate thought from emotion. Useful for skin complaints.

WILD VIOLET

Acceptance and understanding of one's needs and energy to fulfil one's goals. Courage to the timid. Reduction of negative, aggressive tendencies in favour of life-supporting activity. The ability to perceive and live one's own life for personal fulfilment (rather than society's expectations and stereotypes). Adaptation of beliefs to one's own standpoint. Poised self expression. Passionate expression of true potential. Brings love and healing to feelings of confusion and emptiness. Heart chakra.

❈ GREEN MAN TREE ESSENCES ❈

As the image of the Green Man is an interweaving of human features with leaves and tendrils, so is the interaction and interdependence of humankind with the plant kingdom. One cannot be separated from the other. Green Man Tree Essences are a re-affirmation of the link between Man and Nature, acknowledging the healing power of life and the ancient wisdom of the peaceful trees.

Green Man Tree Essences can be used in meditation or to help with self-healing. Each essence holds the vibration of a particular tree species so that, when used, the qualities of the tree become available to you to enhance your life. The essences are prepared from the flowers of trees growing in the British countryside.

GROUP ONE

ALDER

Keyword – Release.

Reduces nervousness and anxiety. Strengthens the abdomen, particularly stomach, liver and gall bladder. Brings clarity of mind and eases physical tension in the muscles caused by stress. Increases life energy available. Speeds effectiveness and absorption of other remedies.

APPLE

Keyword – Detoxification.

Strengthens the immune response of the thumus gland and elimination of toxins through large intestine. Balances sacral, heart and throat chakras which leads to a reduction of tension in etheric body, eases breathing, clears thoughts and releases emotional tension. This in turn allows spiritual energies to enter the emotions.

ASH

Keyword – Strength

Finding one's place in the world. Harmony with the environment. Ability to express freely one's own needs and feelings in a way in tune with surroundings. Flexibility, strength, security. Physically aids skeletal system and its flexibility.

BAY

Keyword – Energy

Brings a deep-rooted vitality to the whole system. This may be too strong for some, especially those with heart conditions. Grounding and strengthening for the physical body, especially the meridian system. May give rise to explosions of energy as blocks release, encourages the expression of anger and other suppressed emotions. Stimulates higher chakras to draw in spiritual energy aligned with Christ Consciousness. (Good to use in conjunction with Apple.)

BLACK POPLAR

Keyword – Solidity

Creates an inner environment where peace is established as a powerful state. Consciousness is raised to a level of detachment where situations are recognised from a spiritual, unifying viewpoint. Brings in universal wisdom and a sense of complete security, at home even in the depths of space. Thymus gland activated which improves immune response and self-confidence. Throat, brow and eleventh chakras opened; fine perception and discernment are aligned with personal Will and expression. A link is created between the soul body and the etheric body, again bringing self-confidence and spiritual security closer to the body. The heart meridian is balanced which allows flow of love and forgiveness.

BLACKTHORN

Keyword – Circulation

Improves efficiency of blood supply, oxygenation of cells and red blood cells. Increases amount of nutrition available to cells. Useful for migraine, PMT, menstrual cramps, restriction of blood supply. Base chakra and heart chakra are activated and also minor chakras at base of arch of feet which stimulate absorption of minerals to stabilise emotions. Increase in hope and joy. Counters the effect of "emotional winter', sadness, solitude, hopelessness. Activates spiritual body in a way that gives protection from non-physical beings.

BOX

Keyword – Clarity

Helps regulate metabolism. Heightens sense of smell and cleanses sinuses. Creates emotional detachment and clarifies thought processes. Helps to clarify communications within the individual and their Higher Self. Strengthens the expression of the will. Eases irrationality, confusion and feelings of alienation from self.

CRACK WILLOW

Keyword – Spiritual sun

Activates throat chakra to be in communication with Higher Self. Strengthens the immune system particularly on the front of the body via thyroid and thymus glands. Has a specific effect on the diaphragm, so useful for hiatus hernia. Gives flexibility on mental and spiritual levels to allow things to happen, to let go, to look at and to accept oneself. Brings a sense of oneness with the world. Linked closely to the planet and from where its sustaining energies are received – the higher vibrations of the sun and Solar Logos.

ELDER

Keyword – Self-worth

Strengthens lungs and lung meridian. Has balancing effect on endocrine system, particularly gonads. Its main function is to calm aggression and intolerance and bring in stability, love and forgiveness. For all issues of understanding, self-worth, self-esteem. Opens heart chakra and minor chakras of chest. Balances astral and emotional bodies. Useful when facing times of transformation and change, especially of a spiritual nature, allowing intuition of the best steps to take. Good for children, fretful babies and toddlers.

GEAN (WILD CHERRY, MAZZARD)

Keyword – Soothing

Increases the effectiveness of the body's natural painkillers, endorphins. Useful for any pain, particularly where there is heat or sensation of heat i.e. fevers, inflammations, irritations, bites. Stimulates the sacral and solar plexus chakras focusing energy into the physical body and stimulating self-healing. Calms and brings peace to the agitated heart and mind. Creates a smooth flow of energy through the subtle nervous system (nadis) and the etheric body and so helps to balance the whole system.

GREAT SALLOW (GOAT WILLOW, PUSSY WILLOW)

Keyword – Soul

Energises solar plexus chakra and the eighth chakra above the head. This creates a link with the soul through which the mind can expand. As this allows greater understanding of one's purpose, tension is released and there is an energising of the whole body. Tension and rigidity in the knees is eased which creates a link to earth energy.

HAWTHORN (QUICKTHORN)

Keyword – Love

Stimulates the healing power of love. Strengthens heart and circulation. Relieves stress on heart centre. Increases trust and ability to love. Brings forgiveness, particularly of the self and helps cleanse the heart of negativity. Balances and aligns all main chakras.

HAZEL

Keyword – Skills

The flowering of skills. The ability to receive and communicate wisdom. Physically stimulates the nervous system, particularly the brain. All forms of philosophy, teaching, information are better received and understood. The mental body becomes integrated with the physical allowing recognition of beliefs and ideas which hold the most truth for each individual. The body's intelligence and wisdom is involved here, which automatically brings more stability and focus on the present. Throat chakra and minor chakra where the collar bones meet are opened. This spiritualises emotions and clears away unwanted debris, particularly outmoded beliefs about the self and problems with the ego. A link to fine levels of creation, particularly earth and plant spirits.

HOLM OAK

Keyword – Negativity

By activating personal creativity and desire to assert oneself in a positive way to increase peace and harmony this essence helps to eliminate restlessness, thwarted expression – anger, envy, greed, jealousy. Helps to express personal power. Releases tension in chest and back from emotional and mental stress. Strengthens bladder and bladder meridian. Activates second chakra. Aligns Higher Self and ego.

LEYLAND CYPRESS

Keyword – Freedom

Activates minor chakras near the wrists that ease hidden fears and anxieties. Unreal possibilities and delusions are let go. A more stable and positive attitude is created where forgiveness, tolerance and compassion for oneself grows, together with a sense of humour. All this creates a sense of freedom and a space to feel comfortable in. Clears the head and shakes off muzziness. Very good for those who are frightened of being on their own.

LILAC

Keyword – Spine

Affects all aspects of the spine, calms inflammations, trapped and pinched nerves, solidification of vertebrae, cleanses spinal fluid, activates energy in spine and all chakras. Helps correct posture and flexibility of the spine. A muscle relaxant. Helps assimilation of calcium, lecithin and B vitamins. The plant has a close link with nature spirits who use lilac to elevate their own consciousness.

ROWAN (MOUNTAIN ASH)

Keyword – Nature

Enhances the ability to tune into the energies of nature. Close link to the deva kingdoms, particularly wood and earth spirits. There is a connection to the "fixed stars", very distant objects, which brings a deeper understanding of the cosmos and the ability to recognise and make use of that energy in a positive, creative way. Enhances mental perspectives for a larger, broader viewpoint.

SCOTS PINE

Keyword – Insight

Activates all energies associated with the third eye. Development of psychic abilities. Brings penetrating insight and allows balanced growth of individual gifts. Increases tenacity and patience. Ability to see the broader aspects of good and bad. Forgiveness.

SILVER BIRCH

Keyword – Beauty

Ability to experience beauty and calmness. Eases harsh judgements of the self and others. Ability to understand and accept other people's views. Brings a state of experiencing quiet and deep beauty and the releasing of old patterns of behaviour. Also for those who find it difficult to express themselves.

SILVER MAPLE

Keyword – Moods

Balances the flow of energy through the body. Balances and regulates moods by normalising blood chemistry. Increases blood flow, absorption of blood sugars and strengthens red and white blood cells. Re-aligns meridian system (useful for acupuncture).

SYCAMORE (GREAT MAPLE)

Keyword – Lightening up

This essence deals with a powerful combination of sweetness and strength. On a physical level it focuses on the assimilation of nutrients through the actions of the small intestine and pancreas. There is also a slight strengthening of the legs. Energy levels are regulated and increased, so useful if lethargy is a problem. The awareness of the sweetness of life which encourages further growth and fulfilment. All meridians are strengthened, particularly bladder and circulation/sex. This increases relaxation and harmony, lifting heavy moods and helping resolution of conflicts. Works with the throat, brow and crown chakras and minor pancreas chakra, which creates emotional stability, calmness and inspiration. Brings all subtle bodies into better alignment with each other, particularly mental and spiritual bodies, helping to channel Higher Self into conscious mind and to contact a deep peace through understanding self and the underlying power of creation.

TREE LICHEN

Keyword – Wisdom

The ability to let go of anything no longer needed, to grow more completely. Knowledge of the cyclical nature of time and events. Knowledge of the Soul outside Time, through integrating mental, causal, soul and spiritual bodies. Access to past knowledge and ancient wisdom. This essence also allows consciousness to move beyond time/space and can be used for interstellar communication. Going everywhere without going anywhere. All main chakras brought into balance and minor chakras in centre of palms which stimulate throat and kidneys and those in the centre of the ears. Physical passageways, nose, sinuses, lungs etc., tend to be cleansed and there is a general process of purification. An ethereal essence that is rooted in physical existence and knowledge of the past. Brings a sense of independence and detachment without isolation.

WHITEBEAM

Keyword – Fairies

Stimulates fine levels of perception. Opens sacral, heart and brow chakras and the minor chakra just above the medulla oblongata, balancing creativity and insight with a keen awareness and alertness. Mental and astral bodies are aligned to work with fine perceptions, so that one can begin to learn how to shift energy levels. A deeper attachment and understanding to the animal and plant kingdoms and the desire to contact and understand the natural world from the level of healing and service. Increases harmony with cosmic energies and opens the heart to recognise the underlying energy that supports all life. It has some effect on the physical system, freeing up hips and legs and helps to clear lungs. Releases emotional energy in upper chest and back, heart and neck muscles.

YEW

Keyword – Protection

All issues of survival and protection. Strengthens blood and immune system, particularly liver. Helps absorption of nutrients. For memory, discrimination, relationship to the planet and solar energy. Protects from harm by activating the highest spiritual values of survival and protection (base and solar plexus chakras).

GROUP TWO

CATALPA

Keyword – Joy

Catalpa helps the stabilisation of the emotions. The small intestine meridian is activated which balances emotions of sadness, sorrow and joy. A minor chakra at the tip of the little finger is stimulated and this helps to stabilise various pulses throughout the body.

This essence helps the mind to find peace and balance. It also can improve the faculty of discrimination and the means of expression.

As Catalpa focuses much of its action on the area of the solar plexus it is an ideal remedy to reduce anxiety and restore emotional balance. Increases sense of peace and self-confidence. Underpins the real spiritual 'raison d'etre' of the individual – though this may not be known to the conscious mind, it will bring a sense of relaxation into one's own true nature and power.

CHERRY LAUREL

Keyword – Balance of mind

Restores balance to the head and mental activities are strengthened on all levels including imagination, inspiration, creative potential. Useful in cases of head trauma.

Brow and crown chakras are energised in a way that opens the individual to underlying universal energies (that increase sense of support and protection) and quietens surface mental activity to a level where more subtle perceptions and insights can be recognised.

Works on very subtle levels of organisation within the organism and will tend to encourage those processes that are evolutionary in nature. The essence stimulates and re-aligns spiritual concepts and belief systems that restrict the orderliness of molecular and cellular integrity. Although it doesn't have direct influence on such things as genetic and free radical damage, this essence may support the biology to make repairs at this level.

CHERRY PLUM

Keyword – Confidence

Reveals the inner security of the self and thus eases tensions that are locked into the muscle system because of fears, mental attitudes and so on.

Helps to combat shyness, by indicating a safe space in which to develop personal potential. The throat chakra is also activated to help expression, communication and intuitive perceptions. Eases one into being happy with the present time and helps to make contact with others on an emotional and feeling level. Emotionally and mentally brings peace and serenity and is useful for those with powerful emotional swings.

ENGLISH ELM

Keyword – Enthusiasm

Knowledge of the beyond. Clear overview of situations. Brings perspective back into balance in situations of lack of control, hysteria, obsession etc.

An increased sense of purpose and direction, a stabilisation of emotions and an understanding of others on a level of feeling, increasing compassion and equilibrium. There is a balance in the heart to act appropriately, particularly when imbalance is due to feeling drained or over-emotional.

Helps to reduce confusion, oppression and fatigue and increases clarity in decision-making and study. There is an increase in enthusiasm, a desire to progress and move onwards. Re-energises the mind when tired and clears the heart.

GIANT REDWOOD

Keyword – Weight of responsibility

Balances, tones and relaxes muscles in the abdominal and pelvic areas.

Helps those who are too hard on themselves and on others. The sacral chakra is stimulated to harmonise with other systems, relaxing to allow energy to flow and accessing wisdom to make correct decisions.

The throat chakra is balanced and this allows change in the manner of communicating and expressing desires and will, both in oneself and others.

Helps to maintain a balance in relationship of self to the outside world. Balances over-involvement with others and likewise a tendency to hold back from sharing.

GORSE

Keyword – Integration

The main function is the integration of heart and mind: Also creating a new synthesis of old truths – re-energising old, established or forgotten patterns of information in a way that expresses the self.

Eases restlessness, frustration and jealousy i.e. discomfort with the present situation and inability to change.

There is a relaxation of the feelings that allows new energy and perceptions to emerge and an increase in the experience of joy from deep within the heart. There is an enhancing of the immune system on the physical level.

HOLLY

Keyword – Power of peace

Acts as a spiritual guide and balance to the mind – clarity. The brow chakra is balanced to reduce irritability and mental chatter and confusion. Peace is given a chance to surface. Feelings of panic, loneliness and unhappiness are eased. The heart chakra is activated to help with self-worth and self-definition. Helps to become more assertive, expressive and passionate in dealing with self-worth, self-love, self-appreciation. This essence brings the active expression of love – an energy that is non-aggressive and peace-loving, yet assertive.

Holly helps to activate and energise the control systems and the systems of intelligence and discrimination within the body and allows a clearer awareness of the body's feelings and survival needs and its quality of life-force.

HORNBEAM

Keyword – Right action

Cleaning away deep trauma to the core energy systems of the body – particularly when these have been instigated by holding views and speaking out against the consensus view i.e. those times when personal expression has been repressed or censored.

There is increased self-confidence and security leading to better decision-making and the ability to work well with others creatively.

A flow of energy is initiated deep within the cellular organism which can stimulate under-energised or stagnant areas and can make internal communication systems more effective (i.e. nervous and endocrine systems).

HORSE CHESTNUT

Keyword – Agitation

Understanding and empathy with others which reduces such feelings as intolerance and impatience. This essence helps to create a flow between differing energies rather than agitation and resistance.

Brings calm and balance to ideas and mental function and peace to an agitated mind. Calming fears and anxieties, this essence also reduces over-rational intellectual or obsessive thought, increasing the flow of intuition. Where there is a build-up of mental 'static', when people are just completely annoying and things 'grate' on us, Horse Chestnut essence opens the energy taps and pressure safety valves so that equilibrium is restored.

ITALIAN ALDER

Keyword – Protected peace

Brings peace, love and protection for delicate energies. Helps when either shyness or over-aggression is a problem. Courage and healing where new beginnings are necessary. Useful for those who feel useless, unworthy, not valued, lacking support etc.

Increased feelings of self-worth via activation of Soul Body releasing guilt and energising the whole physical being. Very deep healing energies are able to enter from other dimensions. There is a protective quality with this essence that helps to strengthen against pollution and all aggressive energies.

IVY

Keyword – Fear

Primarily works on the release of anxiety and the strengthening of personal power. At an emotional level Ivy helps us to face up to fears and discover our true feelings. It allows us to clearly identify emotions and needs. This strengthening of the discriminatory faculties is echoed on the physical level with an enhanced immune system.

Minor chakras at the wrists are energised which help to ease hidden fears and anxieties. The heart chakra and its nadis are also affected beneficially. Ivy essence is a protective and powerful guide through territory which is unknown and scary.

LABURNUM

Keyword – Detoxification

Creates the space and opportunity to allow the release of underlying shocks and imbalances. Aids detoxification by relaxing nervous and muscular tension which also occurs when the mental body is balanced.

Increased ability to communicate with increased discrimination of what can be of use to the body systems, whether that be ideas or nutrients.

Kidney and lung meridians are strengthened which helps detoxification and vital energy transport.

There is an increase in optimism and positivity.

LARCH

Keyword – Will to express

The main energies of this tree focus on the balance and expression of complementary energies, particularly associated with the functions of the throat and sacral chakras, which can be characterised by the Will to express the self and the Desire to experience self with non-self (or 'others').

The sacral or sexual chakra is affected, which controls and directs the physical energy towards expression and exploration of other beings in relationship. Motivates 'joy for life' and healing creativity.

Helps deep healing of shock and trauma, particularly from the past.

There is an aspect of clarity and wise judgement and an understanding of the power of communication and the power of silence.

LAWSONS CYPRESS

Keyword – The Path

Brings energy to base, sacral and solar plexus and brow chakras. In the base, it brings discipline and purpose to direction in life. In the sacral chakra one becomes more creative in achieving desires. The solar plexus chakra is cleared of non-realistic, deluded or fantasised futures. The brow chakra is stimulated to maintain an overview of the 'feelings' activated in the lower chakras. There is a recognition of what actions are required and if changes are needed they can be initiated because this essence allows internal clarity and the ability to project accurately into the future, one's true needs.

LIME

Keyword – Development

Strengthens the endocrine system. Activates the solar plexus and 8th chakra, which allows the creative power necessary to change from one level of activity, or consciousness, or power, to another whilst still maintaining individual balance and personality.

Calms anxieties within the mind and helps ease extremes of emotion, particularly when this is to do with making practical use of one's psychic and healing potential. For those who are unable or unwilling to accept and use their higher faculties. Doubts and fears ease, past-life programming is lessened.

MIMOSA

Keyword – Sensitivity

Physically stimulates the nervous system, particularly increases sensitivity of the system to internal stimuli. Affects the small intestine and large intestine meridians, particularly those issues to do with assimilation of food on a physical level, information and ideas on a mental level and the ability on all levels to let go and release what is not required.

This has a beneficial effect on the emotions with an increased sense of peace. The ability to express one's thoughts and to speak up.

MONTEREY PINE

Keyword – Connectedness

Removal of deep stresses within the system, particularly those related to speaking out against perceived injustices and failure to act when it was necessary. Physical well-being, getting in touch with the body. Confidence in the physical body.

An increase of fine perceptions both in ideas, concepts and in other planes of reality. Past life information. Deep stress is eased allowing increased self-expression and artistic creativity. Artistic blocks lifted.

Information from fine levels, subtle perceptions are able to be evaluated clearly as to their relevance and importance.

NORWAY MAPLE

Keyword – Healing love

Bringing love and acceptance, healing, nurturing energy to emotional shock and trauma. The Triple Warmer and liver meridians are balanced to bring a sense of lightness and a sense of happiness. This essence enables one to take back control of situations where one has felt powerless because of a lack of understanding that everyone has equal status with everything else in creation.

Also helps to find ways to work within current situations. Fears and anxieties ease, joy and comfort increase. At a spiritual level this essence helps to stimulate personal potential and brings it into the awareness – usually as inspiration or imagination – to be able to integrate and develop it.

OAK

Keyword – Manifestation

Absorption and integration of very deep, hidden energy levels from the primal sources of being. Funnelling it through the desire for growth in solid reality and delight in expressing in as many ways as possible.

Calming and unifying. This essence is immensely steadying and stabilising, giving energy to all levels of the individual, though not necessarily realigning them. Whilst anchoring us in the present reality, oak essence will let us experience the huge play of polarities in existence without getting lost in the experience. The ability to manifest possibilities out of 'nothing'.

PLUM

Keyword – Empowerment

Transmutation and transformation of material, physical activity by healing transcendent love. The knowledge and understanding of creation through healing love and the desire to go beyond established boundaries.

Sense of freedom, healing of fears. Helps to counter the enervating emotions of shame and loneliness. Ability to find practical solutions through the strengthening of personal power. Increased feeling of power and belonging.

PRIVET

Keyword – Old wounds

The release of shock from within the subtle bodies. Particularly useful for healing and balancing when there is a need to release blocks caused by physical trauma in this or other lifetimes. Privet creates a harmonious vibration that helps to heal. This essence is not particularly effective on emotional levels – it is more to do with physical, structural programming

Energy is given to the emotional body to understand the need to release patterns and to accept growth and change.

STAG'S HORN SUMACH

Keyword – Meditation

On a physical level there is a release of tension in the neck and throat areas.

Activates the mental body where belief systems, reality models and self-images are held in a way that allows one to determine valid supportive actions ('spiritual direction'). This becomes particularly noticeable when one is in a meditative state.

This essence balances energies for meditation, largely through its action on the brow chakra and related minor chakras. There is a feeling of coolness, a stilling of the mental and emotional processes. With this quietness there is an increased ability to access flows of energy and information and a strengthening of the underlying awareness of reality.

STRAWBERRY TREE

Keyword – Quietude

Energising to the crown chakra increasing potential for healing and personal, spiritual growth. Enhances the qualities of the imagination.

Strawberry tree is excellent for quietening and clearing the mind. Thoughts tend to dissolve away into silence. Allows transformation to come about through stillness and silence: as movement and activity defines form, it requires a cessation of activity and movement in order to effect change. Ceasing to move allows form to become more fluid and less bound by past actions, habits, routine thought and so on.

There is an increase of life-energy in the body via the ears and also a cleansing effect on the nasal sinuses.

VIBURNUM

Keyword – Reassurance

Feeling supported in oneself and one's life. Inner conflicts tend to be understood more clearly and are reduced. There is an increase in ability to perceive clearly.

At a very deep level, where we initiate the tendencies to act in certain ways, there is a clearing of trauma and a re-integration of fragmented energy. Particularly relevant where there have been near-death or life-threatening situations.

Balances causal and mental bodies and thus reduces sense of vulnerability, sensitivity, neuroses, feelings of being unhappy or unsettled. Reassurance and re-evaluation of past experiences in the light of a broader, more positive outlook. A spiritual state of understanding and connection.

GROUP THREE

BEECH

Keyword – Easy-going

Self-creativity – a building up of the self within the self. Healing and accepting oneself.

Physically, helps relaxation of head and solar plexus areas, often associated with tension/anxiety headaches. An increase in hope and confidence. The throat centre is energised also, so a useful essence for those who lack confidence in speaking or have constant sore throats.

Self-awareness problems and blocks eased, particularly in the area of the sexual/reproductive system. Physical and emotional relaxation whilst there is an increase in mental structure and clarity.

BIRD CHERRY

Keyword – Sensuality

Brings about a healing balance and increase of happiness. Relaxation, particularly of body awareness and sensuality.

Feelings of self-righteousness eased by a deeper understanding of oneself.

Emotional indifference is eased. There is a healing of deep hurt which the indifference disguises or covers. The need to love and be loved (i.e. connected to creation), is healing. Feelings of unworthiness, guilt, self-disgust, etc are helped. Increase of energy, forgiveness, fairness.

COPPER BEECH

Keyword – Depression

Relieves depression and brings a deep, enlivening sense of peace and detachment from worry.

Anger and repressed or otherwise inappropriate emotions are expelled in a non-aggressive, positive way. There is more acceptance of deep unconscious emotional tendencies and instincts. Emotional difficulties with relationships are eased. Increase in sense of joy and humour. The emotional body and the emotions themselves are energised and enlivened.

FIELD MAPLE

Keyword – Aching heart

Total security within the self that allows one to be able to love unconditionally (and to receive unconditionally). Acts as a balance to those who desperately seek love without looking inside themselves to discover what may be pushing love away. Brings the high wisdom/love energy from above the crown and establishes it in the solar plexus where it can manifest its power. Physically helps to ease respiratory system and blood flow, mainly through a deep relaxation and clarification of energy use.

Understanding and contentment for those who are overwhelmed by remorse or a sense of being responsible for events and accidents. Rebalance after shocks. Return to centre. Calms over-aggression, passion, anger at oneself or others. An increase in spiritual insight and one's place as part of the whole.

GLASTONBURY THORN

Keyword – Out of the Woods

A clearer direction is found. What feels right to do and be emerges from indecision and chaos. This brings immediate relaxation and release from tension, increasing subtle information and intuition. Claustrophobia.

JUDAS TREE

Keyword – Channelling

Enables completely original thought, as if from nowhere: the seeds of new ideas arising from the finest/deepest levels of information available. Using it in a practical way.

An openness and willingness to accept, peace and calm; listening to one's feelings. Breaking links with past regrets. A willingness to communicate and share as equals. The causal and spiritual subtle bodies are harmonised which helps the development of channelling abilities. Soothes turbulent, passionate and angry states. Enables rational, cool consideration of any situation involving the emotions.

LUCOMBE OAK

Keyword – Creative energy

The main energy is life-supporting creativity, inspiration and ideas. Tolerance and kindness born of wisdom and compassion. Easing and reforming of stressful and life-damaging beliefs. Useful for states of lethargy, confusion and lack of commitment as this essence greatly energises the mental body in a way that increases the desire to act with deep commitment for change and evolutionary growth. Creativity and inspiration increase.

MAGNOLIA

Keyword – Restlessness

For when one feels vulnerable and unclear in oneself and when there is an unsettling restlessness where nothing satisfies.

The heart chakra and its nadis are cleansed of stress and this allows a greater freedom of emotional expression and sense of freedom and relaxation.

The crown chakra is stimulated giving a clearer idea of one's true identity – this has an effect of strengthening the immune system.

This essence helps when there are difficult choices – it balances the heart and mind and allows in calm and happiness to make correct decisions.

MANNA ASH

Keyword – Happy with oneself

Healing the emotions. Recognition of what one needs to establish peace. Increasing the energy flow throughout the meridian system. Self-worth and self-acceptance, clearing emotional blocks in the heart. Good at sorting out unresolved issues, calming of destructive tendencies. Acceptance of how one feels. A quiet, creative level of consciousness is more easily accessed from which to bring greater healing and creativity.

MULBERRY

Keyword – Wrath

Emotional healing: bringing compassion and healing peace and a needed detachment from the source of pain.

Useful for those who decry views that differ from theirs, who will not see deeper truths, who are jaded and cynical about the world.

For those attached to a painful situation or event carrying great remorse, Mulberry essence helps to heal the energy link and bring peace from past pains.

Changes the energy of anger to a more constructive end where it can be mastered and fully expressed through understanding, compassion and awareness of the reality of the underlying situation. Allows full expression but curbs excessive wrathfulness.

OSIER

Keyword – Spiritual void

For when there is a need to let go. To relax the mind and let a deeper wisdom well up.

Strengthens solar plexus, particularly useful when it seems that a void lies behind existence and everything appears shallow and meaningless. This apparent blackness can be, in reality, experience of the unrevealed, hidden or unmanifest levels of creation which has to be understood for what it is: the underlying vibration of life.

A balanced approach to one's relationship with others, neither being too forceful or overbearing, nor too willing to accept others points of view.

Flexibility and creativity in ideas, effective action and correct use of personal power.

PEAR

Keyword – Serenity

Brings clarity of mind, peace and joy. Helps clear nervous system after it has been blocked by past-life experiences and beliefs. This would lead to a relaxation throughout the nervous system – release of tension.

Clarity, simplicity, confidence, inner calm. Increasing feelings of serenity and happiness. Happy to be who you are.

PERSIAN IRONWOOD

Keyword – Alienation

Energising, grounding, earthing. Increases sense of security and emotional stability – especially when dealing with strong drive and emotions.

Helps to bring subtle evolutionary tendencies into the physical: activates fine-level healing.

This essence increases the link to the super-consciousness of the planetary energies as a whole. This is not the same as attunement to the Earth as a planet, more as a link to the Higher Self or potential future Self of Mother Earth. This link brings a strong sense of connectedness, joy and happiness.

There is a greater recognition and understanding of intuitive faculties, an increase in peace, self-worth and ability to share.

Has proved of great benefit for those who are unwilling to fully accept being in physical existence or who have suffered natural disasters such as earthquakes and whose confidence in the solidity of the world is shattered in some way.

PITTESPORA

Keyword – In two minds

Clarity of perception, clarity of mind and the ability to act in an orderly, organised way.

Helps to clarify how one really does feel when one is in "two minds" or unable to determine where one's loyalty lies.

Helps bring creativity into fine levels of the self loosening up anxieties, over-seriousness and lack of humour.

This essence helps the exploration of who one really is. This manifests as clarity of purpose, mental peace and a truly personal, individual way of being alive.

PLANE TREE

Keyword – Fine judgement

Fine judgement – the ability to discern the truth in situations. Wisdom and calm clarity – justice based on a deep tuning into the nature of things. Developing a mental structure to cope with the flow of intuition and information.

Prevents too much introspection and dwelling on sadness. For those prone to over-analysis and melancholy.

Helps to achieve a relaxed, meditative state, calm and detached from anxious organising.

RED CHESTNUT

Keyword – Fear for others

A balance achieved between the mind and the imagination. Fears resolved and phobias eased that were caused by past experiences.

An increase in sense of security and protection. All subtle bodies are effected to balance fears and needs with joy and happiness. Having a more sure awareness of one's own position, it is easier to deal realistically with fears and anxieties.

Problems to do with projection of hopes and fears into the future are eased. An increased ability to live in the present rather than with possible futures.

All this helps to create a better link and relationship to others.

RED OAK

Keyword – Practical support

Energising with practical motivation for the mind, such as the exploration of physically-based spiritual disciplines (Hatha, Chi Kung etc.)

Increases amount of energy to the skeletal system to strengthen and support all aspects of skeleton.

The base chakra is activated to a closer link with the Earth and a deep knowing about one's place and function – the instinctive, right-acting, body personality. "Feeling" what is right to do and be.

The solar plexus is cleared of self-doubt and false self-concepts and beliefs. Healing within all self issues. Encourages the awareness of being loved and supported and helps give practical outlets for spiritual aspirations.

SPINDLE

Keyword – Self-integration

Individuality is attuned to the Higher Self, self-expression in accord with one's true nature without negative egotistical influences of superiority. Understanding the true nature of the self removes any feelings of judgement of others which often manifest as competitiveness, need to succeed, to be "first" etc.

Heart and solar plexus are aligned, helping to feel at home where one is at any time and bringing clarity to purpose and potential.

Ability to look at and understand the deepest, darkest, most hidden parts of the Self. To understand and integrate the shadow self.

Transformation and awareness of what appears negative. Release into the self of those energies suppressed through fear – transformation of negative, stagnant energy into life supporting dynamic energy.

SWEET CHESTNUT

Keyword – The Now

Re-establishes feeling of the Self, centering and focus and stabilises the heart and the energy of sharing. Helps to clear the mind when finding creative ways out of difficult situations. There is an integration between the subtle bodies that reduces disruptive energies and/or tendencies. There is an increase in confidence within the physical body and a sense of well-being. Helps remove the sense of guilt and clarifies personal awareness of right and wrong.

Releases deep guilt, particularly lack of attraction for physical existence, physicality, passions and anything "earthy". Helps to bring the ability to accept change on the physical plane. Is particularly useful for those who feel uncomfortable about physicality as being "unspiritual".

Healing and love. Protection against aggression. Contact with fine levels of healing energy.

TAMARISK

Keyword – Fire of transformation

Understanding one's place at the Centre. Intuiting one's emergence from the Absolute and place within the Absolute even when in the midst of the relative worlds.

Because of this knowledge there is total freedom, total flexibility, complete understanding that all is possible. The divine spark leaping from the central sun of being.

Tunes the solar plexus chakra into intelligent and self-developmental ways to direct the personal Will, life-force, personality and lifestyle.

Cleanses the spiritual body which increases energy. Frees up energies for finding spiritual direction, personal expansion and growth. Deeply cleansing and uplifting.

TREE OF HEAVEN

Keyword – Heaven on Earth

Practical spirituality, practical wisdom. Helps to break through any blocks at the spiritual level – the crown chakra becomes energised and grounded so that its energy is more accessible to other systems of the body. The spiritual is more easily experienced in the physical – the medulla oblongata is stimulated to integrate levels of bliss into the physical.

Minor chakras on the forehead are stimulated to help a clearer understanding of larger truths and ideals, universal concepts and past-life viewing.

The subtle body systems are supported, emotional trauma is eased and there is an ability to bring out new levels of energy.

TULIP TREE

Keyword – Spiritual nourishment

Physically helps bring about cleansing and calming to the abdominal organs and pancreas in particular. Brings relaxation to the abdomen.

Where there is spiritual hunger, a gnawing emptiness, Tulip Tree will bring the means to fulfil the aspirations of the Higher Self.

Strengthens the links with the spirit worlds. Useful as an aid to meditation, creativity and artistic abilities as it clears deep blocks within the throat chakra.

WEEPING WILLOW

Keyword – Ego

Like most willows, Weeping Willow has a deep connection to the solar energies. Its main energy is the balancing of power, which can be both life-giving and life-damaging, like the sun. At its finest it is the spiritual fire, the manifestation of wisdom and beneficial energy to all. Helps deal with the negative ego-based states of cynicism and contempt, both of which originate from a false sense of self-righteousness. Quietens the emotions, increases generosity to others, and calms agitated or bad-tempered states.

Eases contempt that masks a fear that one is perhaps wrong or that one's personal world-view is not unassailable and may be invalid. Positively, it brings on new creative freedom and balance to accept another point of view.

Helps heal the etheric body, particularly those areas where there is a mental/belief system difficulty with that body part or system. Helps heal the underlying breaches in all-accepting love and compassion which can allow serious diseases to manifest. Re-establishing one's true worth and value in creation as equal to all (but superior to nothing).

WHITE POPLAR

Keyword – Starting again

Security from which to grow outwards, express oneself and explore new ways of being and thinking. Having established a sure foundation in one's own worth, exploration of possibilities. Energises and heals heart chakra, so that there is increased determination to recover from setbacks – particularly emotional. Energises relationship to oneself and others, through practical growth and expansiveness.

The ability to make positive changes which are in new directions, perhaps unthought of before, more in line with one's true desires and strengths.

WHITE WILLOW

Keyword – True Self

The Spirit infuses the being – ego is taken out of the equation. Personal influence lessens, one is able to become a clear channel.

The brow chakra is stimulated, increasing mental perception and clarification of communication channels.

The medulla oblongata and forehead centres are stimulated so that one can see a broader perspective of oneself in a greater pattern. The self is brought to a truer balance within itself. There is a clarification and clearing of one's relationship to the universe. A sense of bliss and love wells up – bliss consciousness is brought near.

YELLOW BUCKEYE

Keyword – Devas

A balance between the external environment of Nature and one's own energy systems. A feeling of balance with one's surroundings.

The crown chakra is tuned to experience and understand different levels of communication and thought. Ability to frame new images and concepts in a logical, understandable way. This essence allows easier links to devic energies and access to the wisdom of different levels of consciousness. The tree acts as a focus for devic and elemental awareness and so the essence augments contact with these levels of being.

❀ HABUNDIA FLOWER ESSENCES ❀

The Habundia flower essences are based on the plant medicines used in a shamanic tradition, which has many generations of experience to draw upon. They are divided into three groups: general, spiritual and magical. The general set of essences are designed to help people through the common stresses of life and the lessons normally encountered in our personal development, emotional and mental. The spiritual essences are designed to expand awareness into higher realms to more easily achieve enlightenment, clairvoyance, channelling and inner peace. The magical essences are designed to help with the practical magic of shaping your life and manifesting your desires and help put you in touch with your power. They are all prepared by a shaman in a deep state of communion with the plant spirits.

GENERAL

ALFALFA

Strength, self-worth, earthing and expressing your spiritual spark. Honouring and communicating your own needs, especially spiritual needs. Rooting. Absorbing vitality from the Earth.

BALSAM POPLAR

Cleansing and healing the sexual chakras. Balances the flow of sexual energy. Releases pain and tension from sexual issues.

BEAKED HAWKSBEARD

Connects the solar plexus with the crown chakra, to uplift the emotional body by keeping a spiritual focus. Rising above petty emotions and trusting in one's own destiny.

BRAMBLE

Opening to and understanding love in its deeper levels. Bramble teaches one to approach love with gentleness, care and respect.

CHICKWEED

Being happy with yourself, so you do not need the understanding and appreciation of others and do not need to attract 'draining' relationships.

COWSLIP

Strengthens the solar plexus and settles the emotions. For when you are feeling vulnerable. Comforts and uplifts the emotions.

DANDELION

Centering. Understanding one's emotions and the cause of one's reactions. Helps release hatred and resentment. Allows one to receive nourishment and find the space for healing. Good for liver, pancreas and solar plexus.

FIGWORT

Overcoming judgement towards gross matter. Recognising materiality as an aspect of spirituality. Loving material existence and seeing it as a vehicle for spirit.

FLEABANE

Earths solar energy, to give strength and stability and this gives immunity against parasites on many levels. Provides the quiet vitality that allows one to build health.

HEDGE WOUNDWORT

For healing deep hurts and tapping a source of inner strength. Helps connect with power animals and guardian angels.

HONESTY

Maintains peace and beauty amongst stressful surroundings. Simplicity and faith in who you really are.

GOLDEN SAXIFRAGE

Integrating the Sun into the feminine soul. Understanding the feminine aspect of the solar energy. Opening the heart to give freely.

IVY

Patience, strength, stability, rooting. Gradually growing towards union. Links one to the Earth Mother.

LILY OF THE VALLEY

Safety, by enshrouding the negative tendencies of the subconscious mind that can draw in trouble.

MAYWEED

Integration of different energies. Rising above conflict and stress.

ROSEMARY

Brings clarity when there is great emotional or mental stress, loss of trust, or confusion. Restores harmony by shifting the focus to the underlying perfection in all things. Helps with memorizing and remembrance.

SUNFLOWER

True enthusiasm and balanced masculinity. Softens the ego. For disconnectedness to the feelings, stress and deprivation.

TANSY

Causes one to look at themselves and examine their motives, while providing some protection against outside influences.

WILD ROSE

Bringing out the beauty in your wildness. Overcoming limited conditioned beliefs and finding your true self. Love and appreciation of all things, including self. Acceptance of all Life. Strength through opening the heart to the oneness of nature.

WOOD ANEMONE

Opening the heart to accept love and simplicity. Discriminating from the heart to accept only things of love.

VALERIAN

Red. For emergency use. Dealing with specific shocks. For when one is feeling overwhelmed, by any intense emotion or experience. It is good to follow with white valerian.

White. Calming, soothing. Brings peace and light and enables one to rest. Good for shock and stress.

YARROW

Enhances the aura. Protection. Over identification with other peoples' energies and outside influences.

YELLOW POPPY

Calms emotions and activates the mind. Helps to memorize, synthesize and adapt. Ideas, inspiration, clarity of mind.

SPIRITUAL

BLACKTHORN

Balancing beauty with power. Gives you security in showing your inner beauty, while protecting you and keeping you strong.

ELDER

Wisdom to rise above apparent opposites and encompass dualities. Recognising the importance of all things, each in its own cycle.

MONKSHOOD

Understanding the need for illusion, to protect one's spirit when vulnerable. Gives some protection to the 'psychic gate', when opening. For turning people away from what you wish to keep hidden. For those who feel too 'open', helps draw strength from spirit.

MOSS

Acceptance, non-judgement, transmuting karma by living through it without judgement.

SCARLET PIMPERNEL

Strengthens and nourishes the navel chakra and etheric body. Strengthens against psychic contamination. Aids one to be recharged and nourished through meditation. Replenishes creative and sexual energies. Good to use in meditation. Also helps to bring resentments into the consciousness, particularly linked with sexual issues.

SPINACH

Develops the higher octave of the heart chakra. Shifts the focus from giving on a personal level to a universal level. For growing out of repeated patterns. Strengthens one's spiritual integrity. Oneness.

STINKING HELLEBORE

Balances love and power. Helps break out of conditioning and outer influences which seek to mould' you, while maintaining a state of love. Protects the heart chakra.

THISTLE

Nobility, spiritual value. Develops the crown chakra. Trust in the spirit. Maintaining one's spiritual integrity in spite of undermining company. Strength, protection, unhindered growth. Allows true beauty and gentleness of the soul, without fear.

TREE MALLOW

Develops the spiritual heart. Soothes pain, gives strength and allows rapid growth through adversity.

WATER FORGET ME NOT

Balancing of water and air. Brings air qualities to watery types and vice versa. Tempers the ego and allows one to express oneself gently. Helps bring subconscious fears and repressed feelings to the surface and supports peacefully and gently. Aids connection with the angelic realms.

WATER LILY

Provides an inner sense of space, for detachment, stability and safety. Inner nourishment and connectedness to the source of life.

WHITE ROSE

Purity of heart. Developing your own soul note, without reacting to distracting influences.

WILD PANSY

Developing a strong loving, warm heart. Bringing out the beauty of the soul. Purification of the heart and soul and of the desires.

MAGICAL

BLACK TULIP

Clears the third eye. Clarity, originality. Honouring one's own creative perception, expression and vision, regardless of outer pressures to conform.

COMMON SPOTTED ORCHID

Opening the crown chakra, channelling, contacting devas and angelic kingdoms in a balanced and earthed way.

DEADLY NIGHTSHADE

Powerful third eye stimulator. Psychic purge. Clears one from psychic interference. To be used in single dose as required, rather than repeatedly.

DOG'S MERCURY

Astral projection, path workings and underworld journeys.

DWARF ELDER

Enhances lunar qualities, intuition, subtle power and magnetism.

FIVE LEAVED RED CLOVER

The essence of the magical dynamic of fire, Will, direction, inner strength, purification. (Caution: this essence is volatile and is shaped by your thoughts. Always take it with a clear intention in mind.)

FOUR LEAVED CLOVER

The essence for connecting with Nature Spirits. Puts you in touch with the hidden secrets of nature and expands awareness into new dimensions. The essence of Magic.

FOXGLOVE

For letting go. Releasing anxiety about one's material situation, or what is to come. Seeing the light at the end of the tunnel. Letting go of the material illusion. Aids transition into other planes. Good for trancework and inner journeying. Good for heart and gall bladder.

HAIRY NIGHTSHADE

Encourages one to go forward with sensitivity and awareness, to truly progress on one's real path. Is particularly good for creative visualisations, manifestation work and inner journeying. (Helps those who feel they have lost direction in their lives.)

HENBANE

For understanding death and exploring its realms. Preparing for death initiations. Connecting with spirits who have passed on.

MARJORAM

Restores power and will, deep memory and the knowledge of who you truly are. Strengthens the heart chakra. Marjoram is sacred to the Goddess Venus.

PENNYROYAL

A powerful purifier. Activates the crown chakra. Earths spiritual energies and unconditional love. Encompassing all life without judgement.

PERIWINKLE

Earths, empowers and protects the astral body. Prevents energy leakage. Adds impetus to one's intentions and life expression, by focusing energies and preventing dissipation. Good for recentering after astral experiences.

PRIVET

Connecting with the Tao by understanding the cycle of uniting and dividing, opening and closing. Linked with the Dark Mother and the owl, Silence and Darkness.

THORNAPPLE

'Soulvine'. Aids movement between different planes of existence. Breaking conditioning and limitations of the mind. Seeing the onenesss of life and death. Taken after using the Henbane essence, it can take one deeper into the death initiation. This is a very initiatory essence and should be taken with the utmost respect and with clarity of motivation.

VIPERS BUGLOSS

Understanding primordial powers. Linked with the spider and snake. Very useful for resolving emotional tensions and conflicts which are due to the emergence of subconscious forces. (N.B. This flower will initiate one through these forces, but will not suppress them.)

WILD THYME

Helps to open clairvoyant vision. Enhances feminine power and the feminine will, creative energy and subtle wisdom of the heart. Regenerates the female base chakra. Initiation into feminine power.

YELLOW ARCHANGEL

Aids in contacting and understanding the hidden realms. Helps attune with the angelic intelligences and develops an attitude of acceptance and non-judgement towards all that one may have to face on the path of these planes. Understanding the need for balance of light and dark, all having a divine role and place.

YEW

Connecting with the void through the understanding of opposites. Putting the mind aside and listening to the hidden wisdom of matter.

❀ HAREBELL REMEDIES ❀

Harebell Flower Essences are made in the soft, wild countryside and organic gardens of Southwest Scotland. Mostly they are familiar British wildflowers or, with one or two exotic exceptions, traditional garden plant favourites. The essences are all made with local spring water, non soda glass bottles and best brandy. Great attention is paid to preserving the vibrational quality. To aid holding the plants in mind, there are colour drawings on the labels. First made in the mid 1980's, the number of essences, their descriptions and combinations grow and change with the years. Affirmations accompany the descriptions in the main repertory. Here, the essences are grouped into introductory small sets according to their habitat. A set of combination essences is also included in chapter 9.

COTTAGE GARDEN

CORNFLOWER

For being comfortable with individuality. Protects sensitivity and special gifts. Belonging to oneself and liking oneself. Heals damage from institutions.

FORGET ME NOT

Grounding and emotional balance. Remembering reality. Release of negative thoughts (often through dreams). Trusting inner wisdom and calming irrational fears

GERANIUM (CRANESBILL)

For bringing or allowing a cherished and well grounded plan through to manifestation, e.g. starting a business, getting into print, learning to paint, drive, sing etc.

PANSY

For hardy strength, builds up resistance when feeling low and vulnerable. Overcoming adversity.

POTATO

For coming down to earth. Feeling safe and centred. Calming down over excited states. Enjoying the familiar and commonplace.

RED ROSE-BUD

Opening up to love and sexual feelings. Puberty. New relationships. Feeling safe in giving and receiving love.

SNAPDRAGON

Helps expression of repressed emotions. Good for frustration and speech problems. Irritation (often stuck in the throat or voice), anger, fear or sadness (held tightly in the face, lips and jaw).

WHITE ROSE BUD

For infants and babies in the womb (children and adults too). To help us rest and grow safely in the light of grace. Keeping our sense of heaven on earth.

FAVOURITE GARDEN

CYMBIDIUM

For defiance in the face of undermining influence. Overcoming frustration, lack of confidence and fear of disapproval. Embracing the tiger within.

FLOWERING CURRANT

Is warming and opens the heart, expands and softens the lungs. Strengthens the naturally flowing breath and the capacity to love.

FORSYTHIA

Balancing energy levels. Brings more awareness of how we gain and lose energy. How to absorb or use it better.

JASMINE

A general stimulant. Helps to process, absorb or eliminate. Good for congestion and low self esteem. Learning to be practical, to use or let go of whatever comes our way.

ORIENTAL POPPY

Tendencies toward oblivion. Making the choice to live, to fully be here without escaping, numbing or pretending. Having the capacity to enjoy life as it is.

RED ROSE

For boldness and passion. Being true to your desires and against shame. Living a life of enthusiasm and delight.

RED TULIP

To overcome shyness. To be more outgoing, more daring and vibrant, without losing one's centre. Red Tulip can help us to trust our fire nature and give birth to the whole self.

WHITE NARCISSUS

Letting go of selfconsciousness. Moving from thinking too much to being more aware of feelings and in touch with the spontaneous child within. Being guided by one's heart.

HERB GARDEN

BORAGE

Essentially a tonic. Borage strengthens the heart and eases the emotions bringing encouragement and cheerfulness.

CHAMOMILE

For the release of anxiety and fear. Helps deep relaxation and acceptance of a situation. For high strung, over responsible states. Letting go of worry. Calming and soothing.

COMFREY

Increased sense of integration and wholeness. Good for injury, tiredness, memory loss and for balancing natural cycles. Relaxation, repair and renewal.

HYSSOP

Another tonic which can lessen feelings of anxiety and help the acknowledgement and release of guilt. Owning the true cause of thoughts and actions. Releasing blame.

LAVENDER

Soothes and cleanses. Creates a feeling of peace and space. Stimulates a clear overview. Good for meditation, balancing the emotions, easing conflict and releasing blocks.

MARJORAM

Comforts and protects from harm. Supporting life in times of danger. Aids emotional release especially fear. Helps us to put our trust in creation.

ROSEMARY

Strengthens the heart and mind. Supports trust in friendship, strong bonds and common purpose. Especially good for fear of loss of love and for the freedom and autonomy of the sexes.

SAGE

For the wisdom of not taking oneself too seriously (essential secret of longevity). Awakens the higher self. Aids relaxation and enjoyment of life, affirming one's essential foolishness.

LOWLAND

BUTTERCUP

Connecting with the inner child. Appreciation of life's riches. Able to experience joy and pleasure in the moment.

HEARTSEASE (WILD PANSY)

Brings comfort to an injured heart. To let go of mistaken love and acknowledge sad and lonely feelings. To forgive and move on.

PLANTAIN (RIBWORT)

For turning resignation or a heavy heart into acceptance. Finding strength and joy in being grounded. Renewing the capacity for happiness.

RED CLOVER

'For shock'. Calms and soothes any person, child or animal who has had a fright. Aids the release of fear. Lessens the tendency to panic or react.

SAINT JOHN'S WORT

For protection and containment. Seals the aura and promotes sound sleep. Helps any frightened, anxious or paranoid state. Especially good with children or in stages of certain therapies.

SPEEDWELL

Safe travel, moving with ease, changes, crisis periods, 'more-haste-less-speed' situations. Seeing clearly in new directions.

THISTLE

Keeping integrity and self respect. Staying faithful to our own views and personal truth. Loyal to and supportive of those who share them.

YARROW IN SEA WATER

Can help with the release of vulnerability to environmental dangers such as radiation. Use as a protection or to cleanse after exposure.

OPEN WOODLAND

BLUEBELL (WILD HYACINTH)

Cooling and calming; good after any injury or trauma. For overwrought children, uptight adults and traumatised animals. Useful anytime to promote peaceful, happy feelings.

DAFFODIL

A 'spring clean' essence, helping to banish winter blues. Everyone knows and loves the uplifting Daffodil. Use all year round for depression, self doubt and low self esteem.

LUNGWORT

For the creation of space in the body (lungs) and mind. Encourages deep breathing and clear thoughts.

PRIMROSE

For lightness and cleansing, opening and relief. Help for letting go of tight held back feelings and toxic ailments. Lifting of a weight.

SELF-HEAL

Looking within for healing and nourishment. Releasing self doubt and confusion, developing self love and acceptance. Trusting the healing process.

SNOWDROP

Developing openness and trust. Protecting innocence and simplicity. Healing the inner child. Issues of safety or sexuality.

SWEET VIOLET

For loving. Believing in and practising unconditional love with oneself and others. Being truly loving of self and others and able to receive the love that is around us.

WHITE FOXGLOVE

Liberating the mind of conscious thoughts. Surrendering to a meditative state. Once used 'to induce trance'. Freeing the spirit.

SOUTHERN UPLAND

BROOM

Perseverance. To keep busy and motivated through difficulties. Renewing faith. 'Sweeping clean' and starting afresh. Developing a strong calm will. Steadies the heart.

EYEBRIGHT

Good for a weak brain and memory. Can help us to get things into perspective. Gain some detachment.

HAREBELL

The effect of Harebell is subtle, evoking a true connection with untamed wild nature. The qualities are gentleness, strength and clarity.

HEATHER

Courage to be alone, to face our shadows (the parts of ourselves we do not like). Accepting solitary periods, unknown outcomes and empty spaces.

ROWAN

Evoking soulfulness. Drawing on the rich experience of personal attachment to people, places, nature and culture. Refining the raw materials of life into something valuable.

TORMENTIL

Refusing to be dispirited or overpowered. Springing back with renewed confidence and hope. Having the faith to overcome whatever happens to bring us down.

WILD THYME

Strengthening by purification. Especially of thought, motivation and intention. Can be used to enhance or potentise other essence mixes, also to cleanse crystals or other objects used in healing or divination.

YARROW

Offers protection against negative influences in the environment and in the thoughts and emotions of others. Enhances and strengthens the aura (light/energy field surrounding the body).

WAYSIDE

DANDELION

For relaxation of mental stress and muscle tension (especially neck and shoulders). To stop being overwhelmed and let go of irrational fears. Trust in our ability to cope with life.

ELDER

For protection in situations that are potentially abusive. When we feel invaded or wronged and also feel helpless. Helps us to confront our own fears and say no.

HAWTHORN (MAY TREE)

'Brings hope'. Calms and protects in times of grief or sadness. To know that sorrows are not endless, not damaging, but a natural part of life.

MARSH WOUNDWORT

For fretfulness, old worry and distress. Releasing anxiety, bitterness and discontent from the past. Being open to healing and to the present.

NETTLE

For cold angry states, those who feel apart because of frequent hurt. Arouses warmth and passion in the temperament.

PURPLE FOXGLOVE

Emotional wounds or betrayal. Learning to accept pain as a part of personal growth. Taking some responsibility for whatever has hurt us.

RAGWORT

For trusting, loving and respecting the body. Letting go of overactive mental states. Surrendering thoughts which are not from our wise, body centred self.

ROSE BAY WILLOW HERB

Numbness or 'cut off' toward others. Old defensive patterns that are hard to change. Responding to others without fear.

WILD GARDEN

ALKANET

For deeply centering, balancing polarities, preparing for change and transformation. Gives inner strength.

HONESTY

For confusion or lapses in consciousness. Fosters openness with others and honesty with oneself. Reclaiming memory blanks. Honouring the truth. Being clear about what is real.

IRIS (BLUE FLAG)

'Symbol of power'. Coming into one's own personal power. Releasing blockages to living to full potential. Being our own authority.

JACOB'S LADDER

For being open to receiving or actively seeking help. For those of us who feel we must resolve all problems alone.

LADY'S MANTLE

For the protection and inspiration of wise woman or Goddess energy. Meditation. Prayer. Wonder working. Fertility. Birth.

LILAC

For ease and grace of movement. Opens and connects the chakras. Helps to lessen rigidity in the body (esp. spine) and mind. Surrendering to changes. Flexibility.

MONKSHOOD

'Expels poisons'. For protecting spirituality, identity and purpose. The ability to recognise and banish bad influences from one's life.

RHUBARB

Exhibitionism. For the insecurity of being way off centre. Extrusive behaviour (talking too much etc.) Unaware of boundaries. Allowing feelings and silences.

❀ IMELDA CARROLL – ARD NA NEANTOG ❀ FLOWER ESSENCES

The essences made at Ard Na Neantog to date reflect the needs of the garden and the gardener and are used by both. They are made by Imelda Carroll, the member of the Sí (Gaelic for nature spirit) who deals with essences, the Deva of essences and the Deva of the flower/plant in question, using the sun method, after dawn, before noon.

LAVATERA

Lavatera enhances "the ability to connect with the inner, ancient knowledge".

For those who feel the weight of ignorance a burden.

For those who feel worthless because of lack of perceived or learned knowledge.

NEW ZEALAND FLAX

New Zealand Flax enhances "the ability to divide in order to produce unity and growth".

Strengthens the separate aspects of the personality and therefore the whole.

For those of proud nature who have over stretched themselves.

A great essence for networkers!

SAGE

"Sage enhances the ability to see things as they are, in a grounded way and enhances the strength to accept that truth".

To treat:

Lack of acceptance of reality.

Shock, from bad news, sudden change.

The feeling that you can't carry on in the face of truth.

❀ JEAN JACOB MASTER REMEDIES ❀

FLOWER ESSENCES FROM THE ASCENDED MASTERS

A set of 6 essences of the Ascended Masters: St-Germain – with African Violet and Amethyst, holding the vibration of the violet flame of regeneration from lower to higher vibrations; Sai Baba – with Rose and Gold to personify Unconditional Love; Sananda – with Rose, Moldavite and Rose Quartz, resonating to the heart and Christ consciousness; Melchizedek – with Water Lily and Quartz – he was the Master of Light to bring wisdom and clear thinking; St Michael with Magnolia and Gold – his sword of protection cuts away all the dross giving us strength and power.

All essences have Tachyon water added which contains free energy. To the 5 Masters collection is added Gardenia for peace and purity. These essences are intended for linking with the Masters for meditation and attunement. They were given during the Wesak festival 1996.

SANANDA – (MASTER JESUS)

This essence has been created from the pink rose – Rosa rugosa. It has the highest vibration. The 5 petals are symbolic of Christed Man. It relates to the heart centre.

There is a slight mauvy tinge to the pink which reminds us of the sacrifice. The rose is combined with two crystals – rose quartz, a pale pink and resonates to the heart, it is the crystal of Love. Moldavite is also used – this is a new and rather rare green crystal. All roses have green around the centre and this is also the colour for the heart centre.

This essence is very powerful; it is suggested to take a few drops in a little water before meditation and visualise a pink rose in the heart gently opening to the love of the Christ.

SAI BABA

This essence consists of Rosa centifolia and gold. This rose is a lighter pink with numerous petals, it has a beautiful perfume which immediately raises the vibration. Sai Baba is the personification of Unconditional Love – this is his message. Spiritual love is the pink rose, the red rose is human love. The essence is blended with the essence of gold – the highest vibration of all metals. It represents Wisdom. The golden light pours into the heart bringing us wisdom filled with love.

It is suggested after using a few drops before meditation to visualise Sai Baba holding in his hand a pale pink rose tinged with gold, which he hands to you.

ST. GERMAIN

The African Violet holds a special vibration; it has high spiritual connections often used when opening the 8th chakra. Violet resonates with spirit. It grows high up in the mountains (mountains symbolise the higher levels), the leaves grow in a rosette – collective consciousness – the delicate leaves can easily be broken – we must take great care when raising consciousness. This is the colour of St Germain – the Violet Flame. He is the Master Alchemist, he uses very high vibrations, the work needs much care. Amethyst is the violet crystal resonating to regeneration, we transmute from the lower to the higher self. Visualise the Violet Flame taking you on your journey, become the flame, it holds the power, you can change.

MELCHIZEDEK

The Angel of Angels. We use the water lily, the flower of wisdom, the key. Each petal contains a different aspect of our journey, they open as we progress. The flower opens only when the sun shines. We must have spiritual nourishment for our growth. When man is fully enlightened the thousand petalled Lotus opens in full bloom. Pure, quartz crystal is used with this flower. It gives clarity of mind. Melchizedek is known as the Master of Light to bring us clear thinking, as he has great power, so has the crystal, for it is a Merkaba – original sacred geometry which is pure light. For times when we feel lost tune into the energy of Melchizedek, see him with a water lily at his feet and the whole presence in a great crystal; see the facets reflecting lights pouring onto the flower, become each petal to understand your need – ask and you will receive.

ST MICHAEL

The sword of St Michael cuts away all the dross leaving things pure. Magnolia has a lily like flower which resembles purity. It has pale cream petals tinged with the spiritual mauve. The whole tree resembles purity with its clear lines. It grows high up in the mountains of China where the air is clear and pure. The essence gives strength when one is unsure. Tuning into St Michael will always give strength and power – he is the guardian of the planet. Gold is the purest metal known.

See the magnolia growing in the mountains with its strong lines. Inhale the perfume of the flower. See the golden streaks of light from the Sun pouring down upon the petals. You will gain confidence, strength and power.

GARDENIA

This essence is the only one to be made by moonlight. It resonates to the moon energy. I was guided to the essence by the following experience:

With no outward intention of linking with a Gardenia, just sitting in the silence, I quite suddenly had a visualisation of an aged, Chinese seer who I have known as Shen. He put a bowl of water on the ground, near my feet. As I wondered what it was all about, I perceived a flower floating on the water. On close inspection, I recognised the flower as the Gardenia. Our energies started to blend – the thick, fleshy petals which feel like velvet remind me of flesh. The petals bruise easily and quickly go brown. This is a simile to the person treading the path – the human who can be so easily bruised and hurt with all the transgressions he must face. The petals drop quickly – so man can easily drop out and give up. The flower floats over the water, which is a symbol of the astral – desire. This is where man must strive to rise.

The perfume of Gardenia was overwhelming, it has such strength and power. It is a rather heavy, sensuous perfume, which indicates that it is calling man in his lower, material state, to raise his vibration. The purity of the white petals arranged in circles, brought my mind to the Higher Self. This is the way, the path to what we call enlightenment. The Gardenia represents the Higher Self. Water – the illusion of the desire body. The bowl of water at my feet took me to the foot washing rite of Jesus. He was symbolising getting rid of the dross in order to tread on the path.

So, the Gardenia is given to us for those who are ready to make the journey to raise their vibrations to meet their Higher Selves to come to the Christ Consciousness. It is only for those who are ready, hence the exotic grandeur of the flower. It comes from warm climates, we grow it as a hothouse plant and warmth connects to the fire element – fire is love.

Gardenia is one of the most spiritual flowers on the planet. This essence is for those who find difficulty in overcoming the obstacles on the spiritual path. For those who give up easily. To overcome the desire world of illusion. It is for those who are truly on the path at the door of initiation, so its rareness and difficulty to obtain is readily understood, for only he who is ready can receive.

JEAN JACOB FLOWER ESSENCES

The essences have been made over a ten year period, using the natural, wild flowers locally. They are always blessed and made with spring water, when available, from Glastonbury Well and brandy. They are to help people to raise on all levels to achieve balance and harmony and become as the flowers, at-one with the universe.

AFRICAN VIOLET

Venus.

This plant grows high in the mountains in Kenya. Plants which grow high up have a spiritual significance. The colour also symbolises spirituality. The rosette shape of the growth suggests that it is good to be used in groups. The leaves are fleshy and will break easily, so sensitives can easily be injured with their sensitive make-up and can absorb easily from others.

The tiny, golden stamens are reminiscent of the sun and its golden rays of wisdom.

African violet helps to balance the nervous system, it is associated with the pineal and of use for disharmonies in the mental body. Can help with possessions. The plant has a very powerful aura. It is valuable for those reaching higher vibrations and opening to the spiritual path.

African violet is connected to ultra-violet light which emanates from the sun. Sunlight affects the pineal which contains seratonin and lack of it can produce SAD. It grows among the rocks – on the spiritual path one needs a solid foundation.

BLACKBERRY

Venus. Libra.

Brings causal and spiritual bodies to integrate with the physical. Forgiveness and persistence. Conscious manifestation of creative thought. Awakens love when afraid of dying. Overcome inertia.

BLACKTHORN

Saturn.

Dark night of the soul. Depths of despair. Self opinionated people who are not open. To open the door where one cannot see the light.

BLUEBELL

Venus.

Female depression. Post natal especially with fear and guilt. Helps self-love and kindles re growth for brighter future. Brings joy and colour where there is grief.

BROOM

Mars. Fire/Air.

Renewal. Sweeping out all out-moded and unneeded dross. Opening to the golden light. Perseverance. Protection. Helps depression.

BUTTERCUP

Links to the fairy kingdom. To be childlike and open. 3rd chakra opens to light. Reveals the key to nature.

BUTTERFLY BUSH

When life is empty and barren. Feelings of inertia, without purpose. In need of motivation.

CALIFORNIAN POPPY

Aligns the mental, causal and spiritual bodies. Gives astral, psychic and spiritual balance. Solar Plexus. Psychic vision. For those who can be pulled in the wrong direction who need the spiritual path not psychic deception.

CHICKWEED

Moon and Saturn.

Sharing, uniting kindred spirits – to show us all is one. Balances high and lower energies. Forgiveness over prejudice. Helps to balance 3rd, 4th and 5th chakras to resonance. Star to guide us to the light.

COLUMBINE

Venus.

Opens the 8th/9th chakras. Known as the gift of the Holy Ghost, it raises one to higher consciousness.

COMFREY

Saturn.

Integrates mental and nervous system. Good for memory. Balances left and right brain. Muscular degeneration. Releases sub-conscious tension.

CORNFLOWER

Frees from conditioning. Gives confidence to self.

COSMOS

Aligns the mental and etheric bodies and combines the heart and throat chakras for easier expression. Nervous speech problems when too much information is not absorbed.

CROCUS – YELLOW

Venus.

Saffron – for the navel centre for digesting higher knowledge and processing it.

DAFFODIL

Venus.

Cleansing, removes lack of self-worth. Crown chakra. Raises consciousness, for meditation. Links to the higher self. Good to take when dowsing. Good for emergency in accidents.

DAISY

Venus, Moon, Mars.

Balances 1st, 2nd and 3rd chakras. Aligns the subtle bodies. Alleviates stiffness to be vibrationally flexible. Releases joy through simplicity. Stabilises spiritual seeking.

DANDELION

Jupiter.

Letting go of fear, releases stress. Good for mental body. Aligns etheric, mental and causal. Muscle relaxant, stress in mental body lodges in the muscles.

ELDERFLOWER

Venus, Mars.

Protection for fear of psychic possession. When one feels invaded.

FORGET-ME-NOT

Spiritual relationship of all things. Good for memory. Pineal gland stimulated.

Maintains emotional balance. Aligns mental and emotional bodies so lower influences are closed. Opens the crown. Used for accidents and emergencies. Connects to spiritual guides.

FOXGLOVE

Venus, Mercury, Saturn.

Feelings of being hurt. When there are deep wounds in the heart. Often confused thinking. Wanting a way out. Alba – contacts to the psychic.

FORSYTHIA

Used for sugar addiction. Restores the flow of energy.

FUCHSIA

Repressed emotions which cover up deeper issues.

HAWTHORN

Mars. Saturn.

Heart centre. Activates spiritual properties. Let go of negatives. Good for grief and stress. Clears the etheric and emotional bodies. Eases cancer distribution. For heart breaks. Balances the physical to the subtle bodies.

HONESTY

Moon.

Pituitary. Right brain – feminine – negative attributes. Often secretive in order to assert. Helps to become more open and honest.

HOPS

Mars.

Pituitary. Activates the etheric. Good in groups. Relaxes and calms. Stimulates spiritual growth.

HYSSOP

Moon, Mars, Jupiter.

Releases guilt feelings and being judgmental. Good for groups. Base chakra. Second and third chakras and the etheric bodies are balanced. Helps with sleep when astral travel makes one tired on waking. Helps to assimilate gold.

IRIS

Venus, Moon.

For creativity especially through art. Links to the colour of the soul of nature. The triangle of faith, wisdom and valour. Iris means rainbow – the bridge between spirit and matter, light and dark.

JASMINE

Moon, Jupiter.

For spiritual love. Stimulates the Godspark. It has two devas, male and female. It transmutes physical love to higher levels of spiritual love. It has a very high vibration. Heart centre. Universal Love awakens the fragrance of jasmine. Strengthens the etheric with the physical. Perfume reaches the angels who deal with colour.

LAVENDER

Mercury, Jupiter.

Calms and balances. Crown. Opens lst, 4th, 7th, 8th and 9th chakras. Energises 10th. Gives clear insight and understanding. Helps to hear the music of the spheres. Blends the physical, etheric and astral. Removes karmic blocks. For over stimulated nerves; some spiritual practises and too much meditation can lead to nervous disorders and insomnia.

LADYS MANTLE

Venus.

For protection. Fertility. Alchemy transmutes lower energies into higher. It blends energies into cosmic consciousness of the planet.

LEMON BALM

Sun, Jupiter.

Good for concentration. Aligns the chakras. Helps open 3rd/4th chakras – helps the mental body. For those allergic to cats and dogs. Great healer. Remembering past lives. Comfort to the dying. For groups and spiritual unity.

LILAC

Venus.

Flexibility aligns the etheric, mental and spiritual bodies. Associated with the fairy kingdom. Good for cleansing and all problems connected with the spine. For rigid attitudes.

MALLOW

Moon.

Use for ageing, any stresses or tensions associated with the elderly. Tonic for the endocrine. Pituitary. Invigorates the skin tissue, connections and veins to the brain. Helps to find the warmth of a loving relationship for it attracts love.

MAPLE

Jupiter.

Balances yin and yang. Realigns the meridians. Good with acupuncture.

MARIGOLD

Sun.

When there is too much materiality, denial of spiritual purpose. Strengthening and comforting. Often connected with psychic matters. It is a great protection.

MEADOWSWEET

Jupiter.

Relaxes tension especially in the head. Can uplift. Good in groups. Throat chakra. Perfume expands the possibility to receive love.

NASTURTIUM

Mars.

For energy. Good against negativity. When changes need to be made. To let go of fear. Pituitary. Endocrine. For the over-intellectual which causes depletion. For loose earthly alignment. Depletion of the life force. Good for animals when dying. Useful in colour therapy.

NETTLE

Mars.

Cleansing tonic. High in ferrus. For those who blow hot and cold. Emotional states from a broken home, useful in divorce. For those who feel stung in life.

PANSY

Saturn.

Used for colds and viruses, protection against radiation. Mental body and right brain. Balances resistance. Heartsease – which helps to lighten a sorrowful heart.

PEAR

To ground and strengthen, used with crystals harmonics will activate the creativity of musicians. Harmonious in groups. Aligns mental, emotional and spiritual bodies. Increases elasticity. Balances the spine in conjunction with therapies. Strengthens 3rd and 4th chakras.

PEPPERMINT

Jupiter, Venus, Mercury.

Clarity of vision. Struggle between upper and lower selves. Metabolic/digestive. Regulator-craving for food which makes one sluggish, so the metabolism is unbalanced. Third chakra. Links to the higher nature.

PETUNIA

Crown. Links to the higher self. Anti-depressant. For young children or elderly. Mental body, left brain. Good for stuttering, meditation, visualisation. Can be put on bruises. For public speakers. Etheric and emotional links.

PINKS

Jupiter, sun.

The flower of Zeus. Great healing powers of Sun energy. Gives strength. Grounding.

PRIMROSE

Venus.

Cleansing. Renewal after depressions. Raises the vital force. Five petals represent cosmic man. Clears toxins and mental blockages. Good for the liver. Leaves are used for sleep. A remedy for sensitives.

QUEEN ANNE'S LACE

Mars.

Helps with inner sight, seeing auras. For over intellectualising and those who are confused. Pineal and crown chakra. For mental calm. Bridges the gap between physical and spiritual. Strengthens the rods of the eyes.

RED CLOVER

Mercury.

For shock. For those in a panic and to lose identity with the negative forces. Helps to lead in a crisis. Throat and base chakras. For all emotional issues which cause blockages. Balances right/left brain. Helps oneness with animals.

RIBES

Mars.

To gain confidence. Overcome fear of facing oneself. Third chakra. Releases overall fear. Will provide inner strength.

ROSE

Venus, Jupiter, Mars.

Heart chakra. Spiritual love. Strengthens the etheric, opens 8th chakra. Best used alone. Brings peace and comfort. Links with the higher spiritual forces uniting human and spiritual love. A very high vibration connected to the monad. Gladdens the heart linked to Christ Consciousness.

ROSE BAY WILLOW HERB

Connections to the etheric can become blocked causing one to feel alienated. Removes blockages in the subtle bodies so that energy can move freely.

ROSE GERANIUM

Venus.

Calming, soothing. For those needing to open to love. Heart chakra.

ROSEMARY

When absent minded and forgetful, often when the incarnation is not well-earthed. For psychic protection. When extremities are cold because of lack of warmth from poorly connected etheric/spiritual bodies. Stimulates the pineal and crown chakra to draw down the warmth of the sun to gladden the heart. Transforms, brings joy and light. A stimulator.

RUDBECKlA

Sun.

To confront traumas of the past. Healing forgotten issues which need to be faced. Brings light into darkness.

SAGE

Jupiter.

Connects the mental/spiritual bodies. Second and fourth chakras. For unconditional love/wisdom in that we accept that we do not know everything. Not to take life too seriously, so it promotes long life. A balancer, for too much mental energy makes one agnostic and with too much spiritual energy one becomes a religious fanatic. Great cleanser of negativity of psychic energy. Important in rituals.

SCARLET PIMPERNEL

Gives strength to those who feel taken over by others. Breaks psychic bonds. Helps the kundalini power. Aligns mental/emotional/spiritual bodies. Crown chakra. Assists the loving nature when kundalini awakens.

SELF-HEAL

For taking control of ourselves, trusting in our own inner strength. Crown chakra. For assimilation of spiritual energy. Used with mineral waters when fasting. Strengthens the thermal body. Powerful cleanser of the etheric when it is weakened.

When one has lost confidence in their own capacity for healing.

SPEEDWELL

Jupiter.

More haste less speed. For safe travel and movement. For seeing the way clear.

ST JOHN'S WORT

Sun.

Releases fear from the past. Clears nightmares. Links with the Divine. For sensitive people who are prone to stress and negative elemental forces. Gives light through the darkness. Crown chakra.

SWEET PEA

Venus.

Sweet Pea helps those who do not know where they belong and are always searching, never becoming involved, often outsiders – these people never seem to have roots. They need a homing, a sense of belonging. Sometimes there has been a lot of moving around. Sweet Pea helps one to connect to the earth and relate to others – stop daydreaming. The delicate flower and colour gives a dreamy feeling. The tendrils clinging for support in order to reach the light, tells us we cannot do this until we relate to all that is around us.

RASPBERRY

Venus.

Base and second chakras. Cleanses the etheric. Used for bonding especially with children and the newly born. Releases a sense of fun which children know.

TAGETES PATULA

Sun.

Mental/causal bodies. Psychic abilities, clairaudience. For those who are closed off from the world. For the need to listen.

THYME

Venus.

Etheric/mental bodies. Third, fourth and ninth chakras. Left brain. Alters the time flow of love to the heart. Will speed up remedies being taken. Used in far memory trips. Can travel from the past to the future. Cells carry the blueprints. Thyme helps release information. Gives a sense of direction. Linked to the animal kingdom.

TOADFLAX

Mars.

Deals with connections to the throat or voice. Aligns mental/emotional/causal bodies. For any inability to speak or express. Verbal aggression. When the lower centres are unbalanced the creative expression is not communicated.

VALERIAN

Venus.

For the pathetic. Those who are lost, never having received true love, so they find it difficult to love themselves.

VETCH

To balance yin/yang. When sexual identity is confused.

VIOLET

Venus, Moon.

Links to the 7th ray. For the very sensitive. Yin energy-calming. Strengthens the immune. Purifies the lymphatics. For those who are poor mixers. Those who have a highly refined soul force, who do not want to shine, yet hold back for fear of losing their identity. Often feeling lonely. Appear cool, yet have inner strength. The subtle perfume flows and helps to shift the fears to open and flow with the warmth of others. Very much a new age essence. Protection from radon.

WILD GARLIC

Saturn, Mars, Moon.

Great protection against negative forces. Helps transition at death. Heart chakra. Good for animals. Effects are short-lived. For low vitality, poor immune system. Eases radiation. Rids fears and wards off entities possessing.

YARROW

Venus.

Special protection against radiation and psychic attack. Pink yarrow protects against negative emotions. Gives radiance to the aura. As the spiritual path becomes more open, so there is a need to protect against vulnerable forces which can cause depletion. Yarrow gives a shield of shining light. Very necessary new age essence. One of the oldest plants on earth.

❀ JUDITH HOAD ❀

Sun method essences Eyebright and Self-heal were made in the summer of 1991. Eyebright seemed, intuitively, one that was needed. In meditation three people agreed that it offers an opening for the senses to a clearer, broader view of possibilities available to the individual. Self-heal was made in the same period, on another day, at the request of a friend. This essence offers an opening of the inner view, a sight of the wounds and ways to heal them.

EYEBRIGHT

This remedy appears to impart an ability to see beyond the immediate, to have an overview, as if standing on a mountain top.

SELF-HEAL

This remedy appears to help people who see others' problems better than their own to re-focus and get the 'beam out of their own eye'.

❧ LIGHT HEART FLOWER ESSENCES ❧

As I've been working with these essences the same theme returns constantly and I am sure that this is the theme of all flower essences: that their teaching and inspiration is a call for us to return to love, which is our true expression. I do believe that love heals all and that we are being constantly called to choose love – to unconditionally love ourselves and all that that means practically in our daily choice for integrity and wholeness; and to unconditionally love others and recognise the love which is expressed in everything we see and experience.

These essences are an extension of my healing and are created in partnership with nature and spirit. They are made using the sun method. (The Pussy Willow and Comfrey essences are 'living' essences.)

COMFREY

Blue and pink flowered.

'Infinite patience brings immediate reward'   *Raj*

Positive: For dynamic Patience and Stillness. For being present in the fullness of now. For Meditation. For receiving and communicating information For grounded spiritual and psychic development. For deep connection with the earth and the natural world. For trusting our own unique healing, developmental and creative process. For creating the time and space to heal and be creative. For curiosity and joy. Mental and creative work.

Indications: For feeling limited or restricted by circumstance, fighting or resisting being where you are, inattention and avoidance of being in the now, daydreaming, impatience with the healing process, living for the future, unwilling or unable to experience meaning or good in the now, unable to be still or meditate, not benefitting from experience because of avoiding connecting with situations – sometimes as a result of unresolved previous trauma and fear.

Physical: For recovery from injury to brain, spine, nerves, skeleton and muscles, for degenerative conditions of the spine, for recovery from paralysis and muscle wasting, for recovery from surgery, building fitness and strength, for osteoporosis, for co-ordination of left brain/right brain, for recovery from strokes and comas, for dyslexia, for improving mineral absorption and stimulating the creation of healthy collagen and connective tissue. May help in the treatment of M.S., M.E. and motor neurone disease. Improves memory and detailed memory recall. Regulation of natural cycles. May help reduce excessive and prolonged bleeding in general: from wounds, nosebleeds etc.

Doctrine of Signatures: Comfrey has very deep branching roots, black skinned with white, gummy, mucilaginous, fibrous flesh. It has a rough, hairy hollow stem, 2-3 feet high, much branched, ending in curved racemes of drooping blue, pink, purple, white or yellow flowers. It's lower leaves are abundant, very large, ovate and covered in rough hairs. The stem leaves are smaller. The most noticeable habits of comfrey are it's vigour and abundance, it's ability to renew itself vigorously when cut and to reproduce itself rapidly from a tiny fragment of root, it's ability to draw up minerals and trace elements from the subsoil and the abundant mucilage present in all parts of the plant.

Comfrey essence shows us that Patience is a dynamic state, allowing infinite possibilities of experience in the now of our Being. We get to where we are going by experiencing now, whatever it is, which is the movement of our Being, the unfolding of our Divinity, the creative expression of God. Healing occurs when we become curious to know what opportunity life is offering us in the experience of whatever we are facing. Situations we may be resisting and fighting may offer us a treasure trove of wisdom, joy and tremendous and unforseen potential for development and expansion of awareness. Brings a sense of timelessness and infinity. Deepens meditation. Makes life a living meditation. For giving ourselves the time we need to follow the things that matter to us as individuals – to pursue interests, lines of thought wherever they may take us, to build on our own experience and trust our own unique creative process. For deeper connection with life.

Grounding. Allows us to experience a deep connection to the earth and the physical world, not as something separate from ourselves and our Divinity but as the dynamic, ever new expression of God in All.

Comfrey essence works on a vibrational energy level by creating a fluid matrix, an environment in which creativity and development can occur, connections can be made and information can be received and communicated.

The main physical actions of comfrey essence are regeneration and creation of new cells, connection of cells and the nutrition of cells. It does this by stimulating the production of healthy collagen and connective tissue; and nutritionally, by promoting the absorption and utilization of the minerals and trace elements needed for the repair, regeneration and maintenance of brain, spine, nerve, bone and muscle cells.

It strengthens neural pathways, promotes the creation of new neural connections and greater co-ordination between left and right brain, stimulates the regeneration and restructuring of damaged nerve, bone and muscle cells, soothes traumatized nerves and tissue and helps rebuild and maintain bodily strength, fitness and muscle tone following paralysis, illness, periods of inactivity and sedentary activity. For osteoporosis.

Suggested use – Physical: The action of comfrey essence is greatly enhanced by using it in conjunction with other supportive approaches: take it before and after bodywork treatments such as physiotherapy, cranial osteopathy, educational kinesiology etc, before and after exercise, at the same time as taking nutritional supplements, following meals, as well as morning and evening. Because it's action is that of an ongoing process of creation and connection of cells and maintenance, building one cell to another, it needs to be taken daily throughout the whole healing, strengthening and re-education process in order to gain the maximum benefit. It is safe to use regularly for months at a time. Comfrey essence can be added to baths and massage oils.

Comfrey essence has a specific effective use when one has put one's spine out of alignment. Take 7 drops every 10 minutes initially until pain eases and there is sufficient movement to enable one to lie down. As soon as possible lie in the most appropriate position and continue taking doses every 20-30 minutes until one can feel the vertebrae move into better alignment and the muscles begin to relax – thereafter space the doses until the pain has gone and free and flexible movement is established. (The action of comfrey in this instance is greatly enhanced by taking it in combination with lilac, dandelion and pussy willow flower essences). For general internal use: 7 drops in a 30ml dropper bottle filled with water and brandy – take 7 drops morning and evening, after meals and before and after bodywork and exercise. 14 drops can be placed in a bath and 14 drops can be added to massage oil.

COWSLIP

Positive: Soothing, comforting, gently renewing and restoring. Brings a sense of the 'Divine Mother', a sense of being supported, an awareness that we are not alone. Calming. For self-nurturing. Helps us to give up our burden to God/the Mother/the Source, to cease struggling and listen to our heart and the still voice within. Helps us to ask for and accept, help and guidance: "Show me the way". Comforts and soothes babies and young children, brings a sense of security.

Indications: For those who have been stretched to the limits of their physical and emotional endurance, who have struggled long in difficult and dispiriting circumstances, who are weary and feel alone in their struggle. For those facing long illness, disablement or death, particularly those living alone. For when we feel alone in our troubles and feel the need for support. For when we need mothering, especially if we were deprived of maternal support in childhood. For when we seek attention and sympathy from those around us, sometimes by becoming ill, or by acting the victim ("Poor me"). Cowslip helps us to recognise this desire and encourages us to listen to, love and support ourselves and make positive steps to meet our own needs. For mothers and carers who need to nurture and care for themselves. For worry and over-anxious states. For babies and young children who have been traumatised by a difficult birth, separation from the mother, illness or invasive medical treatment. For children who have been deprived of mothering.

Physical: Exhaustion, weariness. Solar plexus and heart. Digestive problems, particularly those aggravated by worry and exhaustion. Colic. Difficulty assimilating food. (Particularly for babies with digestive problems.) Sleep difficulties when we are over-tired or anxious (combine with Dandelion and Red Clover).

Cowslip essence brings a sense of the presence of the Divine Mother. It is like a soothing mother who comes to comfort and support us; who says "Lean on me, rest and find renewal – you are not alone". It shows us that we are not alone and that we do not have to suffer alone, that love, support and guidance are always available for every one of us. All that is required is for us to hand over our struggle and say "Help!" and then to listen and be open, – to receive the love and the guidance that is always there for us. Often our suffering arises from not listening to the call of our hearts – to the call to love ourselves.

Cowslip is for those who feel alone in their struggle and are longing for support and comfort. For whenever we feel the need for mothering, helps us to listen to our needs and care for ourselves. Helps us to relax and let go of worry, in the knowledge that our needs will be met in whatever situation faces us, – that life supports us when we open ourselves to the Good/God that is always present. For those facing death it brings an awareness of spiritual support.

Suggested Use: In addition to being taken internally, Cowslip essence can be used topically – rubbed directly onto the solar plexus and abdomen, mixed into massage oil or added to bathwater (particularly for babies and children before bed). It can be combined with other essences such as: Dandelion, Pussy Willow, Red Clover etc…

DANDELION

Positive: For the Knowledge that we are invulnerable. For true protection that comes from knowing that nothing can harm us. For deep peace and relaxation and the recognition of God/Good in All. For letting go of defence and releasing fear. For feeling relaxed and secure within the light of one's eternal being.

Indications: For tension, inability to relax, for fearful defence. For locked in fear, trauma, negativity, fear of losing control, or of being overwhelmed by fear or negativity (one's own or someone else's). Vulnerability.

Physical: Solar Plexus. Sacral. Muscles. For releasing tension, fear or strong emotion held in the physical body. For pain of unknown origin and dis-ease arising from tension, trauma or fear. Shock. Trauma recovery – Post traumatic shock syndrome. Panic attacks.

For accident and emergency workers, hospital and psychiatric workers, soldiers, police, aid workers, healers and all those who work in traumatic and stressful conditions (combine with Red Clover essence).

Dandelion teaches us our ultimate 'protection' – the knowledge that we are invulnerable, that nothing can harm us, that God/Good is in all. It shows us that we can 'walk through' our experiences and maintain our sense of wholeness and light throughout. Helps us to understand that resisting our fears and traumas, or other people's emotional energy or fear, creates tremendous tension which locks in the fear and negative feelings. For the understanding that when we let go of fear and defence, we do not make ourselves vulnerable: on the contrary, we let in our peace, our light, our Godhead and the consciousness of our invulnerability.

Acute fear, or strong emotion can become locked into the physical and subtle bodies. This locking in occurs when we put up fearful resistance to experiences, whether in this life or past lives; sometimes as a reaction to traumatic experiences or violent death. This can manifest later as pain or illness, often at times of transition, when an opportunity is created to release this locked in trauma and it's associated mental belief patterns.

Sometimes those who drive themselves hard and strive to keep everything together, with great tension, do so as a defence against losing control. This may be motivated by a deep unconscious fear that if they release their control on life, their deepest fears and emotions will surface and they will become victim to forces beyond their control. Often this unconscious reaction arises from deeply held fear and trauma which has become locked in the astral memory and which continues to echo through into the mental and emotional bodies.

Dandelion is useful for those who are sensitive and who hold tension and fear as a defence against absorbing what they perceive to be 'negative' emotions or traumas – either their own or other people's (including a fear of psychic attack). It can also help to heal phobic or obsessive patterns. It maybe helpful for anyone who is feeling vulnerable, defensive, stressed or fearful.

Suggested Use: Dandelion can be taken at the end of the day to release any tension which has built up over the day and been held in the physical body and memory. It can be put in the bath before bed, for both adults and babies and children, to aid relaxation and the release of tension and fear and can be added to massage oil to help release tension held in in the muscles and physical body. it can also be combined with Red Clover essence and added to water to use as a spray in accident and emergency wards, ambulances, psychiatric wards, hospital wards, consulting rooms etc, to reduce feelings of tension and fear. It can also be taken internally by all those who work in traumatic and stressful situations.

GORSE

> *'Forgiveness is a concept of limitation…in the broader sense of things, no one ever 'did' anything to you. You create your own reality absolutely. Everything in your life you have created, or co-created and you have done so for your greatest spiritual growth, whether or not you accept it as such'.*   P'taah, 'The Gift', channelled by Jani King

Positive: For understanding that true forgiveness is the act of letting go our judgement of ourself and others. A phoenix remedy to build a new way of relating from a centre of unconditional love, understanding and compassion for ourselves and others and the recognition of God/Good in all. For compassion. For healing our desire for justice. For the recognition that each and everyone of us is wholly worthy of love at every moment of our lives, regardless of what acts we have committed.

Indications: For when it is hard to forgive ourselves, or others. For healing conflict and pain in our personal relationships. For hurt feelings, often held for many years. For aggressive defensiveness. For those judged by others to have committed an act that is unforgivable, helps them to release their judgement of themselves and nurture love for themselves as they begin to heal their life. For whenever we feel the victim in our relationship with others. For when we feel we have suffered abuse and cannot forgive those who we perceive to have abused us. Gorse helps us to recognize our part in the story. For whenever we withhold love from ourselves and others because of our judgement. For healing communities where there has been a history of conflict, violence, retaliation and retribution. (Use whilst meditating for peace, reconciliation and healing in these areas. Can also be sprinkled in areas which need healing from past events.) For prison rehabilitation work.

Physical: Heart and mind. May aid the healing process for conditions arising from heat and intense sunlight: dehydration, heat exhaustion, sunstroke, burns and fevers.

May help plants cope with drought and heat: use when watering and transplanting.

Doctrine of Signatures: Gorse bushes provide a first stabilizing shrub cover, (on light coastal and heathland soils), in the natural process of regeneration and reforestation. These spiny bushes become established after forest clearance or fire, covering the soil and providing a sheltering environment in which young trees of silver birch and oak can establish themselves. Gorse survives in very dry soil and hot conditions. Its deep yellow, warmly scented flowers bloom from early spring to August, although one may find bushes in flower almost throughout the year. This inspired the saying:

> *'When Gorse is out of bloom, kissing's out of season'.*

The purpose of Gorse essence is to inspire us to heal our feelings and perception of ourself and others, with unconditional love – to withdraw judgement, to nurture a new way of relating – a fresh start. Often we most judge others when we lack understanding and compassion for ourselves. Sometimes we are afraid to heal our perception of ourselves and others because we do not wish to face the challenge of a greater understanding of who we may be, or of who others may be. When we remove judgements we can no longer maintain a feeling of superiority or inferiority – we realize that we are all the Christ.

Sometimes if we have committed acts which have been judged by others to be unforgivable, or for which we cannot forgive ourselves, we may feel that we can never release this judgement from ourselves and walk wholly in the light. Gorse helps us to recognize our essential innocence and good, to understand that we act without love when we do not recognize love in our lives, that these acts are always a call for love, which is always present – but which we do not recognize. To heal our perception of ourselves and others we need to recognize that we are all continually worthy of love at all times. Gorse teaches us to love ourselves wholly and to hold the light of that love inside ourselves at all times, in the face of the judgement of others and in the face of our own judgement. It will help us to maintain love for ourselves even when we feel completely ostracised by those around us, or society. It encourages us to reach out and give unconditional love to those around us who need to know that they are lovable. When we hold ourselves in love and compassion so we will also heal our perception of others. By withdrawing judgement we release ourselves and others to live in the eternal now of our love and goodness (godness).

Gorse helps us to heal our desire for justice. It helps us to not return to old habits of judgement, but to understand that we choose situations and people who will provide us with the opportunities to honour our integrity, release karma and experience the unity and healing of unconditional love. It is not necessary to muster a huge amount of forgiveness to cancel out what we feel has been a huge act committed against us, or to cancel out an act that we have committed. Forgiveness is quite simply the act of withdrawing the judgement we hold against another or ourselves. It is not about turning the other cheek or choosing to be a victim or pretending that an act was not unloving. It is common sense to say "Don't do that!" and when necessary, to withdraw from situations. We need also to recognize and acknowledge when we have acted without love and take steps to heal our actions; but, it benefits no-one to maintain judgement against ourself or others.

HONESTY

> *'This above all: to thine own self be true and it must follow, as the night the day, thou canst not then be false to any man'.* *William Shakespeare (Hamlet)*

Positive: Honesty without judgement. For allowing ourselves to experience the full depth and range of our feelings, with love and without judgement. For giving ourselves and our inner child the unconditional love, compassion, approval and recognition that we would seek from others. For releasing judgement of ourselves and others. For showing our true face. For understanding that truth is love. For recognising that the greatest gift we can give ourselves and others is the unadorned expression of our human-ness. For being happy to be who we truly are.

Indications: Hiding one's true feelings from oneself, or others, for fear of judgement. Fear of exposure. Suppressed emotion, suppressed grief. Sensitivity to criticism or judgement from others. Self-judgement, self-criticism, low self-esteem, poor body image. For co-dependency in relationships, helps us to recognise when our actions are motivated by our yearning for love, recognition and approval. For when we feel misunderstood – helps us to understand ourself. For those who experienced a deep lack of love, recognition and approval during childhood. For those who deny their own feelings and who feel threatened and are judgmental, when those around them express their feelings and their humanness. For when we are denying our truth and are attempting to live according to the (mis)perceived standards of others or of society. For those who work hard to maintain an image of perfection in order to hide their vulnerability. For stage fright.

Physical: For the heart, solar plexus, thymus, lymphatic system, spine. Cleansing, energy releasing. For loving one's body, one's physical expression. To help heal the patterns of anorexia, addictions, alcoholism, drug addiction (combine with Pussy Willow).

Honesty shows us that it is our deep yearning for love and our fear of being denied that love, which motivates us to hide the truth of who we are from ourselves and from others. We fear honesty because we fear judgement, because we believe that somehow we are not 'good enough' by our own standards, or the standards of others. We judge ourselves and believe that our true human-ness is an expression of imperfection, instead of the expression of the wholeness of our being. If we can 'own' our feelings and develop love and understanding for ourselves, then even our anger can be expressed with love for ourselves, instead of attack of others. Our 'negative' feelings are simply reminders from our true Self, to indicate the ways in which we deny love to ourself and deny our integrity. When we understand this we need no longer fear our painful feelings, recognising them as our inner call to love.

Honesty helps us to open our heart to ourself and to others, without fear of judgement. It helps us to become self-knowing – to lovingly understand what motivates our actions. It helps us to see that whilst we retain judgement of ourselves, we will choose relationships with those who we perceive to judge us, who will mirror our own judgement back to us.

When we unconditionally love the wholeness of the expression of who we truly are, then we see love reflected back to us in all our relationships and we become wholly loving to those around us.

Affirmations: My true expression is a gift of love to myself and others. Truth is love.

Suggested Use: Honesty essence can be taken internally as well as placed in bathwater and applied topically to the areas of the thymus, heart and solar plexus chakras.

PUSSY WILLOW

'Love is the recognition of that which is Real in each and everything.
The most direct route to your Divinity is right through the centre of your humanity'.

Raj

Positive: For deeply loving and nurturing ourselves and our inner child, for knowing we are supported by life, for flexibility born out of responding to the real Flow of life, for self approval, relaxation, abundance, peace, joy and fun. For new beginnings, renewal, cherishing and following inner dreams and talents. To comfort, soothe and nurture the newborn and children.

Indications: For anger, resentment, depression, rigidity, self-denial, self-defence, victim mentality, powerlessness, not honouring one's integrity. For too much doing and never Being, for when we have created difficult stressful situations and bleak lifestyles. For not allowing love, relaxation, abundance, beauty, fun and joy in our lives. For patterns arising from a lack of love and support in childhood or from past lives of poverty and self denial.

Physical: To restore physical flexibility, for arthritis, depression, exhaustion, for spinal problems caused by lack of self-nurturing, feeling unsupported by life, driving oneself too hard and lack of flexibility. For eating disorders, anorexia/bulimia and weight problems: helps us to give ourselves the deep love and nurturing that we need and to let go of the need for control. For infertility in women, where there is a pattern of tension, overwork and denial of inner needs – to love and nurture and listen to the inner child. For rapid healing of wounds, cell regeneration, youthfulness and vigour.

Doctrine of Signatures: Velvet soft pussies (catkins) – nurturing of creativity, soft, comfort, cocooning. Willow is always flexible, healthy and abundant so long as it has adequate water. It roots easily if put in water and renews itself vigorously when cut. When willow dries it becomes brittle and when put on the fire it cracks and spits. If there is too much fire in our lives – too much doing, we become dry and brittle and crack and spit in resentment and anger. So long as we remain connected to the true flow of our Being, the water of life, we remain flexible, healthy and abundant.

If we listen and respond on a daily basis to our human needs, to what is truly comfortable, to our rhythms of activity, rest, nurture and dreaming, to our real sense of inner timing, to what is appropriate, not forced, but which wells up naturally, then we are one with the true Flow of Life, our Divinity, and all our needs will be met, day by day. It is when we deny our integrity and needs that we cut ourselves off from the source of all our love and joy and abundance.

For those who have patterns of self-denial arising from past lives in religious orders and for those who have experienced a lack of unconditional love, support, mothering or parenting during childhood. When we neglect our needs, the needs of our inner child, we experience deep lack and powerlessness, we give away our power to external demands and become angry, resentful, depressed and rigid in fear and self-defence. Over-striving is often a way to avoid experiencing our inner emptiness and fear. This is an essence for those who care for and attend to the needs of others and neglect their own needs.

For children who have suffered trauma, lack of love, nurturing and parenting – to comfort and soothe, to help them feel safe enough to be children, for joy and laughter and play. For babies, to help them to relax and settle and feel secure.

This essence was made on Valentine's day. The key to awakening is LOVE and until we can truly love, support, nurture and understand ourselves we cannot release our defence and truly love others. To be able to follow the flow of our Being and our love every day, as a basis for reality, we need to know that life supports us when we support ourselves. Pussy willow helps us to consciously connect with the flow and infinite abundance of our Divinity and to know that nothing is denied us, that we only deny ourselves.

Suggested use: for internal use – 8 drops in a 30ml dropper bottle with spring water and brandy – take 8 drops morning and evening. Can also put 8 drops in the bath: for adults, children and babies. Can also be gently rubbed on the solar plexus and soles of feet (combine with Cowslip essence to soothe babies and calm digestion).

This essence is a 'living essence' – it was made by tying down a stem of the willow so that the twigs and catkins were immersed in the bowl for the time it took for the essence to be made (2 hours in full sun). The stem was released after that time.

RED CLOVER

There are only ever two choices available for you to experience:- the choice for fear or the choice for love'
        Raj

Positive: For letting go of fear, for breaking the pattern of habitual fear, for recognising that we are never alone and never have been, that we are powerful, not powerless, that we separate ourselves from our birthright of love and healing and ever present good, by our fear. Red Clover helps us to disengage from fear, to let it be and let it go and to allow ourselves to experience a new reality of the complete safety, invulnerability, wholeness and union of our divine expression. For the understanding that we are constantly supported by life, if only we will allow and recognise this in our lives.

Indications: Panic, trauma, terror, accidents and emergencies, mass fear, crowd fear, panic attacks, habitual fears and phobias, fear – both conscious and unconscious, nightmares, faintheartedness, for when we are influenced by fearful images from the media or received fears from society, i.e: fear of the outcome of illness or accident, fear of cancer/Aids, fear of being alone, fear of annihilation, fear of abandonment, fear of violent attack, fear of food poisoning etc.

Physical: Kidneys, adrenals, heart, mind. All chakras, but especially the base, sacral, solar plexus and heart. Panic attacks. Any condition accompanied by fear and feelings of powerlessness.

For accident and rescue workers, hospital and psychiatric staff, soldiers, police, aid workers, healers and all those who work in traumatic and stressful conditions (combine with Dandelion essence).

Red Clover is for when we are fearful and long to live without fear but are afraid to face our fears because we feel we will need tremendous courage to react differently in situations in which we have felt habitually terrified, panic stricken, powerless and unsupported. It is for when we say "I can't". It helps us to see that if we go through the fear, what lies beyond is love and always has been; that by our fear we have denied ourselves the experience of our divine expression of everpresent love, authority of knowing, perfect health and union with all.

Red Clover is calming and soothing and enlightening. It helps us to have the courage to detach ourself from both our own fears and the fears of those around us and society. It helps us to stay at peace and in light and not energise fear when those around us are in fear. It is particularly useful for those with physical conditions which are (mis)perceived to have an inevitable 'negative' development and outcome, or which are seen to be incurable. Red Clover helps us to allow 'unreasonable' and immediate healing and love into our experience at any time. It helps us to awaken from our dream of inevitable suffering to the reality of our wholeness and perfection. It helps us to refuse to join in joint agreements with others about fearful situations or 'inevitable' outcomes and it helps us to stop passing on our fears to others. It can be used to calm and comfort children when they are fearful.

Red Clover can be taken in acute fear situations such as accidents, or when encountering phobic triggers but it can also be used to help uncover the roots of our fears – fear of annihilation, fear of separation, a deep fear of being alone and unsupported, feelings of abandonment. Fear can become a security, it protects us from the challenge of addressing our worst fears. Red Clover shows us that it is safe and utterly reasonable to live without fear; that all that we experience is God whether we perceive it as that, or see it "through a glass darkly".

Suggested Use: Red Clover essence can be combined with Dandelion essence and used internally as well as placing in bathwater, massage oils and creams. It can be used in a spray with dandelion essence for use in accident and emergency wards, ambulances, hospital and psychiatric wards, consulting rooms etc, to reduce feelings of fear and tension. It can be taken internally by all those who work in traumatic and stressful situations and it can be sprayed in areas which need healing from past traumatic events.

Affirmation: The following affirmation can be used for healing, it confirms our authority and helps us to recognise the ways in which we inhibit our healing:

"It is the intent of my body to identify the purpose of my individuality perfectly.

I authorise my body to release whatever is not necessary to its perfect functioning and I withdraw any prior conscious or unconscious authorisation to the contrary".

"My body is a perfectly fluid energy form, there is no material resistance to its realignment".   *Raj*

❀ THE LORD AND LADY FLOWER ESSENCE SET ❀

The Lord and Lady Flower Essences have all been made in the sacred landscape in and around Glastonbury, the ancient isle of Avalon. They have been made in a deeply attuned state with spiritual guidance. Local holy well water has been used in their creation. Some essences needed both sunlight and moonlight to potentise.

BLACKTHORN

Coping with fears, facing one's dark/shadow inwardly and in external environment.

BUGLE

Helping to develop unconditional love. Manifesting inner creativity onto physical level.

BUTTERBUR

Overcoming anxiety. Release of excess energy.

CALENDULA

Releasing sadness by understanding its cause. Earths and balances emotions.

CHAMOMILE

Brings energy and activeness in relaxed way, without causing stress. Helps to develop self discipline.

COLTSFOOT

Working with and attunement to animals. Shamanically working with animal allies. Brings a loving attitude.

COWSLIP

Connecting with the inner child. Accessing inner truth and innocence. Communicating inner truth.

CYPRESS

Overcoming loneliness by connecting to inner self. Bringing oneness (oneness opposite to loneliness).

DAISY

All kinds of emotional release. Helps person to speak and express their emotions.

DANDELION

Oversensitivity, emotional imbalance.

DOGS MERCURY

Releases blocks in root and sexual centres.

EYEBRIGHT

Increasing perception and psychic abilities. Helps to see what needs to be done in one's life.

FLEABANE

Lethargic and apathetic states. Gives life and vitality in gentle way. Overcoming parasitic auric energy (draining people etc.).

GOAT WILLOW

Balancing inner masculine energy and masculine sexuality. Helps in working with dreams.

GOLDEN ROD

Works on ego bringing it into balance by either stabilising an overemphasised ego or increasing self confidence and self worth when these are lacking.

GREEN ALKANET

For being gentle with oneself and others by understanding and accepting who you are and where others are coming from.

HAWTHORN

Balancing inner feminine energy and feminine sexuality.

HAZEL

Access to trance states. Balanced integration of male and female energies within self.

HOLY THORN

Deep contact with subconscious. Releases deep rooted patterns and memories. Attunes to higher soul energies and purpose of incarnation.

IVY

Grounding and stabilising. Brings out intuition.

LADY'S SMOCK

Attunement with personal guides and higher soul self. Connection with personal power in balanced way.

LESSER CELANDINE

Increasing mental faculties, concentration and memory.

LORDS AND LADIES

Balances inner masculine and feminine energies. Good for couples, people working together to take at same time to harmonise energies.

LUNGWORT

Assimilation of vital force (chi, prana etc.). Ideal for use with breathing techniques. Releases blockages and deep feelings within lower chakras to be consciously worked on.

MARSH MARIGOLD

Calmness and relaxation, helps with meditation.

MARSH ORCHID

Overcoming mental restrictions. Releasing negative thought forms and belief patterns.

Overcoming worry.

MISTLETOE

Balances sexual energy with love. Helps one to be an individual within groups.

NETTLE

Increases will power and resilience. Helps to develop patience. Overcoming unwanted habits.

PRIMROSE

Balancing the energy centres.

PURPLE LOOSESTRIFE

Channelling and connection to higher levels. Helps to release grief, good with bereavement and separation.

RAGWORT

Forgiveness of self and others.

RED CLOVER

Lack of focus,confusion, indecisiveness.

RED DEAD NETTLE

Releasing and understanding suppressed anger.

ROSEMARY

Releasing stuck emotions. Cleanses and purifies energy system.

SPINDLE

Overcoming frustration and aggressive tendencies.

STINKING HELLEBORE

Releasing negative energies from aura. Helps with flow of energy through meridians. Brings flow to life, overcoming rigidity.

THYME

Attunement with devas. Helps to connect to inner joy. Brings back a sense of humour to serious people.

TREE MALLOW

Developing visualisation enhancing the ability to manifest on earth plane.

TULIP

Clears blocks in heart centre. Brings an open and loving energy to all aspects of life.

VIOLET

Releasing depression. Connection to inner inspiration.

WHITE FOXGLOVE

Developing sensitivity. Helps in getting in touch with feelings. Helps to release blockages to communication. Sensitivity to others feelings.

WILD ROSE

Helps to develop love. Brings understanding of one's own and others loving needs. Helps to discover where in life one is lacking in love.

YARROW

Protecting and strengthening aura.

YELLOW FLAG IRIS

For stress and bad nerves.

YEW

Deep healing. Letting go of what is no longer needed. Brings soul back to body.

❀ LOVING NATURE ESSENCES ❀

Loving Nature Essences came about by the plants themselves communicating their loving intention to assist us in our journey back to wholeness. The messages are very clear. That by being willing to connect with nature we can learn more about ourselves. We can learn more about our own nature through the use of flower essences. Like the petals of a flower, as they open to the light they reveal their perfectness and divinity. The same will be true for us.

ENGLISH ESSENCES

BLUE GERANIUM

Effect of taking essence: Acceptance of change, especially in menopause, going with the flow of life's cycles and rhythms. Can remove resistance to the change from life creation to creating a life. To help mentally adjust to this new life opportunity. Helps the passage through menopause. The physical changes that come about at menopause (the change of life) can be helped with this essence.

Presenting conditions: Emotional and physical upset predominantly due to the change of life during menopause, i.e. hormonal imbalance, erratic periods. Where there is a resistance to letting go of the fear of not being a woman.

PLANTAIN

Effect of taking essence: A wonderful confidence building essence. Helps give a sense of our uniqueness and divinity, there is a feeling of being surrounded in a halo of light. Accepting your own divine qualities and that everyone is at a different level.

Presenting condition: Feels inferior, feelings of deep hurt especially when you perceive you are being rejected. Can't make the grade, not good enough, seen but not seen,therefore feelings of hurt and rejection.

Helps external wounds heal, as without,so within; healing the wounded child.

REDSHANK

Effect of taking essence: Helps to see the inherent good in oneself. Allows you to take responsibility for one's own health and well-being. You ARE important. Realisation that it is not selfish to look after yourself.

Presenting condition: There is a sense of bitterness towards self, low self-worth. Being subservient and self sacrificing only adds to the feeling of bitterness. Putting others before self, feelings of "I don't count. On a physical level may have circulation problems, diabetes or gall bladder problems, due to internalising the bitterness.

IRISH ESSENCES

BIRDS FOOT TREFOIL

Effect of taking essence: Helps change one's perception of Self, recognising one's value oneself. Not needing to get it from others. When own value is recognised it allows achievement without trying, in all areas and hence recognition.

Presenting conditions: Feels lacking in recognition. Tries to please by doing too much. Feels small and insignificant and lacks focal point. Disperses energy in many directions 'running around like a headless chicken'. Tries to be all things to all people instead of being true to self.

BOG ASPHODEL

Effect of taking essence: Balances up male sexual drive (the male impatience) the change from need, to a loving expression. Also aids diversion of male sexual drive to other creative activities. A lifting of the kundalini energy from base/sacral chakras to the higher chakras (hearth/throat etc.). It can balance the need for release. It can aid in spiritualizing sex, allows openness, removes shame and guilt.

Presenting condition: Preoccupation with sex. Very needy, demanding affection, comfort, release. Looks to others for gratification and reassurance of worthiness.

BOG HYPERICUM

Effect of taking essence: Aids transitions. Helps to move through the pain and fear of showing who we truly are. Pain and suffering can come from resistance. This essence will ease the flow of life past or through the resistance to bring joy.

Presenting conditions: Hiding behind a mask. Fearful of showing true self to the world. Anxiety, unease, or general sadness about inability to move through fear, so hides behind a mask. Particularly when pressures build in our everyday lives. The sadness of hiding – not being able to reveal inner self with joy.

LOOSESTRIFE

Effect of taking essence: Focuses energy to where it is needed. Improves circulation. Balances the energy of the body so the life force flows throughout, from Crown to soles of feet. Grounds in reality. Lifts the veil of our day dreams and returns us to reality to create the world of day dreams.

Presenting condition: Being in your head – feeling detached from reality and the rest of humanity. Seeming to be in a dream. Withdrawing or escaping from the reality of what being human is about. Off with the fairies (or leprechauns). Especially when being used as an escape or distraction from the day to day problems of being human.

SELF HEAL

Effect of taking essence: Cleanses the systems both physical, mental and spiritual, on all levels. Part of a convalescence after a dis-ease. Will give a really good spring clean. It will balance the feeling of 'phew – there's a lot going on for me'. Helps neutralise unqualified energies. A good tonic restoring spirit as well as body to bring back a sense of well-being and reconnection with our divinity. Revitalises. Works well in combinations.

Presenting condition: When the body feels under pressure from illness. Also when body is in need of a tonic, because of wrong diet etc. When convalescing, feeling lethargic or a lack of connection to higher self or divine source.

SUNDEW

Effect of taking the essence: Helps with awareness of possible opportunities for growth. Some opportunities are taken and others are passed by. Often when opportunities are not taken we can live in regret of that "missed opportunity". This essence helps to release these feelings of regret and therefore allows us to be alert to all future opportunities as they present themselves.

Sundew can also help with discerning the most appropriate opportunity at this particular time. It will increase our sensitivity within our discernment and increases the potential for one's synchronistic development.

On a physical level, it helps with glandular problems, especially in early teens and at the start of adulthood. At this time we are unsure of ourselves, our independent life is just beginning. If we have not had the appropriate support in childhood we can feel emotionally insecure to go out into the world. We may be unequipped for the opportunities that will present themselves. These feelings of being overwhelmed by having to make our own decisions lead to a real feeling of lack of "support" which can be turned inwards.

Presenting condition: Nothing seems to work for me, insecurity because of living in regret of missed opportunities, can dwell in the past. Lack of childhood support resulting in a lack of confidence and an indecisive nature.

❀ MIDDLE EARTH FLOWER ESSENCES ❀

The Middle Earth Flower Essences were made in Cornwall during the Summer of 1988 by Ian Woods, Freya Sherlock and a group of their friends.

DEVELOPING CONSCIOUSNESS

CELANDINE

This essence is connected with the throat. It is good for singers, lecturers and all occupations that require transfer of information as it is the communication remedy. It is good for communication on all levels including that with spirit guides and also communication of energies between partners, as it stimulates the tantric experience.

Planets – Mercury, Venus, Uranus, Neptune

Chakras – 5th

FORGET ME NOT

This essence is useful for people who have a bad memory. Continued use will improve the memory so that it can be relied on again. It is particularly useful in connection with remembering dreams as it helps to bring up problems that are trapped in the subconscious (forgotten). These problems are then worked out in the form of dreams which will be easy to remember, particularly if the essence is taken before sleeping.

Planets – Moon, Mercury, Saturn, Uranus

Chakras – 7th

PINK CAMPION

This essence has a very spiritual effect on the consciousness, giving a clear lucid state of mind that allows one to receive spiritual guidance and help from spirit guides and other great souls who are operating on this level. It operates on levels above the main seven chakras.

Planets – Venus, Jupiter, Chiron, Pan

Chakras – 6th, 7th and higher

SAGE

This essence aligns the mental and spiritual bodies bringing a balance between the two. It awakens interest in spiritual matters, psychic and mediumistic abilities. It also stimulates laughter. Sage helps the digestive system by producing enzymes and it is a good essence to take whilst fasting.

Planets – Jupiter

Chakras – 3rd, 4th

SCARLET PIMPERNEL

This essence works mainly on the etheric levels. It is useful for people working with releasing kundalini energies, as it helps to activate the chakras and increases understanding of what is going on. It also helps people who have trouble with their father image and men who have trouble relating to women.

Planets – Mercury, Uranus, Pluto

Chakras – 4th, 6th, 7th

SNOWDROP

This is the essence of inner awakening at the end of a long period of darkness or dormancy. It helps to awaken the energies and prepares for new things, like the light at the end of the tunnel, it offers new hope and a new way forward.

Planets – Sun, Saturn, Pluto

Chakras 1st, 7th

DEVELOPING THE MIND

ALKANET

This essence is connected with the energies of transformation. It acts as a catalyst to facilitate deep changes, working from a firmly rooted base. This can help to transform opposing energy patterns that may have been caused originally by incompatible parental energies in childhood. It works on the mother/father within, affecting the internal male/female energies at the same time.

Planets – Pluto, Moon, Saturn

Chakras – 3rd

CALENDULA

This essence is concerned with cleansing the mind to bring clarity in areas of visualization. The heart/mind link is enhanced allowing one to visualise, without clouding by an overly intellectual approach. Inspirational information in the form of vision can then occur.

Planets – Jupiter, Uranus

Chakras – 4th, 6th

DAISY

This essence is useful if you need to collect scattered information into a cohesive form to make sense of it. It works by spiritualizing the intellect allowing one to gain an intuitive grasp of what is going on. It gives one a clarity of mind which helps you to understand what your feelings are on a particular topic.

Planets – Mercury, Saturn

Chakras – 3rd, 7th

PINK YARROW

This essence gives emotional strength and balance, helping to overcome emotional oversensitivity and reactiveness. It is useful if you act like a psychic sponge absorbing negative or draining energies that happen to be around. This remedy is also a useful defence against psychic attack as it strengthens the aura, acting like a shield so you don't get caught up in the negative energies.

Planets – Moon

Chakras – 1st

WHITE YARROW

This is another remedy that strengthens the aura. It creates a shield of white light around you, giving protection from negative environmental things, such as background radiation or pollutants. This essence is really good if you are over sensitive or feeling vulnerable.

Planet – Moon

Chakra – 3rd

MENTAL PROBLEMS

BLACKBERRY

This essence helps the fears of a dying person or a fear of death in general, whether it be for the self, or fear that someone else is going to die. It is also good for manifesting thoughts and ideas into the tangible world, or if one is feeling stuck it gets things moving again.

Planets – Saturn, Chiron, Pluto

Chakras – 5th

BORAGE

This essence lifts the spirits up, it can turn feelings of discouragement into enthusiasm. Borage makes the heart grow glad, as it expands the heart energies. It gives strength and courage when facing challenging circumstances.

Planets – Jupiter

Chakras – 4th

BUTTERCUP

This essence helps you to discover your hidden talents, whatever they may be. Once you have done this it enables you to share these gifts with others. This is extremely useful if you are in a situation with a group of people and you feel a need to contribute. It will help to overcome shyness as you will know what it is you have to offer.

Planets – Mercury, Saturn

Chakras – 2nd

FENNEL

This essence is of value in calming the mind. It helps to clear muddled thoughts, thus allowing the mind the clarity needed to focus and concentrate. This remedy can be very useful in meditation, as it brings the background 'babble' of thoughts under control.

Planets – Mercury, Pluto, Chiron

Chakras – 5th

PINK FLOX

This essence is for connecting the child to the adult, allowing the child within to manifest more in the adult world. It helps us to balance our inner child needs with our responsibilities, so that we can achieve a balance of work and play.

Planets – Moon, Jupiter, Saturn

Chakras – 3rd, 6th

SPEEDWELL

This essence is the travellers remedy as it enables you to go from one place to another with a sensation of effortless ease. No sooner than you have set off it appears that you are arriving. It is useful if you have a lot of small journeys to undertake e.g. delivering messages, or a long journey.

Planets – Sun, Mercury, Jupiter

Chakras – 3rd, 4th

TORMENTIL

This essence is helpful to ease the tormented mind. If you are experiencing a lot of mental pain and are needing a rest from it for a while, tormentil will shut things down allowing you to rest. It won't necessarily deal with the problems but will give respite. It could be very useful if someone is on a 'bad trip' and would like to close down the mind for a while.

Planets Moon, Mercury, Neptune

Chakras – 3rd, 7th

YELLOW LOOSESTRIFE

This essence brings up problems which are stored in the subconscious. The dis-ease associated with these problems is brought into focus in the mental body. Spiritual help is then received and the issue is brought to rest, working through the levels until it is discharged into the earth. As the name implies, it is for letting loose strife.

Planets – Moon, Mercury, Pluto

Chakras – 1st, 6th, 7th

EMOTIONAL ISSUES

AUBRETIA

This essence is for bringing up and clarifying emotions that have been suppressed, so that they can be dealt with. It can throw new light on a situation that one feels trapped in. Deep breathing is facilitated with this essence therefore useful in such therapies as rebirthing.

Planets – Moon, Neptune, Pluto

Chakras – 2nd, 3rd, 6th

DANDELION

This essence helps to relieve deep physical and emotional tensions that are manifesting as muscular tensions in the body. The essence can be taken in liquid form both orally and in a bath. It can also be mixed with a massage oil to be applied directly to the tense region. It is also helpful in removing deep emotional blockages that may exist.

Planets – Sun, Jupiter

Chakras – 1st

OPIUM POPPY

This essence is mainly useful in dealing with emotional states that can lead towards drug dependency. Also the states caused by drug dependency, particularly by opium based substances. It helps to break the dependency and will help to clear the residual effects both in the etheric and on the physical level. It is good for waking you up from any unreal dream state that you may create to avoid emotional issues.

Planets – Neptune, Moon, Mercury, Sun

Chakras – 5th, 6th

RED STRAWBERRY

This essence helps to calm emotional turmoil that threatens to engulf one. It allows you to look at the root of the problem and communicate it rather than be caught up in the surface turbulence. Also allowing the release of blocked emotions in a controlled way.

Planets – Moon, Mercury, Jupiter

Chakras – 2nd, 3rd, 7th

DEVELOPMENT OF HEALING ENERGIES

ROSE OF SHARON

This essence gives access to past life information and teachings. It is particularly useful when there is a blockage towards manifesting this knowledge, as it involves a release of power which the individual may find difficult to handle. It enables us to manifest this power in a safe way. This remedy can help to develop or retrieve knowledge of healing through the hands.

Planets – Sun, Mercury, Venus, Pluto, Chiron

Chakras – 4th, 5th

STONECROP

This essence is connected to the wounded child that needs to feel part of a family. It is the child within us that wants to feel warmth and protection with a group of people that feel like a family. Stonecrop can help us to find our own healing family where we feel secure and loved. It also helps to promote group healing and can be used by a group to focus healing energy, to someone either in the group or absent.

Planets – Moon, Chiron

Chakras – 3rd, 4th

TUTSAN

This essence opens us up to the flower kingdom allowing us to tune into these subtle energies, making us aware of any flowers that may be needed. By bridging the gap between the human and the plant kingdom we can heal the wounds wreaked upon nature by man and at the same time heal our own personal wounds.

Planets – Sun, Mars, Pan

Chakras – All are involved

TREES AND BUSHES

ASH

This flower essence is for balancing male/female energies in oneself and in relating.

Wherever there is an imbalance, disharmony or a need to connect with the anima/animus this essence would be appropriate. Its signature is that the tree contains both male and female flowers.

Planets – Sun, Moon

Chakras 3rd, 7th

BUDDLElA (ORANGE/YELLOW)

This essence is the 'rainbow bridge' remedy. It enables us to link up with angelic forces and spirit guides, specifically for helping to clear up past life emotional wounds, which are hindering our development.

Planets – Sun, Moon, Chiron

Chakras – 2nd, 3rd, 6th

ELDER

This essence allows one to travel safely and gently into the dark depths of the subconscious, allowing these areas to be lit up and brought to life. For very deep emotional blockages that need healing slowly and gently.

Planets – Moon, Venus, Uranus, Pluto

Chakras – 3rd, 4th, 5th

FUCHSlA

This essence helps in the understanding and awareness of blocked emotions. This can be blocked emotions that are causing tension and psychosomatic illness. It is also good for anyone wanting to change a low opinion of himself.

Planets – Moon, Saturn, Neptune

Chakras – 3rd, 4th

HAWTHORN

This essence can be used for treating precancerous emotional states and can help to check the spread of tumours. It is very useful when there is a feeling of broken heartedness, extreme stress after the passing of a loved one. It is useful in connection with a raw food diet used as a cancer therapy.

Planets – All planets are affected

Chakras – All

LAVENDER

This essence connects people to their higher selves, to remove karmic blockages that are hindering progress. It increases visionary states and can be used to bring emotional balance, as it brings harmony to the feelings. It is also good for people who suffer from nervous oversensitivity.

Planets – Uranus, Neptune

Chakras – 7th

LILAC (WHITE)

This essence mainly influences the spinal column, working on many things associated with the spine. It also improves posture and gives increased flexibility to the spine. Lilac opens up all the chakras and activates the kundalini energy which travels up the spine.

Planets – Mercury, Jupiter

Chakras – All

PEAR

The pear flower helps to bring harmony to groups involved with spiritual endeavours. It integrates the mental, emotional and spiritual bodies putting things in proper perspective. It is also connected with music, amplifying the creative process for musicians.

Planets – Pluto, Chiron

Chakras – 2nd, 3rd, 5th

SNAPDRAGON

This essence is for treating the vocal cords, lips, jaw, facial tissues and muscles. It also treats allergies that manifest as spots on the skin. It helps one to express feelings when there is difficulty, such as in the case of stuttering. It can help one to release anger that has been held back.

Planets – Mercury, Venus, Mars, Jupiter

Chakras – 7th

The following two essences were made in Southern Ireland by Freya Sherlock in the summer of 1990. She makes many essences for her own use and for the welfare of her family and animals.

BLUEBELL

For attuning to devic energies when working in the garden or working with nature.

DAFFODIL

For connecting with one's higher self in a powerful and fearless way. Helps to establish a strong inner connection so that one is able to resolve issues in which fear has previously blocked progress.

❀ MIDDLE EARTH ROSE ESSENCES ❀

These essences were made by Ian Woods in Somerset during the summers of 1988 – 1989.

The rose flowers are a very important system by themselves. They are the English equivalent of the lotus flower and are very much connected with the opening and purification of the heart.

DEEP PINK ROSE

This essence is a 'love' essence and works on the heart, opening it up to a feeling of warm intoxicating and spiritual love. Continued usage of this flower will gently unfold the heart, just like the flower itself opening and move one towards a state where one feels love for all people and all things. It is the essence of universal love.

Planets – Moon, Venus, Neptune, Chiron

Chakras – 4th, 7th

DEEP RED ROSE

The essence of 'pure' passion. It grounds and purifies passionate feelings of the heart. It is useful in allowing us to express sexual feelings in a pure way, through the heart. It releases negative mental thoughtforms connected with blockages and frustrations of these energies.

Planets – Sun, Venus, Mars.

Chakras – 1st, 4th

MOSS ROSE (DUSKY RED)

This essence is good for linking with the animal kingdom, thus enabling us to contact our instinctual feelings. It can help us to contact our power animals allowing us to manifest their energies. It can bring clarity in relationships by linking our conscious to the subconscious, giving a deeper understanding of our true needs and allowing them expression.

Planets – Sun, Moon

Chakras – 3rd, 4th

PALE PINK ROSE

This essence helps us to re-connect with the faery realms. Working with the higher chakras it acts as a bridge to help us to cross to subtler realms where we can perceive and feel the workings of the elementals and devas. It is useful for those people who have grown too 'adult' and need to connect with their magical child within.

Planets – Chiron, Neptune, Pan

Chakras – 7th and higher

RED/ORANGE ROSE

This essence enables one to tune into the heart's vision/wish. It stimulates the pineal gland enabling one to visualise the heart's ideals in a clear way. It helps to deal with wounds stemming from the parents, which impair the vision; by bringing the mother/father inside into a state of harmony. Freeing oneself to follow one's vision.

Planets – Mercury, Venus, Chiron, Neptune

Chakras – 3rd, 7th

WHITE ROSE

This essence attunes one to the pure white light within. It is good for purifying the mental state and giving receptivity to spiritual guidance from higher realms. There is a pure white angelic form attached to this flower. Good for clarity of vision in meditation, especially when wishing to meditate on the white light.

Planets – Jupiter, Chiron, Mars

Chakras – 6th, 7th, 1st

YELLOW ROSE

This essence is concerned with cleansing as preparation for opening channels to the higher self, for the receiving of inspirational creativity to give out to the world. It also helps in opening oneself to trusting in the nourishing and sustaining energies of the universe. When this process has taken place one is able to communicate love and beauty from the heart.

Planets – Mercury, Venus, Chiron, Neptune

Chakras – 3rd

❀ NATIVE TREE ESSENCES ❀

(Dr Helen Ford)

Every tree is an individual, just as we are and every tree also has its source in Spirit. Trees give us life and breath, they fertilise the land and bring up nutrients from deep under the ground where the surface plants cannot penetrate. Trees, especially the older ones, also give us clear, lasting and most beautiful evidence of the true nature of Love.

I have come to believe that each kingdom in Nature – whether plant, animal or mineral – offers us a whole view of Love. This whole view is made up of many individual types within that kingdom, each one of which represents the perfected material expression of one particular aspect of Love.

Just as one view of a hologram represents one particular aspect of a whole while also containing the connection with every other part of that whole, so we can come to know Love both by looking around us oat each individually perfected material being as well as by seeking inwards to the depths of any one individual to reach its source… which is the Source of all.

So it is that if we desire to connect with some particular aspect of Love, either to understand it, to restore it within ourselves or simply for the pleasure of the connection, the trees are there. They are there whether we notice them or not and they give out what they are whether we appreciate them or not. They also keep on being and giving out what they are even if their material forms are damaged or destroyed. (There is no revenge in perfect love!)

These tree essences have been made by placing the water (and brandy!) in the direct line of flow of the tree's life force and asking for the gift of that tree's spirit to flow into the water. They have all been made by people who truly love the trees. Nothing can replace the contact with the tree itself… but if you cannot be with those you love, sometimes it is good to have something to remind you of them.

All the money which is made by the sale of these essences will go back into the growing, planting and caring for trees.

Here is a brief description of the individual essences:

ALDER For the calm and steadiness which come with the direct and open expression of truth right from the core of the inner being. For the fearlessness to face truth and to be truthful in the inner certainty that this steadiness in truth is the surest way to allow every difficulty to work its way out. Helps those who have become bogged down in lying or evasion, for whatever reason, to experience the peace and the relief of stress which always comes when truth is finally openly and wholly expressed.

APPLE For the giving out of the pure sweetness of love without reserve or holding anything back. Helps to understand that this total giving of pure love will not only bring fulfilment but will also always be returned in abundance.

ASH For ecstasy of being, for the pure pleasure in existence and absolute contentment with each moment which comes through total openness to the streaming light of Creation. Helps those who find their world dull, grey and full of drudgery and ugliness. (The E of trees!?)

BIRCH For the grace of being which comes with the free and natural expression of the feelings as they flow direct from the soul. Helps those who feel inhibited or awkward about expressing what they really feel in front of others.

BLACKTHORN For integrity, self respect and the trust that the giving out of individual truth will always bring the return of love. For the strength to resist pressure and manipulation, especially coming from those who claim that the giving and receiving of love automatically involves being or doing what others want rather than staying true to the self. Helps those who have come to believe that doing what feels right to them will automatically alienate them from everyone else. Helps them to understand that it is only by truth that anyone can really belong.

ELDER For universal love. For the true appreciation of the self and of the contribution of every other being. For happiness and contentment in being part of a beautiful and satisfying whole. Helps those who have been taught to see one way of being as better than another to relax into a warm appreciation of all ways and the understanding that every way has its own value and beauty and its own right place in the whole.

HAWTHORN For the lightness of heart which comes with knowing that it is always possible to do anything which is a true heart's desire. To help with the tendency to be discouraged or give up on these desires and with the trust to hold them steadily within the heart and keep on going until they are fulfilled.

HAZEL For relaxed ease of being, for acceptance, warmth and humour. For trust that there is a place for everything, that all experience is food for the soul's growth and every situation an opportunity to express love. Helps those who judge themselves and others for imperfection and tend to take things seriously and/or personally.

HOLLY For gladness of heart, for going through life pouring out love and joy wherever you go, like a happy traveller singing for pure pleasure along the way. For the steady flow of joy in love which makes light of any burden and a pleasure of any task. Helps restore joy to the hearts of those who have come to feel weary of their life and angry or resentful in the belief that others are getting off lightly and/or not doing a fair share.

OAK For trust in the strength and depth of Love. For the generosity of spirit which gives steadily and consistently of the self. Helps with the ability to maintain this giving despite apparent adversity, because of the inner knowing that no matter what happens on the surface, Love's resources are so vast that strength can always be found by tapping deeply inwards to the source of your own being.

ROWAN For the trust which knows that all is well. For knowing that by simply enjoying being what you are and doing whatever feels pleasurable to you to do, all your needs will always be met. Helps with the belief that we have to 'try' to meet some external standard and with the fear that we will not be able to obtain what we need unless we do this.

WILLOW For resilience, for the absolute determination to create the dream of the heart and the knowing that as long as that commitment is there, all the resources which are needed to recover from or overcome difficulties will always be made available. Helps those who have let go of their own dream to return to creating it for themselves. Then they can easily let go of any hatred or resentment they may have felt towards those they have seen as having an easier or 'luckier' life than their own.

YEW For the certain knowing that the soul is free and then taking immense pleasure in the choice to have a material form. Helps those who feel trapped by material form or circumstance to truly enjoy and utilise every experience rather than waste energy in frustration.

❀ PETALTONE ESSENCES ❀

Petaltones are a unique and exciting new form of flower essence. They work via evaporation into the auric field and are capable of multi-level healing. They can also be used to heal animals, interact with crystals and change the energy of buildings. Petaltones work at the deepest and most subtle levels of energy and thus are useful to access deeper levels. However, their application is simple and can be mastered quickly by anyone who can use a pendulum.

The Petaltones are not a static set of essences, but a living, growing system of healing which all users become a part of creating. New discoveries are made all the time; different and exciting ways of working. Check out how they work with crystals and try the space-clearing essence 'Crystal Clear' which can rid your home of negative energies and even entities or ghosts! The 'Elements' listed are the ones through which the essence works, rather than the ones it works on in the client. The 'levels' refer to the aspects of the client which can be affected. The 'colours' referred to are the ones through which the essence works and are actually INNER LEVEL COLOURS. These are a 'higher plane' of colour and can be worked with to good effect.

AMORTHYST

General Use: Spiritual healing. (Don't use when under the influence of alcohol.) Positive futures.

Elements: Earth 100% Fire 100% Ether 100%

Colours: Blue 75% Indigo 100% Violet 95% White 98% Silver 95%

Physical level: Soothes nervous system, Parkinsons, cancer.

Emotional level: Releases suppressed positive emotion.

Mental level: Grounding mental energies, structuring.

Etheric level: Releases blocks in energy flow. Heals etheric.

Astral level: Helps clear pathways to the FUTURE. Adventurousness.

ANKH

General Use: Stamina, fire, anti-depressant, masculine power. Motivation.

Elements: Fire 100% Ether 75%

Colours: Red 100% Orange 85% Yellow 90% Green 85%

Physical level: Lethargy. M.E. Not to be used on physically fragile!

Mental/Etheric level: Stimulates mental activity. Don't use it if 'hyper'. Awakens the sluggish mind. Re-energises depleted etheric. Best used when fully awake, rather than at the start or end of the day.

Psychic level: Cleanses, purifies. Energises depleted chakras. Good to use with fire-orientated cleansing processes.

Creative level: Masculine aspect, physical level, motivation.

Spiritual level: Breaks down kundalini blocks. Positive self-belief, higher self connection.

Polarity: Heals low energy masculine aspect.

Crystals: Can be applied via crystal. Awakens their masculine aspects. Crystal can become a wand for catabolic operations, or a flame for the removal of negative energies.

ALSO: Clears fire meridians in the body.

AURA BLUE
General Use: Clears negative thought forms.
Elements: Earth 90% Air 75% Fire 100% Water 75%
Colours: Yellow 10% Green 25% Blue 100%
Physical level: Assists with breathing problems to some extent.
Mental level: Freedom of thought. Helps one who feels stifled. Enthusiasm.
Etherlc level: Breaks down negative thought forms: powerfully effective.
Creative level: Removal of creative blocks, creative stamina. The strength to go on.
Sexual level: Clears self-demeaning attitudes.
Buildings: Can be used to clear out negative thought forms (use plant mister).

AURA FLAME
General Use: Psychic attack, clearing, revitalising.
DO NOT USE IF ANGRY OR OVER-STRESSED
Elements: Water 30% Fire 75%
Colours: Red 100% Orange 100% Yellow 100% Green 90%
Emotional level: Helps in de-cording, especially negative ties. Revitalises depleted energy. Frustration, too laid back. Helps attract a mate/partner.
Psychic level: Psychic attack, fends off negativity, protects auric field. Cutting ties.
Spiritual level: Releases blocks on very deep levels. Assists with acceptance.
Crystals: Can be applied via crystals.

CLEAR STAR
General Use: Breaks down outmoded structures. Clears dark emotions. Jealousy.
Elements: Earth 100% Air 25% Fire 95% Water 100% Ether 25%
Colours: Orange 10% Yellow 25% Green 75% Blue 100% Pink 100%
Mental level: Assists mental clarity.
Emotional level: Clears darker emotions, hate, jealousy, anger, depression etc. Claiming back one's power. Fear of one's own power.
Astral level: Acts to break down structures holding negative energies and entities.
Creative level: Removal of outmoded creative approaches. Frees energies stuck in old creative patterns.
Crystals: Clears crystals very well.
Buildings: Cleanses atmospheres. Affects fire and water elementals.
Polarity: Clears blocks in masculine energy. (Fears from past abuse by/of masculine energy.)

CLEAR TONE
General Use: Cleansing etheric, tie cutting.
Elements: Earth 100% Fire 50% Water 25% Ether 75%
Colours: Green 25% Blue 60% Indigo 100%
Mental/Etheric level: Excellent cleanser. Clears negative thought forms. Use in sequence with Aura Blue.
Astral level: Cleanses negative energies via fire element. De-energises negative astral entities, cuts negative ties generally.

Spiritual level: Can be used to purify negative karma and ward off misfortune.

Creative level: Assists higher inspiration.

Polarity level: Masculine aspect: assertiveness.

Crystals: Can be used via crystal. Especially useful for dispersing negative thoughtforms.

CRYSTAL CLEAR

General Use: This amazing essence cleanses crystals and also clears negative energies from building. To cleanse crystals/minerals, evaporate a few drops into them from a close distance or soak them in water with a few drops for 5-10 minutes (dowse how many drops for how long). To clear buildings, use four drops in a plant mister half full of water. Leave for one minute, then spray around fairly liberally. Notice the difference! Excellent for healers also, to clear the workspace in between clients.

Elements: Earth 100% Air 77%

Colours: Orange 3% Yellow 25% Green 80% Blue 90% Indigo 100%

Physical levels: Helps strengthen heart. Hay fever, cancer, tumours, boils and spots, aeration of the body.

Emotional and Astral level: Release chakra blocks and negative emotions relating to current lifetime, seals aura against negative invasion. Cleanses lower-mid astral.

Psychic level: Bridges gap between the psychic and the spiritual (7th chakra). Physical protection. Can be used in the bath (a few drops).

Crystals: Cleanses these beautifully. Can also erase their programmes if used with this intent. So be clear!

Spiritual level: Connects psychic to spiritual. Encourages existing aspirations.

Creativity level: Assists in the expansion of creative vision. Direction and goals.

Polarity: Powerful boost for the masculine aspect of both men and women (7th chakra).

FIRE CLEAR

General Use: A clearing essence. Don't use with kidney/liver problems.

Elements: Fire 100%

Colours: Red 94% Orange 55% Yellow 70% Green 100% Blue 100% Indigo 93% Violet 100% Pink 60%

Physical level: Debility. Energy boost, M.E. Old age. Cold sweat, rashes and burns. Clears liver (when this is strong), helps cancer.

Emotional level: Releases suppressed anger. Fear problems (e.g. fear of death, flying, reality, success, paranoia). Motivation and enthusiasm.

Sexual level: Helps shift deep-rooted sexual problems/blocks. Can be used to assist tantric energies, raising level.

Spiritual level: Clearance of negativity, release blockages concerned with group-work. Helps bring a non-aware person toward the spiritual path. Energies of Geburah.

Crystals: Can be applied via crystals.

GOLDEN LIGHT

General Use: Bathes aura in golden light.

Elements: Earth 95% Air 95% Water 100% Ether 100%

Colours: Orange 100% Yellow 90% Green 90% Gold 100% Silver 70%

Physical level: Bruising, blood problems, cholesterol, bad circulation, urinary disorders (not infections), weak bladder.

Emotional level: Transmutation of lower emotions. Over emotional. Flowering, growth. Contacting higher level emotions.

Psychic level: Decording, unhooking from people and past.

Spiritual level: Unconditional love, growth, flowering, setting foot on spiritual path, links with spiritual teachers. Adds positive energy to all chakras and whole energy system.

Crystals: Cleanses and bathes them in golden light. Prepares crystal for healing work.

JASMINE

General Use: Positive self-image, clears depression. Beauty. Birth.

Elements: Earth 90% Fire 88% Water 86% Air 90% Ether 96%

Colours: Red 90% Orange 90% Yellow 80% Green 90% Blue 50% Pink 85% Indigo 100% Violet 87% Gold 87%

Physical level: Assists clearing of the liver and useful in pregnancy.

Emotional level: Positive self-image, clears self-demeaning emotions, self-expression blocks, depression. Clears heart centre.

Astral level: Opens astral doorways. Clears some negativity at this level.

Psychic level: Assists flow of healing energies.

Sexual level: Appreciation of beauty. Heart centre openness.

Creative level: The completion phase of the creative cycle.

Polarity: Strengthens feminine aspect.

Buildings: Clears atmospheres of depression.

Crystals: Can be applied via crystals and some other minerals.

ALSO: Assists when giving birth, helps the incoming soul to have a less traumatic birth.

METTA

General Use: Compassion, accepting the support of others.

Elements: Earth 100% Air 199% Ether 90%

Emotional level: Unconditional love of oneself and others. Receptivity to the compassion of others. Relating to ones own vulnerability. Relaxation.

Sexual level: Female sexual identity. Gay males; balance and polarity.

Spiritual level: Unconditional love, accepting oneself as finite and imperfect.

Crystals: Can be applied via a crystal, which will also be healed by this essence.

ORANGE CHALICE

General Use: Aligning to the Divine Will.

Elements: Fire 5-20% Water 75% Air 75% Air 25% Ether 100%

Colours: Red 100% Orange 100% Yellow 100%

Emotional level: Helps establish boundaries in relationships. Self-demeaning emotions. Shock (7th chakra).

Mental level: Issues related to the will. Weak/strong willed.

Spiritual level: Helps align will to the Divine Will. Helps in receiving of spiritual guidance. Assists feminine aspect of the spiritual (chalice).

Crystals: Helps heal crystals which have been mis-used. Increases level of compassion that crystal can conduct and transmit.

PINK ANGEL

General Use: Emotional healing, compassion.

Elements: Earth 100% Water 100%

Colours: Red 100% Yellow 70% Pink 100%

Physical level: Wounds, boils, spots, kidney disorders.

Emotional level: Heals wounds, broken hearts, wounded healers. Also karmic wounds. People who do not realise their own worth.

Mental level: Clarity of thought, innovative thought, inspiration.

Psychic level: Generally assists development of psychic faculties. Access of Akashic records of persons/buildings.

Creative level: Opens to true worth, to higher octaves of creativity. Assists birth and structuring of creative ideas.

Crystals: Charges crystals with the above properties and can be applied in this way. Heals the crystal too.

RELEASE

General Use: Release of blocks.

Elements: Earth 100% Air 100% Water 100%

Colours: Blue 80% Silver 50%

Physical level: Blood health, congested arteries, lymphatic system, oxygenation, energy from breath, impotence.

Emotional level: Release of deep seated emotions (possibly from deep past) e.g. guilt, grief, terror, hatred, shame, regret, rigidity. General heart chakra and emotional expression. This essence is particularly subject to the intention. Also good for those born under Libra.

Mental level: Assertiveness and development of the will. Communication skills, sales/marketing.

Sexual level: Deep blocks. Impotence.

Psychic level: Very good protection. Seems to work by awakening personal Spirit Protector.

Astral level: Helps with dreams and dream-memory, symbolism and protection.

Buildings: Use a few drops in plant mister to awaken Spirit Protector of building/place. (Use 'Crystal Clear' first.)

SILVER GENIE

General Use: Mental structure, business, discipline. Dreams. Fears.

Elements: Earth 90% Water 97% Ether 96%

Colours: Green 40% Blue 100% Indigo 100% Violet 100% Gold 100% Silver 100%+

Physical level: Leukemia, bone problems, growing bones. Diseases of nervous system. Cools fevers, soothes nerves. Womb health, kidneys.

Emotional level: Helps relationships between individuals and groups. Physical defensiveness. Nurturing, release of tears, deep seated blocks about money. Victim, child abuse, negative female archetype problems.

Sexual level: Releases sexual blocks. Sexual shyness. Magnetism.

Subconscious level: Fears: of the unknown, subconscious fears. Helps bring out hidden intent (3rd and 5th chakra). Fear of masculine tyranny. Fear of the dark. Drug abuse. Aids general access to subconscious and helps deal with it.

Mental level: Mental laziness. Assists generally with business, management, mental structural processes. Analysis. Science, esoteric disciplines and studies (e.g. numerology, astrology). Blocks about money. Passing exams. Academia.

Psychic level: Mindreading (2nd, 3rd and 5th chakras). Realms of Anubis and Isis. Dreams: helps to confront issues in dreams. Dream answers to questions asked before sleep, protection in dreams (2nd chakra before sleep). Dowsing, psychic intuition.

Creative level: Assists the RECEIVING phase of the creative cycle. To accept the rewards of work done. Group work/play.

Spiritual level: Mental side of spiritual discipline, grounding spiritual energies. Providing structures for the higher energies to flow through.

Crystals: Telepathy by crystals. Crystal 'answerphones'. Charges crystals with the essence's properties and can be applied this way. Helps heal a physically damaged crystal. Intercommunication of crystals.

SILVERY MOON

General Use: Sleeping/dream problems.

Elements: Earth 75% Fire 95% Ether 100%

Colours: Green 80% Silver 100%

Emotional level: Contacting feelings/emotions. Clears anger. Image related issues. Assists in projecting one's real self.

Sexual level: Assists with image issues.

Psychic level: Feminine aspect, waxing moon, full moon, scrying. Helps dream work, finding astral pathways, astral projection and protection (via silver light). Dream memory, the realms of Anubis. Sphere of Yesod. Clears negative psychic influence. Helps understanding of refection, symbolism.

Astral level: As psychic level.

Crystals: Cleanses crystals beautifully: a few drops in water, soak for a few minutes.

SOUL STAR (Crystal Charge)

General Use: Can be used after Crystal Clear to CHARGE crystals with powerful positive loving energies. Evaporate a few drops into crystal, or add a few drops to water (can use same water as for 'Clear').

Elements: Earth 100% Fire 50% Ether 80%

Colours: Green 5% Blue 35% Indigo 100% Violet 100% White 95% Pink 75%

Physical level: Assists with energising.

Emotional and Astral level: Disperses depression and self-demeaning emotions. Assists to prevent nightmares. Connects to the higher astral, closes doors to the lower astral. Assists contact with the Angelic realms and more spiritualised aspects of the astral.

Sexual level: Assists more spiritual connections between partners.

Spiritual level: Awakens contact with higher self. Guidance.

Polarity: Boosts the masculine aspect in both sexes.

Crystals: Charges crystals very powerfully with healing energy.

SPIRIT GROUND

General Use: Grounding.

Elements: Earth 90% Fire 100% Water 95%

Colours: Red 100% Orange 90%

Physical level: Assists: Low energy, M.E., bad circulation and arthritis. Rheumatism, strengthens heart and arteries/veins.Loss of blood, period pains, leukaemia, new blood cells, prostate gland.

Emotional level: Assertiveness, self image. Victim syndrome, victims of sexual abuse (this lifetime), violence. Suicidal tendencies. Release of anger. Post natal depression (4th chakra). De-cording (strong ties). Bereavement. Sense of brotherhood/family. Humour.

Sexual level: Assists male erection problems,confidence. Gay men: assists raising level of vibration and reduces negative psychic effects.

Creativity level: Grounding of ideas into form and structure in the world. Good for creative artists generally.

Spiritual level: Fear of one's own power/giving power away (1st and 12th chakras). Contacting the fire elementals. Spiritual energies grounding to earth level. Enhances sense of brotherhood of man. Humour.

Crystals: Will imbue crystal with the above properties.

STANDS ALONE

General Use: Maintain individuality whilst with the crowd. Valuing personal uniqueness. Regression.

Elements: Air 90% Water 100%

Colours: Violet (Pale Violet) 100%

Physical level: Air in bloodstream. Endocrine system, some malfunctioning glands. Benign tumours, stones, blisters and chilblains. Strengthens heart.

Spiritual level: Assists maintaining spiritual centre whilst with the mass. Helps cope with lonely aspects of spiritual path. Feminine aspect: receptivity without weakness. Strengthens aura. Aids regression and access of Akashic records. Helps to find spiritual path.

Crystals: Will take on some of the properties of this essence.

WHITE LIGHT

General Use: High level purification. Mix with some other essences to bring out higher octaves of these.

Elements: Fire 25% Water 90% Ether 80%

Colours: Green 100% Blue 80% Violet 100% Indigo 95%

Physical level: Clearance, liver.

Mental/etheric level: Destroys negative etheric energies. Good for positive thought.

Spiritual level: High level purification. Higher chakras.

Polarity: Enhances feminine aspect.

Creative level: Clears blocks.

Crystals: Can be applied via crystals. Cleanses these also.

WHITE SPRING

General Use: Pure energy source. Re-charges energies.

Elements: Air 75% Water 25% Ether 90%

Colours: Orange 12% Blue 25% Indigo 100% Violet 100%+ White 100% Pink 90%

Physical level: Energies. M.E. Debility.

Emotional level: Emotional exhaustion.

Mental/Etheric level: Mental fatigue, charges depleted etheric.

Psychic level: Gives extra strength before psychic activities (3rd chakra).

Sexual level: Replaces depleted energy centres (by 25%).

Spiritual level: Assists the 'casting off of old clothes'. Becoming more open to this level.

Crystals: Can be applied via crystals. Will also clear crystal and charge it with healing/love energies.

PETALTONE ESSENCES – TANTRIC LOVE ESSENCES

These beautiful essences are applied via evaporation into the aura during foreplay and lovemaking, enhancing subtle energies and the levels of sensitivity.

Application: Place a few drops in the palm of one hand, rub palms together then evaporate into the indicated chakras for about 20 seconds or so, approximately 4-6 inches from skin.

TANTRIC LOVE ESSENCES FOR COUPLES

Use of these essences can be an excellent way to extend foreplay and lovemaking, enhancing sensitivity and the sense of deep sharing. Feel free to experiment and enjoy. Take your time, raise the energies and let spirit shine through.

BEAUTY

Use in chakras 3 and 4 during foreplay. Enhances overall sensitivity, appreciation of beauty and helps to calm the initial sexual impulse so that the energies may be allowed to rise to a higher level. This essence can also be applied via a neutral carrier oil as a massage.

DEEP SPRING

Use in chakra 2 before and during lovemaking. Assists heart contact, communication with higher self and can sometimes bring awareness of past life connections with partner. Increases the depth of the experience. Can also be used to replenish depleted energy centres, before, during or after love.

PURPLE VALLEY

Use in chakra 5 during foreplay. Assists with receptivity, which is important for both partners in higher sex. Also assists transpersonal contact with the feminine (Goddess) and to derive wisdom from sexual experience.

MOUNTAIN YANG

Women: Use before foreplay begins.

Men: Use during lovemaking.

Evaporate into chakra 4 (heart). Boosts the Yang energies, assists contact with higher self and opens the channels for these energies to flow into lovemaking. Can also be applied via a clean oil burner (use spring water) or via a cleansed crystal (evaporate into crystal): leave crystal near the bed.

WARNING: People with recurrent liver/kidney problems should avoid direct applications of this essence and use the crystal or oil burner application instead.

GOLDEN RIVER

Use over whole aura during foreplay. Fills aura with golden light. Assists with transmutation of lower emotions, soulic union and unconditional love. Also helps to dissolve ties with past partners. Boosts both male and female aspects.

TANTRIC LOVE ESSENCES FOR SINGLE PEOPLE

GOLDEN WAY

Use in chakras 4 and 5, for attuning to and helping to attract the right partner for you at this time. Also will uplift and purify your energies. Walk the golden way, not the path of desperation!

BEAUTY

Use all round the aura, to help bring out your beauty and make you more attractive. Will also help you appreciate your own physical beauty and to feel better about it. Helps to heal your sexuality and feel good about it too.

BRIGHT STAR

Stay true to yourself, own your power, speak your heart and shine! This essence helps you to become more fully yourself and to allow this to bring you into partnership.

REAL LIFE REMEDIES

Real Life Remedies have been created using the pure energy of plants with either flowers or leaves and are kept in alcohol. They are totally original and are not made by using ready prepared aromatherapy oils or other commercial remedies. They work by introducing messages into our physical, emotional and spiritual being, which triggers a natural inherent response, promoting better health. We here at Real Life Remedies, believe that nature holds all the answers required for our best possible health, naturally. We are not the only ones who feel this way. Apart from the known effects of homoeopathy, modern medicine has found natural alternatives too, for the ills of today. (Ewe tree clippings are being collected and tested for a possible cure for cancer and one of our most popular pain relief tables, Aspirin is derived from the bark of a tree). We are constantly developing a growing range of remedies, which show positive results for all kinds of problems that are faced by people on a daily basis. N.B. Remedy names are copyrighted by Marion Davis.

AFRICAN DANCE

Personality profile: Especially for those who dance, or use their bodies in any way. Sports people, actors, yoga practitioners, healers and therapists. For meditation, chanting, listening to music, hypnosis and other altered states of consciousness including channelling or spiritual work of any kind. This remedy is an insurance policy against anything nasty intruding, from past, present or future, while you are opening yourself up. Essentially, it releases the negativity adhering to you from dark forces you may have, knowingly or unknowingly, been in contact with. For best results place up to 4 drops on your palm, rub your hands together then place them for a few seconds on the soles of your feet, before you begin your session.

Emotional effects: Protects, cleanses and releases heavy negativity from the aura.

Meditation: Place a few drops on your crown and heart chakra.

Clearing: Place a few drops on crown and heart chakra, then point 4 clear quartz crystals away from you to the North, East, South and West while holding a rose quartz crystal in your right hand. Warning: Do not burn African Dance in your incense burner or take orally.

ASTRONOMY

Personality profile: This remedy is for people who like to connect with the things and the people around them. They're busy people who've accrued a wealth of experience from life, both good and bad. On the whole they're grounded, practical and like exercise and the outdoors. They're open, giving people, who enjoy sharing things with others.

Physical effects: Releases creativity. Releases blocks on healing abilities. Tunes you to the Universe and Universal power sources. Helps to deal with psoriasis when it is stress related.

Emotional Effects: Helps stabilise fluctuating moods removing depression. Clears spiritual pathways and aids transformation. Releases past traumas.

BEAUTIFUL WORLD

Personality profile: A remedy for ambitious, friendly, kind, considerate and warm people, who want to get on in life. They don't tolerate hangers on but conversely, do have time for others who are deserving of their time. They face many changes in life, often in quite short spaces of time and don't have a problem letting go of the past.

Physical effects: Combats depression. Releases inner strength, especially when facing adversity. Introduces positive powers and intuition. Gives grace and support from higher sources of consciousness. Lets you know you are not alone in the world and that there are others like yourself. Gives a feeling of harmonising with the world around even if you have to travel frequently. Helps alleviate worries and tensions, especially around the neck and shoulders. Combats disturbed sleep patterns and encourages more restful sleep and wonderful dreams.

Emotional effects: A remedy for beauty and appreciation of life. It helps you send thanks from the heart and soul to those you truly love. It can help attract the right sort of people to you at the time you need them. Because you are always giving so much love to others isn't it about time you got some back? Even if you consider it a little late in the day, it's never too late to have fun, a partner and a little romance. For bringing out the best in your artistic creative abilities use a few drops twice a day on your hands and throat chakra. To attract the right people to you use a couple of drops a day on your heart chakra.

Crystals: Clears negative energy from crystals and sends loving, harmonising qualities out from them.

BLUE MOOD

Personality profile: For the type of person who, although they like to meet people and are excellent entertainers, tend to withhold both personal and emotional information from others, often unaware of the internal conflicts and pressures this repression causes them. They are sensitive, with deep seated emotions, intellectual, mathematical, logical, organised and capable. Full of drive and ambition, they may already have achieved a lot, although mainly as a result of their inherent sense of insecurity. Good for children and adults who are talented or hyperactive, physically or mentally.

Physical effects: Deals with the allergic reactions to soaps and foods, eczema, psoriasis and dermatitis. Heals physical wounds and scars with greater rapidity. Dilute and spray on minor sunburn or burns. Helps relieve post-operative effects. Relieves stress, frustrations and improves assertiveness. Wonderful for those who need immediate calming. Cleanses the chakras thus cleansing the aura.

Emotional effects: Helps sort out confusion with your perception of yourself. Spotlights and strengthens the hidden, inner person. Releases frustrations and calms the soul. It also heals emotional scars.

Massage: This remedy when mixed with a little grapeseed oil will help people with skin irritations, eczema, psoriasis, dermatitis (use sparingly).

BOUNTY BEAUTIFUL

Personality profile: For people who haven't exactly had an easy time of it. They've worked hard to give others, especially family, a better life, yet, now that everyone's grown up, they feel unappreciated and nobody seems grateful for all that they've done. Caring so much that they worry about those around them, always ready to sacrifice their own needs to take on other people's problems. This eye opening remedy helps these people to see things from another perspective, so that they can understand themselves and others more fully.

Physical effects: Helps combat and defer the onset of arthritis. Helps to relieve aching bones and joints. Opens the heart chakra.

Emotional effects: Helps to alleviate the negative emotional states that lead to feelings of resentment. Encourages self esteem, a positive outlook and healthy emotional growth. Identifies and challenges feelings of martyrdom. Releases bitterness, worries and fears, especially concerning others. Releases old soul ties.

BRETHREN CHILD

Personality profile: This remedy is for people who have had ups and downs to do with family and relationship problems, but through thick and thin they remain faithful and true to those around them. They enjoy holding on to idealistic nostalgic thoughts even though they know in reality times were not always good.

Physical effects: Cleanses, balances chakras and protects the aura. Good for digestive disorders when related to emotional upsets. Stops viruses multiplying in the early stages of their development. Especially good for combating colds and flu making it easier to recover quickly.

Emotional effects: Releases past traumas, especially those experienced in childhood allowing you to remember the experiences without remembering the pain. You can look into the past, get in touch with your emotional well-being, whilst making positive changes in your life. It assists the re-evaluation of you and your relationships, whilst retaining self-esteem and loyalty to others.

BURNING DESIRE

Personality profile: For people with ambition, drive and talent. A remedy that helps to sort out the thought processes and put them in order. Obviously a benefit to someone who really wants to achieve their goals. Not only does it release all those frustrations caused by never having enough hours in the day, it also makes for a warmer, more approachable demeanour.

Physical effects: Cleanses the aura. Calms, relaxes and energises the body. Helps alleviate weariness. Increases the female libido. When inhaled in boiling water helps to clear eyes and stuffy noses.

Emotional effects: Aids clarity of thought. Encourages talent, ambition and drive. Helps to pinpoint achievable aims and desires. Mitigates harsh attitudes, while retaining strong motivation.

CANDLE LIGHT

Personality profile: This remedy is useful for sensitive people, or for nervous timid types who get worried about anything and everything. Especially good for helping people with mood swings or mild depressives. Good for people who have to be up at night. It can help people who are making positive changes, (or those who would like to) in their lives, through the transitional period, by illuminating their way.

Physical effects: Balances the chakras, cleanses the aura. Gives a stronger sense of right and wrong. Heals bruising, old injuries and deep tissue.

Emotional effects: Gives 100% protection from negative forces at night. Gives a calm sense of well-being. Helps control fear and panic. Good for exam nerves and night studying. Clears deep seated emotional traumas, making you feel that you've lightened your load of emotional baggage so you are ready for a new beginning. Helps you decide what's important in your life and what isn't. Breaks old negative soul ties, whilst strengthening positive ones.

EYE ON BRIGHT

Personality profile: For the type of person who's so 'laid back' they accomplish nothing and are a burden to others. Helpful for people who require inordinate amounts of sleep, or are constantly tired or for people who are affected by the full moon, this remedy is an excellent grounder. Especially effective for anyone who has trouble 'coming down'. For people who suffer from hay fever, or house dust allergies, it will help keep your environment cleaner by totally grounding dust, bugs, germs.

Physical effects: Re-calibrates the physical body by grounding it 100% more firmly in the physical world. Aids sounder, more restful sleep and helps to tune you into the Earth energies.

Cleanses land and buildings. A grounding essence for healers, mediums, psychics, clairvoyants and constant astral travellers.

Emotional effects: Helps identify and deal with problematic emotions, such as hates and fears, that stimulate ill health. WARNING: Do not take this remedy orally.

FREEDOM DANCE

Personality profile: This remedy is good for all types of people, although the people who most need it are talented artistic types or academics. For musicians, painters, singers, writers, dancers, to solicitors, teachers, therapists etc who come under attack wittingly or unwittingly from jealousy, anger, bitterness or any negative emotion, releasing this energy from the past or present, protecting against it also for the future. Also for those who find that family and friends are constantly trying to manipulate, or cajole them into doing things they don't want or like. This manipulation may be in the guise of gentle persuasion, or when those around you say they are doing it for your own good, or because they care they wouldn't want you to do the wrong thing.

This remedy releases you from the limitations of others, leaving you to decide what is right or wrong for you. It releases negative energy that has been sent by others and leaves permanent protection from this kind of attack. In spiritual terms, it removes hexes and curses and protects from them.

Physical effects: Calms the nervous system. Creating inner peace and better self control.

Reduces erratic behaviour, anger and frustrations. Allows contact with the inner soul and reasons for living. In other words it helps you to access your spiritual pathway.

Emotional effects: Releases feelings of fear from external forces. Breaks negative soul ties. Allows feelings of self trust and security. Reduces fluctuating moods and brings about more confident behaviour.

FUCHSIA SUCCESS

Personality profile: This remedy is excellent for every type of person. A definite must for the remedy cabinet. A hypochondriacs nightmare! Helps relieve all kinds of negative mental states, including depression. Mitigates bad childhood memories, physical problems and promotes sensitivity without vulnerability. Reduces feelings of frailty.

Physical effects: Helps the body to retain calcium and is an excellent aid for developing bones in children. Good for aiding the regeneration of bones and teeth, tissue, ligaments, muscles, physical wounds and scars. Beneficial in this respect when used post operatively. Helps eczema, psoriasis, dermatitis and rheumatic problems. Excellent for all kinds of pain, especially period pains, cramps and associated problems. For pain relief, a few drops can be applied to the affected area.

Emotional effects: Cleanses, protects, and strengthens the aura. Helps grounding by 30%.

Carrying the bottled remedy on your person can help give psychic and spiritual protection. Helps to relieve severe mental stress associated with trauma, accidents and injuries of all types, rebalancing and rebuilding, emotionally, from the inside out. Frees the heart chakra from old soul ties, removing fears and blocks in regard to the future. Aids change, growth, prosperity and love. Helps to tune into Earth energies, moon movements and flowing water.

Useful to keep at hand for immediate use at these times. Helps to focus and steady the mind, dissipating negative thought associations.

Crystals: Clears crystals 300%! Charges crystals up to 80% and gives them warm, vibratory qualities.

Massage: This remedy can be mixed with a little grapeseed oil and used for massage for physiotherapy, reflexology and healing. To speed recovery of muscle, bone and ligament strains. For dancers and sports people with or without injury to retain suppleness and warmth.

WARNING: When using Fuchsia Success in your bath do not have the water too hot.

GOLDEN WINDOW

Personality profile: Primarily for people who have not, or feel they have not, had a particularly good or easy life. People who have constantly helped and cared for others to the detriment of themselves but, paradoxically, have never given a great deal of themselves away to others for fear of intrusion. These people have strong feelings and emotions, yet cover them up. They don't give themselves a great deal of credit for their achievements, or may consider they have achieved nothing at all. They're quick to put others before themselves.

Physical effects: Cleanses the aura. Opens the heart chakra. Improves perceptual clarity during therapies, meditation, past and present life regression, especially when dealing with childhood aspects.

Emotional effects: Reduces negative and defensive thinking habits. Reinforces self esteem, positive attitudes and behaviour. Balances the mind. Enables life to be embraced warmly and openly with a brighter outlook.

Crystals: Gives crystals a warm vibratory quality.

HERO

Personality profile: For people requiring courage and strength of any kind, whether physical, mental, or emotional. An aid to post operative recovery, it will encourage physical and emotional strength in those who suffer from debilitating or life threatening illnesses such as AIDS, M.E., glandular fever and meningitis. Additional strength, too for people who find the everyday business of life a struggle to deal with, or who find interviews and career or domestic changes difficult to cope with. For those who lack the courage of their convictions, it promotes faith in their sense of right and wrong, enabling them to stand up for themselves and be true to what they believe. Excellent for creative people and those with affinity for nature, the outdoors and a great affection for animals.

Physical effects: Strengthens the general physical body. Boosts self esteem and self worth. Enhances existing creative talents in artists, chefs, craftsmen, carpenters and gardeners etc.

Emotional effects: Releases traumas associated with bad childhood and adulthood experiences. Combats moral uncertainty and ambiguity. Encourages a stronger sense of right and wrong. Reinforces courage and helps to reduce fears and anxieties like examination nerves, stage fright and interview butterflies.

HONEYMOON

Personality profile: For those who have undergone a heavy loss, or emotional trauma such as a heartache or bereavement. It breaks the ties and emotional attachments that prevent them from moving forward without leaving them bitter and cold hearted, alleviating the tendency to wallow in self pity and self denial. By dealing with mood swings and deep depression, it allows life to be lived and even to be enjoyed.

Physical effects: It helps allergies of all types. Especially good for combating hay fever and throat and chest disorders. For gum disorders, put one drop in boiled water and gargle.

Emotional effects: A wonderful cleanser of chakras, especially the heart, the third eye and base chakras. Helps to release firmly entrenched old soul ties. Breaks negative thinking habits and encourages positive attitudes. Effective when emotional readjustment is necessary after profound upsets such as bereavement, shock or loss, mood swings and heartaches.

KARMIC HELPER

Personality profile: Suited to all types, as we all have some karma to work through, although it is suggested that those who are spiritually aware would benefit the most from this remedy as others may not be able to relate to it and the changes which its use brings about.

Physical effects: Reduces feelings of fear and anxiety, especially when related to known and unknown fears or phobias. Transmutes, or has the potential to transmute, negative bacteria, by breaking down their bodies to harmless substances which then leave the body by the natural waste processes. Reduces the effects of stress on the body.

Emotional effects: Grounds 100%. Reduces feelings of fear and rejection. Brings up past traumas and effects healing for them. Crystallises the importance of relationships and soul ties. Releases 'bad karma' destroying any hold that anyone still has over you, allowing you to stand on your own two feet, firmly. Helps re-adjustment in new situations. Releases trapped nervous energy. Helps guide and channel the right energy to you. For those with terminal illnesses, it helps face the fear of death. Releases the soul from new or old covenants with negative forces. In turn this can heal all kinds of illness of the mind, body and soul.

LANCELOT

Personality profile: Good for people who have many interests and a deep reservoir of knowledge. They have passions and obsessions, are hard working and fastidious, but are not good at unwinding and calming down. Forward thinking, they're constantly concerned about the future, chasing plans around in their minds, sometimes to the point where all they generate is worry and fear. A good remedy for sensitive people, especially those with a love of nature. It releases all kinds of traumas, including those that have roots in either present or past lives, (fears or phobias of spiders, birds, flying, heights etc), even ones that seem irrational and unconnected with any remembered events. A remedy for nervous adults, jumpy children and animals with timid or sensitive natures.

Physical effects: Cleanses all chakras. Cleanses and protects the aura. Helps to deal with psoriasis, dermatitis, eczema, fungal infections and neuralgia. Aids physical grounding.

Emotional effects: Clears the mind of habitual negative thinking, also relieving depression. Relieves past life traumas and bad death experiences. Grounds you emotionally in the present, allowing movement towards the future, unencumbered by the past. It unlocks sexual energy, releases inhibitions and helps your natural creativity flow. Connects and tunes you to the nature spirits, animals, plants and wildlife and assists you in becoming more spiritually aware by increasing sensitivity without increasing vulnerability.

Buildings: Clears buildings and land, returning them to the natural vibration that originally existed.

LOOK LIVELY

Personality profile: For people who get bouts of feeling low, especially during the winter months. People who try to make the best of themselves, but never seem pleased or satisfied with the results. They care about the opinions of other people and become stressed and worried about anything and everything out of all sensible proportion. Occasionally agoraphobic, they are prone to isolating themselves, even while in the company of others, thus protecting themselves. Conversely this protective behaviour can also be flamboyant and outrageous, keeping others at a safe distance. In fact, they may only cultivate one or two close friendships with people they feel are truly trustworthy. Other indicators include nail biting, constant colds and flu and an inability to remain calm for very long.

Physical effects: Calms and revitalises. Helps relieve the effects of M.E. and other long term debilitating illnesses. Gives a lighter, more positive outlook.

Emotional effects: Cleanses the aura. Cleans and unclogs heavy negativity from the chakras. Clears heavy negativity from the mind, combating miserable and depressed states.

Crystals: Clears and charges crystals.

Massage: This remedy can be mixed with a little grapeseed oil to tone tissues and relieve old injuries and muscle strains.

WARNING: Do not burn Look Lively in your incense burner.

LOVE 'N' LIGHT

Personality profile: This remedy is particularly good for calm, sensitive people. It can re charge your spiritual batteries, re-newing your hope and faith in human nature. It aids regressive therapy, helping to take a look at the karma created in this lifetime in an objective and un-emotional way. It helps you make connections that are the most important ones for you now, promoting forgiveness and compassion. Quite literally allowing love and light in, especially when there has been darkness and fear, giving the healing process a massive helping hand.

Physical effects: Helps to break down and destroy bacterial and fungal infections and aids growth of positive cell production.

Emotional effects: Frees the heart chakra of old soul ties, re-balancing mind, body and spirit, suggesting positive growth towards a more harmonious future. Destroys negative thinking.

Crystals: Heals and 'loves' crystals. Charges crystals by up to 80%.

MAGNOLIA

Personality profile: Lots of people, from all walks of life, benefit from this remedy. It is however especially good for people with disabilities or difficulties in life, the elderly or infirm. It helps nervous tension, stiffness, aching joints, respiratory problems and hypertension. It helps those with a lot to do, chain smokers, (or those with cravings or addictions), the fearful or paranoid, jumpy children, adults or animals. For demonstrative, affectionate types, or those who feel hard done by, or denied of life's pleasures.

Physical effects: Cleanses and clears the chakras. Calms the nervous system, releases tension, anger and aggression. Controls respiration. Aids restful sleep and disturbed sleep patterns. Releases past traumas. Controls panic and fear. Good for shock and when accidents occur with adults and children. Aids cellular restructuring even after severe injury. Creates time and space for repair and rejuvenation of body and mind tissues. Promotes feelings of peace and tranquillity allowing the individual to deal with day to day stress, difficulties or adverse situations. Repairs the damage that constant stress and worry causes. Aids time and motion study. Helps ageing bone.

Emotional effects: Brings feelings of well-being. Enhances positive behaviour. Re-directs anger and fear and brings intuitive understanding of situations. Creates a space to receive back a positive response from those you care or worry about. Allows you to love yourself and others more fully and appreciate what or who you have around. Opens your eyes to possibilities and opportunities.

MAJESTIC TRIUMPH – HERALD THE ANGELS

Personality profile: This is an ascension remedy. It would suit intellectuals who want to broaden their width of perception or spiritual people who would like to achieve a higher degree of spiritual knowledge and understanding, or want to rise above their present state of consciousness. Good for connecting higher forms of consciousness whether it be with your own inner or outer guidance or angelic forces. Taking this remedy over a period of time will first help achieve greater wisdom, protection and healing ability and then assist to even higher levels of awareness, hence the remedy having two names.

Physical effects: Cleanses and clears and protects the aura. Transmutes negative bacteria within the body, healing and aiding positive cell production. Destroys negative thought forms and so helps depression or despair. Helps individuals achieve their maximum potential. Helps relieve indigestion and chest pain (heart chakra). Helps form stronger bonds within positive relationships and soul ties. Aids regression. Aids spiritual growth.

Emotional effects: Calms body and mind. Releases feelings of emotional rejection. Deals with fears and phobias. Helps collect thoughts, sort them out, putting them and life in order. Gives a warmer demeanour and outlook.

Crystals: Gives crystals a positive vibratory energy, creating a larger positive area around them incorporating this energy into buildings and land.

MARYLIGHT

Personality profile: Good for sensitive, artistic and creative types. A useful remedy for people travelling to carry for emergencies.

Physical effects: Protects the chakras by 80%. Heals skin and soft tissue, wounds, cuts and abrasions. Helps heal eczema and other skin irritations. Helps heal insect bites and stings by reducing swellings. Helps pain relief including headaches, general aches and pains etc. Helps reduce cramping during ovulation and menstruation. Reduces breast pain associated with menstruation and breast feeding. Can increase female potency by up to 60%. Can help grounding by up to 100% so aiding clarity of thought. Can boost the immune system by up to 50%, thus helping people at risk from reduced immunity including the sick, elderly and those with HIV or AIDS, M.E. etc. Best used in the morning, it can energise by up to 60%. It also releases and protects from negativity.

Emotional effects: Has a calming effect on the nervous system. Works well as an anti depressant, to combat negative states of mind. Aids clarity of thought. Aids positive psychic abilities by opening the third eye safely. Relieves stress and depression. Balances feminine aspects. Can help release past emotional rejection, old soul ties. Heals bereavement.

Crystals: Clears crystals 100%. Charges crystals 60%.

Wood: Cleans and clears wood of all negative energy.

MORNING TIDE

Personality profile: This remedy is well suited to individualists, extremists and activists who can either be cool and laid back or fly off the handle when life becomes difficult. Alternatively it can help those who are up all night turning things over in their heads but are so tired during the day that they are unable to produce their best work. It is also good for those under unusually exhausting emotional or physical pressures from changing circumstance or situations or those prone to panic attacks and asthma.

Physical effects: Effects of the remedy are mild and seemingly unwanted at first glance to those who fit the first personality profile in question. It essentially helps you establish a routine of waking and sleeping at regular times so that your body is receiving the best possible rest and exercise. This in turn results in better productivity and the ability for you to take on more responsibility comfortably, so that you rely on yourself to turn up with the goods when they are required of you.

Reduces the risks to health that long term stress, trauma and injuries (physical, mental and emotional) can cause. Relaxes tissue, muscle and ligament damage. (Ideal for sports and dance injuries).

Emotional effects: Literally calms your reflex action to stressful situations down, by telling you when to calm down, rest and sleep naturally.

Massage: This remedy can be mixed with a little grapeseed oil to tone and comfort strained muscles, release tension and stress. Especially good for active, busy people.

PEACHES AND CREAM

Personality profile: Here's a remedy suited to individuals keen on improving themselves in whatever way they can, whether it be in the arts, intellectually or physically. It unlocks inner wisdom and power. It quite literally welcomes you to the tree of knowledge. It creates sacred energy in those who must answer and fulfil their calling in this lifetime.

Physical effects: Cleanses and clears the chakras. Tunes you to higher consciousness. Releases fears and inner frustrations allowing fulfilment in life. Strengthens intuitive understanding of natural law and order, gives clear and concise indications of your soul's purpose. Attracts you to others like yourself who feel the need in life to create more than the average individuals, who are happy just to let life pass them by. Mothers you by making you feel more special and loved when there has been love deprivation. It helps problem children and animals who suffer with either outlandish or difficult behaviour or are withdrawn or unhappy. Other indications of this may appear as eczema or psoriasis or hair loss – helps also these conditions.

Emotional effects: Helps you love yourself and others more fully. Gives a brighter outlook. Gets rid of depression and destructive behavioural traits. Opens your mind to the bigger picture of things. Helps you take control over your life and your wishes, so that you can enjoy life to the full. Strengthens and improves talents and abilities adding bonuses where bonuses are due. Leaves behind old inhibitions and negative lifestyles where they belong in the past.

PURPLE PARADISE

Personality profile: For the type of person who has difficulty putting their life in order and achieving any kind of balance. It helps them to be more aware of their body's needs, when to rest and when to sleep, making for greater and more positive productivity during waking hours. Promotes earlier and easier waking after deeper, more restful sleep. Especially useful for people with a subliminal fear of the dark who stay out or stay awake at night, using dark clothing and a denial of sleep as a shield against their fear.

Physical effects: Excellent for establishing well structured sleeping and waking patterns.

Releases negative states of mind. Balances chakras. Mild grounding effect. Helps the body combat bacterial and viral infections by breaking down the negative energies that create them.

PURPLE PASSION

Personality profile: For people with a multitude of interests, in the arts, music, food, or travel. So many that they don't know which to sample first. They'd love to actively participate in them, too, but they don't have the energy. For stressed nail biters, it calms the nervous system and prepares them to take more on board. Possessing a mild grounding effect, it enables you to connect with others more effectively. It allows you to understand your physical needs and actively realise and enjoy your own particular talents. For those who work or study at night or for those with a fear of the dark. It also helps people who have to cope with varying degrees of blindness.

Physical effects: Helps the immune system rid the body of harmful bacteria and encourage its natural response to repair and replenish damaged tissue. Enlivens the physical body and encourages productive wakefulness. Helps to identify legitimate wants and needs. Relieves stress caused by undirected, wasted energy expenditure and equalises energy levels and protects the aura. Mild grounding effect for better sleep. Restores the equilibrium of the energy levels. Helps to pace and re-order the thought processes. Aids emotional self awareness. For fear of the dark and night-time studying.

REFRESH YOUR MEMORY

Personality profile: This remedy is not just for those who have a bad memory or poor recollection or are studying. It can help many people many different ways. It can remind you of what you originally set off to do in life. It does not just give you the courage of your convictions; it can lead you gently back on path with the knowledge and the truth with which you came into this life.

Physical effects: Cleanses, clears and balances the chakras. Releases negative behavioural conditioning. Clears nasal membranes and chest cavity. (Place 6 drops in boiling water and inhale the vapour.) Reduces swellings and inflammation, especially when they occur in the legs. Reduces the risk of high blood pressure. Attacks viral and chest infections. Good to combat colds. Lessens the risk of heart disease and pulmonary vascular problems.

Emotional effects: Introduces 'new' positive mind powers. Re-establishes familiar feeling and emotions. Compares integrated relationship patterns with the past and present, helping you resist parent and peer pressures and indoctrination. Fundamentally, assisting you towards your own undertakings and goals.

Crystals: Re-tunes crystals to earth energies.

Land: Re-calibrates land and earth energies after major disruption and upheaval to give a regulated positive earth energy drive.

SACRIFICE NOTHING

Personality profile: This special remedy is a great help for all types of people.

Specific effects: Its qualities as a communicator gives an extra dimension to receiving and sending all types of healing or information of a positive nature to individuals or groups and group consciousness. In other words it gives the opportunity to practice radionics with ease. Use it to instigate self-healing, or to attract to you what you need at this present time in every facet of your life. By spraying a mirror it makes it possible to use it as a purple plate. Excellent for healers, mediums or people who meditate or chant, it sends out the messages you want without any interference from the ether or individuals why try blocking or tuning in and using your skills. It can be used for regression or to tune into deeper levels of consciousness by using it on the third eye or to retrieve lost knowledge of the ancient civilisations while channelling. It will not increase sensitivity or vulnerability thus protecting the soul.

Buildings and land: To attract to buildings and land exactly what the earth energy requires spray twice a day for a fortnight and sit back and wait. You should see changes in wildlife and vibration.

SAFE & SOUND

Personality profile: A special blend of remedies for sensitive types or healers, mediums, therapists, counsellors etc, who always come under attack from negative energy.

Emotional effects: Releases heavy negativity from the aura and chakras, protecting and balancing them. Helps the positivity that is sent out to return. Makes any healing or therapy more effective on all levels.

SAVIOUR

Personality profile: Helps people with decisions to make and risks to take. From business meetings and interviews, buying a home or a car, to building an extension or planning a new venture, this remedy permits clearer thinking and strengthens intuition. For those who are terminally ill, or chronically sick in body, it gives the mental and emotional strength to actively participate in life.

Physical effects: Helps encourage the bodies natural resistance to disease and illness. Especially good for those working with the sick. Cleanses, clears and balances chakras, sending in a vibration of love and harmony. Clears negativity from metals and helps clean it.

Emotional effects: Reinforces positivity. Helps in all uncertain, risk taking situations, whether business or relationship oriented. Lessens blinkered and self destructive attitudes in these regards. Gives a stronger sense of right and wrong, encouraging you to trust your instincts. For psychics, healers, mediums and those involved in like work, it helps to tune you into spiritual guidance, all Earth energies and the Universe. Helps the positivity that you send out return to you. Clears your mental and spiritual pathways for meditation, chanting and the giving of healing. Gives you 100% protection from negative forces by creating an impenetrable deflector shield.

SOLEMN FEAST

Personality profile: Suitable for every personality type.

Warning: Not to be used on children below the age of puberty or pregnant women.

Physical effects: Calms the nervous system, giving a feeling of tranquillity and helps combat disturbed sleep patterns and bad dreams.

Emotional effects: Gives complete protection from external negative forces. Helps to deal with bereavement and loss and the process of sorting out family matters. Helps you to come to terms with being alone, even when in the company of others. Balances the chakras and protects you from negative forces. Stabilises energy and moods. Helps with varying states of mental breakdown. Deals with the symptoms of shock and fear, for example, after car accidents, during hospitalisation, or when facing an operation.

Buildings: Controls shock waves that are the result of negative forces including the above and earth tremors.

WARNING; Do not burn Solemn Feast in your incense burner.

SOUL RETRIEVAL

Personality profile: There is no specific type that would benefit from using this remedy, although it has to be said that if you are not a spiritual person you may not be able to tune into all that this remedy has to offer. It can have a profound effect on your life, making you feel more whole and connected to life itself.

Physical effects: Promotes calm, inner strength, vitality. Relieves stress, boosts the immune system.

Emotional effects: Gives 100% protection from negative forces and promotes positive energy. Creates calm. Helps to balance out of control emotions, upsets and traumas from the past, present and future. That is to say that if we can fear things that have not yet happened and feel a sense of peril or foreboding, it helps tune to the right pathways and actions thus avoiding bad situations.

SUNSET BOULEVARD

Personality profile: For people who need to wind down and relax. They don't have problems with change, but on occasion, have doubts about themselves. They thrive on new causes, but sometimes become too deeply involved with them. They tend to be thinkers, with good ideas, but these can get too muddled to be of practical use. When feeling vulnerable, despondent and depressed, this remedy helps to regulate feelings, emotions, strengths and weaknesses.

Physical effects: Relieves stress and depression. Aids relaxation and restful sleep. Helps to stabilise hormone levels. Balances masculine and feminine aspects, individually and within partnerships. Balances the mind. Cleans the chakras. Aids astral projection. Strengthens the etheric body. Aids meditation.

Emotional effects: Reduces lazy, selfish and self destructive attitudes. Reinforces positive thinking and behaviour. Helps heal deep seated mental traumas. Clarifies masculine and feminine aspects.

WARNING: Do not use Sunset Boulevard in your incense burner.

TIFFANY

Personality profile: This remedy helps those people who, although they're secure in their own lives and don't suffer from depression, may be stressed from their workload or family life. They are in control, but the stress results from those around them; from the people who work with and for them, to family, especially children, who need constant organising. Tiffany helps to define relationships with others, enabling you to perceive them, their strengths and potentials more clearly. It helps with decision making, positivity and energy levels, allowing you to achieve better productivity when long hours are involved.

Physical effects: Can increase energy levels by up to 70%. Can clarify thought processes by up to 30%. Heightens physical senses, hearing, eyesight and the like. Sharpens reactions. A protection against the symptoms of industrial and executive stress. Protects the base chakra. Helps grounding by up to 100%. It is suggested that, to achieve the maximum benefit from this remedy, you bath with it for 30 minutes.

Crystals: Charges crystals by up to 70%.

Buildings: By spraying Tiffany, you can help to alleviate geopathic stress and energise your surroundings.

WARNING: Do not use Tiffany in you incense burner.

TIME IMMEMORIAL

Personality profile: This agile remedy can change you by heightening your perception about life and how you've been living it up till now. It can make you realise what you've been missing, or respect and appreciate what you've got and whether it's good or bad for you. Your thoughts could always be clearer. Does the universe know what you want from life? Come to think of it do you really know what you want yourself? If you could only get yourself straight then things would start to fall into place.

Physical effects: This remedy starts by releasing trapped or blocked energy passages around the body. Reduces swellings and inflammation especially around lower limbs. Increases momentum. Especially good for tiredness when it is unrelated to lack of sleep or heavy work loads. Good for M.E. patients or people suffering from the effects and problems that long term illness can cause.

Emotional effects: Reduces feelings of anxiety, fear or feelings of rejection, replacing them with calmness, relief and a positive outlook. Combats heavy negative states of mind. The main thing about this remedy is that it helps you to sort out the wheat from the chaff, exposing things for what they are and not what you think they could be, allowing you to learn from past experience while not being influenced by it. It crystallises the importance of old soul ties and how they affect or relate to you, preparing you physically, mentally and emotionally to change to a new direction and renew zest for life.

Crystals: Charges crystals 200%.

Buildings and land: Reverts the energy of land and buildings back to nature's positive energy, clearing waterways and lakes etc. of negative vibrational fields and changing external forces i.e. building work, repairs or reconstruction to do with new or old property.

TOWER OF STRENGTH

Personality profile: There is no particular personality type that benefits most from this remedy, but it is a great aid to those who lead active busy lives or those who would like to. Especially good for people who have had long term debilitating illnesses or those who have had severe illness in the past or those suffering from post operative stress syndrome. Good for severe panic situations and stressful experiences, nervous adults and jumpy children. A friend for asthma sufferers.

Physical effects: Helps to strengthen the physical body and retain a constant energy level. It calms the nervous system and lowers the blood pressure to safe limits. (It won't lower blood pressure if it's already low.) Controls respiration and regulates breathing. Releases physical traumas. Clarifies thought processes. Heals insect bites. Helps dermatitis and psoriasis.

Emotional effects: Balances and protects the chakras, releasing heavy negativity from them. Grounds 100%. Breaks spells, curses and the energy envy or jealousy leaves around you.

Strengthens positive emotions. Protects from vulnerability. Re-affirms your belief in your own abilities, when those around you are constantly judging, criticising or trying to influence you. Encourages progress and challenges life and situations, when there has been procrastination or lack of enthusiasm. (Remember your pathway and your soul are your own and not somebody else's to control or live.) Helps tune to earth spirits, energy and nature.

Buildings: Clears buildings/land of negative energy leaving it with positive energy.

❀ ROSIE DEVITT FLOWER ESSENCES ❀

Having realised the wonderful potential of vibrational remedies, by at first using the Bach flower remedies and then moving on to others produced in various parts of the world, I decided to experiment with making some myself.

This I did and slowly became aware of beings on higher levels who at times would give help and guidance. I realised that this was something to share and gradually began to market the essences and give advice to others as to their use.

I have been delighted to hear of good results which various people have obtained, dealing with problems both mental and physical. For myself perhaps the most useful gain has been the ability to become more aware of the difference between what I am experiencing and that which truly I am. I make over 100 essences including my own 'rescue remedy' which contains borage, comfrey, nasturtium and herkimer diamond.

ALMOND
Growth in children.

AMARANTHUS (RED)
Viruses, inflammations.

BANANA
Bone marrow.

BLACKBERRY
Lethargy.

BLEEDING HEART
Heart disease, blood pressure.

BORAGE
Strength, courage, happiness.

BUTTERCUP
Self confidence.

CAMELLIA
Loving attitudes, links to earth energies.

CALENDULA
Communication, joy.

CALIFORNIAN POPPY
Inner balance, psyche.

CELANDINE
Stimulates metabolism.

CLOVER (WHITE)
Balance.

CLOVER (RED)
Calm, peace.

CLEMATIS
Insight, wisdom.

COMFREY
Nervous system.

COSMOS
Linguistic abilities.

DAFFODIL
Vitality, blood pressure.

DAISY
Intellectual relaxation.

DANDELION
Muscular relaxation.

ECHINACEA
Immune system.

ELDER FLOWER
Circulation, mental abilities, past life recall.

EVENING PRIMROSE
Communication.

FRENCH MARIGOLD
Inflammation, e.g. inner ear.

JASMINE
Nasal passages,sinuses, throat and lungs.

HAWTHORN
Tumours, stress.

LILAC
Spine.

LOBELIA
Spiritual qualities, peace.

LUFFA
Skin disorders.

MAGNOLIA
Digestion.

MALLOW
Mental stability.

MORNING GLORY
Nervous system.

MUGWORT
Muscular system, I.Q.

NASTURTIUM
Joy.

ONION
Emotional stress.

PASSION FLOWER
Christ consciousness.

PENNYROYAL
Psychic protection.

PETUNIA
Hyperactive children, meditation.

SNAPDRAGON
Larynx.

SNOWDROP
Energy blocks, cleansing.

SOLOMONS SEAL
Mental relaxation.

SQUASH
Hormonal balance.

STAR OF BETHLEHEM
Trauma.

STINGING NETTLE
Relationships,emotions.

ST JOHN'S WORT
Fear.

SUNFLOWER
Spine.

THYME
Strength, augments other essences.

VIOLA TRICOLOR
Viruses, tiredness after meditation.

WALLFLOWER
Digestion.

WHITE CHESTNUT
Worry.

WISTERIA
Subtle body imbalances.

YARROW
Protection.

ZINNIA
Laughter, humour.

RESCUE REMEDY
Contains borage, comfrey, nasturtium and herkimer diamond.

For stress relief, strength, courage and joy.

❀ SILVERCORD ESSENCES ❀

WELSH FLOWER ESSENCES
Welsh Flower Essences are produced from indigenous flowers growing in the counties of Wales. The flowers in these sets are the accumulation of many years of scientific research and of devic guidance. Each essence was selected for its impact upon mind, body, soul, relationships and are a quintessential capsule of vibrations containing sound, sacred geometry and mineral, chromatically balanced energies. They are prepared with compassion and are keyed in by either the sun method or our unique laser method. We have found that these essences are great complementary catalysts for change and can be used to assist other essences in various applications. The other unique aspect of these Welsh Flower Essences is that they are produced in such a way that they contain the elements of the following: Air, Earth, Fire, Water. The essences are not a substitute for allopathic medicine but are certainly complementary.

SET NO. 1

ALKANET
Physical – This is a good essence for healing of wounds. Can be used in cream base. Also for ulcers.

Psychological – "Maybe I should become the decision maker". Self responsibility.

CORNBINE
Physical – An excellent essence to combine with others for constipation, blood, fevers.

Psychological – Emotional traumas, excessive worry and for letting go.

CREEPING JENNY

Physical – For muscular pain, rheumatic joints.

Psychological – For low self esteem, to help with confidence and self expression.

HONEYSUCKLE

Physical – Use for the lungs and bowel.

Psychological – Energising your femininity and for the inability to love, for clinging to emotions of the past.

LOOSESTRIFE

Physical – Digestive disorders, liver complaints and for the blood.

Psychological – Too many thoughts, sharing with others.

MULLEIN

Physical – This essence is used for male fertility, also for gastritis, neuralgia and rheumatic pain.

Psychological – Feeling you are not living up to your own and others' expectations, trying to change.

PLANTAIN

Physical – An anti-inflammatory, good for the urinary system, cardiovascular system and for toothache and coughs.

Psychological – To be emotionally secure and accepted by other people, fear and guilt.

PYRAMID ORCHID

Physical – To be used for the pineal gland and all renal conditions.

Psychological – Trusting in others and recognising your own sensitivities.

ROSE BAY WILLOW HERB

Physical – Heart, circulation.

Psychological – For grief, renewed hope, relaxing your mind and listening to your heart.

RUE

Physical – Water retention, can be used as a tumour inhibitor.

Psychological – High ideals and compassionate thoughts.

SCARLET PIMPERNEL

Physical – Anaemia, disorders of the liver and gall bladder, skin infections, has a cleansing action. It also aids the intestines to absorb nutrients.

Psychological – Restoring your physical endurance, vague fears, feelings of rejection.

SELF HEAL

Physical – Used for the throat and mouth, external wounds and arthritis.

Psychological – Sensitivity to one's personal and spiritual needs. Contacting your intuition.

SILVERWEED

Physical – For bladder and kidney complaints, throat infections and painful menstruation.

Psychological – For poor self image, feelings of frustration or limitation.

SORREL

Physical – For kidney and liver complaints and acute muscular weakness.

Psychological – Feeling consumed by worry or fear, uncertain about the future.

STRAWBERRY

Physical – This will increase the blood flow. For stomach upsets, various inflammatory disorders.

Psychological – To be open to new ideas, to counteract negative thinking and releases over burdening

TUFTED VETCH

Physical – Circulation problems. Chilblains when used in a cream.

Psychological – Trusting in your feelings, using intuition. Protection from over involvements.

WELD

Physical – To be used for the spinal column and for the vertebrae.

Psychological – For balance, strength, harmony, lack of insight.

WELSH POPPY

Physical – Nervine laxative, constipation, liver complaints.

Psychological – Loneliness, communication of feelings.

WHITE FOXGLOVE

Physical – For heart conditions.

Psychological – Unity, need for spiritual protection, insight, perception.

YELLOW IRIS

Physical – General tonic, also used for jaundice.

Psychological – Enhancing your communication abilities and for tolerance.

SET NO. 2

BLUEBELL

Physical – Used for glue ear, throat, thyroid gland.

Psychological – For independence, but being fearful of the unknown and for unsolved problems.

BUTTERCUP

Physical – For pain relief, pancreatic disorders, central nervous system.

Psychological – To enhance feelings of security, for loneliness or feelings of being alone.

COLUMBINE

Physical – To relax the nervous system, hysteria, liver jaundice, gall bladder conditions.

Psychological – For trust and honour of your intuitive, inner feelings and connecting with your wisdom.

COMMON COMFREY

Physical – A calming essence for gastric conditions. Also a very good essence for painful joints.

It has anti-inflammatory qualities. In cream base can be used for eczema and psoriasis.

Psychological – For those who are over emotionally dependent. "I like to be loved".

COMMON VETCH

Physical – For circulation problems, also for the heart.

Psychological – For feelings of frustration and limitations. Unwarranted criticism.

DOG ROSE

Physical – For coughs, colds, constipation, gall bladder problems, general exhaustion, bladder and kidney conditions.

Psychological – For those who are over emotional.

EVENING PRIMROSE

Physical – A very good essence for skin conditions (ectopic eczema especially in children).

Epstein Barr virus, also for hyperactivity.

Psychological – To halt depression, sharing, communicating and expressing yourself.

FLAX

Physical – Such a gentle essence it can be used quite effectively to remove heavy metals from the body. Gentle upon the stomach and for eczema and shingles.

Psychological – For calming down overactivity and increasing your own perception and for those who hide in a crowd.

HERB ROBERT

Physical – Inflammation of the gums, toothache. Has antiseptic qualities, good for bruises, cuts, boils, if used in a cream base. Also has diuretic qualities.

Psychological – To be positive in thought and action.

MARIGOLD

Physical – For stomach disorders, duodenal ulcers, used in a cream base for eczema, sore skin.

Psychological – Uncertainty of direction in life, for changes and those not motivated

OX EYE DAISY

Physical – Will relax, ease tension and stress, a tonic.

Psychological – Patience, relaxes tensions, increases one's own individuality.

PINK FOXGLOVE

Physical – This essence regulates cardiac function. Also for sore throats, laryngitis.

Psychological – For feeling dependent on others or feeling over burdened by outside dependencies.

PURPLE TOADFLAX

Physical – For chest infections, coughs, bronchia.

Psychological – For being aware of your sensitivities and believing in your own inner guidance, expression of feelings.

SPEEDWELL

Physical – Has diuretic qualities, tonic after illness or operation, will help the tissues to repair.

Psychological – For mental exhaustion, problems with decision making.

STITCHWORT

Physical – Will boost your immune system after trauma, operation, also for skin conditions.

Psychological – To be open minded and ready for new pathways in life, new ideas, new insights.

ST JOHN'S WORT

Physical – For hyperactive children, P.M.T. It is also a sedative.

Psychological – For better communication, more self awareness

VIPERS BUGLOSS

Physical – Used for the blood, epilepsy, throat problems and fertility.

Psychological – To enhance your wisdom, discernment.

WILD CLARY

Physical – Good for digestive problems, useful for psychotherapy, also kidney disease.

Psychological – Reduces outside pressures, to see clearly.

WOOD ANEMONE

Physical – Arteriosclerosis, urinary problems, fevers.

Psychological – For those who suffer with loneliness, or those who isolate themselves from others.

SET NO. 3

BRAMBLE

Physical – Stomach disorders, hypertension. Also for coronary disease, used for skin conditions such as eczema, also mouth and throat infections.

Psychological – For those who like to be by themselves, self protection.

BUDDLElA

Physical – Pineal gland, eyes, blood cells.

Psychological – To focus the mind and help you to meditate.

CHICORY

Physical – This essence is for the liver, gout, also rheumatoid arthritis and is used for gall bladder problems and gall stones.

Psychological – For those mentally stressed due to lack of relaxation.

CINQUEFOIL

Physical – For painful menstruation, piles, sore throat.

Psychological – For those with high ideals and goals in life. "Don't burn yourself out".

CORNFLOWER

Physical – A useful essence for skin conditions, it aids digestion and can be tried for stimulating the hair follicles.

Psychological – "Let me show you how creative and expressive I can be".

CRANESBILL

Physical – Used for problems with veins and capillaries.

Psychological – For protection from over involvements, to develop compassion and sensitiveness.

ELDERFLOWER

Physical – For coughs, colds and as a tonic, hayfever.

Psychological – Excessive worry, or mental confusion. A need for your own space.

KNAPWEED

Physical – For the bladder and kidneys, it is a tonic and diuretic.

Psychological – For using your intuitive faculties and insights as a resource for aiding others.

MALLOW

Physical – Coughs, throat infections, stomach and intestinal conditions, can be used in the bath for abscesses, boils, burns, also used for bronchitis, catarrh and eczema.

Psychological – Loving yourself and accepting love as you love others.

MAYWEED

Physical – Can be used for stomach conditions, can also soothe eczema, lack of flora in the intestines.

Psychological – Feeling unloved, lonely, separated, emotionally detached.

PARSLEY

Physical – used for kidney disease, water retention, flatulence.

Psychological – Over response to emotional stresses, a little more openness to yourself and to new ways of living.

RAGGED ROBIN

Physical – Nerve cells, bronchia, cardiovascular system, arteries, capillaries, brain, spinal cord.

Psychological – "I like to love, be loved and care for others".

RED CLOVER

Physical – Has a dermatological key. It is used for psoriasis, eczema and as a sedative for the lungs.

Psychological – For intolerance of others and for feelings of rejection.

RED PHEASANT'S EYE

Physical – Angina and for heart conditions.

Psychological – Lack of physical energy and for anger.

SPOTTED ORCHID

Physical – Skin disease, also for the lungs, infection and catarrh.

Psychological – Fear of being unloved, emotional traumas.

THRIFT

Physical – Skin blemishes, skin cancer, blood.

Psychological – For emotional support for oneself and others, lack of self acceptance, "Yes you can love yourself".

TREFOIL

Physical – Used for the lungs.

Psychological – To help one to express new ideas and oneself.

VIOLET

Physical – For earache, catarrh, coughs, has anti tumour quality, muscle fibres, pancreas.

Psychological – For those restricted by authority, who have difficulty in trusting others completely.

YELLOW DOCK

Physical – Soothing to the joints, rheumatics.

Psychological – To be optimistic and smile, for those who have been hurt.

YELLOW WOUNDWORT

Physical – Used for gout, cramps, jaundice.

Psychological – Despair or depression, expressing yourself.

SET NO. 4

AGRIMONY

Physical – Use for the liver, stomach and also for rheumatics, gastro-enteritis, gall bladder problems.

Psychological – the light bringer. Will help you to absorb more prana and to bring spiritual awareness so that you may acquire spiritual wisdom.

BETONY

Physical – Nervous asthma, migraine, nerve tonic.

Psychological – Awakens the kundalini, through creative visualization this stimulates the energy that is needed for service.

CENTAURY

Physical – For chronic fatigue syndrome, M.E. and for loss of appetite.

Psychological – Stimulates the feminine intuitive energy and will help you to express this.

CHAMOMILE

Physical – Used for nausea, eczema and as a sedative.

Psychological – Will help to gain insights into conscious levels of past lives.

CLEAVERS

Physical – For the lymph system, cystitis, psoriasis and to lower arterial blood pressure.

Psychological – Will help you to connect with nature in a spiritual way, allowing you states of higher awareness.

FUMITORY

Physical – A cleansing essence, good to use before other essences.

Psychological – Awakens deep intuition, which leads to empathy with others.

KIDNEY VETCH

Physical – Circulation problems, kidney disease.

Psychological – A TRANSFORMATIONAL ESSENCE. Will help you to understand spiritual matters, will allow the user to connect with their soul.

LAVENDER

Physical – Antidepressant, migraine and neurological headaches.

Psychological – Aids contact with own true self and the soul's purpose. Will bring enlightenment.

PERIWINKLE

Physical – Mouth ulcers, sore throats, eye conditions.

Psychological – A TRANSITIONAL ESSENCE. Cleanses the bio energy field, so that you may connect with past lives. Also for those in the transition called death.

PINEAPPLE WEED

Physical – Has sedative qualities, used for pineal gland.

Psychological – Deepens your spiritual connections with nature and to release inner knowledge.

POLICEMAN'S HELMET

Physical – for inflammation of the throat, lungs and for the female sexual organs.

Psychological – Will support you in the process of your spiritual development, will help you to be focused in meditation.

PRIMROSE

Physical – For stomach complaints, rheumatism, insomnia.

Psychological – Will help to develop spiritual compassion. Brings forward wisdom from past lives.

REDSHANK

Physical – Anti-inflammatory, piles, heart problems.

Psychological – Will connect you with the Christos energy and open the user to love, compassion and initiation.

REST HARROW

Physical – Cleanses the urinary system, also the gall bladder.

Psychological – supports the process of reawakening and will encourage spiritual strength

RUSSIAN LETTUCE

Physical – Sinuses, bronchia, throat infections.

Psychological – Encourages the user to find their true philosophy of life and to go with the flow.

SCABIOUS

Physical – For respiratory complaints, coughs, asthma and skin conditions.

Psychological – Helps to find self love and inner peace. Will help you to understand the laws of karma.

SEA LAVENDER

Physical – For coughs, nerves, to ease throat infections, indigestion.

Psychological – A TRANSFORMATIONAL ESSENCE. Spiritual cleanser (to many workshops, lectures.)

TANSY

Physical – Varicose veins, rheumatics.

Psychological – Transforms spiritual ideas into matter. Will help you to connect with inner guidance.

TENBY DAFFODIL

Physical – For muscular weakness, tetany, osteoporosis and a nervine laxative, asthma, eczema and for rheumatoid arthritis.

Psychological – "To attain a deep inner wisdom, use me as a light tool, which gives guidance on which spiritual path to take".

THYME

Physical – Used as a sedative, for coughs, bronchitis and whooping cough. This essence can be used with all essences.

Psychological – HEALING PROTECTION ESSENCE. A support for all the other essences, can be used with all of them.

❈ SUE'S FLOWER ESSENCES ❈

The essences which I have made are a contribution towards fulfilling the current need to access higher levels of energy. for healing both humanity and also the planet on which we have chosen to be at this time. The essences listed here work on different aspects of the personality, releasing blockages to allow the life force to better enter the body. Some of them also work physically. All of them help us to deal with 'real life' issues which can be very challenging and which are presented to us daily in the search for the true essence of our own being. In making the essences I have requested assistance from the particular devas associated with each plant and I have also called upon the Universal Family of Light who assist with their guidance as needed. The essences were made using the traditional Sun method as pioneered by Dr Bach.

ANEMONE

This helps to balance all the major chakras, with a particular focus on the throat and the brow, to help with communication, including telepathy. It helps with difficulties in communication due to an inability to ground the energy properly and helps us to focus clearly on our needs.

DAFFODIL

Daffodil works on all 7 main chakras in the body and also those in the hands and feet. It concentrates mainly on the brow, heart and solar plexus chakras, helping to "see" intuitively. It helps to remove fear so that "second sight" can develop naturally. This allows us to perceive that what we need is around us already.

"Those who have eyes to see, let them see".

DELPHINIUM

A combination of two delphiniums, for those who have fear and anxiety lodged in their heart. It works on the throat and heart chakras to enable the fear to be released through communicating effectively. It is also for those who have trouble in sleeping when the cause is anxiety, allowing to come to the surface that which is needed and giving the strength (with perhaps nasturtium following) to make the necessary changes.

"Open your heart to release what you no longer need".

FRENCH MARIGOLD

Each of us has inside a great 'inner knowing' – a being that knows why we came to be here, that knows why the call to Earth was made. That inner being is our Self – it has the wisdom that we need from day to day, based on many experiences. With this wise being we can realise that we already know the answers from inside ourselves; that has always been the case. French Marigold helps us to access more clearly this deep, loving voice within that knows and loves us – that is us, that helps us to find our way out of the maze of all the things that we create and co-create. When we have listened to ourselves, we are more able to listen to others and to 'hear' them correctly. French Marigold is for listening and understanding the truth on all levels. This includes clairaudience and physical hearing.

GERANIUM

This essence, made from mixed zonal geraniums, relaxes the body. It activates the throat, heart and base chakras to release unwanted energy, helping the life force to enter. It aligns all the major chakras and nadis temporarily allowing the light to enter where there has been darkness and lack of direction generally. Good for depression or releasing negative energy.

HIBISCUS

This essence was made from a beautiful hibiscus tree which grows in the garden of the house in which we lived in Norfolk. The tree must have been there for many years to have grown to its current size and has twice survived having branches removed to erect buildings close by. The essence is very grounding. It clears and balances the emotional body, so is helpful after emotional cleansing. It works on the feet, base, sacral and solar plexus chakras and has some effect on the heart energy. It is made with the love of St. Germain. It is good for people who are 'running away', helping them to realise that there can be no escape, but only continuous transformation in whatever form this takes.

IRIS/DIOPTASE

This essence is made from a yellow dutch iris and dioptase crystal. combined in one bowl when the essence was made. It works on all chakras up to the 12th, aligning and opening them at whatever level is needed at the time. It helps to access all the levels of love within you and also relieves guilt. (Would be good to combine with Phlox for cleansing and self-acceptance.)

"Open to receive the light within you".

LAVENDER

Lavender helps connection with the higher self and to feel inner guidance more clearly. It also helps to integrate spirituality into daily life; this is often an area of difficulty. It eases emotional tension and helps to bring in a state of calm and peace. Good for those who are physically tense and tend to overstimulate themselves physically, mentally or spiritually (or all of these).

NASTURTIUM

Nasturtium invigorates. It draws in light through the crown chakra, opening locked doors and allowing fear to lift or subside. It allows you to do what is needed in the moment, removing fatigue and grounding the light. Works also on the sacral and brow chakras.

ORANGE LILY

The straight, erect stem of the lily symbolises the spine and its strength. The fiery orange colour relates to the base and sacral chakras and the essence helps to open these to release anger and frustration, then allowing the kundalini to rise up the spine in a natural way.

PHLOX

This essence embodies the idea of purity and what this means to us individually and collectively. Many ideas of personal purity in this day and age are misconceived; phlox helps with the change in perception which is needed to help us to love ourselves and to realise that we cannot be perfect in this life but that with love we can accomplish much and accept and understand the need for change. When we accept that we are pure within, the need for self-abuse arising from a feeling of being unclean falls away and we are able to nurture ourselves with what we truly need within the physical. May be helpful with eating disorders and to remove toxins from the physical body.

SUNFLOWER

Sunflower helps to align all chakras from throat to feet, connecting to the earth guardians. It is a balancing essence for those who have too much 'father' energy and helps to remove sun toxicity. Good to take when meditating to connect father sun to mother earth for healing to bring about greater balance and harmony in both of these and all things in between.

❀ SUN ESSENCES – THE LIVING ENGLISH ❀ COLLECTION

The Living English Essences are very special. In their preparation the flowers are held – still living – into the bowl of spring water. This appears to bring a grounded dimension to the potency, yet the remedy remains connected to an ongoing stream of life force. Where possible we have used this mode of preparation in the same bowl as picked flowers and believe this has strengthened the healing potential of these Essences.

KEY

F Flowers floated on spring water, in the sunshine

L Living flowers held in spring water, in the sunshine

H Flowers picked by hand

S Plant material filling bowl of spring water and left out in all types of weather

LIVING FLOWERS – SET 1 – Essences made with living flowers

BLACKBERRY (L,F,H)

Grounds ideas into reality

This essence is indicated when a person has lots of ideas but seems unable to find enough will to bring them into reality, perhaps due to the perceived pain of living. Blackberry can harness power and energy and help one to focus on and attain the goal without distraction.

BLEEDING HEART (L,F,H)

Non-attachment

This essence is useful when there has been neediness or co-dependence within a relationship. If the partnership ends, the pain of lost love is often experienced as unendurable. Bleeding Heart helps one to work through the grief and begin the process of healing the self.

BORAGE (L,F,H)

Lightness of heart

Use Borage when there is great heaviness and sadness in the heart. It can break through the dark to discover an inner lightness which brings support, optimism and renewed courage.

BUTTERCUP (L,F,H)

Recognising one's own uniqueness

This essence is indicated when there is a lack of self-esteem. Buttercup warms and nourishes the being with golden light. It brings an understanding of how special and unique life is, no matter how humble it may seem.

CHAMOMILE (L,F,H)

Calming

Chamomile is useful when there is emotional turmoil which can create stress, sleeplessness and digestive problems. This essence can ease the tension and bring relaxation deep within the body.

COSMOS (L,F,H)

Clear interaction

When an individual is overwhelmed by too many negative thoughts, interaction can become defensive and confusing to others. Cosmos cleanses and clarifies the mind processes, enabling communication to be kind and of greater integrity.

DANDELION (L,F,H)

Relaxes tension in the body

Dandelion is helpful when one's body has become tense due to an over stressed lifestyle. This essence can help one to 'go with the flow', feel more relaxed and able to cope better with the ups and downs of everyday life.

EVENING PRIMROSE (L,F,H)

Nurturing

Evening Primrose is indicated when there is an avoidance and fear of deep personal contact, which can inhibit sexuality and the ability to love. This may be due to emotional deprivation experienced in the womb, at birth or throughout early infancy. This flower can help resolve these internal issues by encouraging the beginnings of self-nurturing.

MARIGOLD (L,F,H)

Kind communication

Marigold is indicated for those aggressive and argumentative types who enjoy provoking a reaction in their contacts with others. This essence helps develop assertive communication, but in a clear and compassionate way.

MORNING GLORY (L,F,H)

Body rhythms

This essence can be useful when one is leading an erratic lifestyle often requiring stimulants to stay alert. Morning Glory can gently regulate the body clock so the need for such habits is released. It becomes easier to wake up and feel refreshed.

MULLEIN (L,F,H)

Inner truthfulness

This essence can bring the courage and strength to be true to the higher self and embrace one's rightful path in life. Mullein can be supportive as one explores a sense of individuality in the face of possible opposition.

NASTURTIUM (L,F,H)

Balancing energy

This essence is helpful for the dry, intellectual types who tend to drift into the realms of thought and detach from feelings. Nasturtium can also help to revitalise the mind after periods of excessive mental work, useful during study.

PANSY (L,F,H)

Strengthens physically

Pansy has a predominantly physical application. Helps strengthen the body's defence mechanisms against viral attack. Excellent topically in creams and oils. Useful alongside Ramsons and Jack by the Hedge.

PEPPERMINT (L,F,H)

Clearing

This flower can help to clear and cool down the thinking processes in times of great emotional strain or extreme mental activity e.g. muzzy or foggy head.

PINK YARROW (L,F,H)

Protection

Pink Yarrow is for those who are empathic and may absorb the negative feelings of others. This can cause confusion and a drain of energy. This essence can strengthen and protect the aura so it is also of great help to therapists working with clients. Useful in a spray.

SAGE (L,F,H)

Wisdom

When looking for a positive aspect on a difficult situation, past or present, Sage can bring a detached view-point. This essence can help distil wisdom from life's various experiences and encourage one to see a new angle on the problem.

SELF-HEAL (L,F,H)

Taking responsibility

Self healing can be used in all healing situations. It re-energises the life force from within, reducing the need to seek support from others. One can then take greater responsibility for healing the self through very difficult life challenges.

SUNFLOWER (L,F,H)

Empowerment

When the male aspects of the personality are under-developed Sunflower can bring greater empowerment. Like the Sun, one feels able to radiate outwards and reach for the peaks of personal achievement. It can balance an overdeveloped ego. Also useful where there are problems with the father figure.

TANSY (L,F,H)

Drive

When there is a lack of motivation, procrastination and a poor sense of self, it becomes difficult to see a way forward. Tansy can help one connect to a solid centre within, bringing an instinctive sense of the right direction, which propels one forward into action.

WHITE YARROW (L,F,H)

Environmental protection

Yarrow can help to protect the aura from negative environmental influences e.g. noise, fumes, pollution, radiation, computers etc and the resultant energy drain. Useful in a spray.

LIVING FLOWERS – SET 2 – Essences made with living flowers

ALKANET (L,F,H)

Calm in a storm

Alkanet can help one to keep positive and balanced in situations which are chaotic or obtrusive. Feelings of support and protection help to hold and focus energy, enabling clear communication and a way through difficult circumstances.

AUTUMN LEAVES (S)

Transition

The colours of autumn are mixed together to give a Natural Earth Essence that reconnects you with nature and the ever changing patterns of life. Today people find themselves living many life-times within one – dying and being reborn like the cycles of nature. This can be a very difficult process. Autumn leaves can be supportive when going through such periods of profound personal change.

BLUEBELLS (Mixed colours) (L,F,H)

Tranquillity

The fresh, uplifting quality of a Bluebell Wood is embodied in this healing essence. The fragrance, colour, stillness and perfect peace can reconnect you with your higher self and the tranquillity this brings is useful in times of stress.

COPPER BEECH S

Grounding

A Natural Earth Essence Copper Beech can help to clear the bodies energies, enabling one to feel balanced and grounded. It can renew the life force and strengthen one's connection to the earth. Useful in a spray around the feet.

DOUBLE DAFFODIL (L,F,H)

Abundance

This essence can allow one to let in feelings of joy and happiness. It releases an often long-term, rigid and constricted attitude, opening the heart to the rich abundance of life.

ELDERFLOWER (F,H)

Integration of the shadow side

Elderflower can help one come to terms with the dark side that is within us all which for many can be a daunting challenge. This flower can encourage deeper understanding of the self, so a balance may be found.

EYEBRIGHT (L,F,H)

Clear sight

Eyebright is indicated when there is a need to live life through someone else, which can be confusing. A sense of identity is lost and it then becomes difficult to see one's own path. This essence can bring a wider viewpoint, so one can clearly see the self, others and new opportunities.

FEVERFEW (L,F,H)

Adaptability

In extreme and difficult situations this essence can help one adapt very quickly, encouraging the quality of flexible thinking. It brings out strength and tenacity when needed e.g. travelling, moving house, stressful work situations.

JACK BY THE HEDGE (L,F,H)

Supports a delicate immune system

For sensitive, fragile and delicate constitutions, prone to infection. This essence can help support the heart connection to the body's defence system, so is ideal when emotional pain e.g. grief, has weakened the constitution. Appropriate with Ramsons in any infection.

LADIES MANTLE (L,F,H)

Honours the female side

This essence can help protect the feeling, sensitive, 'female' side of an individual, especially men struggling to be comfortable with their vulnerabilities and holding back emotions through fear. Whatever one's sexual inclination, Ladies Mantle helps give more understanding and acceptance of the feminine aspect.

LUNGWORT (L,F,H)

Energises auric field

Lungwort connects one with the life-force through the breath which can help re-energise the auric field. This process is gentle as it is in tune with the rhythms of the body and ideal for those of a delicate constitution. Useful in a spray.

MEADOWSWEET (L,F,H)

False persona

Meadowsweet is for those who are concerned about their public image and may put on a false, superficial front. They are usually popular, but their sweet and flattering ways are often a guise for control and an insurance that others will continue to like them. Keeping up a false persona can be so stressful that they often 'take it out' on those close to them. This essence helps balance out such extremes of personality.

ORANGE HAWKWEED (L,F,H)

Releasing blockages

This essence is indicated when negative emotional energy starts to affect the physical body. This can be the final result of long-term stressful issues or the immediate effects of shock, operations, accidents, illness, birth for mother and baby etc. Orange Hawkweed can also help clear the effects of negative psychic pollution as this can have a detrimental effect on the physical body. If you feel stuck and don't know why, treatment with this essence might prove beneficial as it can clear the body of old unconscious blocks. Orange Hawkweed can release the life force which brings an expansion of consciousness, clarity and a renewed growth. N.B. Used alone the effects can be strong, for sensitive individuals use along with other essences particularly blue flowers. Partners well with Lungwort.

PRIMROSE (L,F,H)

Lightness to one's inner child

Primrose is indicated when emotional childhood traumas inhibit personal growth. Melancholy and a deep unexplained sadness may be hidden away. This essence can gently nurture the inner child, give what is needed and open up a crushed spirit bringing comfort, hope and release. It's as if one can start anew – pure, unblemished and refreshed to life.

RAMSONS (L,F,H)

Supports the body's defences

By bringing white light into a sluggish, toxic system, this essence can help cleanse the body of toxicity, which if not corrected, can be debilitating and may deplete the immune system. This treatment can raise vitality levels and resistance to infection. Excellent as a spring cleanser, but also as a boost to the body's defences at the beginning of winter.

SCILLA (F,H).

Balancing energy levels

This essence is useful when undertaking work activities that create an imbalance e.g. too much head work, driving, etc. Helps one to be calm, steadfast and clear about what is needed to re balance the energy levels. Useful in spray around head area.

TRINE TREE (F,H)

Synthesis

A rare form of Hornbeam bearing 'leaves like the Oak' hence its latin name. This tree can bring strength and endurance when struggling to harmonise opposing aspects of life i.e. giving equal importance to the diverging needs of the body, mind and spirit. Supports health as it regulates all body systems during times of personal growth, crisis or stress.

VIPERS BUGLOSS (L,F,H)

Balances the love energies

Vipers Bugloss helps to re-align the love energies. When these are extremely out of balance people may become the perpetrator or victim of manipulative patterns in an effort to meet their needs. This flower can help dissolve the distorted patterns, which have become ingrained, thus helping the life force to flow more freely.

WILD DAFFODIL (L,F,H)

Appreciation of one's talents

Wild Daffodil is indicated when one's talents seem insignificant or do not appear to fit into society. This essence can help the recognition of their worth. Once they are used with this positive attitude they can blossom and grow with abundance.

WHITE VIOLET

Acceptance of one's spiritual self

This essence is indicated when one has a strong awareness of the spiritual side of life but through a fear of rejection, denies this aspect of the self. White Violet brings feelings of self-acceptance, truth and trust, so it becomes safer to be open with others. Useful in spray around crown.

Dosage Instructions

Dosage bottles. Fill a 30ml dosage bottle with spring water plus a teaspoon full of brandy. Add two drops of each chosen essence to the mixture and shake. Take 7drops three times a day, morning, late afternoon and evening until the bottle is empty.

Spray bottles. Put 5 drops of stock to 10mls of spring water in a spray bottle. Use as advised or when no specific instructions – as preferred. N.B. Use on skin.

SUN ESSENCE BODY SPRAYS

Most Flower Essences are ideal for topical use, in fact research suggests it is the quickest way to receive the full benefit of the essences as they are put exactly where they are needed. Apparently, once ingested the essence will make its way to where it is most required anyway with a certain loss of energy occurring in the process. Body maps for some sets of essences are available which can give suggestions as to where it is most appropriate to apply the Flower essence – or dowsing for such locations is possible. Applying essences to the chakra areas can also be an approach as these points are connected to all the energy systems of the body and provided the flower is applied to the correct chakra, it will be carried to where it is most required. Daily baths have always been the easiest way of using essences topically and 12 drops of the current treatment bottle to the bath is always recommended. Adding essences to body oils/lotions is another suggestion.

Sun Essences present some of their products for topical use in sprays, creams and oils, their effectiveness being well proven. The Protection Spray is designed for use in the aura and has been very successful. However where possible they are better used directly on the skin. The work on the set of Sun Essence Body Sprays for the Chakras is still in progress but research with the Hawthorn, Redwood and Snowdrop has shown them to be most effective and quick acting. Used night and morning while dressing they fit quite simply into the daily routine.

PINK AND WHITE HAWTHORN

Supports self love

Negative focus: Blocked heart energy – turmoil, confusion, anger, grief, etc. When the heart energy is blocked the result can be distressing inner turmoil. This flower essence spray can create an opening which can restore balance and inner stillness. From this space comes the courage to act appropriately and with self love. Spray directly on skin around heart area and work in with a circular motion. Use twice a day, morning and night.

REDWOOD

Resilience

Negative focus: Vulnerability, easily hurt by others, hooked into abusive situations, fear. Where extreme patterns of self-defeating behaviour create painful vulnerability. There is an inability to take care of oneself and feel supported in life. This flower essence spray can bring feelings of resilience and the ability to stay detached from others and in your own power. Helpful in relationships and supports commitment. Spray directly on skin around lower back and feet, two to three times a day.

SNOWDROP

Enlightenment

Positive focus: Cleansing and purification of blocked, numbed out emotions. Moving you to a place where you can start again. Gives new light on situations and initiates forgiveness and trust. Frees up energies, learning to hang loose and be more enlightened, open and creative. Beginning to hold personal power but being able to let go and connect in loving situations in a different way.

❀ UNITIVE FLOWER ESSENCES ❀

The Unitive Flower Essences are made in England and Wales mostly from indigenous wild flowers. Their fundamental purpose is to promote Unity within and between all levels, i.e. cellular, emotional, mental, whole body, subtle body, relationship and group; on the understanding that illness and dissatisfaction are symptoms of separation.

Maria believes each essence is subtly unique, being influenced by the maker, the flower's environment, planetary configurations etc. On this basis, many of the essences have been prepared in workshops by groups imparting an experience of group unity, whilst providing people with an understanding of particular plants, what flower essences are, and an experience of how they work. It follows, that as mother essences are renewed and consciousness develops, the Unitive Flower Essences will naturally evolve. A range of combination essences (including a trauma remedy) is also available for common 'everyday' experiences. All orders are made individually with the recipient/therapist in mind, to match personal need.

BITTERCRESS

The keyword for Bittercress is 'steadfastness'. This remedy is for people who are loyal companions, who stay with their convictions despite upheavals. These are admirable qualities but bring their own stresses usually in the form of pressure to give way (comparable to a great tree in gale force winds, unable to bend as a young sapling might). Along with these qualities may go a sense of being temporarily unsettled by strangers. Bittercress provides support during times of pressure, bringing inner strength and resilience, confirming one's inner conviction and lightening the sense of being 'weighed down'.

BLACKTHORN

For those who are unconsciously seeking support. Life may be experienced as burdensome, there may be deep feelings of resentment, repressed rage or outbursts of extreme anger. There is a sense of physical tension in the body as if creating an additional support structure to the skeletal system and this may result in back problems especially lower back. Blackthorn helps the recognition that it is not only OK but desirable to be supported by others and by the Universe and that in opening to receive we also give.

BLUEBELL

There are times in life when everything seems to be happening at once. This can feel tremendously exhilarating and/or dangerously overwhelming – a bit like riding rapids. There can be a sense of needing to be in control, which brings frustration, as usually events are moving so rapidly that we have no control and yet, there is another level of control which is required in order to be alert and open to all the experiences and opportunities. This brings a certain amount of inner tension such as a cat poised to leap, but the tension may need to be held over a long period. The whole situation can become quite stressful. Bluebell brings a suppleness to the experience – stamina without rigidity. It's soothing effect in high energy situations also makes Bluebell a useful remedy for over-exposure to the sun.

BORAGE

It is a common condition of Western culture that people fear not having enough and in particular not being able to provide themselves with what they need. There is a loss of trust in the Universe, family, community, environment that one's needs will be met. 'Modern' people live with an increasing sense of isolation where they cannot depend even on close family for support. Borage helps to open the mind to the experience of trusting that one's needs will be provided for. It brings about an increasing sense of 'togetherness', whether with family, friends, community, God or environment and can ease sore throats caused by the stress of not being able to ask for what one needs.

BRAMBLE

Some people go through periods in their lives when the force of physical or mental restrictions are so strong that they are unable to move – they feel debilitated. These restrictions may be imposed by rules, disability or fear, but whatever the limitation, there is a perception of not having any control over the boundaries, or room to manoeuvre. The sense of debility can be accompanied by resistance and struggle or resignation and laziness. Bramble brings a quiet strength, a freeing of the spirit, a sense of expansion which goes beyond the ordinary perception of existence.

BUTTERBUR

Being dependent on external events or validation is not a recommended route to happiness. It's more likely to bring frustration, resentment and an ever increasing lack of trust. Happiness can be viewed as isolated incidents brought on by external events, or a deep continuous undercurrent of inner well-being. Happy people tend to be very open and trusting; they derive pleasure from simple things and are slow to criticize either themselves or others. Butterbur helps to open the senses, to allow experiences of pleasure from sight, sound, taste, touch and smell. These 'gladden the heart' and open the way for an increasing sense of trust.

BUTTERCUP

There are times in life when there is nothing to achieve by 'doing'. It is necessary to wait – for events to unfold, for lessons to be learned. These periods of waiting can be frustrating and it takes great patience and insight to appreciate their value and intrinsic part in the process of life. They are a phase of transition, a period of seeming inactivity which can bring feelings of 'nothing is going to change', associated with a slump in energy and general despondency. It can be tempting to 'give up', to become disillusioned or to fight and attempt to provoke events. Buttercup facilitates a settled energy state whilst awaiting the next phase of development. It brings the qualities of acceptance and joy in the 'here and now'.

CELANDINE

Celandine people are alert; they are acutely aware of sensory information – like seeing a movement from the corner of the eye. But this can make them 'jumpy'/nervous. A high degree of alertness can bring a self-confidence and full participation in life but it can also come with fear and a constantly taut state of being. Celandine helps facilitate a 'relaxed' state of alertness, a poised rather than tense state of being, able to respond to changes in senses and details. This facility comes with an opening of the way internally and externally.

CHICKWEED

When there is a perception of frequently having to move from one environment to another, to adapt one's behaviour and deal with very different issues, a great deal of stress can arise, often manifesting as worry. Chickweed helps to integrate the different environments and needs, to bring the perception that all the environments are part of one larger whole. There comes an increasing sense of being part of a larger community where the self need not be divided and all needs are inter-connected.

COLTSFOOT

This essence comes up for people who 'don't get angry' or are not easily angered. This may be because they were told as children that it was unacceptable to express anger and any provocation will result in guilt, shocked silence or tears. It's as if anger is completely bypassed, almost obliterated from their experience. Anger is a valid emotion and can be expressed safely and respectfully. If it is never expressed or recognised it tends to become repressed and will often result in physical aches and exhaustion and a general numbness and sluggishness of the nervous system. Coltsfoot helps to free the congestion of past repressed anger in a safe way and allows for a freer expression of healthy anger and assertiveness thereby facilitating a sense of quality and will. This results in a release of associated physical problems and an increased alertness to the fast pace and rapid changes of modern life.

DAISY

There is a time to act and a time to be still, but it can be very confusing knowing which is which; one can feel frequently out of synch with events. Daisy helps those who have a fear of being still and it facilitates appropriate responsiveness, but most of all Daisy develops a trust in the connections of life.

DANDELION

Sometimes the difficulties of life can become so overwhelming that any joy or spark of creativity becomes lost. Life, or even one's own body may feel dirty.

Dandelion acts as a purifier; it clears a path through the turmoil, so that a love of life can be seen and felt even amidst the stress and destruction.

FORGET-ME-NOT

As the name says it is very easy to forget about one self – to become distracted by the needs of others. Forget-me-not encourages the user to take some time alone and to enjoy the release of external pressures. In so doing there will be a greater ability to think problems through and to focus on tasks despite sudden disturbances.

GORSE

Gorse is about endurance, knowing no fear and concentration. This remedy can help to strengthen these faculties in times of need such as undertaking a major task which requires stamina, fearlessness and singlemindedness. However, Gorse will also help to lighten up individuals whose life situations have required that they are permanently in this state which then causes undue stress.

HAWTHORN

Change is an essential part of the rhythm and evolution of life. For change to occur all aspects of our lives must grow be they thoughts, beliefs, relationships or life styles and sometimes this can involve letting go of deeply held patterns of behaviour, ideas, people or objects. Hawthorn helps one to understand the patterns of clinginess, or why one might 'hang on' to things. It brings patience which is necessary in the process of letting go as there may be set-backs. But in the letting go of the old Hawthorn also reveals the gifts which become available.

HEART'S EASE

As the name suggests there is a quality of easing the centre of our being with this remedy. More specifically, Hearts Ease helps in situations where one is over-indulging, be that with food or drink, self-pity, self-criticism or worry. Heart's Ease brings an ability to see situations more objectively and to facilitate self-nurturing.

LUNGWORT

In the process of change we learn new ideas and have experiences which bring new understandings. Sometimes when the old patterns are deeply ingrained it is easy to forget these insights. Lungwort helps to reaffirm lessons and new beliefs. It also supports situations where teamwork is required, helping people to work together and share pleasures.

MAYWEED

This herb has one of those smells that is verging on offensive and its healing quality is about opening to what at first glance (or smell) may not seem acceptable. All life is one, all aspects of life are part of the cycle of life. Decay is as much a part of the magic of life as blossoming. Mayweed helps those who feel tormented because they think they are unacceptable, or they are being subjected to unacceptable behaviour by others. It helps to bring a sense of trust.

NETTLE

There is a feeling of having been attacked when stung by a nettle and in the homeopathic tradition of like curing like so the Nettle remedy comes to the rescue in situations where a similar feeling of having been attacked is present. This feeling is often accompanied by feelings of having been knocked off one's feet – 'unearthed' – and of having one's energy 'scattered'.

Nettle helps to restore a sense of balance, enabling restorative action to be taken if necessary.

PINK CHERRY

This essence embodies the qualities of love. It specifically addresses problems some people have with perfection – often they are unable to let go totally into the experience of love because they perceive that they are not perfect. This remedy aids with seeing/accepting blemishes with love (not dismissing the whole for the sake of some damaged parts).

Pink Cherry facilitates the experience of 'oneness' where everything is equal and perfect and a manifestation of love.

PRIMROSE

Primrose is useful in situations where one feels out of one's natural environment. This can bring up feelings of confusion, paranoia and fear and a sense of being in a very confused and disordered environment. Culture shock would be a good example. Primrose helps to provide a sense of inner stability and therefore, aids decision making. It also helps with electrical disturbances in the mouth caused by amalgam fillings which are not part of the mouth's natural environment.

PURPLE COMFREY

This remedy helps people who acknowledge that they have self-abusive behaviour. This abuse may take any form from smoking, to self-denial to self-mutilation. Comfrey plays a fundamental role in herbal medicine and as a flower remedy it plays a fundamental role in self-acceptance and accepting mistakes. There are so many negative messages attached to self-abuse; Purple Comfrey helps to readdress the balance and allow some positivity and creativity to shine through.

RAMSONS

This remedy comes up for people who are having 'problems' with other people, perceiving that it is the other person who has the problems. In these situations it is useful for the person being treated to see how the external situations can be mirrored internally and provide information about the sense of separation within. Ramsons, therefore, aids in a growing sense of self-acceptance and self-responsibility.

RED CAMPION

There are times when we know that in order to move through a particular problem we must talk to someone else. Other times we may know that we are being affected by emotional problems but can't put a finger on exactly what the problem is. Red Campion helps in sharing problems and in the release of emotional problems at a subtle level (not necessarily verbalised or consciously recognised). It is also useful in coming to terms with what we might perceive as failure, i.e. accepting that we don't always achieve what we aim for – the prize may be in the path rather than the goal.

ROSE BAY WILLOW HERB

Another remedy for letting go letting go of the past, of old perceptions. A useful remedy for people who find themselves living in the past through reminiscing. Rose Bay Willowherb helps to move on – to see something familiar in a new way.

SELF-HEAL

Self-heal is appropriate for people who have 'their fingers in a lot of different pies' – giving their attention to many different tasks simultaneously. It feels a bit like juggling with a lot of balls and there is a sense that it is a bit too precarious and may all collapse. Self-heal facilitates a sense of ease with the situation so that there is an experience of smoothness and competence with lightness and fun.

SORREL

Sorrel grows in many forms depending on the conditions in which it grows. The energy of the remedy can match many characteristics; it is useful for those who recognise that their state of being has a tendency to be dependent on their external circumstances. They may feel out of control of their feelings – depending on who they're with or what arrived in the post they can experience wildly varying emotional states from day to day; for example adventurous, angry, vulnerable, worthiness, tenderness. Sorrel helps with the understanding that we are a product of our environment but that we are also self-determining.

SNOWDROP

Snowdrops are the first flowers associated with the beginning of a New Year and this essence was the first made in the Unitive range. It represents aspects of the underlying qualities of the remedies as a whole. Snowdrop facilitates group consciousness, supporting the fundamental aim of the Unitive range to promote Unity within and between individuals, be they cells, organs, people or groups. One of the main contributing factors to distress of any sort is the inability to see beyond the personal and/or individual. Illness, traumas, parts of the body, home, work, play, environment, family etc. tend to be seen in isolation of each other whereas every aspect of our lives and environment are interrelated and can be seen as a whole. A movement of perception from the individual to a wider understanding of the Universe requires trust and an inner peace – Snowdrop brings courage and tranquillity.

SPEAR THISTLE

The purple Spear Thistle has a beautifully lush and delicate flower head atop and surrounded by a formidable construction of thorns. Some people construct and energetically similar barrier around themselves to protect their inner being but this barrier usually causes a deep sense of separation between themselves and others. The barrier may manifest physically as an overweight body, or mentally as a very defensive attitude. The sense of separation can result in a deep unhappiness and lack of self-confidence. Spear Thistle works gently to bring a sense of trust and openness – that I can open my heart and still feel protected. As with Speedwell this issue is deeply rooted and will not be resolved overnight. Spear Thistle supports the intention and brings the experience of ecstasy which comes when the heart is open.

SPEEDWELL

Most people experience at some time a feeling of not wanting to return to ordinary life – maybe after a good holiday or course of study. There is a perception that doing the same daily routine for the foreseeable future will be dull and that nothing exciting will ever happen again. Speedwell lightens this perception bringing an understanding that by living in the moment we can carry a sense of anticipation and newness into daily routines. This is not a one off change in perception – it requires a resolution to change – Speedwell supports this. It is also a useful remedy for those who dislike the cold, which is a related issue in that part of the change in perception which comes with Speedwell is an acknowledgement of the rhythmic nature of life of which the seasonal changes are the most obvious.

TORMENTIL

There are times when a fundamental aspect of one's being rises to the surface and begins to assert itself – it can be seen as the child within asserting itself. This assertion can herald a change in one's being – a gathering of energies to create a new pattern, a new way of being. Tormentil brings a quality of strength and an ability to handle the shift which is being undergone.

VIOLET

Sometimes life can seem like an abstract painting; a collection of random events seemingly unconnected, a disconnectedness with the environment, meaningless sensual impressions. Nothing makes sense, has meaning or a flow of continuity. Violet makes connections, it transcends boundaries including time. With Violet there is a sense of connectedness with past, present and future, possibly an experience of communion with ancient beings and definitely seeing patterns in the Universe.

WOOD ANEMONE

Wood Anemone is concerned with the workings of the mind. It is suited to people who along with a difficulty in concentrating and absentmindedness are able to spot small but vital details. They may perceive the first two traits as being culturally undesirable (although not creating problems in their own lives) and this may bring feelings of insecurity. However, they often fail to recognise their minds are acutely alert in other ways enabling access to avenues not normally explored by everyone else. Wood Anemone supports these uniquely creative individuals.

WOOD SORREL

This essence is suited to people who undervalue themselves, comparing their lack of beauty, strength, character, intelligence or connectedness to that of others. But look a little deeper and they reveal a great strength of character when tested, a settled energy as in meditation and an innate trust in the Universe. Wood Sorrel brings a quiet confidence and self-acceptance.

YARROW

Counselling, psychotherapy etc. help to release the memories, experiences and trauma associated with oppression and violation, but they cannot obliterate or wipe out what has happened. At some point the experience must be integrated into the whole life experience. Yarrow helps with this integration bringing an acceptance of and a release or transcendence from the 'negative' states which initiated the process.

❀ WIGHT FLOWER REMEDIES ❀

All the flower essences here have been made at Ventnor Botanic Gardens or on the surrounding cliffs and downs. The essences presented here are not by any means all those which are available; they serve as a window so you can see how I work and maybe as an encouragement to try and trust your own insight. Some essences have already been outlined by Gurudas and Bach, which my work seems to support, though each plant, being an individual, has its own twist. The other essences are those to which I have been drawn by their sweet silent song. Included in chapter 9 is a clutch of combination remedies which is to be expanded. While I am making essences, the image of a woman is often portrayed to me; she in turn portrays information pertaining to the particular flower being used and you will find references to her in the text which follows.

AGAVE

Accidents, contrary to popular belief, don't happen and it was no accident that at the time I started making flower essences one of the Agaves in the garden started to flower. Because of the climate in the south of the island, especially on the cliffs where the botanic garden is situated, we are able to grow flora which would be killed by frost in other parts of the country. The Agave is a particularly amazing plant which always looks to me like many saw toothed sea mammals bursting out of the ground. It's life cycle is also amazing in that it can take up to thirty years to flower and then seeds and dies; some orgasm! This particular plant was about fifteen years old but had been moved twice in its life, not something a six foot wide succulent plant usually does. This in conjunction with the very hot summer, probably stimulated the flower. The flower spike itself terminated at about eighteen feet and was spectacular in its growth rate. The spike was so charged with energy it was interfering with the air around it. Emitting from it was a deep resonant hum like an organic power station. Being physically able to make the essence was a feat verging on a circus act. This consisted of me climbing a ladder, champagne glass of spring water in one hand, a pair of scissors in the other, supported by the front end loader of a small tractor and two bewildered but congenial fellow gardeners. Our efforts were not in vain. As I cut the first flower it slowly tilted its head towards the water, nectar flowed from it in a slow motion dance and joined the water in a spiralling embrace. The feeling I got at that moment was a beautiful release, like the kiss of the first light of dawn as it is squeezed from the womb of the night. The action of the plant was given to me concisely and clearly, it was so loud and clear that it was almost a shock: **strength in the face of adversity.** Here this reflects the life of the individual plant from which the essence was made, grown in an unnatural location, moved twice in its life and still finding the strength to reach its goal and ultimate expression. This combines with the Agave's attribute of patience as reflected in the life cycle of the species. This combination would be excellent to use with people who are rehabilitating after a long illness, accident or operation, or people who are weary of life's journey, those struggling to see hope for the future.

BELLADONNA

When I made this essence, 'my lady' had a long black cloak in which she wrapped herself. A pervading feeling of quiet introversion, a turning in to look inside and a calmness of mind. This essence could be used for people who are always giving out and never make time for themselves, also those who have trouble sleeping or relaxing. The darkness the cloak represents was not one of fear or foreboding but like the gentle blanket of the night sky calling for a time of rest with a soft, almost womb like reassurance. Over excitement and hyperactivity may also be an indication for this remedy. Hysteria too, but not the kind produced by shock as this may become too internalised.

BUDDLEIA

Buddleia was the catch I hauled in when I baited my mind with the idea of a shock remedy and cast it into the sea of the unconscious. It brought with it the images of war torn London after the Blitz, though it could be any city. In the rubble and devastation even in the brickwork that still stood grew the buddleia. It is one of the first plants to grow and take hold in such a barren site, offering hope, healing and reassurance. It can be used in all cases of shock and trauma, particularly in the cases of miscarriage and abortion. Not only can it be used when a loss has occurred, but being the butterfly bush, it feeds the wings of the life which is born of the transformation – as the saying goes – *"What is death to the caterpillar is birth to the butterfly."* This being so, it can also be used in cases of infertility in both mind and body.

COLTSFOOT

This plant had been calling me for some time, hard to miss its bright yellow blooms held against the dark earth and bare branches of a fading winter. The image I was given was one of my lady first with the flowers growing through her bare feet, then a large bloom over her face and finally she put out her tongue on which was a single flower. The first image is one of grounding, earth energy, getting your feet on the ground and stimulating the chakras there. The second and third images tied in together and are about expression, how we can express with our faces how we feel and how we can vocalise that. I was given the words "allows those to speak who have been held in the silence of winter". The flower on her tongue was definitely brought up from deep inside her allowing it to have expression. This is probably concerned with the past as the flowers come before the leaves and so utilise the energy of the previous season. This has the obvious use of allowing people to express suppressed feelings which are the precursors of many disorders, but also supports them in the process because of the grounding, earthing qualities. The essence can also be used for more simple maladies such as sore throats which often have the same root cause.

DAISY

Daisies have always been for me a symbol of childhood innocence, for summer days and daisy chains . . .why people wish to eradicate them from their gardens eludes me, why would they wish to poison a smile? The signature of the daisy is perfect for its use when unveiled. Each yellow dot in the centre is in fact a flower in its own right, each individual is brought together to form the whole; the perfect metaphor for all creation. The image I was given when connecting with the plant was of a telephone exchange, all the different lines coming in and getting connected. The essence can be used to bring many diverse energies or information together to form a coherent whole and understanding. When we are confused it is usually not because of information we don't have, it's because we need to put what we do have in order so we can discern the pattern. Making this essence gave me great joy, as do they all, but this one in particular was so strong I had little shouts of uncontrolled joy throughout the morning, much to the amusement of visitors to the gardens and staff members alike.

DANDELION

The summer of 1995 was long and hot, 'weeds' were not a problem. Great for a gardener, not so great for the dandelion hunter. My experience so far had taught me that the right plant was waiting for me on the day that felt right to make their essence. So it was that my search led me to an as yet unutilised part of the garden. This area had a seldom used, rough stone road which at one time had led to a farm. On walking up the road I came upon the only dandelions I had seen in a month. They were growing right in the path protected in the shade of a dogwood and wild rose. Their situation was the perfect metaphor for their action. They had set down their tap root in the hardest of materials and had pulled energy up and into the flower, eventually to be released by the wind as seed. This is how the essence affects us. It helps us release knotted energy in our bodies and minds. This action was compounded by these particular plants in that they had been trodden on and probably driven on, but had still been able to flower. Their situation too had been trodden on, as we tread on forgotten feelings until they become the calloused foundation for frustrated lives. The essence was later taken by my dearest friend. She found that at first it created an emotional turmoil because it was stirring emotions, feelings and thoughts that had lain hidden, but after a time this moved on to a state of directed clarity in which she was able to make choices about her life in the light of self honesty.

ELEAGNUS

It was not my intention to make an essence of this shrub when I set out into the gardens early one morning. I sat with the plant I intended to use but couldn't get a 'fix' on it. There was a silent voice in the way pulling me to another part of the garden. After a brief argument with it in which my ego lost abysmally (praise be) I let myself be drawn away until I found myself on a path which was lined with eleagnus, it's small white flowers enveloping me in their fragrance. My mind was drawn to the inner garden where my lady stood, her body completely covered in leaves, apart from her face and a tiny patch on her body. As I watched a single leaf came on the wind and patched the hole perfectly. She told me it was used to mend the outer layers, not so much the skin but the aura which would have a knock on effect on the skin. This reflects the plant as a whole which is used as protection in the garden for more tender plants and in exposed areas as it takes all the punishment that the salt-laden sea winds can throw at it. It would be of use wherever the aura has broken down by debilitating illness, accident, drug abuse, etc. It can also be used to help protect yourself when entering atmospheres of an unbalanced nature which you don't wish to absorb.

EVENING PRIMROSE

With this essence I had a very strong feeling of circulating energy in the area of my digestive organs. It stimulates the digestion through interaction with the solar plexus chakra and can help with disorders from indigestion to constipation. Emotions as with many things play an important role here; this was underlined by the image of a lake in a spent volcano surrounded by evening primrose on it's sloping banks. This would point to the calming of anxiety which often affects digestion through our fight or flight instinct.

MORNING GLORY

From my experience, choosing a particular plant to make an essence seems to honour it in some way. I've come to no firm conclusion as to why, maybe it helps to fulfil its own karmic expression. This action was particularly noticeable in Morning Glory. When I approach a plant I put my hands in amongst it and still myself to an alpha state. I then explain to the plant my intention and it usually reacts by indicating to me which blooms I am to use. In the case of this particular plant I went from one bloom to the next, each one graciously choosing to give the honour to the next flower. This carried on until in the end they chose a flower at the base of the plant which had a petal creased by the wind who did not feel good about itself. This honour it accepted with the same grace the others had shown in choosing it. The action of the essence reflects this support. It helps people who don't feel good about themselves or who have a low self esteem. These people tend to develop nervous afflictions such as stuttering, insomnia or habits such as smoking or drug abuse. So this essence can help in the breaking of such habits by addressing the root cause and offering support at that level.

PHORMIUM

Communication with spirit/higher self. Receiving and transmitting. Stimulates sixth and seventh chakras.

PENNYROYAL

This plant has a strong and forthright energy. When I first communicated with it I had to talk with it for a long time explaining my intention again and again. In the end the only way I could get it to trust me was to let it feel the love I have for it. This now seems obvious and is the way I work all the time, though at that point it was the perfect way for me to experience the plant's abilities. This is not a plant to be swayed by a door to door salesman and this indeed reflects its use as for displacement of negative thought forms. The essence can be used internally or and I recommend this, in a spray form. It seems to touch you like a fresh spring breeze after you've spent the night in a well used public toilet!

PETUNIA

My approach to this plant was at first tentative, though open minded, as it is not a plant which I would choose for my own garden. On first contact however, its approach to me was far from tentative. It came running at me tongue hanging out, tripping over its own tail, banging its head to bounce back up and keep coming. Enthusiastic about the game, but not sure of any rules. This was the first plant in which I noticed an energy change when the sunlight hit the water in which the flower was held. Though a willing participant, the plant didn't understand what I wanted it to do. This was so until the sunshine hit the water, when the flower's energy changed to a deep understanding and knowing, as if it was experiencing a meditative state. This then posed the question of the action of the essence. The power of the sun had brought the plant energy in line with its higher purpose, its higher self. This is the function of the essence. It enables someone experiencing this sort of puppy-like state the ability to see their actions from a higher point of consciousness and for them to be able to be directed in a more constructive manner. This essence, for instance, would be helpful to young people going through adolescence or to old people in a state of senility. I must admit, however puppyish, that after contacting their energy it's hard to resist putting my little finger in their flower, just for the game which I know they enjoy.

PINK YARROW

Pink Yarrow is one of the few plants I've had to look for. Usually they turn up unexpectedly whilst I'm walking or I know where they are in the gardens. As it is with life, the search for one thing reveals many other treasures on the way; the journey is part of the destination. The search for this one led me off the cliff paths laid down by 'authority'; the plants know how to draw me, the silent whispered promise, the glimpse of distant pink on a far bank, which turned out to be century, something which I would not otherwise have found. I was led to a place where the land has slipped and turned up so many new plants it was hard to find a place to sit without sitting on a jewel. On connecting with the yarrow, I got the image of an umbrella which reflects it's use as a shield against negative energy, particularly of an emotional nature. Feeling pleased with myself for finding and connecting with the plant, it had the last word and ticked me off for thinking I had found it when, of course, it brought me to it.

PRIMROSE

The simple primrose, a bunch with which I used to delight my mother when I was a child. This is unfortunately against the law due to over-picking and destruction of their natural habitat This memory being there, I have always had a soft spot for their delicate yellow blooms, though it was a friend's request that pushed the idea over the edge to the actualisation of making the essence. The energy I felt from the plant was like coming home to a warm embrace, it was the softest touch. My lady came to me with open hands, the blooms growing from the chakra points. A feeling of non-judgmental support, the kind you get from stroking a pet that loves you after you have had a bad day. The essence is all about touch, the hands and possibly the tear ducts. My friend who asked me to make the essence is a masseuse and found when taking the essence at she would pick up intuitive information about her clients problems and be drawn to particular areas of the body which would help the client release that energy. It would be useful for people who feel displaced to help them cultivate a sense of home. Sometimes all you need is a hug from someone who knows and loves you; this is what this essence is about.

RED POPPY

Poppy was a symbol presented to me before they bloomed and indeed before the idea of making an essence of them bloomed in my mind. The flower as a symbol was given to me when I was cycling. I'd asked for something to help me up a particularly steep hill and found the visualisation of this bloom gave me new strength in a physical and mental way to help me up the incline. It is this same energy that is held in the essence, one of vitality and strength. The image of my lady lifting dumbbells was a surprising and I must say amusing one, but it was none the less fitting. This is an uplifting essence, stimulating the base chakra and could be used for people of low vitality, either physically or mentally and people convalescing though not after heart attacks as it may be too stimulating. Athletes and those in training could also benefit and because of its base chakra qualities, those who need to manifest their thoughts into action.

ROMNEYA

Opening to higher self. Self beyond gender. Joy, gentleness and love. Enhances meditation.

SILVER BIRCH

This essence started life for me as a dream. It being one of my favourite trees and dreaming about making an essence of it, what else could I do? When I held the tree and asked to feel its energy, the trunk was swaying in a steady tic-toc motion like a pendulum; a steady pulse. It was about balance, but not a static balance, balance in motion, in time. This was tied with the tree's natural pattern of movement in time; it's like walking one foot first, then the next, an ever shifting balance that enables us to evolve. The image my lady presented was that of standing in a cruciform position, the tree growing up through her centre and up out of the top of her head. This too is symbolic of balance but I think more so in subtle energies as she was high in the air and her feet were not on the ground; this would indicate chakra alignment. The tree itself has male and female flowers which reflects it's balancing action. Most of the essences I make in clear glass, but with this particular one, because of the nature and energy of the tree, I made it in two halves of the same crystal geode. I placed the male flowers in one side and the female in the other, then mixing them together whilst decanting them. The essence itself would be useful for people with problems caused by unbalanced subtle energy rhythms which ultimately result in physical ailments.

SWEET PEA

Sweet Pea is an essence I found hard to link with, but this does not seem to be to its detriment. All I could get from the flower itself was that it seemed to be throwing a hood from over its head. It's use as often described is to stimulate the pancreas chakra and to help people come to terms with living in crowded conditions. I gave this essence to a very good friend who has had diabetes for over fourteen years. He found that it affected his pancreas in that it made it more erratic. He described it as like trying to start an engine that has been sitting still for a long time. He felt it would be more effective with people who had milder forms of the condition. At the same time he discovered things about his diet. Because of the diabetes he found he couldn't assimilate vitamin A from beta carotene, the only vegetable source of this vitamin. This is particularly important as he's a vegetarian. In light of this he has been drawn to look at nutrition in much more depth. He has unhooded the situation, much like the flower itself. Not only did he look at his body's nutrition, he also looked at his bank account's nutrition and found this needed a boost as well. He has now taken in a lodger and has come to terms with living in more crowded conditions. So be sure when taking this essence that you have a spare room available!

THORN APPLE

What a powerful plant, as if this wasn't already known. When I was asking about the action, the name Gabriel's trumpet flashed through my head. Sensations started in my abdomen and then went not quite to my ears but in front of them, this then went to my temples. There was an intense pressure there, it was almost uncomfortable, making my eyes wide open and a little starry. Through subsequent use the essence has revealed itself through it's signature. The seed heads are hard and thorny but when ripe split open reveal the new seed. This illustrates the action of the essence in that it helps people unlock their creative potential which may have been protected by psychological barriers put up in childhood, or past harsh experiences.

TOBACCO

Clears the body of nicotine. Helps people deal with dependency on all levels.

Chapter 9

Combination essences

❋ AQUARIUS FLOWER ESSENCES ❋

The Self Improvement Range

This range of flower remedies has been specially formulated for use by those of us who are involved in self-improvement. They can be used alongside any improvement programme or techniques to enhance the results we are seeking. They come in 30ml dropper bottles ready for use and will last 3 to 4 weeks when the standard dose of 4 drops 4 times daily is taken.

HIGHER SELF – ATTUNEMENT

The essences of Daffodil, Petunia and Lavender have been combined in this bottle to allow a greater assimilation of the higher self into the personality. All three have a powerful impact upon the crown chakra, opening us to the spiritual aspects of our being.

JOY

Five essences have been combined to dispel depression and let joy re-enter our lives. Mustard lifts the dark clouds, Borage warms the spirit. Zinnia promotes laughter and humour, Nasturtium brings us out of ourselves and Moon Star encourages us to reflect upon the darker moments so we can better understand the nature of our shadow.

PROSPERITY

The flower essence of Honesty and Moon Cloud aligns the mind to the abundance of the universe, thereby lifting our consciousness above the negative thought patterns centered around poverty and lack.

SELF – EMPOWERMENT

This combination addresses low self-esteem and weak will. The essences of Blackberry and Sunflower help strengthen the forces of will and raise self-esteem in a balanced way, allowing us to feel more in control of our lives. These remedies will also help in the manifestation of our desires.

SLEEPING DRAUGHT

A powerful combination of 4 flower essences to help all of us who seek deeper and more relaxing sleep; Passion Flower and White Chestnut help us mentally to prepare for sleep by letting go of the day. Morning Glory soothes the etheric counterpart of the nervous system and Forget-Me-Not stimulates the subconscious mind so tensions can be released through dreams.

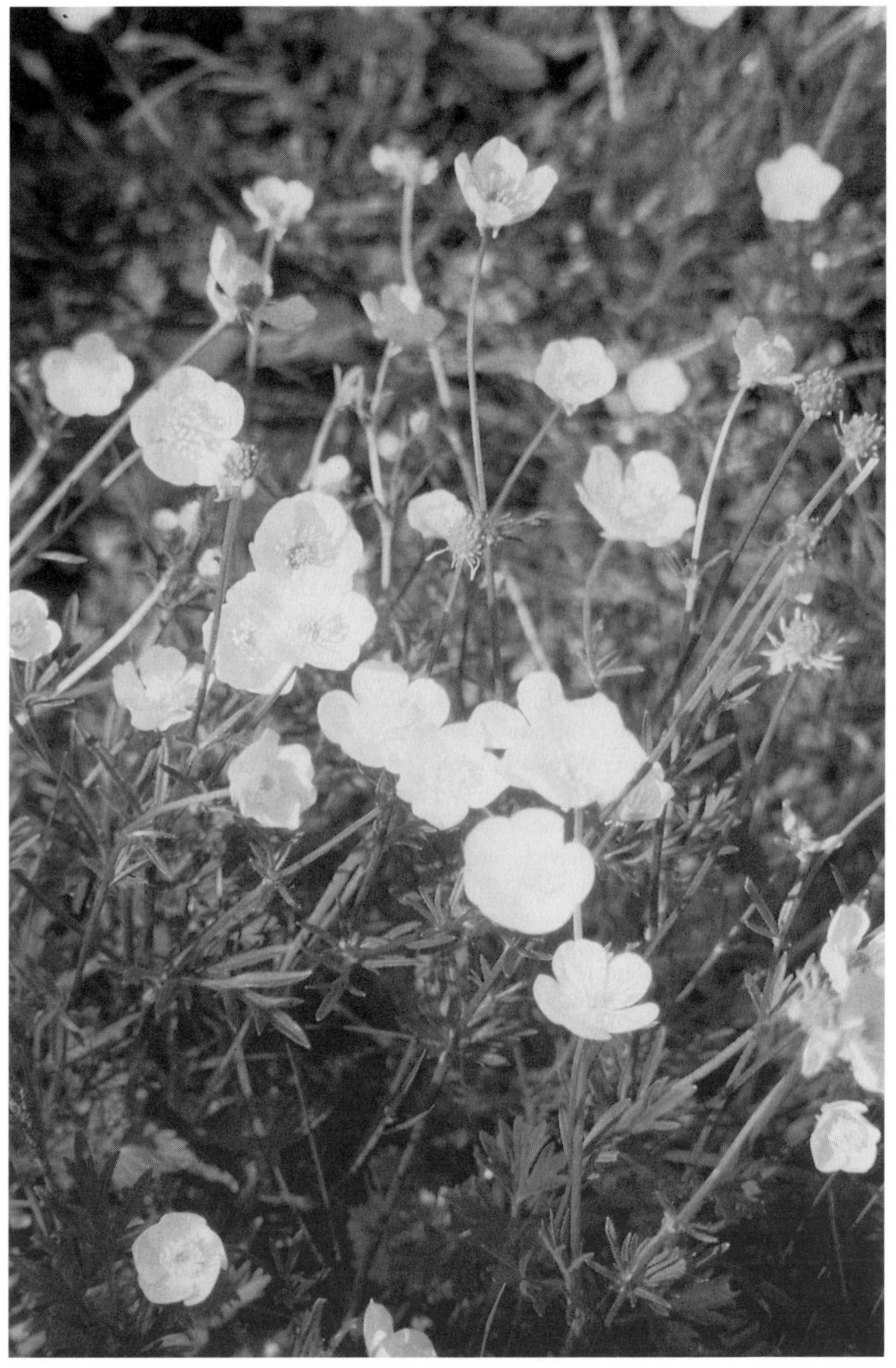

STRESS RELIEF

The essence of Vervain relaxes the over active mind, allowing us to get out of the fast lane and slow down. Dandelion relaxes tensions in the etheric counterpart of the muscular structure and helps us listen more closely to the needs of our body. Thyme alters our perception of time by lifting the mind on to the timeless or eternal plane of consciousness and is therefore an excellent remedy when there is too much or not enough time in the day.

ENERGY BALANCE

Each and every one of us requires balancing on some level, be it physical, emotional, mental or spiritual. Aquarius Flower Remedies have produced a bottle of seven flower remedies to do just this. Energy Balance is a combination of essences which work by aligning the seven major chakras of our auric field.

Contained in the bottle is a mixture of spring water and brandy with the flower essences of Comfrey, Red Dead Nettle, Sage, Passion Flower; Celandine, Nasturtium and Daffodil

❧ BAILEY COMPOSITE REMEDIES ❧

In the following list of essences, those made by alcohol extraction are marked with an asterisk (⋆) before the botanical name. The rest are prepared with the Sun method.

"CHILDHOOD"

Bracken (⋆) *(Pteridium aquilinum)*, Charlock *(Sinapis arvensis)*, Valerian *(Valeriana officinalis)*. This composite is for those who have, for whatever reason, become locked in childhood states. These hangovers prevent the person from fully blossoming in their adult life. These outdated states prevent the full mature adult personality from emerging and fulfilling itself in the world.

Bracken (⋆) is for those who have habitually played this "child" role in life. Perhaps due to parental or other domination whilst a child, the person was never encouraged when growing up, to take increasing responsibility for their life. Because of this lack of self-empowerment, they may try to assert themselves by acting the "child" role, being submissive but often subversive. This subversion is how many children get back at dominant parents. However, playing the subservient role inevitably causes deep resentments. These resentments, when not expressed openly, can lead to feelings of frustration, depression and toxic dejection. The person becomes like a volcano that never blows its top. Because of their inability to handle their own Fire energy, these people may fill with tears when spoken to harshly. The alcoholic extract of Bracken helps to dissolve the influence of these old childish states.

Valerian is the essence for the "lost child". This person may even look rather like a pathetic lost child that is in need of help and support. Instinctively one feels one's heart go out to them – they seem so alone and helpless. In reality, direct help is most likely not needed at all. Usually the original cause of the problem is that the person had a childhood deprived of true love. Although they may put a brave face on things, deep down they feel bereft and unable to love other people. They also know that something within them needs the love, support and encouragement that was previously not available to them. Valerian encourages the development of self-love and self-esteem. This tapers off the need for external support and so progressively reduces the demands placed on others.

Some people however are apparently quite happy to stay with their childhood states. Like Peter Pan, they do not want to grow up. They want to live in a world of make-believe where everything is good and everything is predictable. They tend to have a naive and trusting approach to life and so become prime targets for the world's "con-men". What is needed is for them to leave behind their attachment to childish ways, but without losing the openness of the child-like way of approaching anything new. For this the essence of Charlock is included in the composite. It helps us to see clearly what is really going on in the world around us, rather than what we would like to believe. It shows us that an adult approach to life can be infinitely more rewarding than the restrictions of childhood. Charlock helps to open the door to being a confident, competent, joyful adult with the knowledge that responsibility does not have to mean a heavy way of dealing with things.

"DESPAIR"

Blackthorn *(Prunus spinosa)* and Hawkweed *(Hieracium)*. This composite covers two rather different aspects of despair. The first is that of being in a frozen state with no way of escape, the second is that of being blown about with no way of stabilising one's being.

Blackthorn is for the first state – those who are in a black pit of despair. All seems lost, with both life and death having no meaning. Sometimes the person may feel that they are travelling through the "Valley of the Shadow of Death". This is the ultimate point of the "self-destruct" mechanism of the personality. It is the point where all our illusions have been shattered by the force of outside circumstances. Blackthorn mirrors this feeling with its sharp black thorns everywhere. Yet from these depths a completely new growth into a much lighter way of living is possible – leaving the old destructive ways behind. There is a dawn beyond the darkest night; it is only our fears that block us from seeing the light. The black pit may well have been generated by a strong Ego finding itself in conflict with the force of outside circumstances. It is the conflict between strongly held personal opinions and Truth, (as it is experienced in the person's life) that can finally precipitate the collapse into despair. The Ego can be so powerful that, rather than accept that the strongly held beliefs were incorrect, it will produce despairing or even suicidal thoughts. There is however, always a way out of this despair if the person will accept the challenge and acknowledge that a new way of living is possible. Blackthorn can help to ease the trauma of this change and illuminate the way forward.

The Hawkweed part of the composite is for despair caused by lack of self-confidence. This is not the Blackthorn pit, it is more a feeling of having lost touch with one's original roots. There may be a feeling of being lost in a hellish alien world. Those with particular religious beliefs could well feel that they have been damned and are beyond redemption. In this state there is a sense of being blown about by every wind of change, feeling that one has no means of resisting these forces There can be a total split in the psyche due to these pressures. In this case the personality can change abruptly if the person feels threatened by circumstances around them.

Hawkweed helps to re-establish links with the stabilising Earth energies. From this stable base things can be knitted back together, repairing the damage caused by the extreme emotional states that the person has experienced. In many ways Hawkweed helps the person to be reborn, with a greater sense of balance and wisdom. It can also be beneficial to give other caring and protecting essences such as 'Transition" and Milk Thistle. At a personal level, the unconditional love and support of others can form a vital part of the healing process.

"FEARS"

Betony *(Stachys officinalis)*, Mahonia *(Mahonia aquifolium)*, Greater Celandine *(Chelidonium majus)*.

This composite gets to the roots of many of our difficulties. Fears can inhibit a large proportion of our actions and deny us much freedom and enjoyment in life. Particularly deep-rooted fears operate unseen and often their presence can only be detected by their effects on our life. Deeply conditioned fears may relate back to childhood and the "Childhood" essence can then, with advantage, be given at the same time.

Betony is for unrecognisable and unidentifiable fears. These forces can make us feel unworthy, unloved or unwanted. In extreme cases such fears can drive people to contemplate suicide. These fears cut us off from recognising our own true worth. They may appear as fears of demons, devils, 'The devil within", the shadow side of one's own being. Freud saw the subconscious as a repository of negative suppressed impulses. He did not see that it is also the area of inner wisdom and light. What we need is to be able to compassionately shed light on those inner "demons" and then, see them for what they are – just old thought-forms that have no real substance. Betony helps one to discover this inner truth so that one can go beyond the traps of such negative thinking.

Mahonia helps to free us from the fear of our negative potential. It brings the fragrance of the divine into our life, enabling us to see that it is our fears that inhibit our spiritual progression – not a supposed "evil" within us. Mahonia brings the realisation that our fears are largely fictitious, products of conditionings and imagination. When the burden of fear lifts, there is a great release of the energy which has been held in by the negative thoughts. That energy will then activate unconditional love within the Heart Chakra, love that has been blocked by the fears of the past. A very uplifting essence.

Greater Celandine is for those who fear their spiritual centre. They have put up, however unwittingly, a mental block between themselves and the source of their existence. This can produce many different fears in the mind. There may be a deep-rooted fear of death, or fears of anything to do with the psychic dimensions of life. Fears of this sort may show as a tangled tortured personality. These people may be bitter and self-hating, or they may feel that they have a "mission" in life; perhaps to expose as frauds those people, however genuine, who have conflicting views. This essence has the property of gradually dissolving the inner barriers that have been erected, so that gradually and without opposition a pattern is established that will support the body and the mind. From this secure base inner illumination will then begin to grow, bringing about a total realignment of the body-mind-spirit unity.

"FIRST AID"

Star of Bethlehem *(Ornithogalum arabica)*, Ivy *(Hedera helix)*, Scabious *(Knautia arvensis)*. This is the essence of choice for sudden shock or trauma.

Star of Bethlehem is used as the basic shock essence, taking the initial reaction out of the system. This is vital in severe cases, as the shock effects may even prove fatal. It helps the mind to let go of the immediate traumatic experience and become more detached. This distancing "pulls the sting" from the experience and so greatly reduces the body shock reaction.

Ivy is used to give a strong rooted earth quality. This is necessary for severe shock, as otherwise one may space our' and lose one's contact with the world. Ivy also counteracts the "airy" detachment aspect of the Star of Bethlehem, helping one to root tenaciously into the world whilst remaining detached from the trauma. It brings vital stability to the mind-body system, giving it time to rebalance and adjust to the new situation.

Scabious initiates the healing process after the immediate shock has reduced. It brings a gentle ease, enabling one to accept what caused the shock without resentment or self-recrimination. It helps us to learn from our experience, rather than getting bogged down with any emotional reactions to the situation that caused the shock. Scabious brings ease and comfort and a feeling of inner love.

"GRIEF"

Sheep's Sorrel *(Rumex acetosella)*, Dog Rose *(Rosa canina)*, Yorkshire Fog *(Holcus Ianathus)*, Trailing St. John's Wort *(Hypericum humifusum)*.

All the plants come from Ilkley Moor, gathered in the early morning mist. It was originally created for a friend who suffered from deep shock on the sudden death of her husband. It has since proved to be very helpful in all cases of such separational shock – whether caused by actual death, or by the ending of a close relationship or the loss of a treasured possession. When someone has not been able to fully grieve after such an experience, this remedy can help. The affected person needs to be able to express their inner feelings of grief. They will then find it easier to accept the new changed reality that surrounds them. Grieving can also take place when something (object, event or person) that we have had an investment in, either fails, or is taken away from us. This is a natural human reaction to such occurrences. However, what is needed is for the grieving person to be helped through the process. This means that finally they will be able to accept what has happened, without resentment, anger or bitterness. After such traumatic events in our life, it is in the releasing of these negative reactions that we are healed. It is in these areas that the "Grief" essence can help. As there is often deep shock at such times, it can be very helpful to use the "First Aid" composite to lessen the immediate trauma.

These essences have always been combined to make a composite and are not available separately.

"OBSESSION"

Indian Balsam *(Impatiens glandulifera)*; Ragwort *(Senecio jacobea)*, Gipsywort *(Lycopus europaeus)*.

This essence is for those who have become locked in an endless looping thought. An obsessive thought is like having a constantly repeating tune in the head that will not go away. Indeed the more one tries to make it go away, the more it intrudes. We often feel that by thinking enough about the thought we will be able to resolve it. In the East they say "One cannot cure mind with mind". That sums it up. One needs to disconnect the endless loop so that it no longer feeds on itself. In this, "Obsession" can help. Part of the problem with obsessive thoughts is that they have a big emotional "kick" and can become addictive. This composite essence helps to lessen the craving for such an emotional stimulus. It helps to free us from the tyranny of obsessive thought processes. Once the mind quietens and becomes more detached we will see clearly how we became entangled in the first place and in that insight the entanglements automatically begin to loosen and fall away.

These essences have always been combined to make a composite and are not available separately.

"POSSESSION"

Lesser Stitchwort *(Stellaria graminea)*, White Lilac *(Syringa vulgaris candeur)*, Wild Mallow *(Malva sylvestris)*.

This composite essence is very helpful where outside influences are affecting our attitudes or behaviour. For example if we are under the influence of a very charismatic teacher, they may, without our realising it, have taken control of part of our personality. In a way we become, to a greater or lesser degree, puppets controlled by them. The same thing can happen with some love affairs. The key factor is that we have unwittingly surrendered some of our self-determination and self-control to that other person. What makes the whole scenario more serious is that such manipulation is often at the psychic level where it is far less easy to perceive. The fact that one does not believe in psychic phenomena does not prevent this from happening.

Perhaps more controversially, possession can take place by "discarnate" beings. These are the cases of "possession" that are sometimes reported in the popular press. From my own experience as a healer I can vouch for the fact that such cases do exist, but fortunately they are fairly rare.

In both cases the answer is the same – somehow we need once more to re-establish control of our life.

This essence is designed to help us regain our freedom of self-determination where we are no longer dominated or overshadowed by outside influences. If there is doubt as to whether one is dealing with obsession or possession, then careful questioning should reveal the difference. If the client talks easily about their problem then it is fairly certain to be obsessive thought processes – there is no "hidden agenda". If they become reserved and restive it is much more likely to be caused by possession. In this case the possessing energies will view such probing as an attack on their presence and thus react accordingly.

The things that possess us can be many and various. It may be attitudes and opinions that we have come to believe in. It may be that someone is trying to obtain a dominant position so that they can control our life. Or perhaps we have become so involved with our own possessions that in reality they now possess us, as we endeavour to hold on to them. What we need is to reduce our dependency on things and relationships. When that happens, what we truly need will naturally stay with us and the rest will fall away.

Wild Mallow helps to bring the hidden possessive tensions towards the surface where they can be seen. They can then be identified for what they really are and in that revelation they lose their power. It is as if this essence tightens us up inside so that what is affecting us can be expelled. Rather like wringing out a cloth, the negative possessing energies are "wrung out" by Wild Mallow.

The Lesser Stitchwort part of the composite acts in two ways. First, it helps to dissolve our emotional entanglement with the possessing energies. This means that as Wild Mallow brings things to the surface, they can then be dissolved with the minimum amount of reactive "back-kick". Second, it acts, like a guiding star, to illuminate the path ahead. It also gives us the insight and encouragement to follow that path as it opens up before us.

White Lilac essence helps us to transcend the past influences that have controlled and dominated us. It is the essence of new visions and new beginnings. It helps us to make contact with our true self and brings the peace that comes from disentangling ourselves from old negative influences. It brings a translation of awareness from what has been known before. In many ways it fills in the gaps that are left, as our old emotional entanglements ease away.

"TRANQUILLITY"

Heath Bedstraw *(Galium saxatile)*, Tree Mallow *(Lavatera aroborea)*, Fuji Cherry *(Prunus incisa)*.

As its title suggests, this essence is for promoting Peace and Tranquillity. It is for helping people to relinquish tensions and to come more into the present moment where fears and regrets do not exist. It is the essence for the over-active mind that just will not rest. This mind activity is normally due to one of two causes. Perhaps the person is locked in the past and is worrying about what they did or did not do. Alternatively they may be worried about possible future events over which they have little or no control. The many endless mind-loops that result can have very negative effects. These can range from the extremes of the "workaholic" (who hides from reality by being over-busy), to the "apathetic" (who has become locked in their own thoughts and does very little). It is the essence to choose in all cases where people find relaxation difficult. True relaxation is the state of calm alertness. This essence is not a "tranquilliser" in the normal medical sense. Its action is to help the person come into the present moment, instead of being too involved with things of the past or of the possible future.

We only become tranquil and free when we can work from the present moment, from what exists in the "now". It is our fears that arise from past actions and future possibilities that prevent that vital relaxation occurring in our lives. 'Tranquillity" helps us to centre more easily in the present moment, the "now". In reality, that is the only time that we ever have. We need to make the most of it

These essences have always been combined to make a composite and are not available separately.

"TRANSITION"

Single Snowdrop *(Galanthus nivalis)*, Spring Squill *(Scilla verna)*, Bistort *(Polygonum bistada)*.

Single Snowdrop is for those who are experiencing difficulties in breaking through to new levels of consciousness and awareness. It is the essence for the person who seems to have met a barrier or block on their path towards personal freedom. It may well be that old habitual patterns of behaviour feel that their existence is under threat and so they react in an attempt to remove that threat. The net result is that one's efforts are continually being subverted. There can also be reactions from increasing insight. Seeing things more clearly can, at first, give the impression that it is rather a bleak world that surrounds one (rather like the world which the snowdrop sees as it emerges in the winter). Single Snowdrop helps to reveal the joyful potential of a true and wider vision. Old identities can then be seen for what they really are – apparently comfortable strait-jackets! Single Snowdrop reflects the difficulties that many people face at this period of time. The transition to accepting one's spiritual nature, whilst remaining firmly rooted in the world, is not easy.

Bistort helps those who are at these major change-points in their life. At times of severe personal crisis people may arrive at a point where they may suffer from a "Nervous Breakdown". Their old ways of being are no longer working for them and they can feel very alone and frightened. This negativity can produce a "self-destruct" outlook where people may progressively withdraw from sources of possible help, even becoming suicidal. Bistort helps to support the energies at these times so that a possible breakdown can change into a "breakthrough". It helps to provide an "inner scaffolding" to maintain the basic structure of the personality and also provides loving support during the change processes. It is important to give positive encouragement to people undergoing traumatic changes in their lives. These times are like the pain of giving birth – in this case it can be the birth of a transformed way of living one's life.

For those who are breaking through to these new freedoms there is the need to encourage them to fly free after the old restrictions let go. There is immense joy in realising that one really is free, no longer limited by old ideas and concepts. At such times we may need support for our new found freedoms, yet family, peer groups, "friends" etc, may find our new way of being very threatening. They may well try nearly anything to oppose the changes. Their own belief structures may well feel very threatened by our breakthroughs. It can feel very lonely, flying in freedom, apparently alone.

Spring Squill, relating as it does to the Crown Chakra, can help support our change, even when we meet opposition from those around us. From the viewpoint of freedom, the world is then seen as it is; an amazing workshop for emerging souls. Spring Squill helps us to see more widely and more deeply into the true nature of reality. "Transition" is invaluable at times of breakthrough and "Rites of Passage".

"UNIFICATION"

Forsythia *(Oleaceae intermedia)*, Norway Maple *(Acer platanoides)*, English Oak(*) *(Quercus robur)*, Speedwell *(Veronica persica)*.

One of the greatest blocks to unification of the human psyche is that of trying to find a logical explanation to everything. This can mean rejecting facts just because they do not fit in with our particular model of the universe. Such people often have severe blocks regarding the existence of anything "spiritual" and so deny this essential part of their own nature.

Forsythia helps people to disentangle themselves from these restricted views and eases them into an acceptance of the spiritual dimension of life. This essence also gives support to those who are already on the path of self-realisation, bringing strength and comfort during all the twists and turns of personal growth.

Once we have accepted the spiritual dimension, we may still have difficulties in freeing up our consciousness. Norway Maple helps this to occur and enables the consciousness to move more easily between different levels of perception. This brings in the qualities of airiness and transparency and takes us beyond the restrictions of a too solidly "earthed" way of living. It is then possible to view our multi-dimensional nature with clarity and a lack of emotional reaction. In such revelation, any fear of death disappears, as death is then seen for what it is, merely a gateway between different levels of existence. Such a view is very comforting and stops us from taking our mission in life too seriously It is also helpful in promoting insight within meditation.

It is very useful to develop a quiet detachment in life. For this the alcoholic extract of Oak flowers is included. It stimulates a quiet inner strength and a sense of inner peace. It is as if we can then watch the world with quiet amusement, seeing, perhaps in amazement, just how seriously many people take themselves. It teaches us not to react against the world about us, but to act with freedom to the circumstances around us. We are therefore no longer imprisoned by old reaction patterns which can so often disempower us.

Speedwell is about increasing receptivity. It represents the "all-seeing-eye" of eastern philosophy, bringing insight in such a way that it does not seem like anything special – just another part of life. It is concerned with maintaining our equanimity within meditation so that we do not get emotionally involved with the insights which may be revealed to us. Speedwell enables us to open up to higher levels of consciousness whilst keeping both feet firmly on the ground.

"YANG"

Serbian Spruce *(Picea omorica)*, Yew *(Taxus baccata)*, Nasturtium *(Tropaeolum majus)*, Red Clover *(Trifolium pretense)*.

For balance, the Yang qualities in a person need to fulfill several different aspects. The fundamental property of Yang is concerned with personal power. It is about being able to make one's mark in the world; about going out there and doing things. It is strong, steadfast and protective. These qualities are represented by Serbian Spruce.

Yang can however become too rigid, it needs to be flexible yet strong. Without this ability to yield when necessary, Yang can become domineering and dogmatic. This weakens the organism and makes it vulnerable to opposition. To give this resilience and flexibility the essence of Yew is included.

When Yang needs to make adjustments in its view of the world there can be problems. "Male pride" is a typical reaction against accepting changes, even when those changes are wise and necessary. Nasturtium gives help and support during such times – Yang energy is much more vulnerable than its outgoing quality might suggest at first sight.

Because of this it needs to build bridges with the Yin energies within the being. This is vital for both men and women. It is essential that Yang becomes open to suggestions from the intuitive Yin, which normally sees a much broader picture of what is going on. Without such communication, there will be unease within the being and this will reflect into the outside world as unease in one's relationships with other people. For this aspect of the Yin-Yang partnership, Red Clover is included.

The Yang composite is therefore intended to assist the growth and balance of Yang energies so that they serve, rather than dominate, the being.

"YIN"

Larch (*) *(Larix decidua)*, Marigold *(Calendula officinalis)*, Delphinium *(Delphinium consolida)*, Honesty *(Lunaria annua)*. This essence comprises four flowers that mirror their counterparts in the Yang essence.

The alcoholic extract of Larch is concerned with female power. It is about intuition, feeling for what is going on underneath the surface. It is concerned with knowing how things are. It is also about love and compassion and nurturing. In its purest form it represents the Earth Mother. But this energy needs to be balanced or intuition can be replaced with make-believe.

Where there are difficulties or fears in opening up the Yin, Marigold can be of great assistance. It helps to unblock the power of the Yin energies and then support them In unblocking the channels, it paves the way for Larch to build on secure foundations. Marigold is therefore the opening-up and underpinning essence of the Yin composite.

Without guidance, the Yin insight can be narrow and shortsighted. In this it is like the Male Yang with its tendency to "tunnel vision". Such selective insight can prove to be disastrous. One needs to be able to see the whole picture. Delphinium is concerned with higher levels of insight and enables one to see things from a much wider perspective than might otherwise be the case.

The last essence is Honesty and this helps the Yin to form links with the Yang. In this it mirrors the Red Clover in the Yang essence. Yin can feel very threatened with the self-assurance of the Yang way of looking at things. Intuition, whether in men or women, is often subjugated because of the feeling that the self-assured Yang energy must somehow be right. This can happen repeatedly even though one's inner being knows that it is the intuition that is right. It is therefore vital that the Yin learns to understand the Yang but is not overwhelmed by its outgoing energy.

Note on Yin and Yang essences

The purpose of these two composites is to fully integrate the Yin and Yang qualities that they can grow and develop together. This forms what has been called the alchemical marriage, where neither energy is predominant. This inner harmony will reflect into the outside world, transforming our relationships with other people. We will then no longer be seduced into playing power games at sexual and personality levels. The strength and balance of the Yin Yang partnership brings both self-empowerment and ease into our life.

❀ CHURCH FARM ROSE ESSENCE ❀ COMBINATIONS

Seven combination remedies made from the essences of old roses, grown and prepared at Church Farm house, an old cottage in a tiny Herefordshire hamlet. Each combination covers one of the main bodily systems and one or more of the stages of life and life movements from birth to death. The seven combination remedies support physical, emotional and spiritual well being. These essences are preserved in a vegan base cream to be applied and massaged into the skin.

BIRTH AND RE-BIRTH – ROOT CHAKRA

Essences of: Alba Maxima, Sweet Juliet Mary Rose and Isphan.

A remedy for pregnancy and birth. Adjustment to parenthood and for the new born to bond with parents. Physically relating to both the male and female reproductory systems. Emotionally helps bonding between parents and child and restores balance during any of life's major changes such as puberty, menopause, marriage, divorce and moving house. Spiritually, helps align to the earth energies and for those who find it difficult to stay grounded, also awakening the sense of the Divine Mother within.

CHANGE AND ADJUSTMENT – HARA CHAKRA

Essences of: Pilgrim, Cadfael Louise Odier; Swan and Centifolia.

A remedy for those undergoing life's changes, puberty and the inner child and all the stages of metamorphosis and all traumatic changes. Helps decision making and recovery from physical shock. Physically it relates to the nervous and the digestive systems. Emotionally gives strength, confidence and clarity during times of growth. Spiritually helps one adjust when going through difficult times on the higher journey.

PROTECTION AND HARMONY – HEART CHAKRA

Essences of: Louise Odier; Isphan, Mary Rose, Fishermen and Cadfael.

A remedy for those going through confusion and conflict. Physically it relates to the heart and lung cycles and the blood and immune systems. Emotionally related to all forms of Love, sacrifice and forgiveness. Spiritually opens the heart to acknowledge life's higher purpose.

PURPOSE AND STRENGTH – THROAT CHAKRA

Essences of: Centifolia, Gallica, Sweet Juliet and Alexander.

A remedy for helping those who have difficulty in expressing themselves who feel suppressed. Physically helps with hyper-activity and palpitations, relates to the throat and thyroid.

Emotionally it helps with confidence, depression, anxiety and oppression. Spiritually helps realisation and activation of life's higher purpose.

ANGER AND PAIN – BROW CHAKRA

Essences of: Centifolia, Mary Rose, Pilgrim and Cadfael.

A remedy for those who feel frustration and restriction and who are being prevented from moving forward by strong destructive emotions. Physically helps with all forms of cancer and stress soothing the worried brow. Emotionally helps those suffering from frustration, abuse and injustice. Spiritually it brings awareness of the Divine Light.

RELEASE – CROWN CHAKRA

Essences of: Evelyn, Pilgrim, Isphan, Louise Odier, Swan.

For those who find themselves stuck in a rut and finding difficulty in letting go. Physically related to the bladder, kidneys, skin and bowels. Emotionally helps release suppressed fear. Spiritually helps surrender to the Divine Will.

TRANSMUTATION AND AWAKENING – SOLAR PLEXUS CHAKRA

Essences of: Swan, Church Farm, Mary Rose and Claire.

A remedy to give strength during times of stress such as leaving home, becoming independent, learning to accept ones own strength and power. Helps develop individuality, calming fears and comforting loneliness at times of separation and loss. Physically associated with the liver and spleen and the eyes and head, helping headaches and migraines. Emotionally for anger and resentment and fears associated with separation and loneliness. Spiritually awakening to self realisation.

CRYSTAL HERBS

CHAKRA ESSENCES

These chakra essences are combinations of flower and gem/crystal energies, made through the traditional sun potentisation method using all the elemental forces and the healing power of love.

As the combinations are taken, one may experience a release of old patterns, emotions and fears etc. By visualising or thinking of the colour violet surrounding one's body night and morning, or by calling upon the Angels of the Violet Flame, one can help transmute any misqualified energy the chakras are casting off.

These special combinations are working to clear, open, balance and align the chakras.

HIGHER CHAKRAS Silver, Green Jasper, Convolvulus, Lavender.

CROWN Gold, Sugilite, Lotus, Queen Anne's Lace.

BROW Diamond, Amethyst, Petunia, Nasturtium.

THROAT Lapis Lazuli, Aquamarine, Bluebell, Snapdragon.

HIGHER HEART Rubellite, Sapphire, Rosa de la Hay, Ipomoea.

HEART Ruby, Emerald, Bleeding Heart, Rosa Deep Secret.

SOLAR PLEXUS Pearl, Moonstone, Buttercup, Rose of Sharon.

SACRAL Carnelian, Clear Quartz, Calendula, Squash.

BASE Smoky Quartz, Black Tourmaline, Looestrife, Poppy.

FEET Boji Stone, Bo, Passion flower, Loosestrife.

❄ FINDHORN FLOWER ESSENCE COMBINATIONS ❄

In these combination essences the specific properties of the individual essences have been highlighted in the way they work together to compliment and reinforce the whole.

CLEAR-LIGHT

Broom, Wild Pansy, Birch, Scots Pine, Rose Alba and River Findhorn.

The Clear-Light combination brings about a peaceful state of mind, mental clarity and brightness, which greatly aids in meditation. When heart, body and mind are still and aligned, a clear channel is created whereby the intuition, Higher Self and Higher (or Universal) Mind can be contacted.

Through highest aspiration one can receive inner guidance and help from the Spiritual World and live life in accordance with one's purpose and the Divine Plan.

Broom stimulates mental clarity and concentration.

River Findhorn helps to connect with the Source, freeing the self from personality limitations.

Wild Pansy enhances receptivity and the flow of higher wisdom into the heart.

Birch brings light to the mind and clarity of inner vision.

Scots Pine increases the ability to listen, receive inner guidance and find directions in life.

Rose Alba facilitates the positive, active expression of the guidance received.

FIRST-AID

Scottish Primrose, Thistle, Bell Heather and Daisy.

A soothing combination offering immediate relief in any crisis. Used in cases of stress, trauma or shock on the physical, emotional or mental level, it can help to relieve associated fear and aid in the release of tension and pain.

Daisy brings feelings of calmness, protection and centredness.

Scottish Primrose helps to anchor the life energy in the heart and promotes relaxation and feelings of peace and love.

Bell Heather is stabilising, fostering trust and self-confidence.

Thistle gives courage to take positive action in facing any difficulty or emergency.

HOLY GRAIL

Lady's Mantle, Globe-thistle, Balsam and Rose Alba.

Holy Grail essence enables us to contain and embody spirit in our physical form, hence able to share it with others. We are empowered to empty all that is unreal from the chalice of our being and to integrate and harmonise our physical, emotional, mental and spiritual bodies, bringing them into alignment and synthesis.

When we are attuned on all levels – body, mind and soul – our essential nature is revealed and we become a vessel for the holy spirit.

Lady's Mantle brings awareness of the infinite knowledge and wisdom available to us through the cosmos.

Globe-thistle helps us willingly sacrifice non-essentials in our quest for wholeness.

Balsam allows us to experience love and acceptance of the physical bodies we have chosen to incarnate into as souls. We feel fully present in the world and express love and intimacy in all our relationships.

Rose Alba is the essence of positive outgoing creative expression, allowing us to reflect the power of our true nature in words and action.

KARMA-CLEAR

Birch, Rowan, Holy-thorn and Snowdrop.

This combination aids awareness of the karmic causes of life's predicaments and ailments. Through foresight of future and understanding of past, the cause of suffering is illuminated and attachments which bring about pain, unhappiness and dis-ease may be released. Birch helps to gain insight into the past and future, enabling understanding of the cause of the problem.

Snowdrop gives new hope and facilitates transition into the light through surrender and detachment.

Rowan releases resentment and pain and heals old wounds. It supports the ability to forgive one's self and others.

Holy-thorn opens the heart to love, acceptance, compassion and understanding.

LIFE-FORCE

Gorse, Sycamore, Elder, Valerian and Grass of Parnassus.

Life Force is an excellent combination to help overcome tiredness, apathy and burn-out. It revitalises and strengthens immunity and generates vibrancy and energy.

Gorse brings vitality, enthusiasm and joy.

Elder stimulates the body's natural powers of rejuvenation and renewal.

Sycamore helps to tap into the inner reserves of strength.

Valerian serves to lift the spirits and to rediscover delight and happiness in living.

Grass of Parnassus increases the ability to receive and transform the energies which are available from the universal source.

REVELATION

Stonecrop, Snowdrop, Holy-thorn and Hazel.

Revelation essence facilitates inner change and transformation. As limitations are transcended, it opens the way to a fresh flow of inspiration that restores the inner vitality needed to move forward. Through revealing the mystery of surrender and the highest personal unfoldment of the vision, comes understanding, acceptance, detachment and freedom.

Stonecrop helps to maintain inner stillness whilst in the process of breaking through inertia and resistance to change in the face of imminent transformation.

Snowdrop allows willing surrender to finding the eternal inner light that illuminates the darkness. It brings hope and the ability to behold new vistas.

Holy-thorn opens the heart to love, acceptance, compassion and understanding.

Hazel embodies the spirit of the future. It helps us to let go of the past without grief and inspires a new vision of full creative potential.

SPIRITUAL MARRIAGE

Apple, Holy-Thorn, Mallow and Sea pink

This combination facilitates the integration, control of fluidity and syntheses of the dualities found in every human being – between head and heart, mind and love, will and wisdom, male and female. Stability and balance between the pairs of opposites, achieved through the qualities of cohesion, harmony, expansion and union, releases the potential, freedom and joy of right relationship.

Apple frees the creative willpower.

Holy-thorn opens the heart to love and intimacy and to the expression of the true self.

Seapink brings harmony by balancing the energy flow between all energy centres.

Mallow assists right relationships by the graceful fusion of head and heart, mind and sentience.

❀ GREEN MAN TREE ESSENCE COMBINATIONS ❀

*"THE FOREST ESSENCES"These essence combinations are made from the energy vibrations of particular trees, flowers and wavelengths of light. Initially, they were created to give therapists an effective tool with which they could quickly re-establish balance in their patients' energy state, so allowing much deeper healing work to be safely accomplished.

These essences have been found to be very effective as 'first aid' after stress or trauma – be it physical, emotional, mental or spiritual.

Walking in nature – even a garden or a park – is a relaxing and calming experience. It is so natural we rarely examine what is actually happening in these circumstances. We simply feel refreshed and re-energised. In a similar way each of these essence combinations can be understood as a very particular 'forest walk' which acts on your subtle energies through the types of trees growing around you, the flowers you see and the quality of light falling through the leaves and vegetation.

1. "MERIDIAN ENERGISER"

Developed to help rebalance all 14 major meridian flows in the body. This can be used in post-trauma or shock conditions as first aid and will benefit anyone who is feeling 'out of sorts', for whatever reason. It has been specifically used to prevent the effects of jet-lag. This combination can be used as a tonic to maintain balance of energy.

2. "ENERGY FLOW'

Helps to stimulate the distribution of nutrients and hormones to all the cells of the body. Acts with the lymphatic system to help remove toxins and maintain the effectiveness of the immune system.

3. "STRESS RELEASE"

Stress and tension which has built up over time tends to get locked in the physical body as muscle tension which can reduce efficiency of organs and blood supply. This combination helps to improve the flow of energy in these systems that monitor and regulate stress levels in order to restore normal functioning.

4. "CELLULAR REKINDLER"

A combination to activate and balance very deep energies in the body. There are said to be forty three electromagnetic circuits, that circulate deep in the body tissue. Where there is chronic fatigue, spinal problems, chronic debility and nervous disorders, this combination may help to re establish health promoting energy levels.

5. "STRENGTH"

To encourage sense of personal integrity and validity. For when we feel overwhelmed, lacking in power, unable to achieve success. Increases amount of life-energy available. Activates true potential as individual, self-sufficient beings.

6. "FORGIVENESS"

Encourages happiness and the ability to react out of love and forgiveness. Reduces unhappiness, rage, fury and wrath. The ability to transform a situation in a creative, positive manner – turning self-righteous indignation into a self-creative resolution.

7. "ASSUREDNESS"

Encourages confidence, inner direction, peace and harmony. Counters panic, restlessness, impatience, frustration and sexual indecision and insecurity. Can also be useful for facing fears and phobias.

8. "SELF-WORTH"

Encourages self-worth, humility, tolerance and modesty. When we are sure of our own 'right to exist' it becomes much easier to release the negative patterns of guilt, disdain, contempt, pride, intolerance and prejudice. For all 'bad, dirty and useless' children. If you are absolutely sure you don't need this combination, look again!

9. "TRANQUILLITY"

When there are anxieties about the future this combination will increase confidence and a true sense of security and tranquillity. Contentment and assurance replace the 'black hole' feelings of disappointment, bitterness, greed, disgust and the sense of emptiness.

10. "RELAXATION"

Helps to release us from the failures of the past. The catalogue of our perceived inadequacies – summed up by feelings of regret, remorse, jealousy, sexual tension, stubbornness depression, despair, hopelessness, grief, loneliness and solitude – are gently replaced with a sense of relaxation on all levels, generosity, hope, feelings of elation and lightness.

11. "JOY"

Helps to counter anger, sadness and sorrow by encouraging love, forgiveness and joy. Increases the ability to appreciate and to be appreciated.

❀ HABUNDIA FLOWER ESSENCE COMBINATIONS ❀

CRISIS COMBINATION

Red and White Valerian. For any crisis, shock or trauma. Soothes, calms and centres and allows healing to take place.

CITY COMBINATION

Honesty, Yarrow and Wild Rose. For those living in the city, this combination guards against heavy energies and negativity. Keeps one in harmony without the need to close down one's sensitivity.

VIOLET FLAME

Thistle, 5-leaved Red Clover and Pennyroyal. For works of purification and transformation.

MALE COMBINATION

Sunflower and Water Forget Me Not. The sun does not only produce the golden orb, but also the blue sky. Thus the true male also encompasses the gentle female quality. This essence eases the fear that causes the male ego to react and allows a true radiance and enthusiasm to be expressed, with confidence, clarity and gentleness. Purifies the male expression and tempers the ego.

FEMALE COMBINATION

Black Tulip and Dwarf Elder. Just as the Sun is not complete without the blue sky, the Moon must be balanced by the velvet night sky. This combination consists of silver and indigo. Women are often most damaged in the third eye and base chakra, the former being concerned with clarity, originality and honouring one's own creative perception, expression and vision, regardless of outer pressures to conform. The base chakra is concerned with creativity and self-worth. This combination opens the full female creativity and vision and prevents negative conditioning from the environment.

These two combinations truly spiritualise and perfect the male and female energies.

❀ HAREBELL REMEDIES ❀

ACCEPTANCE – Dandelion, Heather, Marsh Woundwort, Plantain, Sage.
It Is good to change things when we can but in many situations acceptance is a better option. Dandelion for physical relaxation, letting go of all that stress and tension. Whatever we are afraid of Heather gives the courage to face it. Marsh Woundwort is healing where old worries from the past are involved. Plantain turns a grudging acceptance (resignation) into a more positive grounded strength. Finally, Sage awakens a higher self who does not take anything too seriously.

ADDICTIONS – Borage, Chamomile, Forsythia, Hyssop and Red Clover.
This combines Borage for courage and a great tonic, with Chamomile to calm anxiety. Forsythia helps to balance energy levels and Hyssop is an emotional purge. Red Clover adds something for shock and to prevent panic reactions. A mixture

which hopefully will help us stop whatever it is we do not really want to be doing.

MEDITATION – Flowering Currant, Lady's Mantle and White Narcissus.

Flowering currant warms and opens the heart, expands and softens the breath. Lady's Mantle calls for protection and inspiration and White Narcissus helps in letting go of self conscious thoughts. A lovely combination bringing openness and trust.

PHYSICAL TRAUMA – Bluebell Chamomile, Cornfrey and Red Clover.

Bluebell cools, Chamomile calms, Comfrey repairs and Red Clover deals with the shock. A combination which is great after any injury, or operation. (Works well with children and animals too.)

RESISTANCE BUILDER – Jasmine, Pansy, Saint John's Wort, Self Heal and Yarrow.

For building strength and immunity. Jasmine, a stimulant, helps to process and eliminate. Pansy is a great strengthener. Saint John's Wort heals and protects. Self Heal encourages taking control of our own healing and Yarrow strengthens the aura. Use as an emergency protection or as a course of treatment for anyone feeling low or 'run down'.

STRESS RELEASE – Chamomile, Lavender, Red Clover, Sage, Self Heal and Yarrow.

Chamomile calms anxiety and soothes fear. Lavender helps balance emotions and ease conflicts. Red Clover lessens panic reactions. Sage discourages being over serious. Self Heal for taking control, being proactive. Yarrow as protection. Use as a 'rescue' remedy when feeling stressed or as a course of treatment for the nervous system.

TRAVEL ESSENCE – Potato, Speedwell and Yarrow.

A useful combination for any journey. Potato calms down excitement, Speedwell clears the way for new directions, moving with ease through changes, crisis and crossroads. Yarrow to protect from negative influence along the way. (Another good one for children and animals.)

UPLIFT – Bluebell, Daffodil, Hyssop, Primrose and Sage.

Use against depression and low self esteem. Joyful grounded Bluebell and sunny open Daffodil combined are enough to chase away anybody's blues. Hyssop also has a tonic effect. Primrose and Sage gently and humorously to lighten and enlighten.

❋ THE LORD AND LADY FLOWER ESSENCE ❋ COMBINATIONS

INTUITIVE – Ivy, Eyebright, Purple Loosestrife, Tree Mallow, Lady's Smock.
Helps to increase and develop intuitive abilities.

SPIRITUAL – Tulip, Purple Looestrife, Lady's Smock, Eyebright, Holy Thorn.
Helps to bring spiritual qualities into every aspect of one's life.

NATURE SPIRIT – Cowsllp, White Foxglove, Hazel, Thyme.
For attuning to nature spirits and devic forces.

CITY STRESS – Ivy, Red Clover; Stinking Hellebore, Yarrow.

For helping to release stress and stay centred in the fast city environment.

HEAD – Marsh Orchid, Marsh Marigold, Red Clover, Yellow Flag Iris.

For clearing the head, negative thought forms, head stress etc.

HEART – Bugle, Primrose, Tulip, Wild Rose.

For connecting to heart centre and expression of heart in everyday life.

EMOTIONAL – Calendula, Daisy, Forsythia, Lady's Smock, Rosemary, Yarrow.

For stabilising emotions and emotional release.

CLEANSING – Lungwort, Rosemary, Stinking Hellebore.

Cleansing of energy systems and body – good for fasting.

GROUNDING – Ivy, Yarrow, Yew.

Brings soul back to body in times of shock, trauma etc.

CHAKRA – Purple Looestrife, Eyebright, Lungwort, Tulip, Chamomile, Calendula, Ivy.

Balances the chakras.

❀ MIDDLE EARTH COMBINATION ESSENCES ❀

UNICORN ESSENCE

Helps attune to the enchanting and magical state of higher awareness, symbolised by mythological beings such as the unicorn.

Scarlet Pimpernel, Pink Campion, Daisy, Buttercup, Forget-me-Not, Elder, Tormentil.

VISUALISATION MIXTURE

Calendula, Lotus/Deep Pink Rose.

MEDITATION MIXTURE

Fennel, Lotus.

CREATIVE MIXTURE

Pear, Iris.

MASSAGE MIXTURE

Dandelion, Lilac, Lotus and/or Zinnia.

❀ OGHAM IRISH TREE ESSENCES ❀

Ogham Oils and Essences are based on the Ogham alphabet which is a Celtic system of knowledge of the philosophy, language and medicine of the sacred trees. In olden days, the symbols of the Ogham were written on the stones and carried the profound meaning of this ancient medicine. Through a number of intuitive processes and experiences as well as her work with complementary therapies, (reflexology and colour therapy), Roisin Carroll was able to decipher the deepest meanings of the Ogham and develop the oils and essences based on her discoveries. Thus, the resulting products work on the subtle bodies as well as on the physical level. She has identified and created oils and essences from 40 different trees. There are also compounds of three different oils and essences for each of the ten systems of the body. The oils and essences are available as complete sets or individually.

CIRCULATORY SYSTEM

Honeysuckle, Spindle, Vine

Imbalances: Angina, blood pressure disturbances, heart problems, palpitations, phlebitis, poor circulation, thrombosis, varicose veins: Heartache, not allowing love to flow.

Characteristics: Centredness, Love, Nourishment.

Affirmation: 'I allow love to flow freely through me'.

LYMPHATIC SYSTEM

Hazel, Willow, Hawthorn

Imbalances: Blood poisoning, catarrh, flu, glandular fever, mucus in the system, oedema, swollen glands, tonsillitis, varicose veins: Holding onto the old.

Characteristics: Intuition, Empathy, Cleansing.

Affirmation: 'I release that which no longer serves me'.

RESPIRATORY/SKIN SYSTEM

Elder, Ivy, Ash

Imbalances: Asthma, bronchitis, chest infection, emphysema, hay fever, laryngitis, phlegm, pleurisy, sore throat, whooping cough, acne, boils, eczema, ringworm, shingles, skin problems, warts, ear problems, loss of sense of smell: Unable to change with life.

Characteristics: Change, Freedom, Universal Truth.

Affirmation: 'I breath life easily. I speak my truth. I am protected'.

DIGESTIVE SYSTEM

Sycamore, Oak, Beech

Imbalances: Appendicitis, colitis, cold sores, constipation, diarrhoea, diverticulitis, flatulence, gallstones, hernia, indigestion, malabsorption, ulcers: Not taking in life's lessons.

Characteristics: Confidence, Endurance, Tolerance.

Affirmation: 'I let go of old patterns and absorb Life's lessons with wisdom and joy'.

MUSCULAR SYSTEM

Birch, Alder, Sloe

Imbalances: Cramps, frozen shoulder, immobility, lack of energy, lumbago, muscular aches, muscular atrophy, pulled muscle, rheumatism, sprains, stiffness: Stuck in a rut, trapped energy.

Characteristics: Expansion, Expression, Acceptance.

Affirmation: 'I move forward with ease and grace'.

SKELETAL SYSTEM

Holly, Horse Chestnut, Blackthorn

Imbalances: Arthritis, back problems, broken bones, fractures, scoliosis, skeletal problems, slipped disc: Stiffness in mind and body, feeling unsupported.

Characteristics: Strength, Self-Discovery, Surrender.

Affirmation: 'I am supported in life'.

NERVOUS SYSTEM

Furze, Apple, Heather

Imbalances: Anxiety, depression, epilepsy, excessive worry, fear, headache, insomnia, introversion, mental stress, migraine, nervousness, paranoia, phobias, shingles: Feeling out of tune and unable to trust.

Characteristics: Hope, Decisiveness, Simplicity.

Affirmation: 'I am at one with and trust the pulse of life'.

GLANDULAR SYSTEM

Sweet Pea, Lilac, Silver Fir

Imbalances: Fatigue, glandular fever, menopausal problems, mood swings, mumps, poor metabolism, P.M.T., post natal depression, swollen glands: Feeling cut off from the spirit world.

Characteristics: Insight, Inspiration, Vision.

Affirmation: 'I am balanced between spirit and matter'.

URINARY SYSTEM

Copper Beech, White Poplar, Pine

Imbalances: Cystitis, incontinence, kidney problems, water retention, urethritis: Blame, fear, guilt, not going with the flow.

Characteristics: Courage, Faith, Peace.

Affirmation: 'I accept with courage the divine flow'.

REPRODUCTIVE SYSTEM

Wild Rose, The Sea, Yew

Imbalances: Endometriosis, irregular periods, menopausal problems, menstrual cramps, ovarian cysts, prostate problems, sexual problems, thrush: Blockages of feminine/masculine aspects, denying creativity.

Characteristics: Creativity, Resourcefulness, Renewal.

Affirmation: 'I am at one with my creative source.

PANCREATIC SYSTEM

Sweet Pea, Copper Beech, Apple, Furze, Sycamore, Rowan, Honeysuckle

Imbalances: Blood sugar disturbances, diabetes, immune deficiency, disturbances of the pancreas including pancreatitis: Feelings of rejection, loss of sweetness in life.

Characteristics: Insight, Courage, Decisiveness, Hope, Confidence, Protection, Centredness.

Affirmation: 'I accept the sweetness and abundance of life and acknowledge my gifts'.

SINUSITIS

Hazel, Willow, Hawthorn, Elder, Ivy, Ash, Lilac.

Imbalances: Cold, flu, disturbances of the sinuses including sinusitis, loss of sense of smell, tinnitus, vertigo: Irritations, disharmony in the environment.

Characteristics: Intuition, Empathy, Cleansing, Change, Freedom, Universal Truth, Inspiration.

Affirmation: 'I am at one with my environment'.

CANTABILLAE – AURIC

Reed, Grove, Magdalen, Weeping Willow, Rowan, Spiritual Rescue

Imbalances: Accidents, addictions, emotional strain, fatigue, grief, hopelessness, obsessions, personality disorders, pessimism, self doubt, shock, feeling sick and tired, stress, terminal illness, trauma, relationship problems: Avoidance of reality/out of touch with self.

Characteristics: Flexibility, Knowledge, Liberation, Unconditional Love, Protection, Transmutation.

Affirmation: 'I am indestructible. Come what may, I am loved'.

MEESHLA – THE PEACE PERFUME

Pine, Cedar, Elm

Imbalances: Being caught in conflict, carrying hurt from the past, closed down emotionally, feelings of negativity, hard-heartedness, war within the self.

Characteristics: Peace, Compassion, Generosity, Self-Empowerment, Release.

Affirmation: 'I release the need for conflict. I radiate peace from the centre of my being'.

❀ SUN ESSENCES ❀

THE LIVING BLENDS – FOR GROWTH AND TRANSITION

These blends are designed to guide one through the processes of personal growth and bring the being into a state of increased wholeness. They are indicated when there seems to be no progress in any direction.

No.1 – frees up the energy locked into the system.

No.2 – starts the re-integration of the various aspects of the personality in a more balanced way.

No.3 – helps to open the heart and see the need to love the self and others.

No.4 – stills the inner self bringing a deeper realisation of one's true nature.

No.5 – helps establish a stronger connection to the higher self.

The colours of the flowers we use focus healing into the relevant chakras. The vibrations of colour are well known for their curative properties and combined with the healing effects of the living flowers produce powerful and balanced blends.

No.1 RELEASING BLOCKED ENERGY

Contents: Orange Hawkweed, Lungwort, Feverfew, Copper Beech, Jack-by-the-Hedge and Ramsons.

No.2 INTEGRATION

Contents: Ladies Mantle, Elderflower, Sunflower, Trine Tree, Primrose, Vipers Bugloss.

No.3 LOVING THE SELF AND OTHERS

Contents: Bleeding Heart, Meadowsweet, Marigold, Cosmos, Double Daffodil, Hawthorn.

No.4 SELF AWARENESS

Contents: Bluebell, Eyebright, Mullein, Self Heal, Sage.

No.5 STRENGTHENS THE SPIRITUAL CONNECTION

Contents: Golden Yarrow, White Bindweed, White Violet, Wild Daffodil, Trine Tree.

Dosage Instructions: Take 7 drops 3 times a day for two weeks. Allow a further two or three weeks for the healing energy to complete its work.

❋ SUN ESSENCE SOLAR BLENDS ❋

Each Solar Blend is made from a selection of Flower Essences which are designed to balance the various aspects of common emotional problems. The choice of flowers is based on the experience of many years work as practitioners and we also keep the colour of the blooms in mind, so each Blend contains a rainbow. Why? Think of a rainbow, when does it appear? When there is sun and rain. When two things that do not mix exist alongside each other at the same time. The rainbow somehow forms a bridge between them and creates a situation of great beauty and harmony. This theme is quite common throughout our everyday lives as the most stressful situations are often seemingly irreconcilable. The vibration of the rainbow in each Blend assists in creating harmony whenever there is something difficult to come to terms with.

The Blends are ideal for those with little knowledge of Flower Essences as they are user friendly, being easy to choose something helpful without the dilemma of which essences to select from the many sets available. They are safe, non-habit forming and have no side effects, except the ones you want. Ready to take and a complete treatment in themselves, they can be used by all the family.

N.B. Also available in tablet form for people who prefer not to take alcohol.

SOLAR BLEND FOR RELEASING ADDICTIVE HABITS

Are you ashamed that your addiction is a priority in your life?

How much power does it have over you?

Weak-willed? Despise yourself? Use substances to escape?

Compelled to seek the distractions of a hedonistic social life?

Do you want to give up smoking? Chocolate? Alcohol? Caffeine?

This blend can support the self-image and bring calmness, balance, plus the commitment needed to begin the daunting ask of mastering the addiction and stepping into the future without it The urge to actively nourish the self rather than seeking abuse takes root So, despite the inevitable backward steps, you keep the growing belief that there is a way to be released and feel positive about any progress. Depending on the seriousness of your addiction, this blend is designed to be supportive alongside other therapies.

Contents: Agrimony, Cherry Plum, Clematis, Gentian, Morning Glory, Pine, Self-Heal, Star of Bethlehem, Tansy, Walnut.

SOLAR BLEND FOR TRANSFORMATION OF ANGER

Are you ever extremely angry? Intolerant? Bad-Tempered? Critical? Domineering? Cantankerous? Self-righteous?

Do you feel defensive or threatened? Touchy? Behave aggressively? Say unkind things? Ever respond irrationally? Play manipulative games?

Are you unhappy and don't know why? Unable to express powerful emotions positively? Are your children/adolescents argumentative? Contrary?

Anger can manifest in many different ways. This blend can help bring the necessary insight needed to diffuse the energy into a more positive and creative expression. It can initiate the forgiveness process which is an important factor in the restoration of peace and harmony and the start of loving yourself. Strong feelings and their transformation is very much an individual affair depending on the issues involved. Various types of other healing support may be sought to resolve the pent up feelings and this blend is a useful aid at any stage. Anger may be a defence for feelings such as fear, sadness and vulnerability and it might be more appropriate to switch to another blend, returning to the anger blend a week or so after that treatment is completed.

Seven drops in water taken when angry feelings arise may be enough to defuse the energy and bring calm.

Contents: Beech, Cherry Plum, Chicory, Heather, Holly, Impatiens, Marigold, Vervain, Vine, Willow.

SOLAR BLEND FOR COMMUNICATION

Having problems in your relationships? Marital? Parental? At Work?

Is there a breakdown of communication?

Are you immobilised by your feelings? Don't you know the best way to act?

Unable to find a way through your internal confusion?

Feel endless guilt, anger, fear, blame and all the rest?

This blend is an aid for those difficult times in life when more love and acceptance between people is needed. It brings resources to support the communications of everyday life e.g. personal insight, strength, awareness of boundaries and a greater willingness to listen and understand. The qualities of tolerance, kindness and communication bring more love to self and others. This blend may be more effective if partners take it at the same time.

Contents: Beech, Centaury, Chestnut Bud, Chicory, Holly, Pine, Pink Yarrow Red Chestnut, Rock Rose, Willow.

SOLAR BLEND FOR CONFIDENCE

Are you nervous and shy? Do you suffer from low self esteem?

Believe yourself to be an outsider? Fear failure? Do you have an inferiority complex? Everyone suffers from low self esteem at some time or other in their lives and it is thought to be the most common negative condition. This blend can help you to accomplish greater levels of personal power and choice in your life. Positive qualities e.g. courage, confidence and self belief, enable you to tackle new projects, friendships, or just being kind to yourself, thus bringing feelings of fulfilment and wholeness within.

Contents: Buttercup, Centaury, Cerato, Cosmos, Larch, Marigold, Mimulus, Pine, Sunflower, Water Violet.

SOLAR BLEND FOR CRISIS

Are you in a state of shock? Accident? Bereavement? Afraid to go to the dentist? Do you suffer from stage fright? Nervous about public speaking? Exams TODAY? Emotional states, tantrums, arguments or just feeling 'freaked out?'

Crisis blend can relieve shock and trauma, quickly restoring calm and stability. Also ideal for the acute stages of bereavement or loss as the formula is designed to support the heart. Very useful for animals.

Can be used as drops on the tongue, used externally or as a spray, or taken as tablets.

Contents: Bluebell, Borage, Cherry Plum, Clematis, Impatiens, Rock Rose, Star of Bethlehem, Sweet Chestnut.

SOLAR BLEND FOR THE FEMALE CYCLES OF LIFE

Are you going through the menopause? Do you suffer from P.M.S.? Fluid retention? Hot flushes? Cramps? Mood swings? Irritable? Clumsy? How do you cope with these physical cycles of life?

If you are finding these changes uncomfortable and difficult to cope with, this blend may give the necessary emotional and physical support. Eases anxiety, tension, frustration, tiredness, past regrets etc which are all a major part of these inevitable changes. Found to be effective for any life cycle and not just female i.e.puberty, mid-life crisis, retirement, moving house etc.

Contents: Agrimony, Cherry Plum, Crab Apple, Elm, Gentian, Honeysuckle, Impatiens, Morning Glory, Scleranthus, Walnut.

SOLAR BLEND FOR NEW DIRECTIONS

Are you unable to find a fulfilling occupation? Do you dread decision making? Have you lost your direction in life? Want to move house? Find a new interest? Worried about making the wrong choice?

This blend can help you to be decisive and clear when contemplating major decisions. People are generally at their most vulnerable during a period of change. In order to remain successfully in command of all eventualities, these essences have been carefully chosen to provide that vital support. They can also show the presence of any block that might be impeding progress e.g. anger or fear, as our emotions are like the layers of an onion, in which case the appropriate blend can help resolve this, after which the New Directions treatment should be completed.

Contents: Cerato, Larch, Mimulus, Scleranthus, Self Heal, Tansy, Trine Tree, Walnut, White Bindweed, Wild Oat.

SOLAR BLEND FOR LIFTING DEPRESSION

Are you feeling low? Hopeless? Despondent? Gloomy?

Feel as if a dark cloud is hanging over you?

Discouraged and unable to find a way through?

Cut off from the world and inside yourself?

Taking these essences can bring a lighter, more open and objective viewpoint, releasing the need to be focused on the self and personal problems. This new optimistic frame of mind helps life to be more enjoyable, bright and promising. Depression is often a symptom of something deeper i.e. anger. This blend may give insight into other issues and guide one onto the next stage of healing.

Contents: Borage, Cherry Plum, Gentian, Gorse, Heather, Mustard, Sweet Chestnut, Wild Rose, Willow.

SOLAR BLEND FOR ENERGY

Are you exhausted? No get up and go?

Too tired to do the things you generally enjoy?

In conjunction with a healthy lifestyle, this blend can gradually revitalise the system, restoring energy and drive. Useful when the body has been drained and depleted e.g. after illness, childbirth, travelling, shift-work, heavy home commitments, long working hours. If, tired or exhausted, take more doses. If the last evening dose is keeping you awake, take it at tea-time.

N.B. If the fatigue persists it is advisable to see a doctor, as this blend is only an aid to recovery, not a substitute for sleep or medical attention.

Contents: Blackberry, Clematis, Elm, Hornbeam, Morning Glory, Nasturtium, Olive, Pansy, Tansy, Wild Rose.

SOLAR BLEND FOR EVERYDAY FEARS

Do aspects of daily life frighten you? Do you keep your fears to yourself?

Are you nervous? Anxious? Apprehensive?

Scared of spiders? Enclosed spaces? Terrified of crowds or going out?

Do you have irrational fears?

This blend can help reduce your fears to manageable levels by stimulating your own inner strength and courage. As phobic conditions can vary in intensity these essences can be used on their own or as a support with other treatments. Several bottles may be required to effect a lasting improvement as the situation may have taken a long time to develop and may also be a fundamental personality aspect. Letting go of the habit of fear requires effort.

Contents: Aspen, Bluebell, Centaury, Chamomile, Cherry Plum, Honeysuckle, Larch, Mimulus, Rock Rose, Star of Bethlehem.

SOLAR BLEND FOR THE BODY'S DEFENCES

Do you get a lot of colds or flu?

Do you find it difficult to shake them off?

Do you sometimes feel 'rundown' or 'out-of-sorts'?

This blend is designed to support and boost the immune system and is particularly beneficial during the winter months. If susceptible to minor infections e.g.colds, coughs, flu, virus, regular treatments can improve resistance. When having difficulty making a full recovery this blend can speed up the process. If something is coming on, take five or six hourly doses and the infection may be less severe.

Contents: Crab Apple, Gentian, Jack-by-the-Hedge, Lungwort, Oak, Olive, Pansy, Ramsons, Trine Tree, Scleranthus.

SOLAR BLEND FOR RESOLVING LOSS

How long have you been suffering with a broken heart? Family bereavement?

Still pining over the loss of your favourite pet? Does the future seem bleak?

Do you feel the sadness will never ease?

Are you unable to let go of the longings for past, happier times?

This blend can help you feel more comforted and at ease, bringing the hope of new beginnings. It enables you to come to terms with loss in a way that seems appropriate and helps you to find a way forward through the wide range of emotions that are a natural part of the grieving process, e.g. guilt, blame, sadness, despair etc. Response may be rapid and this blend has been called 'happy pills/drops'. However, as grief is a long and drawn out process do not feel discouraged if you feel the need to return to this blend several times.

Contents: Borage, Gentian, Holly, Honeysuckle, Pine, Star of Bethlehem, Sweet Chestnut Walnut, Water Violet, Willow.

SOLAR BLEND FOR MENTAL FATIGUE

Assignments to finish? Exams to take? Study? Revision?

Unable to think clearly? Memory blocks?

Do you spend hours at a computer?

Is your mind fuzzy? Does your brain feel dead?

This combination of flower essences can help to clear your head, improve concentration, revitalise the mind when you have a lot of mental work to do and give you that little boost to cross the finishing line. Follow dosage instructions, but if working under pressure it can be taken as often as required.

Contents: Clematis, Elm, Hornbeam, Morning Glory; Nasturtium, Rock Water; Scleranthus, Tansy, Vervain, White Chestnut.

SOLAR BLEND FOR SLEEP

Do you have problems sleeping? Troubled with night fears?

Are you ever restless? Anxious? Over tired? Are you unable to switch off?

Are your children unsettled at night?

This blend can calm, quieten and soothe the mind and body, encouraging regular sleep patterns. Take three times a day as per instructions until sleeping normally, then just last thing at night Also put seven drops in a little water by the bed in case you wake in the night, sip every five minutes until you return to sleep. Usually quite effective in improving sleep patterns.

Contents: Agrimony, Aspen, Bluebell, Dandelion, Pink Yarrow, Rock Rose, Vervain, Walnut, White Chestnut.

SOLAR BLEND FOR STRESS RELIEF

Do you suffer from stress related complaints? Difficulty coping with the pressure of city life?

Are you tense, irritable – is life a struggle?

Too much to do and not enough time to do it? Do you drive yourself without mercy?

Heading for a nervous breakdown?

A key blend for hectic modern living. Ideal for those with demanding lifestyles e.g parents, carers, students, commuters. Can de-stress the system on all levels (mentally, physically and emotionally) and relaxes the body, thus enabling you to function in a more calm, focused and productive way. Helpful when any illness is caused by stress and can be taken alongside other treatment Psychotropic drugs partly inhibit the effect of flower essences but long-term regular treatment alongside such medication may often prove beneficial.

Contents: Alkanet, Cherry Plum, Dandelion, Elm, Gentian, Hornbeam, Impatiens, Oak, Rock Water, Vervain.

❀ SOLAR BLENDS FOR EXTERNAL USE TO ❀ ACCELERATE HEALING

CRISIS CREAM WITH LAVENDER OIL

Flower essences in a non-lanolin therapy, cream base with peach nut oil, not tested on animals. Useful for cuts, bruises, stings, bites, rashes, aches and pains. Worth trying on any skin problems.

Contents: Bluebell, Cherry Plum, Clematis, Crab Apple, Impatiens, Lungwort, Orange Hawkweed, Rock Rose. Also contains Lavender essential oil.

FLOWER ESSENCE LAVENDER HEALING OIL

To massage or rub in as required, for aches and pains, sprains, bruises, rashes, etc. Contents: Crab Apple, Dandelion, Impatiens, Jack-by-the-Hedge, Lungwort Orange Hawkweed, Pansy, Ramsons, Rock Water, Trine Tree.

SOLAR BLEND FLOWER ESSENCE LAVENDER PROTECTION SPRAY

Is your energy field/aura open and in need of protection?

Do you ever need to cleanse your house or therapy room of negativity?

Sense that you pick up emotional debris from other people?

Are you affected by environment influences? e.g. Cities? Public transport? Pollution?

This blend is specifically for spraying into the aura and around the home or place of work. It contains a selection of flower essences especially chosen for their colour and healing properties to cleanse, protect and clear. Lavender essential oil is added for its fragrance and clearing properties.

Contents: Alkanet, Aspen, Bluebell Copper Beech, Golden Yarrow, Pink Yarrow, Orange Hawkweed, Walnut.

❀ SOLAR BLENDS FOR ANIMALS ❀

Animals like humans suffer from a range of not only physical but also emotional problems. Treatment is available for their physical conditions but there is little on offer for the relief of mental distress. Animals cannot express how they feel and often do not understand what is happening to them e.g. illness, travelling, going to the vet, kennels, change of residence or owner etc. Such things are not familiar to them and reactions can be seen in various ways e.g. fear, withdrawal, aggression etc. Flower essences can help animals cope with these unexpected changes in their routine.

As everyone knows each pet has its own personality and despite receiving the correct care and attention there may still be problems. The following blends have proven to be beneficial for many common problems with pets.

SOLAR BLEND FOR EMERGENCY

Designed for use after accident or trauma.

Crisis situations e.g. after effects of fights, visits to vet, accident, operation, physical abuse.

Contents: Aspen, Bluebell. Elm, Emergency Essence, Mimulus, Oak Olive, Orange. Hawkweed, Walnut, Water Violet.

Dosage for trauma in acute situations: give in a little water or milk every few minutes until calm, then two to three times daily in food and water until recovered. N.B. If the animal is unable to drink, rub the liquid around the mouth or use a spray.

SOLAR BLEND FOR CHANGES

Useful for adjusting to something new, e.g. new owners, house or environment; going to kennels; loss of owners; rescued animals; pet in season; adjusting to new pets in the house. Contents: Borage, Cherry Plum, Chicory, Walnut, Elm, Feverfew, Honeysuckle, Mimulus, Sweet Chestnut, Vervain.

N.B. Should a pet show signs of jealousy, aggression or other problems, try another blend as appropriate, or contact us for advice.

SOLAR BLEND FOR TRAINING

Useful support while training a pet, e.g. any training activities or in re-training. Contents: Alkanet Chestnut Bud, Cherry Plum, Clematis, Eyesight, Feverfew, Sclerenthus, Vervain, Tansy, Wild Oat.

SOLAR BLEND FOR TRAVELLING

Useful for any difficulties when travelling. Helpful for long or short trips.

Contents: Autumn leaves, Chamomile, Emergency Essence, Sclerenthus, Walnut, Feverfew, Honeysuckle, Mimulus, Vervain, Wild Oat.

Dosage – give a dose twice daily and just before trips until pet travels comfortably.

SOLAR BLEND FOR STRENGTHENING

Use as a support during periods of convalescing, e.g. long term illness, old age, pregnancy/lactation.

Contents: Agrimony, Clematis, Dandelion, Elm, Gentian, Walnut, Pink Yarrow, Gorse, Impatiens, Oak Olive, Self-Heal, Wild Rose.

SOLAR BLEND FOR THE BODY'S DEFENCES

When extra resistance to infection is required, e.g. use if pet has a virus, or any other infection e.g. cat flu, if exposed to infection, or general resistance is low.

Contents: Crab Apple, Gentian, Jack-by-the-Hedge, Oak, Olive, Pansy, Ramsons, Scleranthus, Trine Tree.

Dosage – In acute cases or if an infection is just starting, give six hourly doses, then two to three times daily.

N.B. Not a substitute for veterinary care.

SOLAR BLEND FOR STRESS

Brings relief in highly stressful situations. Particularly for show animals in the ring, but also applicable to any acute/stressful situation. Can help to calm down over excited, edgy or frightened animals but encourage an alert frame of mind.

Contents: Alkanet, Cherry Plum, Elm, Gentian, Hornbeam, Impatiens, Mimulus, Nasturtium, Pink Yarrow, Vervain, Walnut.

Dosage – Give doses every five to ten minutes as required.

SOLAR BLEND FOR THE HIGHLY STRUNG

e.g. weight loss, nervous tension, hyperactive, sensitive, jittery etc.

Contents: Agrimony, Aspen, Bluebell, Chamomile, Cherry Plum, Impatiens, Pink Yarrow, Rock Water, Scleranthus, Self-Heal Vervain.

SOLAR BLEND FOR THE OVER AGGRESSIVE

e.g. impulsive, wild, hostile, uncontrollable, stubborn, unmanageable etc.

Contents: Chamomile, Chicory, Emergency Essence, Holly, Honeysuckle, Marigold, Pink Yarrow, Vervain, Vine.

N.B. If there is no response to this blend the pet may in fact be frightened and the aggressive behaviour a defence, in which case an individual blend, especially for animal's particular needs, may be more helpful.

SOLAR BLEND FOR THE TIMID

e.g. frightened, withdrawn, sensitive, shy, lacking in confidence, trembling etc

Contents: Aspen, Bluebell, Buttercup, Centaury, Emergency Essence, Honeysuckle, Mimulus, Pink Yarrow, Water Violet.

❀ UNITIVE FLOWER ESSENCES ❀

THE TRAUMA REMEDY

This is a combination of six Unitive Flower Essences, Blackthorn, Celandine, Nettle, Butterbur, Daisy and Primrose in equal proportions.

The Trauma Remedy is useful for old 'stuff' that wasn't cleared at the time and rears its 'head' when certain new issues are presented. It can sometimes be used as a pre-remedy, one dose given to settle an old trauma so that the current issue can be treated with its appropriate essence. It's energy is about creating a sense of trust – trust that it's OK to move on. There is a quality of deep underlying shock, sometimes repressed anger and a sense of having been completely 'thrown', like not knowing who one is any more or how one can relate to the environment Although the trauma may have occurred a long time ago the sense of inner isolation persists at a very deep level (usually not consciously recognised). The Trauma Remedy brings a healing process appropriate within the context of the individual's life.

❀ WIGHT FLOWER REMEDY COMBINATIONS ❀

REMEDY ONE (HELP!)

Buddleia, Forget Me Not, St John's Wort, Red Clover, Daisy.

This is a combination remedy to help in stressful or emergency situations. It treats shock, confusion and fear. It helps one understand and cope with the situation in a calm, clarified manner.

REMEDY TWO (S.O.S.)

Buddleia, Lavender, Stinging Nettle, Primrose, Snowdrop, Borage.

This remedy is for the emotionally wounded, it helps to soothe the broken-hearted and put the pieces back together. It is applicable in all affairs of the heart including broken homes, bereavement and the ending of love affairs. It gives understanding, support and light at the end of a tunnel.

REMEDY THREE (SNOT)

Jasmine, Pansy, Snapdragon, Coltsfoot

This combination helps with the symptoms and cause of colds and 'flu'. It will help expel the virus from the body, deal with mucous congestion and sore throats.

REMEDY FOUR (SHIELD)

Pink and White Yarrow, Pennyroyal, Eleagnus and Selfheal.

This remedy is to increase auric protection.

REMEDY FIVE (ALPHA COM.)

Romneya, Mugwort; Daffodil, Pimpernel, Californian Poppy, Phormium.

This remedy helps with all forms of meditation and can aid in the development of psychic abilities and guide communication.

Chapter 10

Channelled essences

"Give fully. Give your heart to your brother' and he will live unto eternity Your brother is in everything you see. Be at peace."   *Galaxy M33. Received March 1995*

This chapter has been included by popular request as it is felt that there is a great need to express the information which it contains. All of the essences here are offered with love to humanity and to be shared in any ways which seem appropriate.

❀ 'SILVER STAR' VIBRATIONAL ESSENCES ❀

Julian Perry worked for ten years in the NHS as a clinical scientist but left in 1990 to focus more intently upon the spiritual path. He lectures and runs workshops encouraging people to access their own Divinity, working with the Mother energy to facilitate awakening. Interest in energy and vibrational medicine has blossomed in recent years and he initiated the creation of a series of essences within the 'Silver Star' group that has been running for over twelve years.

Julian is now deputy director of a charity dedicated to bringing a wide range of complementary healing practices in to prisons where he also applies his own skills in vibrational medicine. The idea to create an essence, that could make a valuable contribution to most conditions, arose during 1995. A brief was channelled (see below) whereupon it was described how this essence would function as a relay or trigger.

The decision to create a whole further series of essences occurred during early 1996 in response to an inner prompt to expand the theme of channelled essences and to address specific aspects of the path of transformation. The brief for this series of essences was then channelled together with names.

The essences are activated during the weekly meetings of 'Silver Star' at an appropriate time during the proceedings. Prior to the meeting Julian makes up a receptive base for the Mother Tinctures made either from spring water with 25% cider vinegar as a preservative, or from lactose tablets if the 'Silver Star' remedy is being made. Typically he gathers together six or so bottles for any particular remedy, labels them and places them near the middle of the gathering. At the appropriate time he invokes the energies of the Divine to activate the remedy known as.... The infusion only takes about a minute. Near the end of the meeting, after the Divine Mother blessings, another remedy can be activated if required.

The Mother tinctures are used to make up running or treatment remedies by adding two drops to a base mixture of water with 10% cider vinegar. Alternatively one can activate a tablet version in an 8gm bottle of lactose tablets with one drop of the Mother tincture.

Although these Mother tinctures are initially activated in the 'Silver Star' group, Julian is also able to energise any of the remedies in his hand using the chakras

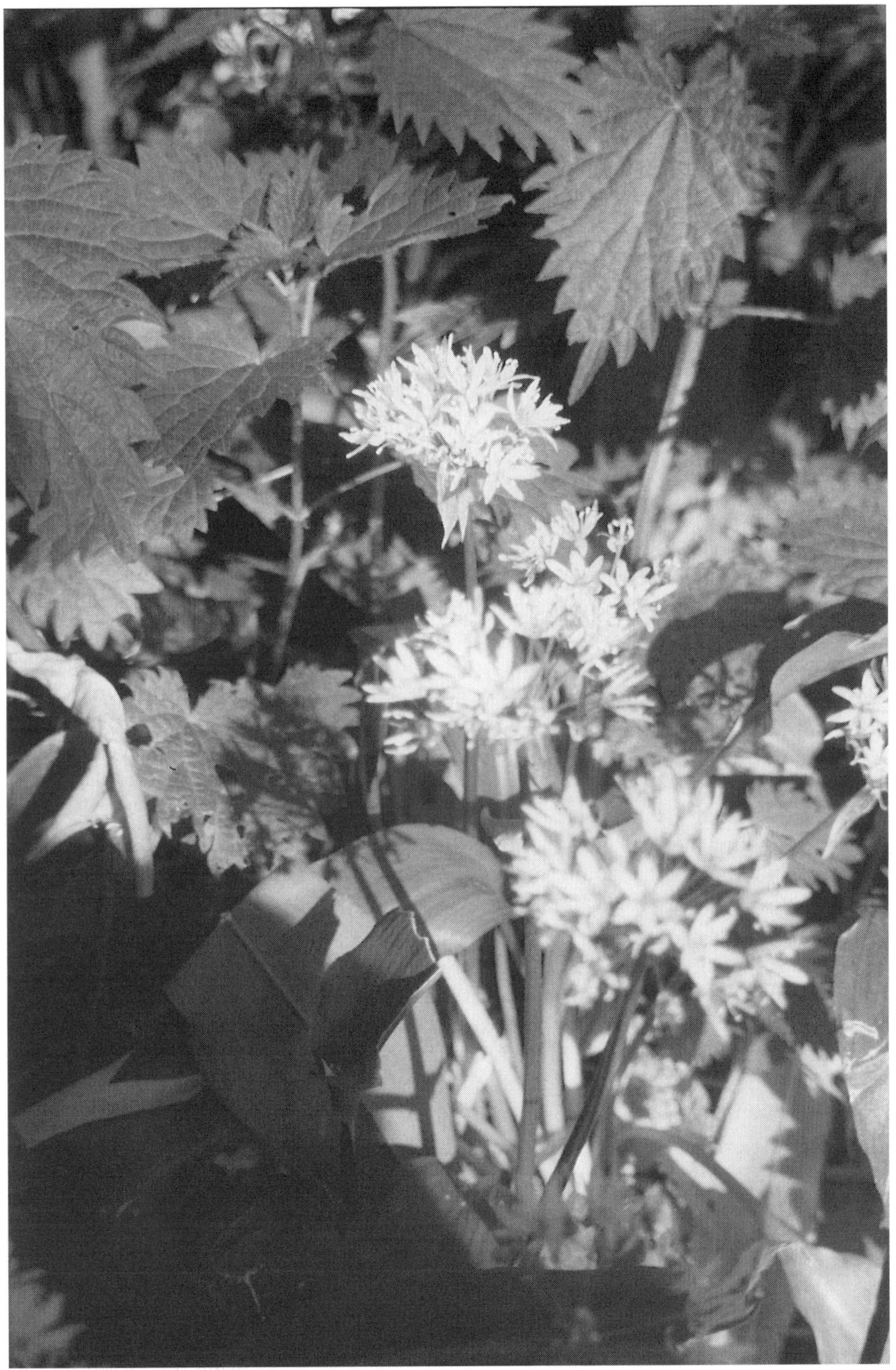

system. However, the vibration brought through will only be that which already exists as a result of the most recent energy brought through the group. In other words, it is very important to continue to generate the essences in the group so as to advance them and to incorporate new and refined qualities in to them. Once a particular one is made the pattern exists and people are able to access and recreate the vibrational pattern through their own energy system.

The essences have been very well received and there are at least six healing centres around the country who are working with complete sets of Mother tinctures so they can prescribe them in their own way.

THE 'SILVER STAR' REMEDY

Brief: 'The remedy that we will create with you will be different from a classical homoeopathic preparation, since in that case one selects a specific remedy and potency to match a specific disorder. In the case of the 'Silver Star' remedy we are harnessing a vibration within the matrix of the lactose tablets that will act as a trigger in the recipient such that they are rendered open to the particular energies of 'Silver Star' that are relevant to them at that time.

'Silver Star' deals with many different energies and qualities, those of the Higher Realms, the Ascended Masters, the Elohim and the Divine Mother amongst others, all with special qualities suited to the moment to moment experience of the group members. There are therefore energies dealing with healing, strength, love, guidance, transformation and so on which would be impossible to encode for each individual in one physical form.

What this remedy will do therefore is to transfer a special pulse of energy to the recipient that will cause their whole being to vibrate in a particular manner that will open them to the full array of 'Silver Star' energies. What they receive will then be determined by their focus and needs at the time as determined and mediated by the Higher Self in that the act of taking the remedy will serve as an inward call for assistance of a particular kind. Each will therefore receive what they truly need in the moment and in highest wisdom; making the remedy particularly powerful in its capacity to cater for a wide range of individuals and needs.

This 'remedy' should be thought of as a complement rather than as a replacement to other more specific treatment that may have already been described, and yet in some cases one may be able to use it as a substitute. Learning to use it intuitively is part of its function, and yet in whatever context it is employed, it is offered with the great Love and Light that emanates from the heart of 'Silver Star'. Take it with reverence and focus when you feel the need and may it bring you health, wholeness and the transformation you seek.'
Julian Perry 1&2.96

Although the original 'Silver Star' (tablet form) or 'Starburst' (liquid form) remedy is a multi-focus aid with powerful capabilities, recently the group have been led to create a wider range of vibrational remedies or essences that serve more specific functions. Due to the increasing rate of expanding consciousness on the planet, it is now considered appropriate to infuse higher dimensional energies directly into the individual to assist activating and integrating one's 'Lightbody'.

To this effect they are now offering a further selection of 12 individual essences and three combination ones that have been infused with specific energies via 'Silver Star' and which may assist in one's spiritual development. These potions are not medicines and no medical use is suggested. Neither do they represent a short cut to spiritual growth but, with the blessings of Divine Grace, they are offered as aids to smooth our passage to greater heights of Divine expression There is also a 'First Aid' remedy and a 'Stress Management' oil.

While the 'Silver Star'/'Starburst' remedy exists in both tablet and liquid form, these potions are energy infusions primarily in liquid form and made from mineral water with some cider vinegar added as a preservative. However, if for any reason one specifically requires an essence in tablet format, then this can be arranged upon request. A dose is two drops and is typically taken twice a day, either directly into the mouth or in a drink of water or juice. While in some cases they may be recommended under 'guidance' as part of a treatment regime, equally they can be selected and used intuitively by anyone. They are available from Julian Perry and are offered free of charge, although contributions towards the cost of bottles, p&p etc. would be gratefully received along with any feedback regarding their effects.

DESCENSION

Assists the assimilation of incoming frequencies and energies into all levels of one's being. In this way it will ease the mutational and descension symptoms that are often experienced and encourage an acceptance and joy in one's transformation.

DIVINE LOVE

Used to help clear and awaken the Heart as a doorway to multi-dimensional experience. Pushes through blockages and defence mechanisms that are resisting the Heart opening and enhances one's capacity to give and receive unconditional Love in all areas of one's life.

FAITH

Together with the quality of surrender, this assists you to open to your Spirit, the inner Light, by dissolving long-term resistances and defence systems created by the ego that oppose its dissolution. This essence helps one to 'let go and let God' so one may embrace awakening more spontaneously and effortlessly.

FREEDOM

Designed to release hurt, the effects of abuse and life's scars. It bridges any schisms between body, mind and spirit so that energy can flow and reconnect the disparate parts into a unified whole. This will help individuals cleave to their Higher Self and Will rather than to substitutes and addictions. It is a powerful healing vibration designed to bring freedom from limitation and control by negative forces.

HAVEN

This essence comprises two components, the first designed to ensure that your home or special place is clear of unwanted energies and residues from the past. The second part seals the cleared space and facilitates the alignment of your inner bodies so that you can engage your spiritual practice unimpeded and with peace and harmony.

KARUNAMAYI

Made from the vibhuti provided by Mother Karunamayi when she visited England in 1996, it offers the Grace of the Divine Mother expressed through this form and aspect of Her consciousness. Focusing primarily on Higher Wisdom and Knowledge, it assists one to open to the Divine Truth within and to embody this within our daily life. (This and 'White Horse' essence were not made by the invocation method previously described.)

LIGHTWORKER

A support for those working for Planetary need and large concerns and who would otherwise risk overloading their spiritual bodies. It encourages greater sensitivity and fluidity of consciousness in keeping with your particular Lightwork and simultaneously eases any discord between the Higher Will and its earthly manifestation.

RAPTURE

Assists one to open more fully to Divine Joy and Ecstasy. It helps align the higher dimensional bodies thereby allowing the qualities of one's Inner Presence to flow into your life. It also smoothes the awakening of the Kundalini force in an appropriate way.

RELATIONSHIP

Helps deal with the shifts required in transforming relationships from the personal to the transpersonal level. Working on both the emotional and physical bodies, it assists in the development of a new perspective on Self and others that is the foundation of fulfilling relationships.

RELEASE

Helps release and express memories: old emotional patterning and karmic parameters stored in the cells and body generally. This can pave the way for new directions on your path that have hitherto been blocked due to ties and experiences from the past. To be used sparingly under guidance.

SHEKHINA

This infusion prepares and assists one to receive the gifts of the Divine Mother. These gifts are those appropriate to enhancing the link with the Christ Consciousness and the 'I AM' Presence such that these may be more easily grounded and manifested

WHITE HORSE

This is a remedy for cleansing of the lower bodies. Dealing particularly with emotion and unwanted energy patterns locked into our system, it carries them both upward and downward out of the system with its vortex of energy. This essence was made from a vortex energised by the Higher Realms, at the White Horse on the downs near Seaford in Sussex, in response to an experiment in conjunction with them.

The three combination essences also available are Descension/Shekhina, Faith/Shekhina and Lightworker/Starburst.

FIRST AID REMEDY

This particular remedy serves to provide for the immediate needs resulting from an accident or event that involves shock, bodily or mental trauma or emotional stress. It brings together many of the qualities of flower essences, homeopathy and other vibrational remedies to assist the patient to heal quickly and to draw upon their own and higher energies for maximum recuperation and the restoration of a normal state of health.

The remedy is activated spring water preserved in brandy and a few drops should be taken directly by mouth as well as being applied directly to the injured area as required. In cases where application by mouth is not possible or not advised, then drops should be applied to the temples, behind the ears or to the wrists. This remedy should not be used as a substitute for medical treatment but rather as a complement.

❈ THE STARSEED ESSENCES ❈

These essences first came about in 1995 in response to prompting from various members of the Universal Family of Light. They were all made by Sue Monk; at the time they seemed to be a natural follow-on from the flower and gem essences which she was making at the time. A couple more have been added since to address the different needs of humanity as the pace of vibrational change increases.

They are offered free of charge to those who feel drawn to them at this time; however any donations towards bottles, postage, etc will be welcomed as will any feedback as to effects. As with the Silver Star Essences, they do not attempt to deal with specific ailments but take a 'broad brush' approach; each person is able to take from the essence that which is right for them at that time in accordance with their Higher Self and Divine Will.

The suggested dose is 3 drops, 3 times daily, directly onto the tongue, unless otherwise guided. The Mother tinctures have 50% brandy added as a preservative.

DOLPHIN

This was made on the Spring Equinox in 1995, in response to a suggestion from St Germain, who presides over the dolphins and other cetaceans who are safeguarding the oceans. The essence started life as a dioptase gem essence made by the sun method, which was further activated by the higher realms. The dioptase is used to focus and accelerate the incoming energy; dioptase is very much a healing stone for the new age and helps one to understand that today is real, and that we all need to live in the moment. It assists in the enrichment of one's life, environment and planet and can help one to hear the silence of the resonance of Earth.

'As you pour out your love for all sentient beings, so you will be helped by this remedy. As you connect with the oceans, the remedy will amplify your own energy. It is for use when you meditate, to send peace to the earth and to every living thing. That includes you all.'

DIOPTASE/SIRIUS

This essence was made on the Summer Solstice 1995, overnight, again in response to a prompt from St Germain. It started life as a lunar essence made with dioptase and distilled water but was energised in particular by the Sirians and the Earth Mother. It is to help to rid our lower chakras, and in particular the base chakra, of all that which is not love, aligning and balancing it; allowing the Earth to replace negativity with Love.

M88

This was made in March 1995 and started life as an amethyst gem essence made by the sun method. Made in response to a request from Melchizedek and with his guidance, it supplies 'the keys to the kingdom' – i.e. it provides various keys to unlock facets of the Lightbody according to what each person is able to accept. In this way it helps to further ground us all within the Earth's newly established Light Grid such that we may each find our Self and within that achieve Oneness. It is a good one to take when meditating.

ANDROMEDA

This essence was prepared with the use of a stargate; it is activated spring water made by the sun method in June 1996. It is about belonging in infinite space and being happy there. With that infinite capacity and trust and grace, one can maintain separateness and also communion. It helps one to understand and to communicate effectively while still maintaining one's own space, to keep a sense of one-ness while retaining one's own boundaries in good grace.

ANGELICLIGHT (SUN AND STARS)

This essence was prepared in June 1996 with the use of a stargate, and incorporates the qualities of both starlight and sunlight, Father Sun and Sister Moon. It is to allow you to become one, and to balance both sides, both the father and the mother, this essence being between these two 'polarities'. It allows you to come home. It is connected to the cosmic Christ, the Family of Light and then to all the things you are, the things you truly own. It connects to all dimensions in which you find your soul.

Chapter 11

Flower essence cross-reference

Using the Flower Essence Cross-reference section

This section covers a broad range of mental, emotional and spiritual issues plus a section devoted to physical ailments, all of which are designed to assist the practitioner and layperson in their selection of flower essences.

After each essence listed is an abbreviation which identifies the maker. Combination essences (more than one essence in a bottle) are printed in bold. The flower essence names listed in this section are as stated by the maker in the A-Z repertory and sets of essences.

It is appropriate when selecting an issue to start with either the positive goal or the pattern of imbalance, sometimes related issues are suggested for further consideration – the issues shown are a mixture of positive and negative indications.

Having established which flower essences may be appropriate, consulting the A-Z repertory and sets of essences will give a more detailed description of the qualities of each essence.

It is also suggested and may be helpful to familiarize oneself with the A-Z repertory and makers' sets of essences, by so doing the reader will know instinctively which makers/sets of essences they are drawn to and would like to work with.

ESSENCE MAKERS ABBREVIATIONS

★Comb. after an abbreviation indicates a combination remedy★

AFE	Artemis Flower Essences
AFR	Aquarius Flower Remedies
ACFR	Aquarius Chakra Flower Remedies
AT	Andrew Tressider
BE	Bailey Essences
BFE	Balleybane Flower Essences
BFR	Bridget's Flower Remedies
CG	Carol Guyett
CFR	Church Farm Rose Essences
CH	Crystal Herbs
DC	Dawn Carol
EE	Earth Essences
FFE	Findhorn Flower Essences
GE	Gaia Essences
GHTE	Glastonbury Holy Thorn Essences
GMFE	Green Man Flower Essences
GMTE	Green Man Tree Essences
HFE	Habundia Flower Essences
HR	Harebell Remedies
IC	Imelda Carroll
JH	Judith Hoad
JJ	Jean Jacob
JW	Wight Flower Essences – Julian Winslow
LHFE	Light Heart Flower Essences
LLFE	Lord & Lady Flower Essences
LNE	Loving Nature Essences
MEFE	Middle Earth Flower Essences
MERE	Middle Earth Rose Essences
OIT	Ogham Irish Tree Essences
PE	Petaltone Essences
RD	Rosie Devitt
RLR	Real Life Remedies
SCE	Silvercord Essences
SE	Sun Essences
SM	Sue Monk
UFE	Unitive Flower Essences

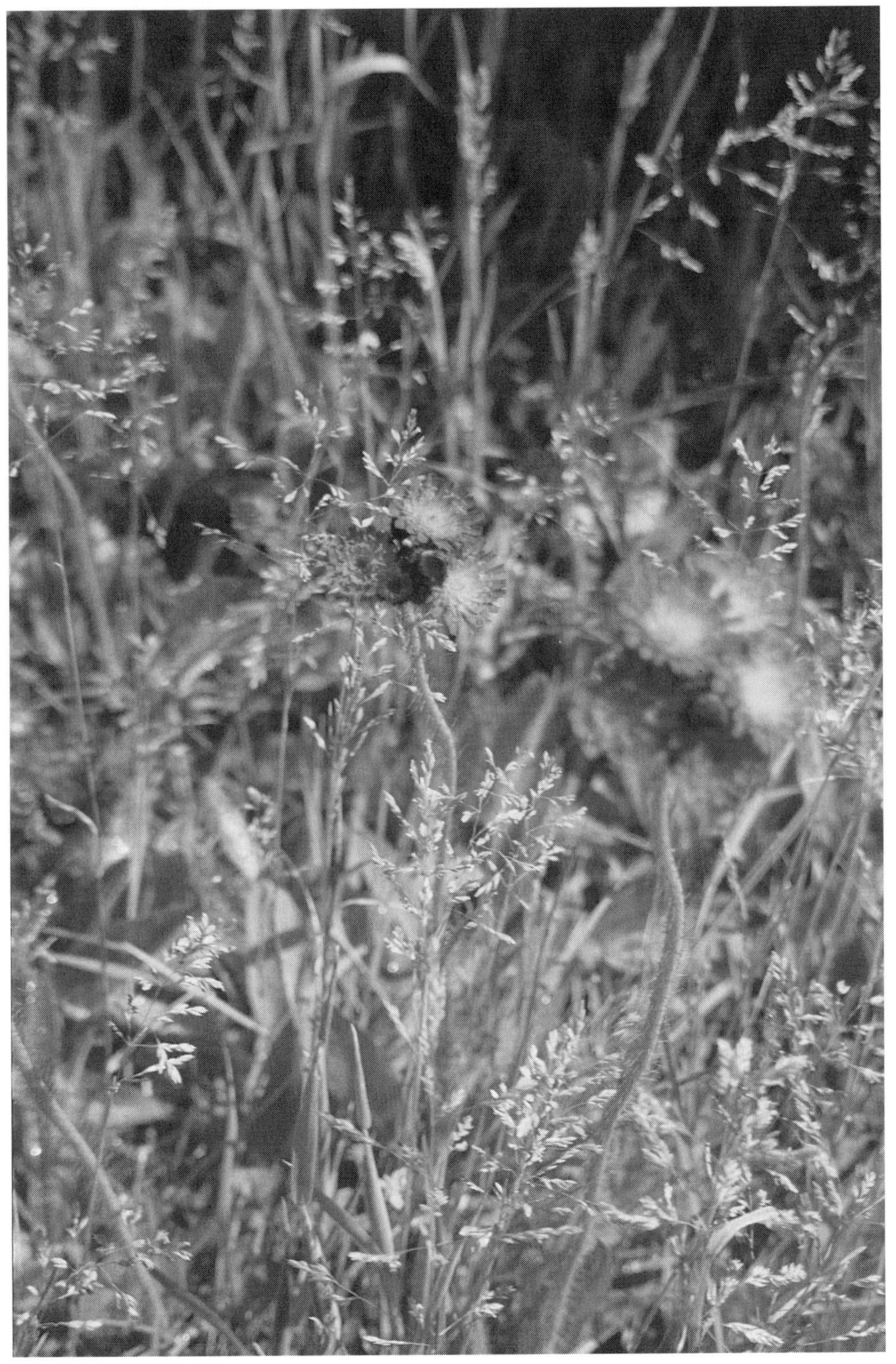

Index of cross-reference issues

EMOTIONAL/MENTAL/SPIRITUAL ISSUES

PHYSICAL ISSUES

Emotional/Mental/Spiritual Issues

*indicates combinations of flower and gem essences

Type in bold represents a combination remedy

ABANDONMENT
See also, Loss/Separation/
Loneliness/Rejection

Universal Suffering (GHTE)
Rose Water Lily (FFE)

ABSENTMINDEDNESS
See also, Forgetfulness/Memory

Wood Anemone (UFE)

ABUNDANCE

Buttercup (HR)
Prosperity (AFR Comb), Honesty (AFR)
Evelyn (CFR)
Silver Genie (PE)
Sea Rocket (FFE)
Double Daffodil (SE)
Borage (UFE)
Pussy Willow (LHFE)

ACCEPTANCE
See also, Understanding

Daffodil – The Crown Chakra (ACFR)
Pilgrim (CFRE)
Onionflower, Osteospermum, Geranium (CH)
Crack Willow, Silver Birch, Lime, Norway Pine, Manna Ash,
Sweet Chestnut (GMTE)
Green Alkanet (LLFE)
Aura Flame (PE)
Chamomile, Self-heal (HR), *Acceptance (HR Comb)*
Wild Rose, Moss, Yellow Archangel (HFE)
Elder, Holy Thorn, Hazel (FFE), **Revelation (FFE Comb)**
Dandelion (EE)
White Violet (SE)
Sweet Pea (JW)
Pyramid Orchid (SCE)
Buttercup, Mayweed, Purple Comfrey, Ramsons, Wood Sorrel (UFE)
Blue Geranium (LNE)

ADAPTABILITY
See also, Flexibility

Feverfew (SE)

AGGRESSIVENESS

Solar Blend Transformation of Anger (SE Comb)
Comfrey – The Root Chakra, Sage –
The Solar Plexus Chakra (ACFR)
Kerria (CH)
Elder, Italian Alder, Field Maple (GMTE)
Snapdragon, Wild Violet (GMFE)
Spindle (LLFE)
Marigold (SE)
Toadflax (JJ)
Gorse (LHFE)

AGITATION

Horse Chestnut (GMTE)

ALIENATION
See also, Loss/Separation/
Isolation

Rose Bay willowherb (HR)
Strelitzia (GE)
Persian Ironwood (GMTE)

AMBITION
See also, Goals

Burning Desire (RLR)

ANGELIC KINGDOM

Angelica (AFR)(CH)
Buttercup, Forget-me-not, Jasmine (JJ)
Gallica (CFR)
Columbine, Deutzia , Dipladenia Yellow, Iris 'Amethyst',
Philadelphus (CH)
See also Holy Archangel Essences (DC)

	Soul Star (PE)
	Yellow Archangel, Hedge Woundwort, Water Forget me not, Common Spotted Orchid (HFE)
	Buddleia (Orange/Yellow)(MEFE), Pale Pink Rose (MERE)
ANGER *See also, Resentment/Bitterness*	***Transmutation & Awakening – Solar Plexus Chakra (CFRE Comb)** Pilgrim (CFR)* ***Forgiveness, Joy (GM Comb)*** *Holm Oak, Copper Beech, Field Maple, Judas Tree (GMTE)* ***Solar Blend Transformation of Anger (SE Comb)*** *Pink & White Hawthorn Body Spray (SE)* *Red Dead Nettle – The Sacral Chakra, Sage – The Solar Plexus Chakra (ACFR)* *Garlic, Rose of Sharon (CH)* *Clear Star, Spirit Ground, Silvery Moon, Fire Clear (PE)* *Orange Lily (SM)* *Red Dead Nettle (LLFE)* *Nettle (HR)* *Willowherb (FFE)* *Snapdragon (MEFE)* *Marigold (GE)* *Euphrasia , Tormentil (BFE)* *Honeysuckle, Passion Flower, Penstemon (AFE)* *Red Pheasant's Eye (SCE)* *Sorrel (UFE)* *Pussy Willow (LHFE)* *Compact Rush (BE)*
ANIMAL KINGDOM	*Whitebeam (GMTE)* *Coltsfoot (LLFE)* *Wild Garlic, Nasturtium, Red Clover, Thyme (JJ)* *Moss Rose (Dusky Red) (MERE)* *Peaches & Cream (RLR)*
ANXIETY *See also, Worry*	*Bells of Ireland (CH)* ***Tranquillity (GM Comb)**, Alder, Leyland Cypress, Ivy, Lime, Norway Maple, Pittespora, Catalpa, Horse Chestnut (GMTE)* *Flowering Currant (GMFE)* *Comfrey – The Root Chakra (ACFR)* *Christmas Rose (BFR)* *Chamomile (CH)(HR)* *Forget-me-not (CH)* *Butterbur (LLFE)* *Delphinium (SM)* *Hyssop, St. John's Wort (HR)* *Foxglove (HFE)* *Scottish Primrose (FFE)* *Hero, Karmic Helper, Time Immemorial (RLR)* *Evening Primrose (JW)* *Cowslip (LHFE)* *Lady's Smock (BFE)* *Bog Hypericum (LNE)*
APATHY	***Life Force (FFE Comb)**, Gorse (FFE)* *Fleabane (LLFE)* *Valerian (JJ)* *Lucombe Oak (GMTE)*
ARROGANCE	*Yellow Archangel (SE)* *Apricot (GE)* *Flowering Red Currant (BBFE)*
ASCENDED MASTERS	***See, Sanada(Master Jesus), Sai Baba, St. Germain, Melchizedek, St. Michael** (Jean Jacob Flower Essences from the Ascended Masters)*

ASSERTIVENESS

Sage – The Solar Plexus Chakra (ACFR)
Spirit Ground, Release, Clear Tone (PE)
Blue Mood (RLR)

ASTRAL TRAVEL/PROJECTION

Bindweed, Mugwort (AFE)
Dogs Mercury (HFE)

ASTROLOGY

Jasmine (AFE)

ATTACHMENT
See also, Co-dependence/neediness

Barley Grains, Bay Buds (AT)
Bleeding Heart (SE)(AFR)(CH)
Wild Iris (CH)
Harebell, Rowan, Snowdrop, Willowherb (FFE)
Hazel (FFE)
Eyebright (SE)
Mulberry (GMTE)
Charlock, Lesser Stitchwort, Leopardsbane (BE)

ATTENTION, & LACK OF
See also, Concentration, Focus

Hairy Sedge (BE)

AURAS

***Solar Blend Flower Essence Lavender Protection
Spray (SE Comb)***
Thistle (CH)
***See also, Crystal Light Essences, Living Rainbow Aura
Essences (DC)***
Golden Light, Stand Alone (PE)
Fleabane, Stinking Hellebore (LLFE)
Yarrow (LLFE)(HR)(HFE)
St. John's Wort (HR)
Field Pansy (EE)
Pink Yarrow (MEFE)(SE)
White Yarrow (MEFE)
Lungwort (SE)
*African Dance, Beautiful World, Burning Desire, Candle Light, Blue
Mood, Fuchsia Success, Golden Window, Lancelot, Look Lively,
Majestic Triumph, Purple Passion (RLR)*
Queen Anne's Lace (JJ)
Remedy 4 'Shield' (JW Comb)
Penstemon (AFE)

AUTHORITY

Blackthorn (JJ)
Violet (SCE)

AVOIDANCE
*See also, Denial, Escapism/
Resistance*

Rowan (FFE)
Marigold (JJ)
Flax (SCE)

BABIES
*See also, Babies(Physical)/
children/childhood issues*

White Rose Bud (HR)
Cowslip, Pussy Willow (LHFE)

BALANCE/BALANCING
See also, Emotions

Alkanet, Scilla, Vipers Bugloss (SE)
Anemone(CH)(SM)
Californian Poppy (JJ)(RD)(CH)
Black Medick, Dandelion, Hawthorn Leaf (EE)
Energy Balance (AFR Comb),
Daffodil – The Crown Chakra (ACFR)
Chamomile, Red Clover (AFR)
Spiritual Marriage (FFE Comb), *Harebell, Sea Pink, Globe
Thistle (FFE)*
Meridian Energiser (GM Comb), *Bilberry, Catalpa, Cherry
Laurel (GMTE)*
Saxifrage, Chamomile, Oriental Hellebore (GMFE)
Amelanchier (BFR)
Sweet Juliet, Arthur Bell, Centifolia (CFR)
*Auricula, Camelia, Chrysanthemum, Gladiolus,
Hibiscus, Mahonia (CH)*
Hazel (LLFE)

	Sunflower (SM)
	Forget me not, Forsythia (HR)
	Stinking Hellebore, Blackthorn (HFE)
	Pink Yarrow, Ash, Lavender (MEFE)
	Golden Window, Love 'n' Light, Morning Tide, Purple Paradise, Sunset Boulevard (RLR)
	Chickweed, Lavender, Maple, Sage, Vetch (JJ)
	White Clover (RD)
	Evening Primrose (AFE)
	Silver Birch (JW)
	Nettle (UFE)
	Firethorn (BE), **Yang, Yin (BE Comb)**
	Crystal Celestial (DC)
	Loosestrife (LNE)
BEAUTY	*Silver Birch (GMTE)*
	Jasmine (PE)
	Freedom Dance (RLR)
BELONGING	*Daisy (EE)*
BEREAVEMENT &	*Strelitzia (GE)*
BEREAVEMENT DEPRESSION	**Solar Blend Crisis (SE Comb), Solar Blend Resolving Loss (SE Comb)**
	Christmas Rose (BFR)
	Purple Loosestrife (LLFE)
	Spirit Ground (PE)
	Honeymoon, Mary Light, Solemn Feast (RLR)
	Blackberry, Forsythia, Snowdrop (CH)
	Harebell, Evening Primrose (AFE)
BETRAYAL	*Universal Suffering (GHTE)*
	Buttercup (BE)
BEWILDERMENT	*Soapwort, Foxglove (BE)*
BITTERNESS	**Tranquillity (GM Comb)**
See also, Resentment	*Marsh Woundwort (HR)*
	Bounty Beautiful (RLR)
	Redshank (LNFE)
BLAME	*Hyssop (HR)*
	Compact Rush (BE)
BLOCKAGE/RESISTANCE/RELEASE	**Living Blend 1 (SE Comb),** *Orange Hawkweed (SE)*
See also, Letting Go	*Red Dead Nettle – The Sacral Chakra (AFR)*
	Fig, Iris 'Bluebeard', Fuchsia (CH)
	Dogs Mercury, Lungwort (LLFE)
	Release (PE)
	Iris (Blue Flag) (HR)
	Ragged Robin, Sea Pink, Scots Pine, Stonecrop, Wild Pansy (FFE)
	Dandelion, Red Strawberry, Elder (MEFE)
	Time Immemorial (RLR)
	Forsythia, Pansy, Primrose, Red Clover (JJ)
	Snowdrop (RD)
	Sweet Violet (GE)
	Honeysuckle (SCE)
	Blue Iris, Holly Buds (AT)
	Forget-me-not, Scarlet Pimpernel, Stitchwort (GMFE)
	Coltsfoot, Red Campion (UFE)
	Early Purple Orchid, Lilac, Wood Anemone, Bracken – Aqueous Extract (BE),
	Unification (BE Comb)
BONDING	**Birth & Re-birth – Root Chakra (CFR Comb)**
	Alba Maxima (CFR)
	Sweet Pea (AFR)
	Raspberry (JJ)

BOREDOM — *Meadowsweet (BFE)*

BOUNDARIES — *Fuchsia (BFE)*

BRAIN (RIGHT/LEFT IMBALANCE)
See also, Brain

Penstemon, St. John's Wort, Witch Hazel, Lemon (AFE)
Honesty, Pansy, Red Clover, Thyme (JJ)
Single White Cherry (BFR)
Campsis, Primrose (GE)
Comfrey (CH)(LHFE)
Petunia (CH)
Daffodil – The Crown Chakra (ACFR)
Bracken – Aqueous Extract (BE)

CALMING
See Stillness/Worry/Stress/Trauma/
Soothing/Tension/Stillness/
Tranquillity/Inner Peace/
Relaxation

Orange (RD)
Harebell, St. John's Wort (AFE)
Bilberry, Horse Chestnut (GMTE)
Golden Crocus, Saxifrage, Snowflake (GMFE)
Bluebell (HR)
Crisis (HFE Comb)
Solar Blend Stress Relief (SE Comb), Solar Blend
Transformation of Anger (SE Comb), *Alkanet (SE)*
Mary Rose, Church Farm Rose, Cadfael (CFR)
Chamomile (CH)(AFR)(HR)
Lavender (SM)(JJ)
Marjoram, Potato (HR)
Yellow Poppy (HFE)
Daisy (FFE)
Fennel (MEFE)
Burning Desire, Look Lively, Majestic Triumph, Marylight,
Morning Tide, Soul Retrieval (RLR)
Hops, Violet (JJ)
Square-Stalked willowherb (GE)
Belladonna (WFR)
Remedy 1 'Help' (JW Comb)
Amaryllis, Hypericum 'Hidcote', Lupin, Peach, Lily (CH)
Red Clover (RD)(CH)(LHFE)
Cowslip (LHFE)

CATHARSIS — *Fuchsia (AFR)*

CELEBRATION — *Arizona Fir (BE)*

CHAKRAS – GENERAL
See also, Spirituality/
Spiritual Growth

Anemone (CH)(SM)
Energy Balance (AFR Comb)
Chakra (LLFE Comb), *Primrose, Rosemary (LLFE)*
See also, Aquarius Chakra Flower Essences, Crystal Herbs
Chakra Essences, Church Farm Rose Combination Chakra
Essences
Cowslip, The Bride, Amelanchier, Christmas Rose, Rosemary,
Canary Bird Rose, Dog Tooth Violet (BFR)
Gallica (CFRE)
Campsis (GE)
Hoya, Lychnis, Philadelphus, Regensberg (CH)
Hawthorn, Leyland Cypress, Tree Lichen (GMTE)
Lilac (GMTE)(HR)(MEFE)
Blackberry, Jasmine, Lemon, Lavender, Penstemon, Tansy (AFE)
Crystal Clear (PE)
Daffodil, Geranium, Iris/Dioptase, Sunflower (SM)*
Sea Pink (FFE)
Scarlet Pimpernel (MEFE)
Beautiful World, Honeymoon, Candle Light, Lancelot, Look Lively,
Blue Moon, Marylight, Magnolia, Refresh Your Memory, Saviour,
Solemn Feast, Tower of Strength, Peaches & Cream,
Sunset Boulevard (RLR)
Lemon Balm (JJ)
Red Clover (LHFE)
Early Purple Orchid (BE)

CHAKRA – FEET
See also, Spirituality/
Spiritual Growth

*Feet Chakra (CH Comb)**
Passion Flower (CH)
Poppy (DC)
Blackthorn (GMTE)
Daffodil, Hibiscus (SM)

CHAKRA – HANDS

Daffodil (SM)
Catalpa, Ivy (GMTE)

CHAKRA – ANKLES

'Orange' (DC)

CHAKRA – KNEES

'Yellow' (DC)

CHAKRA – SPLEEN

'Orange' (DC)

CHAKRA – BASE
also, Spirituality/Spiritual Growth

Aubergine, Calendula, Dahlia, Loosestrife, Periwinkle, Poppy, See
Zucchini (CH)
Birth & Re-birth – Root Chakra (CFR Comb)
Base Chakra (CH Comb)*
Comfrey – The Root Chakra (ACFR)
'Emerald', 'Pink Crimson' (DC)
Blackthorn, Yew, Lawsons Cypress, Red Oak (GMTE)
Mock Orange (GMFE)
Dogs Mercury, Lungwort (LLFE)
Geranium, Hibiscus, Orange Lily (SM)
Honeymoon, Tiffany, (RLR)
Daisy, Hyssop, Lavender, Raspberry (JJ)
Red Poppy (JW)
Red Clover (JJ)(LHFE)
Thrift (BE)

CHAKRA – SACRAL
See also, Spirituality/Spiritual Growth

Balsam Poplar (HFE)
Change & Adjustment – Hara Chakra (CFR Comb)
Sacral Chakra (CH Comb)*, *Calendula, Coral Bells, Dahlia,*
Periwinkle, Zucchini (CH)
Whitebeam, Apple, Gean, Holm Oak, Giant Redwood, Larch,
Lawson's Cypress (GMTE)
Dogs Mercury, Lungwort (LLFE)
Hibiscus, Nasturtium, Orange Lily (SM)
Skullcap (CG)
Daisy, Sage, Raspberry (JJ)
Dandelion, Red Clover (LHFE)

CHAKRA-SOLAR PLEXUS
See also, Spirituality/Spiritual Growth

Auricula, Avocado, Chamomile, Fredontodendron, Cinquefoil,
Mahonia, Marsh Marigold, Pennyroyal, Rose of Sharon, Deep Red
Rose (CH)
Beaked Hawksbeard (HFE)
Buttercup, Californian Poppy, Chickweed, Daisy, Lemon Balm,
Peppermint, Pear, Ribes, Thyme (JJ)
Transmutation & Awakening – Solar Plexus Chakra
(CFR Comb)
Sage – The Solar Plexus Chakra (ACFR)
Cowslip (BFR)(HFE)(LHFE)
'All shades of blue', 'Spring Green', 'Gold' (DC)
Great Sallow, Yew, Catalpa, Lawson's Cypress, Lime, Beech, Osier,
Red Oak (GMTE)
Mock Orange, Sage (GMFE)
Daffodil, Hibiscus (SM)
St. John's Wort (CG)
Scarlet Pimpernel (HFE)
Evening Primrose (JW)
Buttercup, Golden Sage, Passion Flower (AFE)
Dandelion (HFE)(LHFE)
Honesty, Red Clover (LHFE)

CHAKRA-HEART
See also, Spirituality/Spiritual Growth

Basil, Bleeding Heart, Camellia, Catmint, Helianthus, Orchid
'Equestris', Soapwort, Sunflower, Weigela (CH)
Heart Chakra (CH Comb)*

	See also, Crystal Herbs – 'Roses'
	Borage (HR)(SE)(CH)
	Protection & Harmony – Heart Chakra (CFR Comb)
	Heart (LLFE Comb), *Tulip (LLFE)*
	Living Blend 3, Solar Blend Resolving Loss (SE Comb)
	Pink & White Hawthorn Body Spray (SE)
	Passionflower – The Heart Chakra (ACFR)
	Louise Odier, Centifolia, Ispahan (CFR)
	Jasmine (CH)(AFR)(JJ)
	'Rose Pink', 'Amethyst', 'Violet', 'Mother of Pearl Ray',
	Lotus Tree' (DC)
	Universal Suffering (GHTE)
	Blackthorn, Apple, Elder, Whitebeam, Magnolia,
	White Poplar (GMTE)
	Passion Flower (GMFE)(CH)
	Wild Violet (GMFE)
	Jasmine, Release, Pink Angel (PE)
	Daffodil, Delphinium, Geranium, Hibiscus (SM)
	Flowering Currant (HR)
	Wood Anemone, Spinach, Stinking Hellebore, Tree Mallow,
	Wild Rose, Marjoram (HFE)
	Wild Pansy (HFE)(FFE)
	Lavender, Pear, Thyme, Wild Garlic, Chickweed, Cosmos,
	Hawthorn, Lemon Balm, Rose Geranium, Rose (JJ)
	Sage (JJ)(GMFE)
	Fuchsia, pink (AT)
	Deep Pink Rose (MERE)
	Bounty Beautiful, Golden Window, Honeymoon,
	Love 'n' Light (RLR)
	Cowslip, Honesty, Red Clover (LHFE)
	Arizona Fir, Buttercup, Milk Thistle (BE)

CHAKRA-HIGHER HEART
See also, Spirituality/Spiritual Growth

Higher Heart Chakra (CH Comb)★
Daisy (AFR)

CHAKRA-THROAT
See also, Spirituality/Spiritual Growth

Anemone, Geranium (SM)
Celandine – The Throat Chakra (ACFR)
Basil, Bellflower, Bluebell, Baby Bottlebrush, Bellflower, Canterbury Bell, Catmint, Ceanothus, Celandine, Flax, Iris 'Bluebeard', Jonquil, Centaurea (CH),
Throat Chakra (CH Comb)★
Delphinium (CH)(SM)
Purpose & Strength – Throat Chakra (CFR Comb)
Amelanchier (BFR)
'Magenta', 'Blue', 'Gold' (DC)
Apple, Black Poplar, Crack Willow, Hazel, Cherry Plum, Giant Redwood, Larch, Beech, Tulip Tree (GMTE)
Passion Flower (GMFE)(CH)
Chickweed, Cosmos, Meadowsweet, Red Clover (JJ)

CHAKRA-BROW
See also, Spirituality/Spiritual Growth

Anemone, Daffodil, Nasturtium (SM)
Honeymoon (RLR)
Head (LLFE Comb)
Anger & Pain – Brow Chakra (CFR Comb)
Brow Chakra (CH Comb)★, *Columbine, Jonquil (CH)*
Nasturtium – The Brow Chakra (ACFR)
Gallica (CFR)
The Bride (BFR)
Black Poplar, Scots Pine, Sycamore, Whitebeam, Cherry Laurel, Holly, Lawson's Cypress, White Willow (GMTE)
Marsh Gentian (GMFE)
Universal Suffering (GHTE)
'Ruby Rose', 'Gold', 'Blue' (DC)
Deadly Nightshade (HFE)

Phormium (JW)

CHAKRA-CROWN
See also, Spirituality/Spiritual Growth

African Violet, Petunia, Self-heal, St. John's Wort, Scarlet Pimpernel (JJ)
Beaked Hawksbeard (HFE)
Brompton Stock, Carnation, Convolvulus, Gazania, Gladiolus, Magnolia, Iris purple, Jonquil, Sweet Violet (CH),
Crown Chakra (CH Comb)*
Release – Crown Chakra (CFR Comb)
Higher Self (AFR Comb), *Daffodil – The Crown Chakra (ACFR)*
Lavender (AFR)(JJ)
Queen Anne's Lace, Rosemary (CH)(JJ)
Sycamore, Magnolia, Cherry Laurel, Strawberry Tree (GMTE)
Daffodil (GMFE)
Forget me not (GMFE)(JJ)
Columbine (GMFE)(CH)
'Gold', 'Silver' (DC)
Nasturtium (SM)
Universal Suffering (GHTE)
Skullcap (CG)
Thistle, Common Spotted Orchid, Pennyroyal (HFE)
Phormium, (JW)

HIGHER CHAKRAS
Crown & above

Centaurea, Convolvulus, Deadnettle, Guelder Rose, Jonquil, Philadelphus, Regensberg, Brompton Stock (CH)
Bay (GMTE)
Columbine, Daffodil (GMFE)
White Light (PE)
Pink Campion, Pale Pink Rose (MEFE)
Chickweed (JJ)
Crystal Light Rainbow (DC)

CHAKRA – 8TH

Clematis (CH)
Christmas Rose (BFR)
'Emerald' (DC)
Great Sallow, Lime (GMTE)
Lavender, Rose (JJ)

CHAKRA – 9TH

Rosemary (BFR)
Corn Cockle (CH)
'Sapphire' (DC)
Lavender, Thyme (JJ)
Witch Hazel (AFE)

CHAKRA – 10TH

Single White Cherry (CFR)
Corn Cockle (CH)
'Pink Lavender' (DC)
Lavender (JJ)

CHAKRA – 11TH

Cowslip (BFR)
'Crystal Blue White Light' (DC)
Black Poplar (GMTE)

CHAKRA – 12TH

Canary Bird Rose (CH)
'Divine White' (DC)

CHAKRA – 13TH

Deadnettle (CH)
'Purest White' (DC)

CHANGE
See also, Moving on/
Spiritual Growth/Transformation

Bistort (BE)
Black-eyed Susan, Onion Flower, Geranium (CH)
Alkanet (HR)
Speedwell (HR)(EE)
Birth & Re-birth – Root Chakra, Change & Adjustment – Hara Chakra (CFR Comb)
Elder, Sweet Chestnut, White Poplar (GMTE)
Honesty, Gorse (GMFE)
Autumn Leaves (SE)
Fuchsia Success (RLR)

	Revelation (FFE Comb)
	Nasturtium (JJ)
	Marigold (SCE)
	Hawthorn, Tormentil (UFE)
	Leopardsbane (BE)
	Blue Geranium (LNE)
CHANNELLING *See also, Psychic development/abilities*	*Nasturtium (CH)* *Universal Suffering (GHTE)* *Judas Tree (GMTE)* *Purple Loosestrife (LLFE)* *Common Spotted Orchid (HFE)* *African Dance (RLR)* *Azalea 'Wayford Woods' (AT)* *Blackberry, Mugwort, Passion Flower (AFE)*
CHANTING	*Bluebell (CH)* *African Dance (RLR)*
CHEERFULNESS *See also, Joy/Lightness/Humour* *Laughter*	*Borage (HR)(SE)* *Zinnia (CH)*
CHILDREN & CHILDHOOD ISSUES *See also, Inner Child*	*Baby-blue eyes (AFR)(CH)* *Bellflower, Nettle, Cowslip, Genista (Broom), Geum, Melilot,* *Petunia, Speedwell, Maidens Blush (CH)* *Bluebell, Valerian, Monk's Hood, Pine Cones, Rhododendron (BE)* ***Childhood (BE Comb)*** *Alba Maxima, Arthur Bell (CFR)* *St. Johns Wort (CG)(HR)* *Alkanet (MEFE)* *Primrose (SE)* *Beautiful World, Peaches & Cream (RLR)* ***Self-worth (GM Comb)****, Elder (GMTE)* *Petunia, Raspberry (JJ)* *Fuchsia, Creeping Buttercup, Dog Violet, Early Purple Orchid,* *Hawkweed (BFE)* *Thorn Apple (JW)* *Cowslip, Pussy Willow (LHFE)*
CHILDLIKE	*Buttercup (JJ)* *Single White Cherry (BFR)* *Petunia (CH)* *Bracken (BE)*
CHILDISH, NOT WANTING TO **GROW UP**	*Almond (CH)* *Bracken, Charlock (BE)*
CITY LIFE	***City (HFE Comb)*** ***City Stress (LLFE Comb)*** ***Solar Blend Stress Relief (SE Comb)***
CLAIRAUDIENCE *See also, Intuition/psychic development*	*Canterbury Bell, Hyacinth, French Marigold (CH)* *Tagetes Patula (JJ)* *Daffodil (CH)(GMFE)*
CLAIRVOYANCE *See also, Intuition/psychic development*	*Universal Suffering (GHTE)* *Daffodil (SM)(GMFE)* *Wild Thyme (HFE)*
CLARITY	***Clear Light (FFE Comb)*** *The Bride, Amelanchier (BFR)* *Claire (CFR)* *Daisy (CH)(AFR)(MEFE)(GMFE)* *Geranium (CH)* *Alder, Box, Pear, Plane Tree, Pittespora, Holly (GMTE)* *Love-in-a-mist, Pennyroyal, Chamomile, Oriental Hellebore (GMFE)* *Forget me not (CH)(GMFE)* *Pink Angel (PE)*

	Cosmos (AFR)(SE)
	Lavender, Harebell (HR)
	Rosemary, Yellow Poppy, Black Tulip (HFE)
	Guelder Rose Berry (EE)
	Aubretia, Red/Orange Rose (MEFE)
	Burning Desire, Tiffany, Tower of Strength, Sunset Boulevard (RLR)
	Peppermint (JJ)
	Square-stalked willowherb (GE)
	Dandelion (JW)*
	Wild Clary (SCE)
	Witch Hazel (BFE)
	Orange (RD)
	Blackberry, Lemon (AFE)
	Crystal Mercury (DC)
CLAUSTROPHOBIA	*Dog Tooth Violet (BFR)*
CLEANSING (EMOTIONAL)	**Cleansing (LLFE Comb)**
See also, Purification	**Solar Blend Flower Essence Lavender Protection Spray (SE Comb)**
	Cosmos, Snowdrop Body Spray (SE)
	Single White Cherry, Canary Bird Rose (BFR)
	Fisherman's Friend, Claire (CFR)
	Garlic, Centaurea, Poppy, Soapwort (CH)
	Crystal Clear, Clear Tone, (PE)
	Red Clover (AFR)
	Hibiscus (SM)
	Lavender, Primrose (HR)
	Yellow Rose (MERE)
	Daffodil, Primrose (JJ)
	Pennyroyal (JW)
	Lady's Smock (BFE)
	Sea Lavender (SCE)
	Crystal Earth Emerald (DC)
	Self Heal (LHFE)
CLUMSY	**Solar Blend Female Cycles of Life (SE Comb)**
	Witch Hazel (BFE)
CO-DEPENDENCE	*Bleeding Heart (SE)(AFR)(CH)*
See also, Neediness/Attachment	*Monkeyflower (FFE)*
	Eyebright (SE)
	Tobacco (JW)
	Common Comfrey, Pink Foxglove (SCE)
	Butterbur (UFE)
	Marsh Thistle, Pine Cones, Scarlet Pimpernel, Witch Hazel (BE)
	Honesty (LHFE)
COLOUR AWARENESS	*Nasturtium (CH)(JJ)*
COMFORT	*Heartsease (Wild Pansy) (HR)*
	Rose, Lemon Balm, Marigold (JJ)
	Buttercup (AFE)
	Cowslip (LHFE)
COMMUNICATION	*Alfalfa (HFE)*
	Anemone (SM)
	Bilberry, Ash, Cherry Plum, Giant Redwood, Judas Tree, White Willow (GMTE)
	Snapdragon, Marsh Gentian, Scabious (GMFE)
	Purpose & Strength – Throat Chakra (CFR Comb), *Church Farm Rose (CFR)*
	Solar Blend for Communication (SE Comb), *Alkanet, Marigold (SE)*
	Celandine – The Throat Chakra (ACFR)
	Harebell, Campanula, Delphinium, Flax (CH)
	Celandine (CH)(MEFE)

	White Foxglove (LLFE)
	Release (PE)
	Spotted Orchid, Lady's Mantle, Broom (FFE)
	Pink Oxalis (EE)
	Yellow Iris, St. John's Wort (SCE)
	Scarlet Pimpernel (BFE)
	Calendula, Evening Primrose (RD)
	Comfrey (LHFE)
	Early Purple Orchid (BE)
COMPASSION	*Borage (AFR), Passionflower – The Heart Chakra (ACFR)*
	Ruby Red (CH)
	Metta, Pink Angel (PE)
	Holy Thorn, Scottish Primrose (FFE)
	Meeshla – The Peace Perfume (OIT Comb)
	Apricot (GE)
	Rue, Cranesbill, Primrose (SCE)
	Lucombe Oak, Mulberry, English Elm (GMTE)
	Honesty, Gorse (LHFE)
	Buttercup, Leopardsbane (BE)
COMPETITIVENESS	*Spindle (GMTE)*
CONCENTRATION	*Broom (FFE)*
See also, Lack of attention/	*Comfrey – The Root Chakra (ACFR)*
Focus/Study	*Lesser Celandine (LLFE)*
	Fennel (MEFE)
	Lemon Balm (JJ)
	Primrose (GE)
	Meadowsweet (BFE)
	Penstemon, St. John's Wort (AFE)
	Wood Anemone (UFE)
CONDITIONING	*Cornflower (JJ)*
	Lungwort (UFE)
	Thorn Apple (HFE)
CONCERN & LACK OF	*Wild Iris (CH)*
See also, Worry	*Bird Cherry (GMTE)*
CONFIDENCE	*Bell Heather (FFE)*
	Buttercup (RD)
	***Assuredness, Tranquillity (GM Comb)**, Black Poplar, Catalpa, Cherry Plum, Beech, Pear, Sweet Chestnut, Hornbeam (GMTE)*
	Snowdrop, Snowflake (GMFE)
	Solar Blend Confidence (SE Comb)
	Sage – The Solar Plexus Chakra (ACFR)
	Flax, Geum, Harebell (CH)
	Golden Rod (LLFE)
	Cymbidium, Tormentil (HR)
	Cornflower, Ribes (JJ)
	Self-Confidence (DC Comb)
	Ground Ivy (EE)
	Brethren Child (RLR)
	Forget-me-not (BFE)
	Creeping Jenny (SCE)
	Wood Sorrel, Spear Thistle (UFE)
	Charlock (BE)
	Plantain (LNE)
	White Leaved Oak (GHTE)
CONFLICT	*Bell Heather, Mallow (FFE)*
	Protection & Harmony – Heart Chakra (CFR Comb)
	Sycamore (GMTE)
	Flowering Currant (GMFE)
	Mayweed, Vipers Bugloss (HFE)
	Meeshla – The Peace Perfume (OIT Comb)

<table>
<tr><td></td><td>Ragged Robin (BFE)</td></tr>
<tr><td></td><td>Nettle (UFE)</td></tr>
<tr><td></td><td>Gorse (LHFE)</td></tr>
<tr><td>CONFUSION</td><td>Birch, Broom, Wild Pansy, (FFE)</td></tr>
<tr><td></td><td>Protection & Harmony – Heart Chakra (CFR Comb)</td></tr>
<tr><td></td><td>Cowslip, The Bride (BFR)</td></tr>
<tr><td></td><td>Church Farm Rose (CFR)</td></tr>
<tr><td></td><td>Box, Lucombe Oak (GMTE)</td></tr>
<tr><td></td><td>Pennyroyal (GMFE)</td></tr>
<tr><td></td><td>Red Clover (LLFE)</td></tr>
<tr><td></td><td>Honesty, Self-heal (HR)</td></tr>
<tr><td></td><td>Pink & White Hawthorn Body Spray (SE)</td></tr>
<tr><td></td><td>Blue Mood (RLR)</td></tr>
<tr><td></td><td>Foxglove, Queen Anne's Lace (JJ)</td></tr>
<tr><td></td><td>Remedy 1 'Help' (JW Comb)</td></tr>
<tr><td></td><td>Creeping Buttercup (BFE)</td></tr>
<tr><td></td><td>Elderflower (SCE)</td></tr>
<tr><td></td><td>Holly Buds (AT)</td></tr>
<tr><td></td><td>Primrose (UFE)</td></tr>
<tr><td></td><td>Daisy (UFE)(FFE)</td></tr>
<tr><td></td><td>Foxglove, Soapwort (BE)</td></tr>
<tr><td>CONNECTEDNESS</td><td>Violet (UFE)</td></tr>
<tr><td>CONSIDERATION</td><td>White Clover (EE)</td></tr>
<tr><td>CONTENTMENT</td><td>Bay Buds (AT)</td></tr>
<tr><td></td><td>Bluebell (HR)(BFE)</td></tr>
<tr><td></td><td>Chickweed (HFE)</td></tr>
<tr><td></td><td>Valerian (FFE)</td></tr>
<tr><td></td><td>Sea Campion (BE)</td></tr>
<tr><td>CONTROLLING/CONTROLLED
See also, Dominating</td><td>Hazel, Rose Alba (FFE)</td></tr>
<tr><td></td><td>Vipers Bugloss (SE)</td></tr>
<tr><td></td><td>Scarlett Pimpernel (JJ)</td></tr>
<tr><td></td><td>Possession (BE Comb)</td></tr>
<tr><td></td><td>Pussy Willow (LHFE)</td></tr>
<tr><td>COURAGE
See also, Inner Strength</td><td>Agapanthus, Handel, 'Yellow' (CH)</td></tr>
<tr><td></td><td>Agave (JW)</td></tr>
<tr><td></td><td>Black-eyed Susan (JJ)</td></tr>
<tr><td></td><td>Borage (HR)(SE)(AFR)(RD)</td></tr>
<tr><td></td><td>Solar Blend Confidence (SE Comb)</td></tr>
<tr><td></td><td>Mullein (SE)</td></tr>
<tr><td></td><td>Amelanchier (BFR)</td></tr>
<tr><td></td><td>Bud Essence, (GHTE)</td></tr>
<tr><td></td><td>Wild Violet (GMFE), Italian Alder (GMTE)</td></tr>
<tr><td></td><td>Tormentil (HR)</td></tr>
<tr><td></td><td>Thistle, Rose Water Lily (FFE)</td></tr>
<tr><td></td><td>Hero (RLR)</td></tr>
<tr><td></td><td>Snowdrop (UFE)</td></tr>
<tr><td></td><td>Red Clover (LHFE)</td></tr>
<tr><td>COUNSELLING/PSYCHOTHERAPY</td><td>Onion (AFR)</td></tr>
<tr><td></td><td>Wild Clary (SCE)</td></tr>
<tr><td>CRAVING
See also, Addiction</td><td></td></tr>
<tr><td>CREATIVITY</td><td>Azalea 'Wayford Woods' (AT)</td></tr>
<tr><td></td><td>Bellflower, Bluebell, Iris purple, Rosemary, Thrift (CH)</td></tr>
<tr><td></td><td>Blackberry (JJ)</td></tr>
<tr><td></td><td>Broom (FFE)</td></tr>
<tr><td></td><td>Comfrey – The Root Chakra, Red Dead Nettle –</td></tr>
<tr><td></td><td>The Sacral Chakra (ACFR)</td></tr>
<tr><td></td><td>Evelyn, Louise Odier (CFR)</td></tr>
<tr><td></td><td>Bud Essence (GHTE)</td></tr>
<tr><td></td><td>Bugle (LLFE)</td></tr>
</table>

Daffodil – The Crown Chakra, Passionflower –
The Heart Chakra (ACFR)
Relaxation (GM Comb), *Copper Beech (GMTE)*
Solar Blend Depression (SE Comb)
Christmas Rose (BFR)
Dill, Potato (CH)
Petunia (CH)(AFR)
Violet (LLFE)
Soul Star, Jasmine, Ankh (PE)
Daffodil (HR)
Geranium (SM)
Primrose (HR)(JJ)
Majestic Triumph, Peaches & Cream, Sunset Boulevard, Astronomy,
Candle Light, Marylight, Freedom Dance, Fuchsia Success,
Honeymoon (RLR)
Field Scabious (BFE)
Evening Primrose (SCE)
Yucca (GE)
Lavender (SCE)
Blackberry, Penstemon (AFE)
Uplift (HR Comb)
Bluebell (BE)(JJ)
Bistort, Bracken (BE)
Pussy Willow (LHFE)

DESPAIR
See also, Hope/hopelessness/
Sadness

Blackthorn (JJ)(BE)
Relaxation (GM Comb),
Universal Suffering (GHTE)
Pilgrim (CFR)
Buddleia, Yellow Rattle (CH)
Gorse (AFR)
Majestic Triumph, Honeymoon (RLR)
Dog Violet, Lady's Smock, Purple Loosestrife (BFE)
Despair & Despondency (DC Comb)
Tormentil (MEFE)
Yucca (GE)
Yellow Woundwort (SCE)
Despair (BE Comb)

DESTRUCTIVENESS
See also, Abuse

Anger & Pain – Brow Chakra(CFR Comb)
Peaches & Cream (RLR)

DETACHMENT

Water Lily (HFE)
Mallow, Wild Pansy (FFE), ***Revelation (FFE Comb)***
Sweet Pea (JJ)
Mulberry (GMTE) Saxifrage (GMFE)
Solomon's Seal, Pink Purslane, Rhododendron (BE)

DEVAS
See also, Nature awareness

Nature Spirit (LLFE Comb), *Thyme (LLFE)*
Carnation (CH)
Hazel, Rowan, Whitebeam, Yellow Buckeye (GMTE)
Common Spotted Orchid, Four Leaved Clover (HFE)
Tutson, Bluebell (MEFE)
Lancelot (RLR)

DIRECTION
See also, Lack/Uncertain of Direction

DISAPPOINTMENT

Tranquillity (GM Comb)
Hazel (FFE)
Compact Rush (BE)

DISCERNMENT

Bilberry, Yew, Catalpa, Laburnum, Plane Tree (GMTE)
Snowdrop (GMFE)
Tansy, Wood Anemone (HFE)
Petunia (JW)
Vipers Bugloss (SCE)

	Change & Adjustment – Hara Chakra (CFR Comb) **Emotional (LLFE Comb)**, *Calendula , Cypress, Dandelion, Rosemary (LLFE)*

Change & Adjustment – Hara Chakra (CFR Comb)
Emotional (LLFE Comb), *Calendula , Cypress, Dandelion, Rosemary (LLFE)*
Red Dead Nettle – The Sacral Chakra (ACFR)
Baby Blue Eyes, Chamomile, Onion (AFR)
Evening Primrose (AFR)(AFE)
Christmas Rose, Dog Tooth Violet (BFR)
Corn, White Fuschia, Fuschia, Guelder Rose, Kerria, Mahonia, Pulsatilla, Rudbeckia, Auricula, Avocado (CH)
Golden Light, Amorthyst (PE)
Cowslip (HFE)
Coltsfoot (JW), **Remedy 2 'SOS' (JW Comb)**
Bluebell, Sloe (BBFE)
Catalpa, Lime, Copper Beech, Manna Ash, Mulberry (GMTE)
Chamomile, Flowering Currant, Honesty, Rue (GMFE)
Sorrel (UFE)
Honesty (LHFE)
Cornbine, Honeysuckle, Dog Rose, Spotted Orchid, Thrift, Yellow Dock (SCE)
Stinging Nettle (RD)
Jasmine (AFE)

EMPATHY
See also, Compassion

Passionflower – The Heart Chakra (ACFR)
Globe Thistle (FFE)
Flowering Red Currant (BFE)
Fumitory (SCE)

SELF-EMPOWERMENT
See also, Personal Power/Purpose/ Potential

Willowherb, Monkeyflower, Rose Alba (FFE)
Lady's Smock, Flowering Red Currant (BFE)
Redwood Body Spray, Sunflower (SE)
Self-heal (JJ)
Meeshia – The Peace Perfume (OIT Comb)
Snowflake, Plum (GMFE)
Lungwort (UFE)
Wild Thyme (HR)

ENCOURAGEMENT

Lesser Stitchwort (BE)

ENHANCEMENT OF VIBRATIONAL REMEDIES

Orchid 'Oncidium' (CH)
Thyme (CH)(AFR)(JJ)(SCE)(RD)
Alder (GMTE), Camphor (GMFE)
Blackberry (AFE)

ENTHUSIASM

Gorse (FFE)
Witch Hazel (BE)
Scabious (GMFE), English Elm (GMTE)

ENVY
See also, Greed/Materialism

Holm Oak (GMTE)

ESCAPISM
See also, Denial, Avoidance

Birch (FFE)
Tansy (AFR)
Oriental Poppy (HR)

EXPECTATIONS

Firethorn, Rhododendron (BE)

EXHIBITIONIST

Rhubarb(HR)
Balsam (FFE)

EXPRESSION
See also, Communication

Alfalfa (HFE)
Bluebell (CH)
Purpose & Strength – Throat Chakra (CFR Comb)
Holm Oak, Silver Birch, Catalpa, Mimosa, Magnolia (GMTE)
Wild Violet, Snapdragon, Rue, Golden Crocus, Mock Orange (GMFE)
Holy Thorn (FFE)
Toadflax (JJ)
Coltsfoot (JW)
Creeping Jenny, Welsh Poppy, Evening Primrose, Purple Toadflax,

Cornflower, Trefoil, Yellow Woundwort (SCE)
Bracken, Lilac (BE)

FAILURE
See also, Rejection/Confidence

Solar Blend Confidence (SE Comb)
Relaxation (GM Comb)
Purple Loosestrife (BFE)
Mullein (SCE)
Red Campion (UFE)

FALSE PERSONA
See also, Rejection/Confidence

Blackthorn (JJ)
Meadowsweet (SE)

FAMILIES

Sweet Pea (CH)
Spirit Ground (PE)

FANTASIES

Nasturtium – The Brow Chakra (ACFR)

FATHER AND FATHERING
See also Parenting/
Masculine consciousness

Birth & Re-birth – Root Chakra (CFR Comb)
Arthur Bell (CFR)
Cowslip (CH)
Sunflower (CH)(AFR)(SM)
Scarlet Pimpernel (MEFE)

FEAR/FEARLESSNESS

Bindweed, Black Medick (EE)
Release – Crown Chakra, Transmutation & Awakening –
Solar Plexus Chakra (CFR Comb), Cadfael, Mary Rose (CFR)
Solar Blend Fear, Solar Blend Crisis,
Solar Blend Sleep (SE Comb)
Comfrey – The Root Chakra (ACFR)
Fig, Peace, Pink Rose (CH)
Garlic (CH)(AFR)
Leyland Cypress, Horse Chestnut, Ivy, Lime, Norway Maple,
Red Chestnut (GMTE)
Flowering Current (GMFE)
Blackthorn (LLFE)
Silver Genie, Fire Clear (PE)
Delphinium (SM)
Nasturtium (SM)(JJ)
St. Johns Wort (CG)(HR)(GMFE)
Chamomile, Marjoram, Rosemary (HR)
Dandelion (HR)(JJ)(LHFE)
Water Forget-me-not (HFE)
Harebell, Scottish Primrose, Thistle, Balsam (FFE)
Fear (DC Comb)
Purple Passion, Time Immemorial, Peaches & Cream (RLR)
Bluebell (SCE)(JJ)
Ribes (JJ)
Remedy 1 'Help' (JW Comb)
Field Scabious, Scarlet Pimpernel, Sloe, Witch Hazel,
Purpose Loosestrife (BFE)
Plantain, Scarlet Pimpernel, Sorrel, Spotted Orchid (SCE)
Honeysuckle, Passion Flower, Harebell (AFE)
Wood Anenome, Bracken – Aqueous Extract, Double Snowdrop,
Flowering Currant, Marsh Thistle, Milk Thistle, Moss (BE),
Fears (BE Comb)
Gorse (UFE)
Red Clover (LHFE)

FEAR OF DYING
See also, Death/Fears

Blackberry (JJ)(AFR)(CH)(MEFE)
Lady of the Night (CH)
Chrysanthemum (AFR)
Snowdrop (FFE)
Karmic Helper (RLR)

FEMININE CONSCIOUSNESS
See also, Mother & Mothering/
Parenting

Birth & Re-birth – Root Chakra Chakra (CFR Comb)
Female Comb. (HFE Comb), *Golden Saxifrage,*
Wild Thyme (HFE)
Silvery Moon, Stand Alone, Silver Genie, Jasmine, Orange Chalice,

	White Light (PE)
	Hawthorn, Hazel, Lords & Ladies (LLFE)
	Lady's Mantle (HR)
	Balsam (FFE)
	Dwarf Mallow (EE)
	Lady's Mantle (SE)
	Honesty (JJ)
	Honeysuckle, Centaury (SCE)
	Quince (GMFE)
FLEXIBILITY/INFLEXIBILITY	*Buttercup, Dandelion (EE)*
	Digitalis (CH)
	Ash, Crack Willow, Osier (GMTE)
	Honesty (GMFE)
	Globe Thistle (FFE)
	Feverfew (SE)
	Daisy (JJ)
	Cantabillae-Auric (OIT Comb)
FICKLENESS	*Sloe (BFE)*
FREEDOM	*Arizona Fir, Double Snowdrop (BE)*
FOCUS	*Fennel (MEFE)*
	Pulsatilla, Cranesbill, Valerian (CH)
	Anemone (SM)
	Red Clover (LLFE)
	Geranium – Cranesbill (HR)
	Self heal (JH)
	Fuchsia Success (RLR)
	Square-stalked willowherb (GE)
	Buddleia (SCE)
	Pussy Willow (AT)
	Sweet Chestnut (GMTE), Daisy (GMFE)
	Forget-me-not (UFE)
FORGETFUL	*Rosemary (JJ)*
See also, Memory/Absentmindedness	*Sloe (BFE)*
FORGIVENESS	*Blackberry, Chickweed (JJ)*
	Protection & Harmony – Heart Chakra (CFR Comb)
	Joy, Forgiveness (GM Comb), *Bird Cherry, Hawthorn, Elder,*
	Scots Pine (GMTE)
	Golden Crocus (GMFE)
	Sweet Violet (CH)(GE)
	White Violet (CH)
	Ragwort (LLFE)
	Snowdrop Body Spray (SE)
	Orange Azalea (AT)
	Golden Sage (AFE)
	Gorse (LHFE)
FRUSTRATION	*Hazel (FFE)*
	Anger & Pain – Brow Chakra (CFR Comb)
	Assuredness (GM Comb) *Gorse (GMTE)*
	Single White Cherry (BFR)
	Cymbidium (HR)
	Spindle (LLFE)
	Orange Lily (SM)
	Snapdragon (HR)
	Brethren Child, Peaches & Cream (RLR)
	Dandelion (JW)
	Silverweed, Common Vetch (SCE)
	Sloe (BFE)
	Bracken (BE)

FUTURE LIVES	*Thyme (CH)*
GENEROSITY	***Relaxation (GM Comb)***
	Meeshla – The Peace Perfume (OIT Comb)
GENTLENESS	*Grass of Parnassus (FFE)*
	Pink Oxalis (EE)
	Harebell (HR)
GOALS	*Apple (FFE)*
	Meadowsweet (BFE)
	Oriental Hellebore, Wild Violet (GMFE)
GRACE	*Stonecrop (FFE)*
GRATITUDE	*Ispahan (CFR)*
GREED	***Tranquillity (GM Comb)***
See also, Envy/Materialism	*Holm Oak (GMTE)*
	Apricot (GE)
	Witch Hazel (BFE)
GRIEF	*Basil (CH)*
See also, Sadness/Hope/lessness	*Bleeding Heart, Jack-by-the-Hedge, Pink & White Body Spray,*
	Hawthorn (SE)
	Bluebell (JJ)
	Relaxation (GM Comb)
	Passionflower – The Heart Chakra (ACFR)
	Christmas Rose, Single White Cherry (BFR)
	Louise Odier, Centifolia (CFR)
	Purple Loosestrife (LLFE)
	Hawthorn (HR)(MEFE)(JJ)
	Heartsease (Wild Pansy) (HR)
	Release (PE)
	Hedge Woundwort, Tree Mallow (HFE)
	Snowdrop (FFE)
	Rosebay willowherb (SCE)
	Scarlet Pimpernel (BFE)
	Harebell (AFE)
	Spear Thistle (UFE)
	Honesty (LHFE)
	Grief (BE Comb)
GROUNDEDNESS/GROUNDING	*Copper Beech (SE)*
	Alfalfa, Pennyroyal (HFE)
	Anemone (SM)
	Blackberry (SE)(AFR)
	Birth & Re-birth – Root Chakra (CFR Comb)
	Grounding (LLFE Comb), *Ivy (LLFE)*
	Comfrey – The Root Chakra (ACFR)
	Dipladenia White, Hoya, Loosestrife, Poppy, Sweet Pea, Valerian,
	Ageratum (CH)
	Bay (GMTE)
	Spirit Ground (PE)
	Hibiscus (SM)
	Eye on Bright, Ruchsia Success, Lancelot, Marylight, Tiffany, Tower
	of Strength (RLR)
	Meadowsweet (BFE)
	Pear, Pinks (JJ)
	Primrose (GE)
	Coltsfoot (JW)
	Hyacinth (AT)
	Golden Sage, Lavender, Passion Flower (AFE)
	Loosestrife (LNE) (CH)
	Speedwell (UFE)
	Crystal Galaxy (DC)
	Thrift (BE)
	White Leaved Oak (GHTE)

GROUP EXPERIENCE/WORK/ ATTUNEMENT
See also, Communication

African Violet, Hyssop, Hops, Lemon Balm, Meadowsweet (JJ)
Mullein, Harebell, Flax, Pink Rose H.F. (CH)
Mistletoe (LLFE)
Fire Clear, Silver Genie (PE)
Pear (MEFE)(CH)(JJ)
Buttercup, Stonecrop (MEFE)
Snowdrop, Lungwort (UFE)

GUILT
See also, Shame

Basil (AFR), Passionflower – The Heart Chakra (ACFR)
Self-worth (GM Comb)
Single White Cherry, Canary Bird Rose (BFR)
Hyssop (CH)(AFR)(HR)
Judas Tree (CH)
Release (PE)
Iris/Dioptase★ (SM)
Iona Pennywort (FFE)
Bluebell (JJ)
Plantain (SCE)
Rock Rose, St. John's Wort (AFE)
Wood Anemone (BE)

HALLUCINATIONS

Nasturtium – The Brow Chakra (ACFR)

HATE
See also, Jealousy/Anger

Clear Star, Release (PE)
Dandelion (HFE)
Lady's Smock (BFE)
Penstemon (AFE)

HEALING

Hazel (EE)
Lychnis, Himalayan Poppy (CH)
Gean (GMTE)
Yew (LLFE)
Amorthyst, Pink Angel (PE)
Yellow Loosestrife (MEFE)
Self-heal (SE)(JJ)
Sacrifice Nothing, Saviour (RLR)
Lemon Balm, Pinks (JJ)
Phormium (JW)
Thyme (SCE)

HIGHER SELF

Higher Self (AFR Comb)
Clear Light (FFE Comb), *Lime, Rose Alba (FFE)*
Living Blend 5 (SE Comb), *Bluebell (SE)*
Daffodil, Golden Rod (CH)
Box, Crack Willow, Holm Oak (GMTE)
Lady's Smock, Purple Loosestrife (LLFE)
Soul Star (PE)
Lavender (AFR)(SM)
Skullcap (CG)
Sage (HR)
Hawthorn Leaf (EE)
Yellow Rose (MERE), **Unicorn Essence (ME Comb)**
Peaches & Cream (RLR)
Gardenia, Petunia, Peppermint, St. John's Wort (JJ)
Phormium, Romneya (JW)
Self-heal (LNE)

HONESTY
See also, False Persona

Campanula (CH)
Honesty (HR)(JJ)
Fuchsia (BFE)

HOPE/HOPELESSNESS
See also, Despair/Sadness

Agave (JW)
Relaxation (GM Comb)
Solar Blend Depression (SE Comb)
Pilgrim (CFR)
Chionodoxa, Wintersweet, Yellow Rattle (CH)
Gorse (AFR)

	Tormentil (HR)(BFE)
	Snowdrop (MEFE)
HUMOUR *See also, Joy/Laughter/Cheerfulness*	*Zinnia (CH)* *Bud Essence (GHTE)* *Leyland Cypress (GMTE)* *Thyme (LLFE)* *Spirit Ground (PE)*
HUMILITY	***Self-worth (GM Comb)*** *Gallica (CFR)* *Daisy (AFR)* *Silverweed, Willowherb, Globe Thistle (FFE)* *Apricot (GE)*
IDEALISM	*Fuchsia (BFE)* *Rue (SCE)*
IDEAS *See also, Inspiration*	*Blackberry (SE)* *Groundsel (CH)* *Geranium – Cranesbill((HR)* *Yellow Poppy (HFE)* *Laurel (FFE)* *Strawberry, Trefoil (SCE)* *Witch Hazel (AFE)* *Mimosa, Judas Tree, Lucombe Oak (GMTE)* *Saxifrage (GMFE)*
IDENTITY CRISIS	*Canary Bird Rose (BFR)*
ILLUSION	*Honesty (CH)* *Leyland Cypress (GMTE)* *Monkshood (HFE)* *Iona Pennywort (FFE)* *Ornamental Crab Apple (AT)* *Pink Purslane (BE)*
IMAGINATION	*Snowdrop (GMFE), Cherry Laurel (GMTE)*
IMPATIENCE *See also, Patience*	***Assuredness (GM Comb)**, Horse Chestnut (GMTE)* *Lady's Smock (BFE)*
INADEQUACY	*St. Johns Wort (CG)* ***Relaxation (GM Comb)*** *Forget-me-not (BFE)* *Pine Cones (BE)*
INDECISION *See also, Uncertainty*	*Bell Heather, Scots Pine (FFE)* ***Change & Adjustment – Hara Chakra (CFR Comb)*** ***Solar Blend New Directions (SE Comb)*** *Cowslip (BFR)* *Wild Orchid (CH)* *Red Clover (LLFE)* *Speedwell (SCE)* *Penstemon (AFE)* *English Elm, Hornbeam (GMTE)* *Primrose (UFE)*
INDEPENDENCE	*Tree Lichen (GMTE)* *Bluebell (SCE)*
INDIVIDUALITY	*Ox-eyed Daisy (SCE)* ***Transmutation & Awakening – Solar Plexus Chakra (CFR Comb)*** *Stand Alone (PE)* *Golden Rod (AFR)* *Cornflower, Harebell (HR)* ***Strength (GM Comb)***

INERTIA
See also, Procrastination/Avoidance

Blackberry, Butterfly Bush (JJ)
Stonecrop (FFE)
Scarlet Pimpernel (BFE)

INFERIORITY COMPLEX

Solar Blend Confidence (SE Comb)
Plantain (LNE)

INFLEXIBILITY
See also, Flexibility

INJUSTICE

Anger & Pain – Brow Chakra (CFR Comb)
Elder (HR)
Monterey Pine (GMTE)

INNER CHILD
See also, Childhood Issues/
Children

Bracken (BFR)
Buttercup, Snowdrop, White Narcissus (HR)
***Change & Adjustment – Hara Chakra (CFR Comb)**, Alba*
Maxima (CFR)
Cowslip (LLFE)
Pink Flox, Pale Pink Rose, Stonecrop (MEFE)
Hawthorn (BFE)
Bindweed, Passion Flower (AFE)
Pussy Willow (LHFE)
Plantain (LNE)

INNER PEACE
See also, Calming/Stillness/
Tranquillity/Relaxation

Assuredness (GM Comb), Holly, Italian Alder, Mimosa,
Pear, Persian Ironwood (GMTE)
Yellow Archangel (SE)
Magnolia, Brethren Child (RLR)
Lady's Smock (BFE)
Grass of Parnassus (FFE)
Fuchsia – red (AT)
Scabious (SCE)
Red Clover, Lobelia (RD)
Honeysuckle (AFE)
Crystal Celestial (DC)
Dandelion (LHFE)

INNER STRENGTH

Agave (JW)
Alfalfa (HFE)
Alkanet, Cymbidium, Rosemary, Harebell (HR)
Bindweed, Oak Acorn (EE)
Bistort (BFR)
Change & Adjustment – Hara Chakra, Transmutation &
***Awakening – Solar Plexus Chakra (CFR Comb)**, Alexander,*
Fisherman's Friend (CFR)
Borage (RD)
Buttercup (RD)(HR)
Himalayan Poppy, Ladies Bedstraw, Agapanthus (CH)
Ash (GMTE), Mock Orange, Pennyroyal (GMFE)
Fleabane, Hedge Woundwort, Ivy, Wild Rose, Tree Mallow, Five
Leaved Red Clover (HFE)
Thistle (HFE)(FFE)
New Zealand Flax (IC)
Sycamore, Snowdrop, Globe Thistle, Bell Heather (FFE)
Pink Yarrow (MEFE)
Trine Tree (SE)
Freedom Dance, Hero, Soul Retrieval (RLR)
Pear, Pinks, Ribes (JJ)
Strelitzia (GE)
Weld (SCE)
Bittercress, Bramble, Gorse, Tormentil (UFE)
Bog Asphodel, Flowering Currant (BE)
White Leaved Oak (GHTE)

INSECURITY
See also, Security

Baby Blue Eyes, Rosemary (AFR), Daffodil – The Crown
Chakra (ACFR)

Feverfew, Lily (CH)
Plantain (SCE)
Assuredness (GM Comb)
Wood Anemone (UFE)
Sundew (LNE)
Sea Campion (BE)

INSPIRATION
See also, Ideas

Nasturtium – The Brow Chakra (ACFR)
Wintersweet (CH)
Violet (LLFE)
Yellow Poppy (HFE)
Spotted Orchid (FFE)
St. John's Wort (AFE)
Lucombe Oak, Cherry Laurel (GMTE), Columbine (GMFE)
Welsh Poppy (BE)

INSTABILITY
See also, Stability

INTEGRATION

Hyacinth, Lupin (CH)
New Zealand Flax (IC)
Rowan (HR)
Crystal Venus (DC)
Gorse, Spindle (GMTE)
Yarrow (UFE)

INTEGRITY

Thistle (HR)
Silverweed, Willowherb, Mallow (FFE)
***Strength (GM Comb)**, Golden Crocus, Pennyroyal (GMFE)*
Pussy Willow (LHFE)

INTELLECTUALISM

Cowslip (BFR)
Coreopsis (CH)
Nasturtium (SE)(JJ)
Queen Anne's Lace (JJ)
Daisy (RD)
Horse Chestnut (GMTE), Daisy (GMFE)
Foxglove (BE)

INTIMACY

Holy-thorn, Balsam (FFE)

INTROSPECTION

Lime (FFE)
Plane Tree (GMTE)

INTROVERSION

Christmas Rose (BFR)
Cosmos (AFR)
Belladonna (JW)
Golden Sage (AFE)

INTOLERANCE
See also, Tolerance/Acceptance/Flexibility

Red Clover (SCE)
Horse Chestnut (GMTE)
***Self-worth (GM Comb)**, Elder (GMTE)*
Solar Blend Transformation of Anger (SE Comb)
Lime, Mallow (FFE)

INTUITION
See also, Clairaudience/
Clairvoyance/Psychic development/
abilities

Broom, Scots Pine, Rose Alba (FFE)
Nasturtium – The Brow Chakra, Daffodil –
The Crown Chakra (ACFR)
Ivy (LLFE)
Silver Genie (PE)
Daffodil, French Marigold (SM)
Dwarf Elder (HFE)
Freedom Dance (RLR)
Euphrasia (BFE)
Campsis (GE)
Weld, Self-heal, Tufted Vetch, White Foxglove, Knapweed, Fumitory,
Tansy (SCE)
Cherry Laurel, Field Maple (GMTE)
Daisy, Pansy, Snowdrop, St. John's Wort (GMFE)
White Leaved Oak (GHTE)

Daffodil (JJ) (GMFE)
Chamomile, Forget-me-not, Marsh Gentian (GMFE)
Stag's Horn Sumach, Tulip Tree (GMTE)
Comfrey (LHFE)
Solomon's Seal (BE)

MEMORY/MEMORIES

Fig, Magnolia (CH)
Forget-me-not (MEFE)(CH)(JJ)(AFE)
Yew (GMTE)
Holy Thorn, Lesser Celandine (LLFE)
Comfrey (JJ)(HR)
Eyebright (HR)
Forget-me-not (AFR)
Rosemary, Yellow Poppy, Marjoram (HFE)
Thyme (JJ)
Primrose (GE)
Lady's Smock (BFE)
Honeysuckle, St. John's Wort (AFE)
Hairy Sedge (BE)

MENTAL FATIGUE
See also, Fatigue/Exhaustion/
Tiredness/Energy

Solar Blend Mental Fatigue (SE Comb)
Yucca (GE)
Red Poppy (JW)
Peppermint (SE)
Hawthorn (BFE)
Tansy (AFE)

MENTAL GROWTH

Primrose (CH)
Silver Genie (PE)
Lesser Celandine (LLFE)
Elderflower (RD)
Thorn Apple (AFE)
Pansy (GMFE)

MERIDIANS

Meridian Energiser (GM Comb), *Bay, Elder, Holm Oak, Silver*
Maple, Sycamore (GMTE)
Lungwort, Rosemary, Stinking Hellebore (LLFE)
Maple (JJ)
Wisteria (CH)
Blackberry, Bindweed, Golden Sage, Lemon, Penstemon, St. John's
Wort, Thorn Apple, Witch Hazel (AFE)

MODESTY

Self-worth (GM Comb)
Grass of Parnassus (FFE)

MORALITY

Hero, Candle Light, Saviour (RLR)

MOTHER AND MOTHERING
See also, Parenting/
Feminine Consciousness

Birth & Re-birth – Root Chakra (CFR Comb)
Alba Maxima (CFR)
Cowslip (CH)

MOTHER EARTH
See also, Earth Healing

Trillium (CH)
Yew (GMTE)
Ivy (HFE)
Daisy, Ground Ivy (EE)
Sweet Pea (JJ)
Camelia (RD)
Comfrey (LHFE)

MOTIVATION & LACK OF

Gorse (FFE)
Butterfly Bush (JJ)
Ankh, Fire Clear (PE)
Tansy (SE)
Burning Desire (RLR)
Marigold (SCE)
Golden Sage, St. John's Wort (AFE)

MOVING ON
See also, Change/Spiritual Growth

Cantabillae Auric (OIT Comb)
Broom (JJ)

	Change & Adjustment – Hara Chakra (CFR Comb) *Primula, Begonia (CH)* *Stinking Hellebore, Hairy Nightshade, Papaya (HFE)* *Rose Water Lily (FFE)* *Sweet Violet (GE)* *Forget-me-not (BFE)* *White Poplar, Rosebay willowherb (UFE)* *Charlock, Marsh Thistle, Soapwort (BE)*
MUSIC *See also, Singing*	*Pear (MEFE)* *Fuchsia (BFE)* *Bluebell (CH)*
NARROWMINDEDNESS	*Silverweed (FFE)*
NATURE AWARENESS	*Tutsan (MEFE)* *Buttercup (JJ)* ***Nature Spirit (LLFE Comb)*** *Sweet Juliet (CFR)* *Rowan, Whitebeam. Yellow Buckeye (GMTE)* *Four Leaved Clover (HFE)* *Balsam (FFE)* *Autumn Leaves (SE)* *Bells of Ireland (CH)* *Cleavers, Pineappleweed (SCE)* *Comfrey (LHFE)*
NEEDINESS *See also, Co-dependence/* *Attachment*	*Barley Grains, Bay Buds (AT)* *Bleeding Heart (SE)(AFR)(CH)* *Bog Asphodel (LNE)* *Hawthorn (UFE)*
NEGATIVITY	*St. John's Wort (CG)* ***Anger & Pain – Brow Chakra (CFR Comb)**, Claire (CFR)* *City (HFE Comb)* ***Head (LLFE Comb)**, Marsh Orchid, Stinking Hellebore (LLFE)* *Daffodil – The Crown Chakra (ACFR)* *Digitalis, Pennyroyal, Deep Red Rose (CH)* *Holm Oak (GMTE)* *Crystal Clear, Fire Clear, Clear Star, Aura Blue, Clear Tone (PE)* *Geranium (SM)* *Forget-me-not, Snapdragon, Yarrow (HR)* *Sycamore, Snowdrop (FFE)* ***Meeshla – The Peace Perfume (OIT Comb)*** *Time Immemorial, African Dance, Look Lively, Love 'n' Light,* *Marylight, Purple Paradise, Refresh your Memory, Saviour, Solemn* *Feast, Soul Retrieval (RLR)* *Nasturtium, Sage, Wild Garlic (JJ)* *Sweet Violet (GE)* *Strawberry (SCE)* *White Yarrow (MEFE)(SE)* *Cosmos, Pink Yarrow, Orange Hawkweed (SE)* *Purple Loosestrife (BFE)* *Witch Hazel, Lemon (AFE)* *Holly Buds (AT)* *Yarrow (UFE)* *Crystal Earth Violet (DC)* *Dandelion (LHFE)* *Buttercup, Bluebell (BE)*
NERVOUSNESS *See also, Anxiety*	***Solar Blend Confidence (SE Comb)*** *Mary Rose (CFR)* *Harebell, Morning Glory (CH)* *Alder (GMTE)* *Forget-me-not (BFE)* *Monkeyflower (FFE)* *Lavender (MEFE)*

**PERSONAL POWER/PURPOSE/
POTENTIAL**
*See also, Individuality/
Empowerment*

Iris (Blue Flag), Red Rose (HR)
Marjoram (HFE)
Apple, Monkeyflower (FFE)
Daisy (FFE)(EE)
Self-heal (JJ)
Snowdrop Body Spray (SE)
Bull Thistle Buds, Lily 'Stargazer', Nasturtium Leaf (AT)
Golden Sage (AFE)
*Ivy, Lawson's Cypress, Norway Maple, Osier, Pittespora, English
Elm (GMTE)*
Wild Violet, Snowflake, Golden Crocus, Mock Orange, (GMFE)
Confrontation of Truths (DC Comb)
Red Clover (LHFE)
Forget-me-not (UFE)
Bird Foot Trefoil (LNE)
Early Purple Orchid, Bluebell, Butterbur, Sumach (BE)

PESSIMISM

Spotted Orchid (FFE)
Cantabillae-Auric (OIT Comb)

PHOBIAS
See, Fears

Assuredness (GM Comb)
Majestic Triumph (RLR)
Dandelion, Red Clover (LHFE)

PLANTS
See also, Nature awareness

Harebell, St. John's Wort (AFE)
Gorse (LHFE)

POSSESSIVENESS

Claire (CFR)
Cleaver (CH)
Harebell (FFE)
Firethorn (BE)

POSSESSION

Possession (BE Comb), *Lesser Stitchwort, Scarlet Pimpernel (BE)*

POSITIVITY

Spotted Orchid (FFE)
*Time Immemorial, Soul Retrieval, Sunset Boulevard, Saviour,
Refresh your Memory, Golden Window, Look Lively, Freedom
Dance, Bounty Beautiful, Magnolia (RLR)*
Herb Robert (SCE)
Forgiveness (GM Comb), *Laburnum (GMTE),*
Pennyroyal (GMFE)
Purple Comfrey (UFE)
Bistort (BE)
Witch Hazel (BFE)

PREJUDICE

Self-worth(GM Comb)
Lime (FFE)
Chickweed (JJ)

PRIDE
See also, Ego/Selfishness

Self-worth (GM Comb)
New Zealand Flax (IC)

PROCRASTINATION
See also, Inertia/Procrastination

Cosmos (AFR)
Laurel, Hazel (FFE)
Tansy (SE)
Tower of Strength (RLR)

PROTECTION
See also, Psychic Attack

Angelica (AFR)
Solar Blend Flower Essence
Lavender Protection Spray (SE Comb)
Mary Rose (CFR)
Blackthorn (HFE)(GMTE)
Yew (GMTE)
Crystal Clear, Release (PE)
St. Johns Wort (CG)(HR)
Yarrow (AFR)(HFE)
Marjoram, Elder (HR)
Monkshood (HR)(HFE)
Tansy, Blackthorn, Thistle (HFE)

	Tufted Vetch, White Foxglove (SCE)
	Lady's Mantle, Marigold, Rosemary, Broom (JJ)
	Candle Light, Brethren Child, Fuchsia Success (RLR)
	Cantabillae Auric (OIT Comb)
	Bramble, Cranesbill, Thyme (SCE)
	Pennyroyal (RD)
	Buttercup, Honeysuckle, Lemon, Mugwort (AFE)
	Dandelion (LHFE)
	Crystal Earth Violet (DC)

PSYCHE
Californian Poppy (RD)

PSYCHIC ATTACK/SHOCK
See also, Protection

'5' Blackberrys (AT)
Solar Blend Flower Essence
Lavender Protection Spray (SE Comb)
Orange Hawkweed (SE)
Hibiscus (CH)
Pink Yarrow (CH)(MEFE)
Yarrow (AFR)
Silvery Moon, Aura Flame, Crystal Clear (PE)
St. Johns Wort (CG)
Scarlet Pimpernel, Deadly Nightshade (HFE)
Boletus Edulus (AT)
African Dance, Brethren Child, Safe & Sound (RLR)
Elderflower, Yarrow (JJ)
Pennyroyal (GMFE)
Nettle (UFE)

**PSYCHIC DEVELOPMENT/
ABILITIES**
*See also, Intuition/Clairaudience/
Clairvoyance*

Californian Poppy (JJ)(AFR)
Fig, French Marigold (CH)
Scots Pine (GMTE)(FFE)
Eyebright, Lady's Smock, Tree Mallow (LLFE)
Orange Chalice, Pink Angel (PE)
Daffodil (SM)
Queen Anne's Lace, Tagetes Patula (JJ)
Campsis (GE)
Remedy 5 'Alpha Com' (JW Comb)
Lavender, Mugwort, Passion Flower, Thorn Apple (AFE)
Comfrey (LHFE)
Thrift, Bracken – Aqueous Extract (BE)
White Leaved Oak (GHTE)

PURIFICATION/PURITY
See also, Cleansing (Emotional)

Violet Flame (HFE Comb)
Wild Rose, Wild Pansy, Five Leaved Red Clover, Pennyroyal (HFE)
Tree Lichen (GMTE)
White Light (PE)
Ragged Robin, Watercress (FFE)
Dandelion (UFE)
Wild Thyme (HR)
White Leaved Oak (GHTE)

REBIRTHING
Aubretia (MEFE)

RECONCILIATION
Rowan, Lady's Mantle (FFE)
Flowering Red Currant (BFE)

REGRET
Relaxation(GM Comb)
Release (PE)
Forget-me-not (BFE)
Sundew (LNE)

RE-INTEGRATION
See also, Integration

Living Blend 2 (SE Comb)

REJECTION
Evening Primrose (AFR)
Karmic Helper, Time Immemorial, Majestic Triumph (RLR)
Hawkweed (BFE)
Scarlet Pimpernel, Red Clover (SCE)
Plantain (LNE)

RELATING

Scarlet Pimpernel (MEFE)
Sweet Pea (JJ)
Hawthorn (BFE)

RELATIONSHIPS

Solar Blend Communication (SE Comb)
Galtonia, Nettle (CH)
Red Rose Bud (HR)
Scottish Primrose, Mallow (FFE)
Orange Chalice, Soul Star, Silver Genie (PE)
Forget-me-not (AFR)
Moss Rose (Dusky Red), Nettle (JJ)
Cantabillae Auric (OIT Comb)
Remedy 1 'SOS' (JW Comb)
Stinging Nettle (RD)
Evening Primrose (AFE)
Honesty (GMFE) (LHFE)
Gorse (LHFE)

RELATIONSHIPS/CHILDREN
See also, Parenting/Mother &
Mothering/Father & Fathering/
Childhood Issues

Broom, Galtonia, Nettle (CH)

RELAXATION/SEDATING
See also, Calming/Stillness/Soothing

Rosebay willowherb, Ox-eyed Daisy, St. John's Wort,
Pineappleweed, Thyme (SCE)
Sycamore (GMTE)
Chamomile (HR)
Geranium (SM)
Marsh Marigold (LLFE)
Metta (PE)
Purple Loosestrife (BFE)
Daisy, Solomon's Seal (RD)
Evening Primrose, Harebell, Rock Rose (AFE)
Dandelion (RD) (LHFE)
Celandine (UFE)
Rhododendron (BE)

RELEASE
See also, Blockages/Letting Go

Bramble (UFE)

RENEWAL

Broom (JJ)(HR)
Evening Primrose (AFR)
Elder (FFE)
Strelitzia (GE)
Speedwell (EE)
Copper Beech (SE)
Forget-me-not (BFE)
Cowslip (LHFE)

RESENTMENT

Dandelion (HFE)
Transmutation & Awakening –
Solar Plexus Chakra (CFR Comb)
Rowan (FFE)
Bounty Beautiful (RLR)
Passion Flower (AFE)
Pussy Willow (LHFE)
Compact Rush (BE)

RESIGNATION

Plantain – Ribwort (HR)

Redwood Body Spray (SE)
See also, Inner Strength   *Bittercress, Gorse (UFE)*
Yew (BE)
White Leaved Oak (GHTE)

RESISTANCE/RELEASE
See also, Blockages/Letting Go

Stonecrop, Grass of Parnassus (FFE)
Wild Fuchsia (AT)
Coltsfoot, Red Campion, Yarrow (UFE)
Marigold (BE), ***Unification (BE Comb)***
Blue Geranium (LNE)

	See also, Petaltone, Tantric Love Essences *Red Rose Bud, Snowdrop (HR)* *Scarlet Pimpernel (EE)(HFE)* *Celandine, Deep Red Rose (MEFE)* *Evening Primrose (SE)* *Burning Desire, Lancelot (RLR)* *Vetch (JJ)* *Lavender (AFE)* *Bog Asphodel (LNE)* *Tufted Vetch (BE)*

SHAMAN — *Mugwort (AFE)*

SHAME
See also, Guilt

Basil (AFR)
Release (PE)
Rowan, Iona Pennywort (FFE)
Purple Loosestrife (BFE)
Plum (GMTE)

SHYNESS

Solar Blend Confidence (SE Comb)
Harebell (CH)
Cosmos, Mallow (AFR)
Red Tulip (HR)
Buttercup (MEFE)
Golden Sage (AFE)
Oriental Hellebore (GMFE), Cherry Plum, Italian Alder (GMTE)

SINGING
See also, Music

Bluebell (CH)

SOFTENING — *Grass of Parnassus (FFE)*

SOOTHING
See also, Calming/Stillness

Crisis (HFE Comb)
Gean (GMTE)
Chamomile, Lavender (HR)
White Valerian (HFE)
Rose Geranium (JJ)
Cowslip, Red Clover (LHFE)

SORROW
See also, Grief

Grass of Parnassus (FFE)
Ruby Red (CH)

SOUL ISSUES

Ageratum, Ragged Robin, Geranium (CH)
Holy Thorn, Yew (LLFE)
Fuchsia (AFR)
Elderflower (SE)
Peaches & Cream (RLR)

SPIRITUAL INDEPENDENCE

Yellow Archangel (SE)
Vetch (CH)

SPIRITUALITY
See also, Spiritual Growth/
Crown/Higher Chakras

Agrimony, Rest Harrow, Tansy (SCE)
See also, Jean Jacob Ascended Master Essences
Bilberry (GMTE)
Bittercress, Hawthorn Flower, Hawthorn Leaf (EE)
Anger & Pain – Brow Chakra, Release – Crown Chakra,
Transmutation & Awakening – Solar Plexus,
Chakra (CFR Comb)
Spiritual Marriage, Holy Grail (FFE Comb),
Sea Pink, Rose Water Lily (FFE)
Spiritual (LLFE Comb)
Comfrey – The Root Chakra (ACFR)
Louise Odier, Ispahan (CFR)
Brompton Stock, Deadnettle, Gladiolus, Iris Brown/Gold, Marsh
Marigold, Passion Flower (CH)
Universal Suffering (GHTE)
Orange Chalice (PE)
Lavender (SM)
Thistle, Wild Rose, Alfalfa (HFE)

	Hawthorn, Rose, Gardenia, Californian Poppy (JJ) *Celandine, White Rose (MEFE)* **Unicorn Essence (ME Comb)** *Cotoneaster Berry (AT)* *Crystal Sun Gold, Crystal Life Rainbow (DC)*
SPIRITUAL GROWTH *See also Spirituality/Crown/* *Higher chakras*	*Sage (MEFE)* *African Violet, Blackthorn, Gardenia (JJ)* *Brompton Stock, Cyclamen, Himalayan Poppy, Penstemon,* *Rhododendron, Sage, Black Eyed Susan (CH)* **Change & Adjustment – Hara Chakra, Purpose & Strength** **– Throat Chakra (CFR Comb)**, *Church Farm Rose (CFR)* **Living Blend 5 (SE Comb)** *Comfrey – The Root Chakra (ACFR)* *Majestic Triumph (RLR)* *Hops (CH)(JJ)* *Stand Alone (PE)* *Spinach, Thistle, Tree Mallow (HFE)* *Silverweed (FFE)* *Policeman's Helmet, Russian Lettuce (SCE)* *Lavender, Love in a Mist, Marsh Gentian (GMFE)* *Strawberry Tree, Tulip Tree, White Willow (GMTE)* *Comfrey (LHFE)* *Lesser Stitchwort, Nasturtium (BE),* **Unification (BE Comb)**
STABILITY/INSTABILITY	*Bell Heather (FFE)* *Baby blue eyes (AFR)* *Church Farm Rose, Arthur Bell (CFR)* *Elder, Sycamore (GMTE)* *Ivy (LLFE)(HFE)* *Water Lily (HFE)* *Mallow (RD)* *Evening Primrose (AFE)* *Primrose (UFE)* *Thrift (BE)*
STEADFASTNESS *See also, Inner Strength/*	*Bittercress (UFE)*
STILLNESS *See also, Calming/Worry*	*Yellow Archangel, Bluebell (SE)* *Square-stalked willowherb (GE)* **Clear Light (FFE Comb)** **Tranquillity (GM Comb)**, *Silver Birth (GMTE)* *Scottish Primrose (FFE)* *Amaryllis (CH)*
STRESS *See also, Trauma/Shock/* *Emergency/Injury*	**Cantabillae-Auric (OIT Comb)** *Bell Heather, Sycamore (FFE),* **First Aid (FFE Comb)** *Bluebell, Morning Glory (SE),* **Solar Blend Crisis, Solar Blend** **Stress Relief (SE Comb)** **Anger & Pain – Brow Chakra (CFR Comb)**, *Church Farm* *Rose, Louise Odier (CFR)* **Stress Release (GM Comb)**, *Alder (GMTE)* **Stress Release (HR Comb)** **Head (LLFE Comb)**, *Yellow Flag Iris (LLFE)* *Comfrey – The Root Chakra, Sage – The Solar Plexus Chakra* *(ACFR),* **Stress (AFR Comb)** *Dandelion (CH)(AFR)(HR)(JJ)* *Hawthorn (AFR)(JJ)(BFE)* *Honesty, White Valerian, Mayweed (HFE)* *Blue Mood, Fuchsia Stress, Purple Passion, Tiffany (RLR)* *St. John's Wort (JJ)* **Remedy 1 'Help' (JW Comb)** *Ox-eyed Daisy, Wild Clary, Chicory, Cinquefoil, Parsley (SCE)* *Onion (RD)*

	Buttercup, Golden Sage, Honeysuckle, Lemon, Rock Rose, Tansy (AFE)
STUBBORNESS	*Cinquefoil (CH)*
	Stonecrop (FFE)
STUDYING	*Primrose (CH)*
See also, Concentration/Memory	*Daisy (AFR)*
Learning Difficulties/Focus	*Golden Sage (AFE)*
SUBTLE BODIES	*African Violet, Blackberry, Petunia, Peppermint, Queen Anne's*
See also, Auras/Chakras	*Lace, Thyme, Rosemary, Rose-bay willowherb, Self-heal, Scarlet Pimpernel, Raspberry, Toadflax, Cosmos, Daisy, Dandelion, Forget-me-not, Hawthorn, Hyssop, Hops, Jasmine, Lilac, Tagetes Patula, Californian Poppy (JJ)*
	Beaked Hawksbeard, Periwinkle, Scarlet Pimpernel (HFE)
	Orchid 'Oncidium' (CH)
	Apple, Hazel, Black Poplar, Elder, Sycamore, Gean, Tree Lichen, Whitebeam (GMTE)
	White Light, Clear Tone, Amorthyst (PE)
	Hibiscus (SM)
	Field Pansy (EE)
	Sage (JJ)(MEFE)
	Pear (JJ)(MEFE)
	Sunset Boulevard (RLR)
	Holy Grail (FFE Comb)
	Lavender (JJ)(AFE)
	Bindweed, Buttercup, Golden Sage, Mugwort, Tansy, Thorn Apple, Witch Hazel (AFE)
	Wisteria (RD)
SUPPORT	*Alkanet, Borage (SE)*
	Buddleia (CH)
	Water Forget-me-not (HFE)
	Primrose (JW)
	Viburnum, Red Oak (GMTE)
	Blackthorn, Lungwort, Speedwell (UFE)
	Sundew (LNE)
	Cowslip, Red Clover (LHFE)
	Bistort, Lilac (BE)
SURVIVAL	*Yew (GMTE)*
See also, Protection	
TELEPATHY	*Anemone (SM)*
See also, Intuition/	*Artemisia (CH)*
Clairvoyance/clairaudience	
TEMPERAMENTAL	*Nettle (JJ)*
TOLERANCE	*Silver Birch (GMTE), Golden Crocus (GMFE), **Self-worth (GM***
See also, Intolerance/Acceptance	***Comb)***
Flexibility	*Dandelion (EE)*
	Yellow Iris (SCE)
TRANCE STATES	*Hazel (LLFE)*
	Foxglove (HFE)
TRANQUILLITY	*Crystal Celestial (DC)*
See also, Calming/Soothing/	***Tranquillity (BE Comb)***
Stillness/Inner Peace/Relaxation	*Snowdrop (UFE)*
	Strawberry Tree (GMTE)
TRANSFORMATION	*Alkanet (HR)(MEFE)*
See also, Change/Moving-on/	***Violet Flame (HFE Comb)***
Spiritual Growth/Purification	*Cyclamen (CH)*
	Universal Suffering (GHTE)
	*Watercress, Stonecrop (FFE), **Revelation (FFE Comb)***
	Astronomy (RLR)
	Comfrey (BFE)

	Kidney Vetch, Sea Lavender (SCE)
	Spindle, Tamarisk (GMTE)
	Crystal Light Turquoise (DC)
TRANSITION *See also, Change/Moving-on*	*Alkanet, Autumn Leaves (SE)*
	Angelica (AFR)
	Birth & Re-birth – Root Chakra, Change & Adjustment – Hara Chakra, Transmutation & Awakening – Solar Plexus Chakra (CFRE Comb)
	Transition (BE Comb)
	Stonecrop (FFE)
	Bog Hypericum (LNE)
TRAUMA *See also, Stress/Injury/Emergency/Shock*	*Black-eyed Susan, Redbeckia (JJ)*
	Bell heather (FFE), ***First Aid (FFE Comb)***
	Bluebell, Red Clover (HR), ***Stress Release (HR Comb)***
	Buddleia (JW)(CH)
	Meridian Energiser (GM Comb)
	Crisis (HFE Comb)
	Solar Blend Crisis (SE Comb)
	Church Farm Rose, Centifolia (CFR)
	Rosemary (AFR)
	Sweet Violet (GE)
	Astronomy, Magnolia, Soul Retrieval (RLR)
	Sage (IC)
	Cornbine (SCE)
	Star of Bethlehem (RD)
	First Aid (BE Comb)
	The Trauma Remedy (UFE Comb)
TRAVEL	***Travel Essence (HR Comb)***
	Speedwell (MEFE)(JJ)
TRUST *See also, Acceptance*	*Beaked Hawksbeard (HFE)*
	Baby Blue Eyes (AFR)
	Elderflower, Osteospermum (CH)
	Hawthorn (GMTE)
	Jacob's Ladder, Rosemary, Snowdrop (HR)
	Hazel, Sea Rocket (FFE)
	White Violet, Snowdrop Body Spray (SE)
	Brethren Child (RLR)
	Self-heal (JJ)
	Columbine, Pyramid Orchid, Purple Toadflax, Violet (SCE)
	Borage, Mayweed, Spear Thistle (UFE)
	Comfrey (LHFE)
	Butterbur, Double Snowdrop, Lily of the Valley (BE)
TWINS/TWIN ENERGY	*Sweet Juliet (CFR)*
UNBALANCED ERRATIC BEHAVIOUR *See also, Emotions*	*Single White Cherry (BFR)*
	Kerria (CH)
	Sweet Pea, Fuchsia (AFR)
	Peaches & Cream (RLR)
	Yellow Archangel (SE)
UNCERTAINTY	***Uncertainty (DC Comb)***
	Saviour (RLR)
	Sorrel (SCE)
	Wild Orchid (CH)
UNDERSTANDING	*Bittercress (EE)*
	Buttercup, Elderflower (SE)
	Karma Clear, Revelation (FFE Comb)
	Day Lily, Primula, Sage, Trillium, Wintersweet (CH)
	Elder, Rowan, Great Sallow, Hazel (GMTE)
	Daisy (AFR)
	Delphinium (SM)
	Dandelion (HFE)

WORRY

Birch (FFE)
Solar Blend New Directions (SE Comb)
Hypericum 'Hidcote' (CH)
Mary Rose (CFR)
Marsh Orchid (LLFE)
Marsh Woundwort (HR)
Candle Light, Bounty Beautiful (RLR)
Flowering Red Currant (BFE)
Cornbine, Sorrel, Elderflower (SCE)
White Chestnut (RD)
Copper Beech (GMTE)
Chickweed, Heart's Ease (UFE)
Cowslip (LHFE)

YEARNING

Lily of the Valley (BE)

Physical Issues

ABDOMEN

Cone flower (CH)
Alder (GMTE)
Hawkweed (BFE)

ABORTION

Buddleia (JW)

ABUSE
See also, Sexual Abuse/Stress/
Trauma/Destructiveness

Anger & Pain – Brow Chakra (CFR Comb), *Evelyn (CFE)*
Sage – The Solar Plexus Chakra (ACFR),
Evening Primrose (AFR)
Calla, White Chicory (CH)
Silver Genie (PE)
Dog Violet, Hawthorn, Lady's Smock (BFE)
Gorse (LHFE)
Purple Comfrey (UFE)

ACNE
See also, Skin

Lemon (AFE)

ADDICTION

Addiction (HR Comb)
Solar Blend Releasing Addictive Habits (SE Comb)
Amelanchier (BFR)
Forsythia (JJ)
Morning Glory (JW)
Poppy 'Papaver'(CH)
Tobacco (CH)(JW)
Nettle (LLFE)
Silver Genie (PE)
Globe Thistle (FFE)
Cantabillae-Auric (OIT Comb)
Opium Poppy (MEFE)
Magnolia (RFR)
Witch Hazel (BFE)
Thorn Apple (AFE)
Pennnyroyal (GMFE)
Purple Comfrey (UFE)
Honesty (LHFE)

ADRENALS
see also, Endocrine

Borage (AFR), Comfrey – The Root Chakra (ACFR)
Red Clover, (LHFE)

AGEING

Almond, Helleborus (CH)
Mallow (CH) (AFR) (JJ)
Fire Clear (PE)
Petunia (JJ)
Field Scabious (BFE)

ALLERGIES

Tower of Strength, Honeymoon, Eye on Bright, Blue Mood (RLR)
Snapdragon (MEFE)
Lemon Balm (JJ)
Euphrasia (BFE)
Corn, Fredontodendron, Oil Seed Rape (CH)
Betony (SCE)

ALZHEIMERS DISEASE

Canary Bird Rose (BFR)
Caster Oil Plant (CH)

AMALGAM FILLINGS
See also, Teeth

Primrose (UFE)

ANAEMIA
See also, Blood

Scarlet Pimpernel (SCE)

ANGINA
See also, Heart

<table>
<tr><td>ANOREXIA NERVOSA
See also, Eating Disorders</td><td>Cowslip (BFR)
Honesty (LHFE)</td></tr>
<tr><td>APPENDIX</td><td>Red Dead Nettle – The Sacral Chakra (ACFR)</td></tr>
<tr><td>APPETITE</td><td>Centaury (SCE)</td></tr>
<tr><td>ARTERIOSCLEROSIS</td><td>Canary Bird Rose (BFR)
Wood Anemone (SCE)</td></tr>
<tr><td>ARTHRITIS</td><td>Red Dead Nettle – The Sacral Chakra (ACFR)
Canary Bird Rose (BFR)
Spirit Ground (PE)
Bounty Beautiful (RLR)
Self-heal, Tenby Daffodil, Chicory (SCE)
Pussy Willow (LHFE)</td></tr>
<tr><td>ASTHMA
See also, Allergies</td><td>Scabious, Tenby Daffodil (SCE)
Jasmine (AFE)
Nettle (GMFE)</td></tr>
<tr><td>AUTISM</td><td>French Marigold (AFR)</td></tr>
<tr><td>BABIES</td><td>Bellflower, Woodruff (CH)
White Rose Bud (HR)
Elder (GMTE)
Cowslip, Pussy Willow (LHFE)</td></tr>
<tr><td>BACTERIA</td><td>Jasmine (AFE)</td></tr>
<tr><td>BED-WETTING</td><td>Sea Campion (BE)</td></tr>
<tr><td>BILE</td><td>Sedum (CH)</td></tr>
<tr><td>BIRTH</td><td>Birth & Re-birth – Root Chakra (CFR Comb)
Lady's Smock (BFE)
Campion (CH)
Jasmine (PE)
Skullcap (CG)
Lady's Mantle (HR)
Lavender (AFE)
Cowslip (LHFE)</td></tr>
<tr><td>BLADDER
See also, Urinary Organs</td><td>Holm Oak (CH)
Silverweed, Dog Rose, Knapweed (SCE)</td></tr>
<tr><td>BLEEDING</td><td>Comfrey (LHFE)</td></tr>
<tr><td>BLOOD
See also, Circulation/Veins/
Capillaries</td><td>Blackberry, Red Clover (AFR), Passionflower – The Heart
Chakra (ACFR)
Protection & Harmony – Heart Chakra (CFR Comb),
Fisherman's Friend (CFR)
Rosemary, Single White Cherry, Dog Tooth Violet (BFR)
Cone Flower, Japanese Quince, Maltese Cross, Salvia (CH)
Blackthorn. Silver Maple, Yew (GMTE)
Golden Light, Spirit Ground, Release (PE)
Mallow (JJ)
Cornbine, Loosestrife, Ragged Robin, Thrift, Cleavers, Vipers
Bugloss, Buddleia (SCE)</td></tr>
<tr><td>BLOOD PRESSURE</td><td>Bleeding Heart (RD)
Magnolia, Refresh Your Memory, Tower of Strength (RLR)
Bramble (SCE)
Passion Flower, St. John's Wort, Golden Sage, Honeysuckle,
Mugwort, Thorn Apple (AFE)
Daffodil (RD)</td></tr>
<tr><td>BONES
See also, Joints</td><td>Banana (RD)
Clover (CH)
Fisherman's Friend (CFR)
Silver Genie (PE)
Fuchsia Success (RLR)</td></tr>
<tr><td>BOWELS</td><td>Release – Crown Chakra (CFR Comb)</td></tr>
</table>

	Rose-Bay willowherb, Strawberry, Tufted Vetch, Common Vetch,
	Kidney Vetch (SCE)
	Passionflower (AFE)
	Elderflower (RD)
	Blackberry, Honeysuckle, St. John's Wort (AFE)
	Redshank, Loosestrife (LNE)
CLAUSTROPHOBIA	*Glastonbury Thorn (GMTE)*
CLEANSING (PHYSICAL)	*Watercress (FFE)*
	Welsh Poppy, Flax, Scarlet Pimpernel, Fumitory (SCE)
	Christmas Rose, Single White Cherry, Canary Bird Rose (BFR)
	Claire (CFR)
	Chrysanthemum, Lamb's Tongue, Garlic (CH)
	Apple (GMTE)
	Blackberry, Thorn Apple (AFE)
	Cleansing (LLFE Comb)
	Solar Blend Flower Essence
	Lavender Protection Spray (SE Comb)
	Ramson (SE)
	Single White Cherry, Canary Bird Rose (BFR)
	Fisherman's Friend, Claire (CFR)
	Tree Lichen (GMTE)
	Fire Clear, White Light (PE)
	Jasmine, Lungwort, Primrose (HR)
	Lilac, Primrose, Nettle (JJ)
	Self-heal (LNE)
	Honesty (LHFE)
	White Leaved Oak (GHTE)

CONSTIPATION
See also, Bowels

Passion Flower (AFE)

COUGHS & COLDS
See also, Respiratory system/
Sinuses/Catarrh

Beautiful World (RLR)
Sea Lavender, Thyme (SCE)
Jasmine (AFE)

CRAMPS

Solar Blend Female Cycles of Life (SE Comb)
Yellow Woundwort (SCE)

DEHYDRATION

Canary Bird Rose (BFR)
Sea Rocket (FFE)
Tormentil (BFE)
Gorse (LHFE)

DIABETES

Sage – The Solar Plexus Chakra (ACFR)
Redshank (LNE)

DIARRHOEA
See also, Bowels

Streptocarpus (CH)
Honeysuckle (AFE)

DIET
See also, Mineral & Vitamin
absorption/Nutrition

Hawthorn (MEFE)

DIGESTIVE SYSTEM

Change & Adjustment – Hara Chakra (CFR Comb),
Swan (CFR), Cedar (CH)
Sage – The Solar Plexus Chakra (ACFR)
Majestic Triumph, Beautiful World (RLR)
Digestive System (OIT Comb)
Evening Primrose (JW)
Peppermint (JJ)
Common Comfrey, Loosestrife, Mullein, Marigold. Wild Clary,
Cornflower, Mayweed, Parsley, Agrimony, Sea Lavender (SCE)
Magnolia, Wallflower (RD)
Golden Sage, Lemon, Lavender (AFE)
Cowslip (LHFE)
Sage (GMFE)

DIURETIC

Herb Robert, Speedwell, Knapweed (SCE)
Rock Rose (AFE)

DYING
See also, Death/Fears of Dying/
Fears/Bereavement

Wild Garlic (JJ)
Strelitzia (GE)
Harebell (AFE)
Cowslip (LHFE)

DYSLEXIA
See also, Learning Difficulties/
Concentration/Focus/Memory/
Studying/Brain – right/left imbalance

Campsis (GE)
Lady's Mantle (FFE)
Thorn Apple (AFE)
Cowslip (LHFE)

EARS
See also, Tinnitus

Californian Poppy (AFR),
Nasturtium – The Brow Chakra (ACFR)
Dog Tooth Violet (BFR)
Ligularia, Toadflax, Vipers Bugloss (CH)
French Marigold (AFR)(SM)
Bluebell, Violet (SCE)
Strawberry (GMTE)

EATING DISORDERS
See also, Anorexia Nervosa

Pussy Willow (LHFE)

ECZEMA

Angelica (AFR)
Cowslip, Dog Tooth Violet (BFR)
Blue Mood (RLR)
Common Comfrey, Mallow, Mayweed, Chamomile,
Tenby Daffodil (SCE)
Lemon (AFE)

EMERGENCY

Bluebell (HR)
Buddleia (JW)
Meridian Energiser (GM Comb)
Crisis (HFE Comb)

ENDOCRINE

Blackberry (AFR)
Nasturtium – The Brow Chakra (ACFR)
Mallow, Nasturtium (JJ)
Glandular System (OIT Comb)
Dog Tooth Violet, Amelanchier (BFR)
Elder (GMTE)
Stand Alone (PE)
Sundew (LNE)

ENERGY
See also, Exhaustion/Fatigue/
Lethargy/Tiredness

Meridian Energiser (GM Comb)
Canary Bird Rose (BFR)
Geum, Lychnis, Canna 'President', Poppy (CH)
Great Sallow, Alder, Sycamore (GMTE)
Butterbur, Chamomile (LLFE)
Soul Star, Spirit Ground, Fire Clear, Aura Flame,
White Spring (PE)
Forsythia (HR)
Dog Rose, Red Pheasant's Eye (SCE)
Yucca (GE)
Lungwort (SE)
Burning Desire (RLR)
Red Poppy (JW)
Nasturtium (JJ)
Sun Silver Diamond Light (DC)
Welsh Poppy (BE)

EPILEPSY

Angelica (AFR)
Vipers Bugloss (SCE)
Witch Hazel (AFE)

EXHAUSTION *See also, Fatigue/Tiredness/* *Lethargy/Energy*	*Life Force (FFE Comb)* **Solar Blend Energy (SE Comb)** *Fisherman's Friend (CFR)* *Calendula (CH)* *White Spring (PE)* *Sycamore (FFE)* **Cantabillae(Auric) (OIT Comb)** *Hawkweed (BFE)* *Speedwell (SCE)* *Cowslip, Pussy Willow (LHFE)*
EYES	*Californian Poppy (AFR), Nasturtium – The Brow Chakra (ACFR)* **Transmutation & Awakening – Solar Plexus** **Chakra (CFR Comb),** *Pilgrim (CFR)* *Tiffany (RLR)* *Dog Tooth Violet (BFR)* *Euphrasia (BFE)* *Hemp Nettle, Lobelia, Pheasant's Eye (CH)* *Queen Anne's Lace (CH)(JJ)* *Periwinkle, Buddleia (SCE)* *Penstemon, St. John's Wort (AFE)*
FASTING	*Cistus (CH)*
FATIGUE *See also, Exhaustion/Energy/* *Lethargy/Tiredness*	*Sage – The Solar Plexus Chakra (ACFR)* *The Bride (BFR)* *Burning Desire (RLR)* *Agave (JW)* *Bluebell (BFE)*
FEET	*Dog Violet (BFE)*
FERTILITY *See also, Infertility*	*Buddleia (JW)* *Red Dead Nettle – The Sacral Chakra (ACFR)* *Hazel (EE)* *Mullein, Vipers Bugloss (SCE)* *Zucchini (CH)* *Lady's Mantle (HR)(JJ)*
FEVER *See also, Inflammations*	*Gean (GMTE)* *Dandelion (AFR)* *Silver Genie (PE)* *Cornbine, Wood Anemone (SCE)* *Gorse (LHFE)*
FLEXIBILITY	*Pussy Willow (LHFE)*
FLUID RETENTION	**Solar Blend Female Cycles of Life (SE Comb)** *Jasmine (AFE)*
FRIGIDITY	*Balsam (FFE)*
GALL BLADDER	*Sage – The Solar Plexus Chakra (ACFR)* *Alder (GMTE)* *Dog Rose, Scarlet Pimpernel, Columbine, Chicory, Rest Harrow,* *Agrimony (SCE)* *Redshank (LNE)*
GOUT	*Chicory, Yellow Woundwort (SCE)*
GROWTH	*Almond (RD)* *Hops (CH)* *Foxglove (HFE)*
HAEMORRHOIDS	*Cinquefoil, Redshank (SCE)*
HAIR	*Cornflower (SCE)* *Dog Tooth Violet (BFR)* *Peaches & Cream (RLR)* *Cedar (CH)* *Penstemon (AFE)*

	Energyflow (GM Comb), *Crack Willow, Yew (GMTE)*
	Resistance Builder (HR Comb)
	Solar Blend Body's Immunity (SE Comb), *Jack by the Hedge,*
	Ramsons (SE)
	Passionflower – The Heart Chakra (ACFR)
	Single White Cherry (BFR)
	Lewisia, Lily (CH)
	Pansy (HR)(SE)
	Fleabane (HFE)
	Garlic, Violet (JJ)
	Stitchwort (SCE)
	Love 'n' Light, Mary Light, Purple Passion, Saviour,
	Soul Retrieval (RLR)
	Echinacea (RD)
	Jasmine (AFE)

IMPOTENCE — *Release (PE)*

INFECTION — *Bergamot (CH)*

INFERTILITY
See also, Fertility

Buddleia (JW)
Red Dead Nettle – The Sacral Chakra (ACFR)
Zucchini (CH)
Fuchsia (BFE)
Pussy Willow (LHFE)

INFLAMMATIONS

Amaranthus Red (RD)
Cowslip (BFR)
French Marigold (CH)
Time Immemorial (RLR)
Plantain, Common Comfrey, Strawberry, Redshanks (SCE)
French Marigold (RD)

INJURY
See also, Emergency/Shock
Stress/Trauma

Jasmine, Thorn Apple (AFE)
Physical Trauma (HR Comb), *Bluebell, Comfrey (HR)*
Amelanchier (BFR)
Cantabillae-Auric (OIT Comb)
Magnolia (RLR)
Early Purple Orchid, Witch Hazel (BFE)
Cherry Laurel (GMTE)

INSOMNIA
See also, Sleep Problems

Sleeping Draught (AFR Comb)
Solar Blend Sleep (SE Comb)
Sweet Juliet (CFR)
Lavender (JJ)
Square-stalked willowherb (GE)
Feverfew, Forget-me-not, Passion flower (CH)
Delphinium (SM)
Morning Orchid (JW)
Early Purple Orchid (BFE)
Primrose (SCE)
Harebell, Tansy (AFE)

I.Q. — *Mugwort (RD)*

INVIGORATION — *Nasturtium (SM)*

JAUNDICE
See also, Liver

Yellow Iris, Columbine, Yellow Woundwort (SCE)

JAW
See also, Mouth

Snapdragon (GMFE)

JET LAG
See also, Travel

Meridian Energiser (GM Comb)
Sage (CH)

JOINTS
See also, Bones

Magnolia (RLR)
Comfrey (BFE)
Potentilla, Clover (CH)
Creeping Jenny, Common Vetch. Yellow Dock (SCE)

KIDNEYS	***Release – Crown Chakra (CFR Comb)**, Evelyn (CFR)* *Chrysanthemum, Cone flower, Kidney Vetch (CH)* *Silver Genie, Pink Angel (PE)* *Stinging Nettle (AFR)* *Silverweed, Sorrel, Dog Rose, Wild Clary, Knapweed, Parsley, Kidney Vetch (SCE)* *Red Clover (LHFE)*
KNEES	*Great Sallow (GMTE)* *Sloe (BFE)*
LARGE INTESTINE	*Red Dead Nettle – The Sacral Chakra (ACFR)* *Swan (CFR)*
LEGS	*Whitebeam (GMTE), Love in a Mist (GMFE)*
LETHARGY *See also, Exhaustion/Fatigue/Energy/Tiredness*	*Blackberry (RD)* ***Solar Blend Energy (SE Comb)*** *Fleabane (LLFE)* *Ankh (PE)* *Yucca (GE)* *Morning Glory (AFR)* *Lucombe Oak, Sycamore (GMTE)* *Self-heal (LNE)*
LEUKAEMIA	*Dandelion (AFR)* *Silver Genie, Spirit Ground (PE)*
LIBIDO *See also, Sexuality*	*Snapdragon (GMFE)*
LIVER	***Transmutation & Awakening –*** ***Solar Plexus Chakra (CFR Comb)**, Pilgrim (CFR)* *Sage – The Solar Plexus Chakra (ACFR)* *Cowslip, Single White Cherry (BFR)* *Chrysanthemum, Erthrina (CH)* *Yew, Alder (GMTE)* *Jasmine, White Light (PE)* *Dandelion (HFE)* *Primrose (JJ)* *Loosestrife, Scarlet Pimpernel, Sorrel, Welsh Poppy, Columbine, Chicory, Agrimony (SCE)* *Blackberry (AFE)*
LUNGS *See also, Respiratory system*	***Protection & Harmony – Heart Chakra (CFR Comb)**,* *Alexander (CFR)* *Passionflower – The Heart Chakra (ACFR), Stinging Nettle (AFR)* *Cone flower(CH)* *Elder, Tree Lichen, Whitebeam (GMTE)* *Stinging Nettle (AFR)* *Flowering Currant (HR)* *Red Clover, Spotted Orchid, Trefoil, Policeman's Helmet (SCE)* *Honeysuckle (AFE)(SCE)* *Jasmine (RD)*
LYMPHATIC SYSTEM	***Energyflow (GM Comb)*** *Amelanchier, Single White Cherry (BFR)* *Release (PE)* *Violet (JJ)* ***Lymphatic System (OIT Comb)*** *Cleavers (SCE)* *Thorn Apple (AFE)* *Honesty (LHFE)*
M.E.	***Cellular Rekindler (GM Comb)*** *Spirit Ground, Ankh, Fire Clear, White Spring (PE)* *Hero, Look Lively, Time Immemorial (RLR)* *Centaury (SCE)* *Lavender, Thorn Apple (AFE)* *Comfrey (LHFE)*

	Comfrey (HR)
	Betony (SCE)
NERVOUS SYSTEM	*African Violet (JJ)*
	Angelica, Forget-me-not (AFR)
	Californian Poppy (AFR)(CH)
	Change & Adjustment – Hara Chakra (CFR Comb), *Cadfael, Centifolia (CFR)*
	Cellular Rekindler (GM Comb), *Hazel (GMTE)*
	Stress Release (HR Comb)
	Celandine – The Throat Chakra, Daffodil – The Crown Chakra , Chamomile, Cowslip (BFR)
	Comfrey (CH)(JJ)(RD)
	Erthrina (CH)
	Morning Glory (CH)(AFR)
	Silver Genie, Amorthyst (PE)
	Lavender (JJ)
	Campsis (GE)
	Buttercup, Columbine (SCE)
	Brethren Child, Solemn Feast, Tower of Strength (RLR)
	Nervous System (OIT Comb)
	Evening Primrose (AFE)
NEURALGIA	*Golden Sage (AFE)*
NIGHTMARES	*St. John's Wort (CH)(CG)(JJ)*
	Soul Star (PE)
	Red Clover (LHFE)
	Scarlet Pimpernel (GMFE)
	Sea Campion (BE)
OBESITY	*Christmas Rose (BFR)*
OSTEOPOROSIS *See also, Bones*	*Tenby Daffodil (SCE)*
	Honeysuckle (AFE)
	Comfrey (LHFE)
PAIN CONTROL/RELIEF *See also, Neuralgia*	*Fuchsia Success, Mary Light (RLR)*
	First Aid (FFE Comb)
	Gean (GMTE)
	Mullein, Buttercup (SCE)
	Buttercup, Lavender, Passion Flower, St. John's Wort (AFE)
	Dandelion (LHFE)
PALPITATIONS	***Purpose & Strength – Throat Chakra (CFR Comb)***
PANCREAS	*Sage – The Solar Plexus Chakra (ACFR), French Marigold (AFR)*
	Cistus (CH)
	Dandelion (HFE)
	Sweet Pea (JW)
	Buttercup, Violet (SCE)
	Pancreatic System (OIT Comb)
	Tulip Tree (GMTE)
PANIC ATTACKS	*Red Clover (CH) (JJ) (LHFE)*
	Scottish Primrose (FFE)
	Assuredness (GM Comb), *Holly (GMTE)*
	Candle Light, Magnolia, Tower of Strength (RLR)
	Witch Hazel (BFE)
	Dandelion (LHFE)
PARKINSONS DISEASE	*Amorthyst (PE)*
	Witch Hazel (AFE)
PELVIS	*The Bride (BFR)*
	Early Purple Orchid (BFE)
PHOBIAS *See also, Fears*	
PHYSICAL STRENGTH *See also, Vitality/Energy*	*Scarlet Pimpernel (SCE)*

PINEAL
See also, Endocrine

African Violet, Queen Anne's Lace, Rosemary, Forget-me-not (JJ)
Red/Orange Rose (MEFE)
Pyramid Orchid, Buddleia, Pineappleweed (SCE)
Scarlet Pimpernel (GMFE)

PITUITARY GLAND
See also, Endocrine

Ribes (CH)
Nasturtium, Honesty, Hops, Mallow (JJ)
Scarlet Pimpernel (GMFE)

POST-NATAL DEPRESSION

Bluebell (JJ)
Spirit Ground (PE)
Jasmine (AFE)

POST-OPERATIVE RECOVERY

Agave, Red Poppy (JW)
Physical Trauma (HR Comb)
Fuchsia Success, Blue Mood, Hero, Tower of Strength (RLR)
Hawthorn (BFE)
Speedwell (SCE)
Comfrey (LHFE)
Self-heal (LNE)

PREGNANCY

Birth & Re-birth – Root Chakra (CFR Comb)
Campion (CH)
Jasmine (PE)

PRE-MENSTRUAL SYNDROME
See also, Menstruation/Sexual &
Reproductive Organs/Menopause

Solar Blend Female Cycles of Life (SE Comb)
Evening Primrose, Pulsatilla (CH)
Bluebell (BFE)
Blackthorn (GMTE)
St. John's Wort (SCE)
Ragged Robin (BFE)

PSORIASIS
See also, Skin

Astronomy, Blue Mood (RLR)
Common Comfrey, Cleavers (SCE)
Lemon (AFE)

PSYCHOSOMATIC ILLNESS

Cowslip (BFR)

PUBERTY

Solar Blend Female Cycles of Life (SE Comb)
Red Rose Bud (HR)

RADIATION/UV

Rosemary (BFR)
Sunflower (AFR)
Yarrow (JJ) (AFR)
Yarrow in Sea Water (HR)
White Yarrow (MEFE)(SE)
Pansy, Violet, Wild Garlic (JJ)
Harebell (AFE)

REJUVENATION
See also, Skin

Strelitzia (GE)
Forget-me-not, Hawksweed, Tormentil (BFE)

RESPIRATORY SYSTEM
See also, Sinuses/Catarrh/Breathing

Passionflower – The Heart Chakra (ACFR), Jasmine,
Stinging Nettle (AFR)
Single White Cherry (BFR)
Alexander (CFR)
Pansy (CH)
Burning Desire, Magnolia, Refresh Your memory,
Tower of Strength (RLR)
Dog Violet (BFE)
Plantain, Dog Rose, Pink Foxglove, Purple Toadflax (SCE)
Remedy 3 'Snot' (JW Comb)
Respiratory/Skin System (ME Comb)
Elderflower, Mallow, Violet, Russian Lettuce,
Scabious, Thyme (SCE)
Jasmine, Snapdragon (RD)
Field Maple (GMTE)

RHEUMATISM

Red Dead Nettle – The Sacral Chakra (ACFR)
Spirit Ground (PE)
Fuchsia Success (RLR)

TEMPERO-MANDIBULAR JOINT DISORDER	*Snapdragon (GMFE)*
TENSION *See also, Anxiety/Worry/Stress*	*Balsam Poplar, Rowan, Vipers Bugloss (HFE)* **Stress (AFR Comb)** **First Aid (FFE Comb)** **Stress Release (GM Comb)**, *Holm Oak, Laburnum, Glastonbury Thorn (GMTE)* *Oriental Hellebore (GMFE)* *Hyssop, Evening Primrose, Petunia (CH)* *Lavender (SM)* *Fuchsia (MEFE)* *Dandelion (SE)(GMFE)(LHFE)* *Freedom Dance (RLR)* *Comfrey, Meadowsweet (JJ)* *Purple Loosestrife (BFE)* *Ox-eyed Daisy (SCE)* *Bluebell (UFE)*
TESTICLES *See also Sexual/Reproductive organs*	
THROAT	**Purpose & Strength – Throat Chakra (CFR Comb)** *Alexander (CFR)* *Single White Cherry (BFR)* *Flax, Snakeshead Fritillaria, Vipers Bugloss (CH)* *Snapdragon (CH)(HR)* *Celandine (MEFE)* *Toadflax (JJ)* *Coltsfoot (JW)* **Remedy 3 'Snot' (JW Comb)** *Self-heal, Silverweed, Bluebell, Pink Foxglove, Sea Lavender, Vipers Bugloss, Bramble, Cinquefoil, Periwinkle, Policeman's Helmet, Russian Lettuce (SCE)* *Jasmine (RD)*
THYMUS *See also, Lymphatic system*	*Rosemary (BFR)* *Passionflower – The Heart Chakra (ACFR)* *Apple, Black Poplar, Crack Willow (GMTE)*
THYROID *See also, Endocrine*	*Borage (AFR), Celandine – The Throat Chakra (ACFR)* **Purpose & Strength – Throat Chakra (CFR Comb)** *Single White Cherry (BFR)* *Ceanothus, Celandine (CH)* *Crack Willow (GMTE)* *Hawthorn (BFE)* *Bluebell (SCE)* *Evening Primrose (AFE)*
TINNITUS *See also, Ears*	*Penstemon (AFE)*
TIREDNESS *See also, Energy/Exhaustion/ Fatigue/Lethargy*	*Nasturtium (CH)* *Comfrey (HR)* *Time Immemorial (RLR)*
TOUCH	*Primrose (JW)*
TOXICITY/TOXAEMIA	**Energyflow (GM Comb)**, *Apple (GMTE)* *Canary Bird Rose (BFR)* *Phlox, Sunflower (SM)* *Primrose (HR)(JJ)* *Ragged Robin (FFE)* *Ramsons (SE)* *Buttercup, Passion Flower, Thorn Apple (AFE)*
TRAUMA	*Buddleia (JW)* **Meridian Energiser (GM Comb)** **Crisis (HFE Comb)**

Physical Trauma, Stress Release (HR Comb)
Tower of Strength (RLR)

TUMOURS

Rue, Violet (SCE)
Hawthorn (RD)

ULCERS

Hypericum 'Hidcote' (CH)
Sage – The Solar Plexus Chakra, Daffodil –
The Crown Chakra (ACFR)
Dog Tooth Violet (BFR)
Alkanet (SCE)
Lavender (AFE)

URINARY ORGANS

Release – Crown Chakra (CFR Comb), Evelyn (CFR)
Comfrey – The Root Chakra, Red Dead Nettle –
The Sacral Chakra (ACFR)
Golden Light (PE)
Urinary System (OIT Comb)
Plantain, Wood Anemone, Cleavers, Rest Harrow (SCE)
Blackberry (AFE)

VARICOSE VEINS

Amelanchier (BFR)
Hawthorn (BFE)
Tansy (SCE)
St. John's Wort (AFE)

VEINS
See also, Blood/Circulation

Lily Pink (CH)
Cranesbill (SCE)

VIRUSES

Amaranthus Red (RD)
Rosemary, Single White Cherry (BFR)
French Marigold (CH)(AFR)
Jasmine (CH)(AFR)
Lily (CH)
Pansy (CH)(AFR)(SE)(JJ)
Beautiful World, Purple Paradise (RLR)
Evening Primrose (SCE)
Viola Tricolor (RD)
Lavender, Golden Sage (AFE)

VITALITY
See also, Physical Strength/
Rejuvenation

Blackberry, Primrose (JJ)
Alfalfa (HFE)
Life Force (FFE Comb), *Gorse, Wild Pansy (FFE)*
Meridian Energiser (GM Comb), *Bay (GMTE)*
Scarlet Pimpernel (SCE)(EE)
Sage – The Solar Plexus Chakra (ACFR), Garlic, Rosemary (AFR)
Canary Bird Rose (BFR)
Fleabane (LLFE)(HFE)
Lungwort (LLFE)
Yucca (GE)
Bluebell (BFE)
Ramsons (SE)
Look Lively, Soul Retrieval, Tiffany, Purple Passion, Tower of
Strength (RLR)
Red Poppy (JW)
Daffodil (RD)
Pussy Willow (LHFE)
Self-heal (LNE)

VOICE/VOCAL CHORDS

Canary Bird Rose (BFR)
Celandine, Petunia (CH)
Snapdragon (HR)(MEFE)
Toadflax (JJ)

WARTS
See also, Skin

Passion Flower (AFE)

WATER RETENTION
See also, Diuretic

Rue, Parsley (SCE)

WEIGHT PROBLEMS
See also, Diuretic

WOUND HEALING

Pussy Willow (LHFE)

Bergamot (CH)
Pink Angel (PE)
Fuchsia Success, Blue Mood, Mary Light (RLR)
Herb Robert (SCE)
Pussy Willow (LHFE)
Plantain (LNE)

Flower Essence Suppliers

N.B. Overseas enquiries: For those readers who live outside the U.K. and who require information from the essence makers and suppliers in this appendix, please send with your request, an International postal coupon (or equivalent) to the value of approx £1.00. sterling.

ESSENCE SUPPLIERS

Ard Na Neantog. Co Creative Garden

Imelda Carroll, St Johns Point, Dunkineely, Co Donegal, Eire.
Tel: * 073 37325

Flower Essences and medicinal herbs by post. Culinary herbs, vegetables, plants and holistic fertilisers available direct from the garden. For sale or barter or Irish LETS. Visitors please phone first – tours can be organised.

Artemis Essences.

Kay Harrison . 'Healthcare at the Grange'. Clyst Heath, Woodwater Lane, Exeter, Devon, EX2 7HW
Tel: 01392 446354

Contact Kay for a listing of over 100 essences and for further information on Personalised Combination Essences.

Aquarius Flower Remedies.

Simon French, Threpwood Hill Cottage, Birtley, Hexham, Northumberland NE48 3HL
Tel: 01434 230499

Promethean Flower Essences. Moon Flowers, Chakra Flower Essences, Self Improvement Range (Flower Essences Combinations), Energy Balance, Guide to Chakra Flower Essences (Book)

The Doctor Edward Bach Centre

Mount Vernon, Bakers Lane, Sotwell, Wallingford, Oxfordshire. OX10 0PZ
Tel: 01491 834678. Fax: 01491 825022

Advice, information and education on Doctor Edward Bach's work and information regarding suppliers of the Bach Flower Remedies.

Bailey Essences.

Arthur Bailey, 7/8 Nelson Road, Ilkley, West Yorks LS29 8HN
Tel: 01943 432012. Fax: 01943 432011

Bailey Essences make and stock a range of 48 Flower Essences and 12 Composite remedies. Please send A5 S.A.E. for broadsheet of information and price list.

Church Farm Roses.

Val St Clair, 34 Newland St, Eynsham, Oxford. OX8 1LA
Tel: 01805 881320

The vibrational essences of roses preserved in a vegan base cream

Crystal Herbs.

Waveney Lodge, Hoxne, Suffolk IP21 4AS
Tel: 01379 642374. Fax: 01379 642374

Crystal Herbs make and supply a range of flower, gem and crystal essences, including the traditional English Remedies, Karmic Essences, Angel Essences, Chakra and Self-treatment Combinations, and Light Body Essences.

Earth Essence.

Mary Harris, Home Farmhouse, North Burlingham, Norwich NR13 4SX

Earth Essence is offered to individuals as part of an holistic, diagnostic and healing process, and may currently be obtained only from Mary Harris. Practitioners and therapists wanting further information should please contact Mary Harris direct..

The East Anglian Flower and Vibrational Essence Forum

Brackendale, Mill Lane, Brandeston, Woodbridge, Suffolk IP13 7AP

The East Anglian Flower and Vibrational Essence Forum is a group of Flower and Vibrational Essence makers and therapists who work together sharing information, research and resources to further understanding and development of healing with vibrational essences. The Forum produces a joint mail order vibrational essence catalogue for practitioners, containing detailed descriptions of the different sets of essences. The Forum supplies the following sets of essences:-

Sun Essences (Vivien Williamson and Jane Stevenson)

Light Heart Flower Essences (Rose Titchiner)

Gaia Essences (Rosemary Potter)

Loving Nature Essences (Patricia Staines)

Sue's Flower Essences (Sue Monk)

New Moon Essences (Paul Burry)

The Forum encourages practitioners to provide feedback from their experience of using essences – Members of the Forum jointly and individually run day and weekend courses and conferences in Flower and Vibrational Essences, Vibrational Essence Therapy and healing.

Findhorn Flower Essences

Marion Leigh, Wellspring, 31 The Park, Findhorn Bay, Forres, Morayshire. IV36 0TY

Tel: 01309 690129 / Fax: 01309 690300

Glastonbury Holy Thorn Flower and Bud Essences

Barbara Mockett, 133 The Crescent, Andover, Hants, SP10 2LN
Tel: 01264 323888

Also available from Chalice Well Gardens, Chilkwell St, Glastonbury, and Pendragon, The Glastonbury Experience, Glastonbury.

Green Man Tree Essences.

Simon and Sue Lilly, 2 Kerswell Cottages, Exminster, Exeter EX6 8AY
Tel: 01392 832005

Green Man Tree Essences make and supply a range of more than 70 Tree Essences, over 30 Flower Essences, 11 Combination Remedies and 11 Light Essences. Please send A5 S.A.E. for catalogue and price list.

The Guild of Vibrational Medicine.

Waveney Lodge, Hoxne, Suffolk IP21 4AS
Tel: 01379 642374. Fax: 01379 642374

The Guild of Vibrational Medicine has a register of qualified practitioners throughout the Country. Please write or phone for details.

Habundia Flower Essences.

Peter Aziz, PO Box 90, Totnes, Devon TQ11 0YG

There are three sets of Habundia Flower Essences: General Healing, Spiritual, and Magical. Send A5 S.A.E. for catalogue and price list.

Harebell Remedies.

Ellie Web, PO Box 7536 Dumfries DG2 7DQ SW Scotland
Tel: 01387 261962

Supply of 64 + Flower Essences. Illustrated stock bottles. Small introductory boxed sets. Practitioner and trade discounts. For information from within Britain, please send A5 size SAE. Enquiries from abroad, please send international reply coupons (from your PO) to cover postage.

Mary Harris.

Home Farmhouse, North Burlingham, Norwich NR13 4SX

Mary Harris occasionally holds workshops in Norfolk. Please contact her direct for details..

Healing Herbs

Julian Barnard. The Flower Remedy Programme, PO Box 65, Hereford. HR2 0UW

International Flower Essence Repertoire

The Working Tree, Milland, Nr Liphook, Hants. GU30 7JS
Tel: 01428 741 572

Bailey Flower Essences, Healing Herbs, Findhorn Flower Essences, Also wide range of International Flower Essences.

Irish Flower Essences (Ballybane Flower Essences).

Bridget Meagher, Ballybane East, Ballydehob, W Cork, Eire.
Tel: ★ 353 (0) 28 37462

Jean Jacob's Flower Essences.

Crablands Cottage, Drift Lane, Selsey . PO20 9BG
Tel: 01243 604687

Essences of the Ascended Masters in Tachyon Water.

Light Heart Flower Essences.

Rose Titchiner, The Duke, Chediston Green, Halesworth, Suffolk. IP19 0BB
Tel: 01986 785 242

Please send S.A.E. for leaflet and price list or £1.50 for handbook with detailed descriptions. Light Heart Essences are also available from the East Anglian Flower and Vibrational Essence Forum.

The Living Rainbow Aura Essences,

Dawn Carol, Glebe House, Church Lane, Wilcot, Pewsey, Wiltshire, SN9 5NS
Tel: 01672 562298

Also the New Age Remedies, Holy Archangel Essences, Crystal Light Essences, The Silver Light Dimensional Essences, The Golden Light Lateral Essences, The Aura Gems.

Loving Nature Essences.

Patricia Staines, 6 Nursery Cottages, Thorington, Halesworth, Suffolk. IP19 9JF
Tel: 01502 478282

Send S.A.E. for leaflet and price list. Loving Nature Essences may also be obtained from the East Anglian Flower Essence and Vibrational Essence Forum.

Native Tree Essences

Dr Helen Ford, Penrhyn Natural Health Centre, 11 Church Street, Penrhyn, Eudraeth, Gwynedd, Wales. LL48 6AB.
Tel: 01766 770700

Dr Helen Ford has made a set of Native Tree Essences – send S.A.E. for leaflet. (Profits from the sale of these essences go to tree planting and tree preservation). The Penrhyn Natural Health Centre acts as a health information service and can order Flower Essences.

The Ogham Apothecary

Roisin Carroll, Carlingford, Co Louth, Ireland
Tel: * 353 (0) 42-73793

Essence ranges made and/or supplied.

Phoenix Apothecary

The Park, Findhorn Bay, Morayshire, Scotland. IV36 0TX
Tel: 01309 691044 Fax: 01309 690933 e.mail.dhoyle@findhorn.org

Phoenix apothecary stocks Findhorn Flower Essences, Nelson's Bach Flower Remedies, Healing Herb Essences, plus a wide range of Flower Essences from around the world and flower essence books. Mail order catalogue available upon request. Orders sent throughout UK and World Wide.

Real Life Remedies – Marion Davis.

Real Life Remedies, PO Box 398, Edgeware HA8 8PH
Tel: 0181 905 4614

Real Life Remedies create and supply a range of powerful healing essences for adults, children and animals, effective also in promoting positive energy in land, building, crystals etc. Please send A5 S.A.E. for information booklet.

Revital Health Shop

35 High Road, Willesden, London. NW10 2TE

Revital Health Place

No 3A The Colonnades, 123 Buckingham Palace Road, Victoria, London. SW1
Tel: Freefone – 0800 252 875 for placing orders.

Revital are specialist suppliers of flower essences and vitamins for practitioners. They run a mail order distribution service.

Rosie's Essences.

Rosie Devitt, 20 Glencraig Park, Holywood, Co Down BT18 0BZ
Tel: 01232 422628

Rosie makes and supplies a range of over 100 flower and gem essences. Please send an A5 S.A.E. for catalogue and price list.

Silver Star Essences

Julian Perry, 'Ashdene', College Lane, East Grinstead, W Sx. RH19 3LY
Tel: 01342 311807

A range of 16 meditatively created 'Silver Star' essences for general well-being, transformation and empowerment.

Silvercord Essences

Colin Kingshot. Turnpike Cottage, Chawleigh, Chumleigh, Devon. EX18 AEU
Tel: 01769 580913

Welsh Flower Essences, Sentient Tree Essences, Fungi Essences, Grass Essences, Chromosol Essences, Combination Essences, Precious Stone Mineral Essences, Gem and Flower Cream and Pills, Gem Sprays. Made using traditional sun method, also lasers.

Sue's Flower Essences.

Sue Monk
Tel: 01954 789852

Please phone for leaflet and price list. Sue's Flower Essences are also available from the East Anglian Flower and Vibrational Essence Forum.

Sun Essences.

Vivien Williamson, Studio 3, 25 – 27 Muspole Street, Norwich NR3 1DJ

Tel: 01603 761128. Fax: 01603 861317. e.mail Solarblend@aol.com
Solarblends for Stress in the Nineties, Solarblends for Pets, The English Collection , Set 1 – Traditional Essences, Sets 2 & 3 – Living Essences, Body Sprays. Also available from The East Anglian Flower and Vibrational Essence Forum
Please send three first class stamps for colour brochures and if from overseas, international reply coupons to the value of approx. £1.00 sterling.

Dr Andrew Tressider

Yarn Barton, Sea, Ilminster, Somerset. TA19 0SB
Orange Azalea, Blue Iris and Hyacinth Stocks available.

Unitive Flower and Life Essence Range

Maria Maw, Cynlas, Rhos Isaf, Caenarfon, Gwynedd LL54 7NL
Tel: 01286 882556

Veda Essences

Richard Gonzalez Lic. MH.
No 2 Combe Head Cottages, Combe St Nicholas. Chard, Somerset. TA20 3LY
Tel: 01460 64098

Wight Flower Remedies.

Julian Winslow, 4 Undermount, Bonchurch Village Road, Ventnor, Isle of Wight
PO38 1RG
Tel: 01983 856157
Wight Flower Remedies make and supply a wide range of flower essences and gem elixirs. Please send A5 S.A.E. for information and price list.

Willow Aromatic Shop.

Pamela Kendall, Wyndley Garden Centre, Lichfield Rd, Sutton Coldfield, West Midlands.
Tel: 0121 323 4637
Stocks: Julian Barnard's Healing Herbs.

EQUIPMENT SUPPLIERS

Above and Beyond – *Distinct Images of Nature*

Vivien Williamson. Studio 3, 25 – 27 Muspole St, Norwich. NR3 1DJ
Tel: 01603 761128 Fax: 01603 861317 e.mail Solarblend @aol.com
Visual Aids for Essence Workshops and Talks. Range of slides, posters, prints for books, brochures etc.
Send three first class stamps for brochures and price lists. For overseas, international reply coupons for £1.00 sterling.

Brightstar – *Creative Consultancy*

Richard Osbourne. No 6, 35 Park Lane, Norwich. NR2 3EE
Tel: 01603 762189 Fax: 01603 762719 email:brightstar@paston.co.uk
Professional graphic design, but in the manner of flowers.

Bristol Bottle Company.

Ashmead Trading Estate, Ashmead Rd, Keynsham, Bristol. BS18 1TZ
Tel: 01179 869667
Range of bottles.

Essentially Oils Ltd

8, 9, 10 Mount Farm, Junction Rd, Churchill, Chipping Norton, Oxfordshire. OX7 6NP.

Tel: 01608 659544 Fax: 01608 659566 e.mail essentially.oils.ltd@dail.pipex.com
Essential oil suppliers to Aromatherapy professionals.

French Flint and Ormco Ltd 'The Glass Container Specialists'.
61 St Thomas St, London SE1 3QX
Tel: 0171 4031733. Fax: 0171 4075877
Bottle suppliers.

Homoeopathic Supply Co.
Fairview, 4 Nelson Rd, Sheringham. NR26 8BU
Tel: 01263 824683 Fax: 01263 821507. E.mail homsup@paston.co.uk.
Stock dropper bottles, screw cap vials, unmedicated tablets, carrying cases, boxes.

International Flower Essence Repertoire
The Working Tree, Milland, Nr Liphook, Hants. GU30 7JS
Tel: 01 428 741 572
Cobalt blue bottles with dropper tops.

Johnson and Jorgenson
15 Jessie Street, Polmadie, Glasgow. G42 0PG
Tel: 0141 423 3066
Bottle suppliers.

Quinessence
1 Birch Ave, Whitwick, Leicester. LE67 5GB
Tel: 01503 838358
Aromatherapy oils, cream bases, base oils, etc.

Wains of Tunbridge Wells
Chapman Way, North Farm Rd, Tunbridge Wells, Kent. IN2 3DU
Tel: 01892 521666
Range of blue, amber and clear bottles and jars.

THERAPISTS

Peter Aziz.
4 Bossell Park, Buckfastleigh, Devon TQ11 0DX
Tel: 01364 643127
Peter Aziz is a Homoeopath and Shaman. He works with plant spirits to release emotional traumas and inspire changes in consciousness.

Arthur Bailey
8 Nelson Road, Ilkley, West Yorks LS29 8HN
Tel: 01943 602177
Healer and flower essence practitioner.

Marion Bielby
17 Bristol Road, Ilkeston, Derbyshire. DE7 5HD
Tel: 01159 323373
Kinesiology, Herbal Medicine and Flower Essences.

Janet Brown
Member of the Society of Holistic Practitioners.
Walnut House, St Ninian's Road, Alyth, Blairgowrie, Perthshire PH11 8AP
Tel: 01828 633599. e mail Reiki Jan @aol.com
Reiki, Reflexology, Therapeutic Massage, Aromatherapy and Flower Essences.

Dawn Carol

Glebe House, Church Lane, Wilcot, Pewsey, Wiltshire. SN9 5NS

Tel: 01672 562295

Spiritual Healing, Aura Essences, Bach Remedies, Reiki, Colour Healing, Chakra Balancing, Aura Cleansing, Cleansing and Clearing, Absent Healing, Line Cutting.

Marion Davis (Real Life Remedies)

Real Life Remedies, PO Box 398, Edgeware HA8 8PH

Tel: 0181 905 4614

Marion Davis gives talks, lectures and workshops in 'How to Transform the Negative into Powerful Positive', karma release, soul retrieval, healing, bonesetting and trance channelling.

Roisin Carroll

The Ogham Apothecary, Carlingford, Co. Lough, Ireland.

Tel: ★ 353 (0) 42 73793

Hand Ogham (therapy based on the medicine of the trees), Reflexology, Colour Therapy, Tree Oil Therapy, Crystals Therapy.

Anne Mari Clarke

61 Granville Road, Limpsfield, Oxted, Surrey. RH8 0BY

Tel: 01883 715977

Flower Essence Therapy, Spiritual Healing, Crystal Healing, N.L.P.

Bridget Craig

'Little Foxes', Briar Court, Appledore Road, Tenterden, Kent. TN30 7AY

Tel: 01580 763334

I specialise in the use of both Bach and 'Briar Court' Flower Remedies granting friendly informal consultations, holistic counselling and whole body approach conducted in a very healing relaxed environment.

Marion Davis

C/O Real Life Remedies. PO Box 398, Edgeware. HA8 8PH

Tel/Fax 0181 905 4614

Healing, Bone Setting, Spiritual Guidance, Trance Channelling, Psychic Readings. By appointment.

Rosie Devitt

20 Glencraig Park, Holywood, Co Down BT18 0BZ

Tel: 01232 422628

Flower and Gem essence therapy.

Margaret Gallier

19 Maxwell Drive, Hazlemere, Bucks. HP15 7BX

Tel: 01494 715745

Flower Essence Therapy, Counselling and Healing.

Dr Helen Ford

9 Red Hill, Stourbridge, West Midlands. DY8 1NA

Tel: 01384 379740

Flower Essences, Homoeopathy, Healing, Spiritual Counselling and Aura Diagnosis.

Kestrel Gerrard

Flat 2, 7a St Benedict Street, Glastonbury, Somerset, BA6 9NE

Tel: 01458 833775

Kestrel is a full healer member of the N.F.S.H. and the College of Healing, he has an ITEC

Diploma in Massage. He offers the following healing and therapies:- Spiritual healing with sound, Healing regression, Guidance and direction (Higher perception readings) Holistic massage (he offers reduced rates for low/unwaged people)

Maureen Godden.

8a Rochester Terrace, Camden. NW1 9JN
Tel: 0171 284 3429

Uses Kinesiology as a diagnostic tool to find the required therapy. This can come in the form of nutrition, structural work and electro-magnetic therapy (this comes in the form of Flower Essences and Gem elixirs).

Richard Gonzalez LIC. MH.

No. 2 Combe Head Cottages, Combe St. Nicholas, Chard. Somerset. TA20 3LY
Tel: 01460 64098

I offer full Herbal consultations. Treatment with Vibrational Essences, either as a distant healing as in radionics or as a bottled prescription by post. Treatment with essences also includes animals and places.

Juin Gurney

25 Wideatts Road, Cheddar, Somerset, BS27 3AD
Tel: 01934 741306. Mobile: 0370 896422

Flower Essences. Reiki Master. Kinesiology. Counselling.

Uses Kinesiology, Oriental Diagnosis or Counselling as appropriate.

Kay Harrison

Healthcare at the Grange, Clyst Health, Woodwater Lane, Exeter, Devon. EX2 7HW
Tel: 01392 446354

Reflexology, Crystal Healing and flower essences.

Clare Harvey

Middle Piccadilly Natural Healing Centre, Holwell, Nr Sherborne, Dorset. DT9 5LW
Tel: 01963 23468 / 23038

or The Hale Clinic, 7 Park Crescent, London. WIN 3HE
Tel: 0171 637 3377

Clare Harvey (author of the Encyclopaedia of Flower Essences – Thorsons) is a Flower and Gem essence Therapist and is available for consultations at the above address. She also teaches a 2 year Professional Diploma in Vibrational Medicine (see courses)

Patricia L Higgins BSYA (FL.ESS.)

69 Copperfields, Lydd, Romney Marsh, Kent. TN25 9UU
Tel: 01797 320496

Flower Essence Therapist and Healer, Home visits.

Judith Hoad Dip. SHEN TAO, I.T.E.C.

Room for Healing, Inver, Co Donegal, Republic of Ireland.
Tel: ★ 353 (0) 36406

Vibrational Medicine Practitioner. Shen Tao Acupressure and/or Flower Essences offered in treatment session by appointment only.

Jean Jacobs

Crablands Cottage, Drift Lane. Selsey, Sx. PO20 9BG
Tel: 01243 604687

Meditation and healing with colour and crystals. Astrology the Spiritual Path. Lectures on the spiritual and esoteric life of flowers.

Mary Kendall

44 Lake Avenue, Park Hall, Walsall, West Midlands, WS5 3PA
Tel: 01922 62349

Reiki and Crystal Healing, Hypnotherapy and Regression, Stress Management, Magnotherapy, Aromatherapy, Vibrational Medicine, Indian Head Massage, Nutrition, Metamorphic Technique, Reflexology, Yoga, Counselling, Back Care, Reflexology, Remedial Sports Injuries.

Colin and Diana Kingshott

Turnpike Cottage, Chawleigh, Chulmleigh, Devon. EX18 7EU
Tel: 01769 580913

Vibrational Medicine, Zone Therapy, Crystal Sound Therapy, Regression, Element Diets.

Phillippa Lee

20 Tynedale Terrace, Hexham, Northumberland. NE43 3JE
Tel: 01434 607926

Flower Essence Practitioner, Reiki 2nd Degree, Postal Consultations for Flower Essences.

Sue Lilly

2 Kerswell Cottages, Exminster, Exeter EX6 8AY
Tel: 01392 832005

Sue Lilly uses Tree and Flower essences as part of her Health Kinesiology practice.

New Light

76 Parkville Road, Withington, Manchester. M20 4TZ
Tel: 0161 445 7199

A group of therapists offering Kinesiology and Flower Essence Therapy.

Maria Maw

Cynlas, Rhos Isaf, Caenarfon, Gwynedd LL54 7NL
Tel: 01286 882556

Maria is a Unitive Kinesiologist, astrological counsellor and flower essence therapist. (Maria is available to run day & weekend courses).

Bridget L Meagher D.Bth. M.R.H.

Ballybane East, Ballydehob, West Cork. Eire.
Tel: ★ 353 (0) 28 37462

Medical Herbalist.

Barbara Mockett

133 The Crescent, Andover, Hants, SP10 3BN
Tel: 01264 323888

Flower Essences, Counselling, Healing, Aromatherapy, Lymphatic Massage, Working with Animals

Sue Monk

Tel: 01954 789852

Flower and Gem Essence Therapy, Reiki Attunements and Healing.

Mark Mordin

The Milton Natural Health Centre, 33 Milton Avenue, Highgate, London. N6 5QF
Tel: 0181 340 7062

Nutrition, Flower Essences, Shiatsu, Bio-magnetic Therapy, Kinesiolgy, Reflexology.

Yana Nilsson MISPA ITEC RSA CERT TP

Little Fosters, Martinstown, Dorchester, Dorset. DT2 9JP
Tel: 013305 889945

Flower and Gem Essences, Counselling, Aromatherapy.

Ann Parker B.A.

11a Westgate, Ripon, North Yorks. HG4 2AT

Tel/Fax 01765 604947

Health Kinesiology Therapy and Training. Essences – Flower, Crystal, Tree, Light and Sea.

Penrhyn Natural Health Centre

11 Church Street, Penrhyn, Eudraeth, Gwynedd. LL48 6AB
Tel: 01766 770700

Offers a variety of natural health therapies including healing, homoeopathy, and flower and tree essence therapy.

Julian Perry

Ashdene, College Lane, East Grinstead, W Sx. RH19 3LY
Tel: 01342 311807

Works with channelled vibrational remedies and energies tailored to the individual's needs and encourages the patient to acknowledge and open to their potential for health, harmony and well being.

Rosemary Potter

Brackendale, Mill Lane, Brandeston, Woodbridge, Suffolk IP13 7AP
Tel: 01728 685 446

Flower and Gem Essence Therapy. Reiki Healing, Aromatherapy.

Sylve Provot

165 Robin Hood Road, Norwich. NR6 4BX
Tel: 01603 440674

Graphology, Stress Management Techniques and Flower Essences. Health and Happiness Fairs.

Maire Pullar

19 Millcroft, Norwich NR3 3LS
Tel: 01603 425419

Personal power work using Flower Essences (Sun Essences) and Louise Hay.

Jill Richardson

Jasmine Cottage, Street Farm, The Street, Topcroft, Bungay, Norfolk. NR35 2BL
Tel: 01508 482677

Jill Richardson (R.G.N., M.I.P.T.L., MWSH and Healer) has been involved in the caring and healing professions all her adult life, first as a registered nurse and then as a therapist. Her involvement in the healing arts of complimentary medicine arose out of her need and desire to heal herself. Her medical knowledge, therapeutic skills and personal experience give her a rare quality as a healer. Jill includes in her practise a wide variety of flower and gem essences which she has made herself in England and America (see also under courses).

Gail Shaw

93 Station Road, Hayling Island, Hants. PO11 0EE
Tel: 01705 462250

Flower Essences and Reflexology

Gay Slater

5 Yeoman's Meadows, Sevenoaks, Kent. TN13 2LS
Tel: 01732 451297

Reiki, Chakra Healing, Homoeopathy, Flower and Gem Essences.

Patricia Staines

6 Nursery Cottages, Thorington, Halesworth, Suffolk. IP19 9JF
Tel: 01502 478282

Flower Essence Therapist, Reiki Master/Teacher of Living Nature Essences.

Val St Clair

34 Newland St, Eyncham, Oxford. OX8 1LA
Tel: 01865 881320

Diagnosis for Health and Life Issues.

Jane Stevenson

Studio 3, 25 – 27 Muspole Street, Norwich NR3 1DJ.
Tel: 01603 615328 / 761128

Flower Essences postal and individual consultations with dowsing for people and animals.

Peter Tadd

Foilnamuck, Ballydehob, County Cork, Ireland.

Tel: ★ 353 (0) 28 37540

Clairvoyant Therapist, Healer and Lecturer. He offers individual consultations on life and health questions.

Liz Thompson

27 Sutherland Road, Brighton. BN2 2EQ
Tel: 01273 697373

Intuitive Healing, Flower Essences.

Liz came to healing through a serious illness that took her out of an old life and allowed her to enter a completely different one. As her own healing progressed, aided by regular flower essence therapy, and through meeting many healers herself, she found that she too was able to channel healing to others. Liz works with intuition, seeing the blocks in the aura and body, both past-life and present, and allowing them to be released. This process is often supported with Flower Essences which Liz intuits for the highest good of that particular client.

Rose Titchiner

The Duke, Chediston Green, Halesworth, Suffolk. IP19 0BB
Tel: 01986 785242

Flower Essence Therapy and Healing.

Claire Tomlins

Harmony, 78 Victoria Park Drive South, Scotstoun, Glasgow. G14 9NX
Tel: 0141 401 2470 or 0141 401 1369

Alexander Technique, Kinesiology, Allergy Testing and Flower Essence Therapy

Ellie Web

PO Box 7536, Dumfries, SW Scotland. DG2 7DQ

Flower Essence 'readings'. From a letter and brief description of your present situation, Ellie offers dowsed combinations of her remedies and personal confidential help with their interpretation. Fee includes 25ml remedy plus P/P. For information please send A5 size sae.

Julian Winslow

4 Undermount, Bonchurch Village Road, Ventnor, Isle of Wight PO38 1RG
Tel: 01983 856157

Julian uses a range of diagnostic techniques to get to the root of the problem, then applies this information to choose the appropriate gem, flower, or combination remedy.

TRAINING AND WORKSHOPS

Bach Flower Remedies. Seminar Programme

Broadheath House, 83 Parkside, London. SW19 5LP
Tel: 0181 780 4200

Arthur Bailey (Bailey Essences)

7/8 Nelson Road, Ilkley, West Yorks LS29 8HN
Tel: 01943 432012. Fax: 01943 432011

Day and weekend courses in dowsing and flower essences.

Marion Bielby

17 Bristol Rd, Ilkeston, Derbyshire. DE7 5HD
Tel: 01159 323373

Flower Essences and Touch for Health and Kinesiology weekend and day courses.

Dawn Carol

Glebe House, Church Lane, Wilcot, Pewsey, Wiltshire.SN9 5NS
Tel: 01672 562295

Aura Essence Workshop (weekend). Includes vibrational medicine generally.

Healing Workshop (includes Flower Essences).

Anne Maire Clarke

61 Granville Road, Limpsfield. Oxted, Surrey. RH8 0BY
Tel: 01883 715977

Healing Development (NFSH healing training). 1 day Flower Essences introductory courses. Further training in Flower Essences is available. Meditation for beginners and advanced.

Rosie Devitt

20 Glencraig Park, Holywood, Co Down BT18 0BZ
Tel: 01232 422628

Occasional one day workshops on flower and gem essence making, and therapy.

Kestrel Gerrard

Flat 2, 7A St Benedict Street, Glastonbury, Somerset. BA6 9NE
Tel: 01458 833775

Kestrel offers day and weekend courses in:-

Developing Higher Perception and Guidance. (day workshop)

Healing the Past, Empowering the Present (a weekend workshop for healers).

The Guild of Vibrational Medicine.

Waveney Lodge, Hoxne, Suffolk. IP21 4AS
Tel: 01379 642374 Fax: 01379 642374

Flower, Gem and Crystal Essence Therapy. Diploma Course leading to a Qualification in Vibrational Medicine.

Kay Harrison

'Healthcare at the Grange', Clyst Heath, Woodwater Lane, Exeter, Devon. EX2 7HW
Tel: 01392 446354

Workshops available in a variety of subjects including: Basic Astrology, Chakras and Subtle Energies, Crystals, Dowsing, Protection and Support, Subtle Reflexology and Shamanic Work.

Clare G Harvey

Middle Piccadilly Natural Healing Centre, Holwell, Nr Sherborne, Dorset, DT9 5LW
Tel: 01963 23468/23028

Clare Harvey runs the International Federation for Vibrational Medicine, Flower and Gem Essence two year professional diploma course (Diploma in Vibrational Medicine). Clare also runs introductory weekend courses in flower and gem essences.

Judith Hoad Dip. Shen TAO. I.T.E.C.

Room for Healing, Inver, Co. Donegal, Republic of Ireland.
Tel: *353 (0) 73 36406

Workshops include

Wandering through the Weeds – an exploration of the medicinal and nutritional values of mostly, wild plants, including ways to convert them into medicines. e.g. tinctures, decoctions, ointments etc.

Balanced Rebirthing – a series of workshops showing how Shen Tao and Flower Essences can be used to enhance the natural process of pregnancy, birth, early infancy and parenting. For parents, midwives, G.Ps, and obstetricians.

Therapeutic Loving Care – self-help techniques in Shen Tao, Flower Essences, Meditation, Visualisation and Qi Gong for Carers to use for themselves and those for whom they care by bringing the healing process back to the individual.

Essence and Intention – using and making Flower Essences, including dowsing and kinesiology as methods for choosing essences.

International Flower Essence Repertoire

The Working Tree, Milland, Nr Liphook, Hants. GU30 7JS
Tel: 01428 741 572

Developers from overseas, coming on average once a month.

Simon and Sue Lilly

2 Kerswell Cottages, Exminster, Exeter EX6 8AY
Tel: 01392 832005

Day workshops and seminars exploring the energy of tree and tree spirits through the use of tree essences. Longer courses also available.

Maria Maw PhD

Cynlas, Rhos Isaf, Caernarfon, Gwynedd, Wales. LL54 7NL.

Maria is a Natural Health Therapist and Flower Essence maker. She works with Flower Essences, Kinesiology, Herbs and Astrology.

Maria runs workshops in making flower essences, herbal tinctures, ointments, and oils, working with astrological charts using colour, energy patterns and sub-personalities. She uses Kinesiology (muscle testing with a question and answer technique) as the basis for much of her work.

New Light

Pamela Corin, Joy Fernandes, Ann Banks.

76 Parkville Road, Withington, Manchester. M20 4TZ
Tel: 0161 445 7199

Key – In Foundation Course. 2 day courses in Kinesiology including how to choose the best remedies for any individual through the use of kinesiology.

Rosemary Potter

Brackendale, Mill Lane, Brandeston, Woodbridge, Suffolk. IP13 7AP
Tel: 01728 685 446
Introductory day and weekend courses in Flower Essences. Reiki attunements.

Maire Pullar

19 Millcroft, Norwich. NR3 3LS
Tel: 01603 425419
'You Can Heal Your Life' Study groups. Personal power work using Flower Essences and Louise Hay.

Carol Richardson

Farend, Pyebush Lane, Acle, Norwich. NR13 3QZ
Tel: 01493 751544
Courses in Natural Flower Essences.

Carol Rudd and Jutta Gassner

The Dancing Man, Burgh Hall, Aylsham, Norfolk, NR11 6TD
Tel: 01263 732523 Fax: 01263 731777
One Year Flower Essence Practitioner Certification Programme

Gail Shaw

93 Station Road, Hayling Island, Hants. PO11 0EE
Tel: 01705 462250
Introductory weekend courses in Flower Essences.

Silvercord Essences.

Turnpike Cottage, Chawleigh, Chumleigh, Devon. EX18 7EU
Tel: 01769 580913. Fax 01769 580292
Holistic apothecary of Essences – Two year Practitioners Course.
Week courses , Introductory.

Patricia Staines

6 Nursery Cottages, Thorington, Halesworth, Sfk. IP19 9JF
Tel: 01502 478282
Flower Essence Workshops and Reiki Attunements.

Peter Tadd

Foilnamuck, Ballydehob, County Cork, Ireland.
Tel: * 353 (0) 28 37540
'The Healer's Path' is a year long training in intuitional development with Peter Tadd, clairvoyant therapist, healer and lecturer.
Weekend seminars with Peter Tadd, especially designed for Flower Essences practitioners, are promoted by the Flower Essence Repertoire.

Dr Andrew Tresidder MB BS MRCGP

Yarn Barton, Sea, Ilminster. Somerset. TA19 0SB
Teaching in the Health Professions.

Ellie Web

Harebell Remedies, PO box 7536, Dumfries, SW Scotland. DG2 7DQ
Tel: 01387 261962
Occasional day workshops or short residential courses.

Vivien Williamson. Cert Ed

Sun Essences. Studio 3, 25-27 Muspole Street, Norwich. NR3 1DJ
Tel: 01603 761128
Weekend Workshops on English Flower Essences.
Introductory one day courses, held in people's homes.

Suggested Reading List

FLOWER AND VIBRATIONAL ESSENCES
An Astrological Study of The Bach Flower Remedies – *Peter Damian: Neville Spearman 1986*
Australian Bush Flower Essences – *Ian White: Findhorn Press 1991*
The Collected Writings of Edward Bach – *Dr. Edward Bach: Flower Remedy Programme 1987*
Bach Flower Remedies – *Mechthild Scheffer: Thorsons 1990*
The Encyclopaedia of Flower Remedies – *C. Harvey & A. Cochrane: Thorsons 1995*
The Essential Flower Essence Handbook – *Lila Devi: Masters Flower Essences 1996*
Flower Essence Repertory – *P. Kaminski & R. Katz: Flower Essence Society 1994*
Flower Essences and Vibrational Healing – *Gurudas: Cassandra Press 1989*
Flower Remedies – *Peter Mansfield: Optima 1995*
Flower Remedies Handbook – *Donna Cunningham: Sterling 1992*
Flower Remedies for Women – *Christine Wildwood: Thorsons 1994*
A Guide to the Bach Flower Remedies – *Julian Barnard: C.W. Daniel 1993*
The Healing Herbs of Edward Bach – *J. & M. Barnard: Flower Remedy Programme 1988*
Heal Thyself – *Dr. Edward Bach: C. W. Daniel Co Ltd. Saffron Walden, Essex*
The Medical Discoveries of Edward Bach Physician – *Nora Weeks: C. W. Daniels Co Ltd. Saffron Walden, Essex*
A New Perception – Flower Essences of New Zealand – *Mary Garbely, N.Z. Flower Essence Co-op 1990*
The Original writings of Edward Bach: *C. W. Daniel Co Ltd. Saffron Walden, Essex*
Patterns of Life Force – *J. Barnard: Flower Remedy Programme 1989*
Plant Spirit Medicine – *Eliot Cowan: Swan, Raven Co 1995*
Starlight Elixers and Cosmic Vibrational Healing – *M. Smulkis & F. Rubenfeld: C.W. Daniel 1992*
The Twelve Healers and Other Remedies – *Dr. Edward Bach: C. W. Daniel Co Ltd. Saffron Walden, Essex*

HEALING, HEALTH AND EMOTIONAL THERAPY
Ageless Body – Timeless Mind – *Deepak Chopra: Random House 1993*
Cutting the Ties that Bind – *Phyllis Krystal: Samuel Weiser 1993*
Cutting More Ties that Bind – *Phyllis Krystal: Samuel Weiser 1993*
The Dance of Anger – *Harriet Goldhor Lerner: Pandora 1989*
Dare to Connect – *Susan Jeffers: Piatkus 1992*
Dowsing for Health – *Arthur Bailey: Quantum 1990*
Forgiving and Moving On – *Tian Dayton: Health Communications Inc 1992*
Hands of Light – *Barbara A Brennan: Bantam 1988*
How We Work – Understanding the Human Body – *P. Whitfield & S. Greenfield: Marshall Edns 1997*
Light Emerging-Journey through Personal Healing Process – *Barbara Brennan: Bantam 1993*
Love is in the Earth – A Kaleidoscope of Crystals Update – *Melody: Earth-Love Publishing 1995*
Map. The Co-Creative White Brotherhood Medical Assistance Program (Second Edition) – *Machaelle Small Wright: Perelandra, Ltd*
Modern Herbal – *Mrs. M. Grieve: Dover 1971*
The New Holistic Herbal – *David Hoffman: Element 1983*
Opening our Hearts to Men – *Susan Jeffers: Piatkus 1987*
The Parents' Book – *I. Sokolov & D. Hutton: Thorsons 1988*
The Power is Within You – *Louise Hay: Eden Grove Edns 1987*
Prescribed Drugs and the Alternative Practitioner – *S. Gasgoigne Energy Medicine Press 1992*
Quantum Healing – *Deepak Chopra: Bantam 1989*
The Spiritual Properties of Herbs – *Gurudas: Cassandra Press 1988*
Subtle Aromatherapy – *Patricia Davis: C. W. Daniel 1991*
Trees for Healing-Harmonizing with Nature for Personal Growth and Planetary Healing – *Pamela Louise Chase and Jonathan Pawlik: Newcastle Publishing Co. Inc. 1991*
Understanding Disease – *John Ball: C. W. Daniel 1993*
Vibrational Medicine – *Richard Gerber MD: Bear & Co 1996*
You Can Heal Your Life – *Louise Hay: Eden Grove Edns 1987*
The Yoga of Herbs-An Ayurvedic Guide to Herbal Medicine – *Dr. D.Fawley & Dr.Vasant Lad*

SPIRITUAL/NEW AGE

Answers – *Mother Meera: Rider 1991*
Behaving as if the God in all Life Mattered – *Machaelle Small Wright updated and revised: Perelandra Ltd 1997*
Bhagavad Gita,chapters 1-6 – *tr. Maharishi Mahesh Yogi: Penguin 1969*
Book of the Beyond – *Arthur Conan Doyle: White Eagle 1994*
Bringers of the Dawn – Teachings of the Pleiadians – *Barbara Marciniak: Bear & Co 1992*
Buddhism – *Christmas Humphreys: Pelican 1951*
The Celestine Prophecy – *James Redfield: Bantam 1994*
A Course in Miracles: *Arkana 1985*
Earth-Pleiadian Keys for a Living Library – *Barbara Marciniak: Bear & Co 1995*
From the Heart of a Gentle Brother – *Bartholomew: High Mesa Press 1987*
God and Man – *Masahisa Goi: Byakko Press 1983*
I Come as a Brother – *Bartholomew: High Mesa Pr 1986*
The Imitation of Christ – *Thomas A Kempis: Collins 1957*
Meditations for Women Who Do Too Much – *Anne Wilson Schaef: Harper S.F 1990*
Opening to Channel-How to Connect with your Guide – *S. Roman & D. Packer: H. Kramer Inc*
Pearls of Consciousness – *Christa F. Burka, Broth'hd of Life Inc 1987*
The Pleiadian Agenda-A New Cosmology for the Age of Light – *Barbara Hand Clow: Bear & Co 1995*
P'taah 'The Gift' – *Channelled by Jani King: Triad Publishers Inc 1995*
The P'taah Tapes 'Act of Faith' – *Channelled by Jani King: Triad Publishers Inc 1991*
The P'taah Tapes 'Transformation of the Species' – *Channelled by Jani King: Triad Publishers Inc 1991*
The Quiet Mind – Sayings of White Eagle: *White Eagle Publishing Trust 1972*
A Quiet Mind Companion – *Jenny Dent: White Eagle Publishing 1993*
The Raj Tapes – *NWFFACIM, P.O box 1490 Kingston, W.A.98346 USA*
Reflections of an Older Brother – *Bartholomew: High Mesa Press*
A Return to Love – *Marianne Williamson: Thorsons 1992*
Sevenfold Journey-Reclaiming Mind,Body and Spirit through Chakras – *A. Judith & S. Vega: Crossing Press 1993*
Signet of Atlantis-War in Heaven Bypass – *Barbara Hand Clow: Bear & Co 1992*
Taming Our Monkey Mind – *Phyllis Krystal: Sam Weiser 1994*
The Tao of Leadership – *John Heider: Gower 1986*
The Tenth Insight – *James Redfield: Bantam 1996*
Time is an Illusion – *Chris Griscom: Fireside 1986*
To Hear the Angels Sing – *Dorothy MacLean: Lindisfarne Press 1980*
The Vortex – *D. Ash & P. Hewitt: Gateway 1991*
The Way of the Wizard – *Deepak Chopra: Rider 1995*
Wings of Light – White Eagle: *White Eagle Publishing Trust 1991*

NATURE AND GARDENING

The Englishman's Flora – *Geoffrey Grigson: Paladin 1975*
The Findhorn Garden – *Findhorn Community: Turnstone 1975*
Folklore and Symbolism of Flowers, Plants and Trees – *E. & J. Lehner: Tudor, New York*
The Golden Web – *G. Armstrong Fraser: Findhorn Press 1995*
Journey into Nature – *Michael J. Roads: H. Krama Inc 1990*
Nature Spirits and Elemental Beings – *Marko Pogacnik: Findhorn Press 1997*
Perelandra Garden Workbook I (Second Edition) – *Machaelle Small Wright: Perelandra Ltd*
Perelandra Garden Workbook II – *Machaelle Small Wright: Perelandra Ltd*
The Secret Life of Plants – *P. Tomkins & C.Bird: Allen Lane 1974*
The Secret Life of the Soil – *P. Tomkins & C. Bird: Arkana, Penguin Group 1992*
To Honor the Earth – *D.MacLean & K. Thormod Carr: Harper SF 1995*

HISTORY AND MEDICAL HISTORY

Ancient Mesoptomia-Portrait of a Dead Civilisation – *A.Leo Oppenheim: Univ of Chicago 1977*
The Encyclopaedia of Ancient Egypt – *Margaret Bunson: Facts on file 1991*
Encyclopaedia of Medical History – *Roderick McGrew: Macmillan 1985*
The Hermetic and Alchemical Writings of Paracelsus the Great – *ed. A. E.Waite: Shambhala*
How We Work-Understanding the Human Body – *P. Whitefield & S. Greenfield: Marshall Edns 1997*